Dacie and Lewis
Practical
Haematology

Commissioning Editor: Serena Bureau
Project Development Manager: Francesca Lumkin
Project Managers: Ian Stoneham, Cheryl Brant
Design Manager: Jayne Jones
Illustration Manager: Mick Ruddy

Dacie and Lewis Practical Haematology

Edited by

S Mitchell Lewis BSc, MD, FRCPath DCP FIBMS
Emeritus Reader in Haematology and Senior Research Fellow, Department of Haematology,
Hammersmith Hospital, Imperial College School of Medicine, London, UK

Barbara J Bain FRACP, FRCPath
Reader in Diagnostic Haematology and Honorary Consultant Haematologist,
Department of Haematology, St Mary's Hospital Campus, Imperial College School of Medicine,
London, UK

Imelda Bates MD, MRCP, MRCPath, DTM&H
Senior Lecturer in Tropical Haematology, Division of Tropical Medicine,
Liverpool School of Tropical Medicine, University of Liverpool, Liverpool, UK

NINTH EDITION

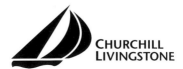
CHURCHILL
LIVINGSTONE

LONDON EDINBURGH NEW YORK PHILADELPHIA ST LOUIS TORONTO 2001

CHURCHILL LIVINGSTONE
An imprint of Elsevier Science Limited

First edition 1950
Second edition 1956
Third edition 1963
Fourth edition 1968
Fifth edition 1975
Sixth edition 1984
Seventh edition 1991
Eighth edition 1995
Ninth edition 2001
Reprinted 2001, 2002 twice

A 012727

WH 100

ISBN 0 443 06377 X
ISBN 0 443 06378 8 International Student Edition
Reprinted 2001, 2002 (3 times)

British Library Cataloguing in Publication Data
A catalogue record for this book is available from the British Library

Library of Congress Cataloging in Publication Data
A catalog record for this book is available from the Library of Congress

Note
Medical knowledge is constantly changing. As new information becomes
available, changes in treatment, procedures, equipment and the use of
drugs become necessary. The editors, contributors and the publishers have
taken care to ensure that the information given in this text is accurate and
up to date. However, readers are strongly advised to confirm that the
information, especially with regard to drug usage, complies with the latest
legislation and standards of practice.

Existing UK nomenclature is changing to the system of Recommended
International Nonproprietary Names (rINNs). Until the UK names are no
longer in use, these more familiar names are used in this book in
preference to rINNs, details of which may be obtained from the British
National Formulary.

your source for books,
journals and multimedia
in the health sciences
www.elsevierhealth.com

The
publisher's
policy is to use
**paper manufactured
from sustainable forests**

Printed in China

Contents

Contributors

Roger J Amos MA MD, FRCPath
Consultant Haematologist
Department of Haematology
Homerton Hospital
London
UK

Barbara J Bain FRACP FRCPath
Reader in Diagnostic Haematology and Honorary
Consultant Haematologist
Department of Haematology
St Mary's Hospital Campus
Imperial College School of Medicine
London
UK

Imelda Bates MRCP, MD, MRCPath, DTM&H
Senior Lecturer in Tropical Haematology
Liverpool School of Tropical Medicine
University of Liverpool
Liverpool
UK

Daniel Catovsky FRCP, FRCPath, DSc, FMedSci
Professor of Haematology
Academic Haematology and Cytogenetics
Royal Marsden Hospital
The Institute of Cancer Research
London
UK

Jaspal S Kaeda PhD, FIMBS, GiBiol
Research Associate
Leukaemia Research Unit
Department of Haematology
Hammersmith Hospital
Imperial College School of Medicine
London
UK

Sue M Knowles BSc, MBBS, FRCP, FRCPath
UK National External Quality Assesment Scheme
for Blood Transfusion Laoratory Practice,
Watford General Hospital
Watford
UK

Mike Laffan DM FRCP FRCPath
Senior Lecturer and Honorary Consultant in
Haematology
Department of Haematology
Hammersmith Hospital
Imperial College School of Medicine
London
UK

D Mark Layton
Consultant Haematologist and Honorary Senior
Lecturer Department of Haematology
Hammersmith Hospital
Imperial College School of Medicine
London
UK

S Mitchell Lewis BSc, MD, FRCPath DCP FIBMS
Emeritus Reader in Haematology and Senior
Research Fellow
Department of Haematology
Hammersmith Hospital
Imperial College School of Medicine
London
UK

Richard A Manning BSc, FIBMS
Chief Biomedical Scientist
Department of Coagulation
Hammersmith Pathology Centre
Hammersmith Hospital
London
UK

Estella Matutes MD, PhD, FRCPath
Reader in Haematological Malignancies
Institute of Cancer Research
Royal Marsden Hospital
London
UK

Ricardo Morilla MSc
Senior Scientific Officer
Department of Academic Haematology
Royal Marsden Hospital
The Institute of Cancer Research
London
UK

Marion Newlands BA, FIMLS
Training co-ordinator
Department of Blood Transfusion
Hammersmith Hospital
London
UK

Fiona Regan MRCP, MRCPath
Consultant Haematologist
Hammersmith Hospital
London
UK

David Roper FIBMS, MSc
Chief Biomedical Scientist
Department of Haematology
Hammersmith Hospital
London
UK

David M Swirsky FRCP, MRCPath
Consultant Haematologist
Haematological Malignancy Diagnostic Service
Department of Haematology
Leeds General Infirmary
Leeds
UK

Thomas J Vulliamy BA, PhD
Clinical Scientist and Honorary Lecturer
Department of Haematology
Hammersmith Hospital
Imperial College School of Medicine
London
UK

Barbara J Wild PhD, FIBMS
Principal Clinical Scientist
Department of Haematological Medicine
King's College Hospital
London
UK

Mark Worwood BSc, PhD, FRCPath, FMedSci
Professor of Haematology
Department of Haematology
University of Wales College of Medicine
Cardiff
UK

Preface

The first edition of *Practical Haematology* was published in 1950. This was a slim book of ten chapters in 170 pages, written by J.V. Dacie (now Sir John Dacie) who, in his preface described it as 'a little book on Practical Haematology which had its origin in notes on haematological technique and interpretation prepared for students taking a one year course for the London University Diploma in Clinical Pathology. The methods outlined are those of which I have had experience, and they are in routine use in the Haematology Laboratory of the Postgraduate Medical School of London'.

This book became a success far beyond the original intended readership, reprinted one year later, with a second edition in 1956. For the third edition, in 1963, Dacie invited S M Lewis to be his co-author, and this partnership saw the book through six editions, ever increasing in size and contents as the practice of laboratory haematology expanded, with advancing technology, advent of DNA techniques as applied to haematological problems, replacement of manual methods by instrumentation and automation, computers and a changing pattern of laboratory practice with increasing awareness of the importance of laboratory organization and management.

This new volume has been exetensively revised to take account of these developments, and also the value of standards, reference reagents and recommendations for standardized methods from the International Council for Standardization in Haematology, the British Committee for Standards in Haematology and other authoritative bodies. The role of the laboratory in support of near-patient or point-of-care testing is recognised, as is the increasing use of commercially available ready-to-use kits for many laboratory tests. We have also attempted to provide for all levels of laboratory practice from reference centres using sophisticated technology to primary health centres where only a few diagnostic tests can be carried out; one chapter is devoted to the essential requirements for a laboratory service where resources are limited. To include these various developments without excessively increasing the size of the book has meant that obsolescent tests have been omitted, as have some older or rarely used tests for details of which readers are referred to previous editions.

The 9th edition marks the retirement of Sir John Dacie, and I have been fortunate in having two new co-editors, Dr Barbara Bain and Dr Imelda Bates, with whose support and understanding Practical Haematology will continue to maintain the objectives of the book which are as relevant today as they were when Dacie first stated them in his preface fifty years ago:

> 'I think every laboratory worker feels that the burden of routine investigation is often too great and that too much time and energy are expended on the normal, with the result that abnormal conditions are not properly investigated and general technical standards are lowered. It is clearly desirable to make the most effective use of bench space and personnel..... It is most important that all those concerned with laboratory work should understand what is the significance of the tests they carry out, the relative value of haematological investigations and the order in which they should be under-taken. I hope that this book will make more interesting the essential work that is done.'

This volume is dedicated to Sir John Dacie with affection and appreciation.

S Mitchell Lewis
London, 2001

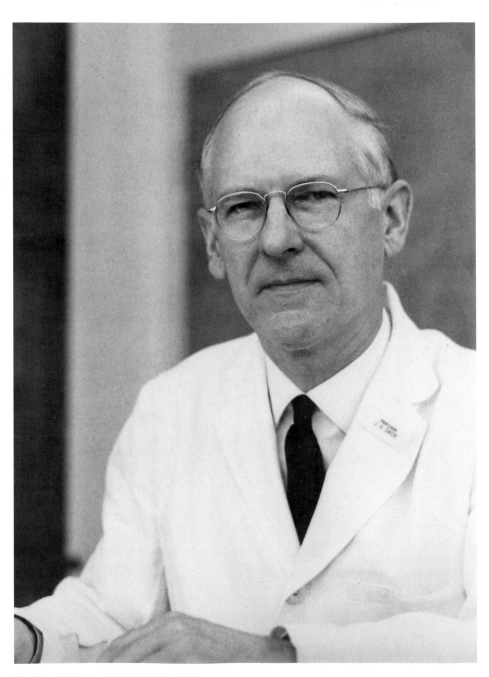

Sir John V Dacie MD FRCPath FRS

Editorial note

In keeping with recommendations from the International Organization for Standardardization (ISO), the World Health Organization (WHO) and other international authorities we have used the Système International (SI) for expressing quantities and units (see p. 606). Concentration of solutions is expressed either in mol/l (for substance concentration) or g/l (for mass concentration), whichever is more appropriate. Whilst we are aware that in some countries g/dl is still in common use for expressing haemoglobin concentration, in keeping with the internationally agreed convention we have expressed Hb in g/l.

Where details of *Methods* are given we have indicated the source of a reagent, kit or special equipment if there is a single manufacturer or if a specific make is recommended. If no source is indicated suitable material will generally be available from different suppliers.

Collection and handling of blood

S. Mitchell Lewis

In investigating physiological function and malfunction of blood, it is essential that, as far as possible, tests do not give misleading information because of technical errors. It is therefore important to avoid faults in specimen collection, storage and transport to the laboratory. Venous blood is preferred for most haematological examinations. Peripheral capillary samples can be almost as satisfactory for some purposes if a free flow of blood is obtained (see p. 3), but in general they should be restricted to children and to some direct 'point-of-care' screening tests.

BIOHAZARD PRECAUTIONS

When collecting a blood sample, the operator should, wherever possible, wear disposable plastic or thin rubber gloves*, especially if he or she has any cuts, abrasions or skin breaks on the hands. Care must be taken to prevent injuries when handling syringes, needles and lancets. Disposable syringes, needles and lancets should be used if at all possible, and they should not be re-used. They should be placed (without separating needles from syringes) in a puncture-resistant container for disposal or subsequent decontamination (see p. 557). Specimens should be sent to the laboratory in individual closed plastic bags, separated from the request forms to prevent their contamination should there be any leakage from the specimens. Tubes which minimize the risk of leakage are described on page 557.

---

*Some individuals may have an allergic reaction to either plastic or rubber gloves.

STANDARDIZED PROCEDURE

The method used for blood collection may affect the sample. The constituents of the blood may be altered by a number of factors as listed in Table 1.1. It is thus important to have a standard procedure for the collecting and handling of blood specimens.

Recommendations for standardizing the procedure have been published.[1,2]

Table 1.1 Causes of misleading results from discrepancies in specimen collection

Precollection
Toilet within 30 min
Meal within 2 h
Smoking
Physical activity (including fast walking) within 20 min
Stress

During collection
Different times of day: diurnal variance
Posture: lying/standing/sitting
Haemoconcentration from prolonged tourniquet pressure
Excessive negative pressure when drawing blood into syringe
Capillary or venous blood

Handling of specimen
Insufficient or excess anticoagulant
Inadequate mixing of blood with anticoagulant
Patient and/or specimen identification error
Delay in transit to laboratory

VENOUS BLOOD

It is now common practice for specimen collection to be undertaken by specially trained phlebotomists, and there are published guidelines which set out an appropriate training programme.[1,3]

Blood is best withdrawn from an antecubital vein by means of either an evacuated tube or a disposable plastic or glass syringe. The needles should not be too fine or too long; those of 19 or 21G* are suitable for most adults, and 23G for children, the latter especially with a short shaft (about 15 mm). It is usually recommended that the skin should be cleaned with 70% alcohol (e.g. isopropanol) and allowed to dry before being punctured; however, some doubts have been expressed on the utility of this practice for preventing infection at the venepuncture site.[4] Care must also be taken when using a tourniquet (see below) to avoid contaminating it with blood.[5]

When a series of samples is required or when the blood sampling is to be followed by an infusion, it is convenient to collect the blood by means of an intravenous cannula or winged ('butterfly') needle connected to a length of plastic tubing attached to the patient's arm by adhesive tape.

Except in the case of very young children, it should be possible with practice to obtain venous blood even from patients with difficult veins. Successful venepuncture may be facilitated by keeping the subject's arm warm, applying to the upper arm a sphygmomanometer cuff kept at approximately diastolic pressure and tapping the skin over the site of the vein a few times. In obese patients, it may be easier to use a vein on the dorsum of the hand, after warming it by immersion in warm water. When the hand is dried and the fist clenched, veins suitable for puncture will usually become apparent. If the veins are very small, a 23G needle should enable at least 2 ml of blood to be obtained satisfactorily. Vein punctures in the dorsum of the hand tend to bleed more readily than at other sites. The arm should be elevated after withdrawal of the needle and pressure should be applied for several minutes before an adhesive dressing is placed over the puncture site.

---

*The International Organization for Standardization has established a standard (ISO 7864) with the following diameters for the different gauges: 19G = 1.1 mm; 21G = 0.8 mm; 23G = 0.6 mm.

If possible, compression of the vein should be completely avoided so as to prevent haemoconcentration. In practice, it is usually necessary to use a tourniquet. This should be loosened once the needle has been inserted into the vein. The piston of the syringe should be withdrawn slowly and no attempt made to withdraw blood faster than the vein is filling. After detaching the needle, the blood should be delivered carefully from the syringe into a container and, if it is desired to prevent coagulation, it should be promptly and thoroughly but gently mixed with the anticoagulant. It is convenient to use as containers for blood samples disposable glass or plastic flat-bottomed tubes fitted with caps; except for coagulation studies, the choice between glass and plastic is a matter of availability or personal preference. Because of the possibility of infection of personnel when blood has leaked from the container or when removing the cap causes an aerosol discharge of the contents, it is essential to use containers designed to minimize these risks, e.g. an evacuated tube system or a container with a pierceable cap through which the blood can be sampled.

Haemolysis can be avoided or minimized by using clean apparatus, withdrawing the blood slowly, not using too fine a needle, delivering the blood gently into the receiver and avoiding frothing during the withdrawal of the blood and subsequent mixing with the anticoagulant.

The most common disposable containers available from commercial sources contain dipotassium or tripotassium or disodium ethylenediamine tetra-acetic acid (EDTA) as anticoagulant and are marked at a level to indicate the correct amount of blood to be added (see p. 5). Containers are also available containing trisodium citrate, heparin or acid citrate dextrose.

Evacuated tube systems are becoming increasingly popular. They consist of a glass tube (with or without anticoagulant) under vacuum, a needle and a needle holder which secures the needle to the tube. The main advantage is that it is not necessary to remove the stopper to fill the tube. The vacuum controls the amount of blood which enters the tube, ensuring an adequate specimen for the subsequent tests and the correct proportion of anticoagulant, when this is present. Evacuated tube systems can be used for routine coagulation screening tests; activation of coagulation factors is prevented by using siliconized tubes: special precautions for collecting blood for coagulation tests are described on p. 349.

Design requirements and other specifications for evacuated and non-evacuated specimen collection containers have been described in a number of national and international standards, e.g. that of the International Organization for Standardization (ISO 6710).

Ideally, blood films should be made immediately the blood has been withdrawn. In practice, blood samples are often sent to the laboratory after a variable delay. Films should be made in the laboratory from such blood as soon as is practicable. After careful and thorough mixing of the blood, a glass or plastic capillary can be used to take up a sample and deliver a drop of the right size on to a slide so that films can be made. The differences between films made of fresh blood (no anticoagulant) and anticoagulated blood are dealt with on page 6.

CAPILLARY (PERIPHERAL) BLOOD

Capillary blood is liable to give erroneous results[6] and there is greater likelihood of contamination and risk of transmission of disease than with venesection. It should be a used only with infants under 1 year or when it is not possible to obtain venous blood.

Collection of capillary blood[7]

Skin puncture is carried out with a needle or lancet. After use, they should be placed in a puncture-resistant container for disposal or subsequent decontamination (see p. 558), and they must never be re-used on another individual. In infants, satisfactory samples can be obtained by a deep puncture of the plantar surface of the heel in the area shown in Figure 1.1. As the heel should be really warm, it may be necessary to bathe it in hot water. The central plantar area and the posterior curvature should not be punctured in small infants to avoid the risk of injury to the underlying tarsal bones. In an older child and adult, the blood can be obtained from the distal digit of the third or fourth finger on its palmar surface, about 3–5 mm lateral from the nail bed.

A free flow of blood is essential, and only the very gentlest squeezing is permissible; ideally, large drops of blood should exude slowly but spontaneously. If it is necessary to squeeze firmly in order to obtain blood, the results are unreliable. If the poor flow is due to the part being cold and

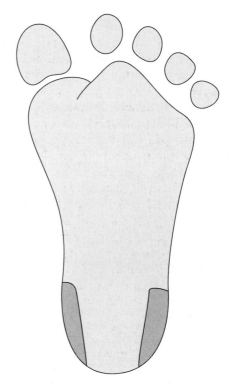

Fig. 1.1 Skin puncture in infants. Puncture must be restricted to the outer medial and lateral portions of the plantar surface of the foot where indicated by the shaded area.

cyanosed, too high figures for Hb[†] red cell count, and leucocyte count are usually obtained.

Clean the area with 70% alcohol (e.g. isopropanol) and allow to dry. Puncture the skin to a depth of 2–3 mm with a sterile disposable lancet. Wipe away the first drop of blood with dry sterile gauze. If necessary, squeeze very gently to encourage a free flow of blood. Collect a sample directly onto a reagent strip or by a 10 μl or 20 μl micropipette for immediate dispensing into diluent. There are also methods for collecting the blood into a capillary tube fixed into the cap of a microcontainer to allow the blood to pass by capillary action into the container[8] (e.g. Microtainer*; Microvette**). In another system (Unopette*), a calibrated capillary is completely filled with blood

---

† Throughout the book, Hb is used as an abbreviation for either *haemoglobin* or *haemoglobin concentration* where appropriate.

* Becton Dickinson; ** Sarstedt.

and linked to a pre-measured volume of diluent.[9] An adequate puncture with a free flow of blood can also enable a larger volume to be collected, drop by drop, into a plastic or glass container.[7]

DIFFERENCES BETWEEN CAPILLARY AND VENOUS BLOOD

Venous blood and capillary blood are not quite the same, even if the latter is freely flowing, and it is likely that free-flowing blood obtained by skin puncture is more nearly arteriolar in origin. The packed cell volume (PCV), red cell count (RBC) and Hb of capillary blood are slightly greater than in venous blood. The total leucocyte and neutrophil counts are higher by about 8%, the monocyte count by about 12%, and in some cases by as much as 100%, especially in children.[10,11] Conversely, the platelet count appears to be higher in venous than in capillary blood; this is on average by about 9% and in some cases by as much as 32%.[10,11] This may be due to adhesion of platelets to the site of the skin puncture.

SERUM

Blood collected in order to obtain serum should be delivered into sterile tubes or screw-capped bottles and allowed to clot undisturbed for about 1 h at room temperature.* Then loosen the clot gently from the container wall by means of a wooden stick, or a thin plastic or glass rod. If it is roughly treated, lysis is certain to follow. Close the tube with a stopper and centrifuge for 10 min at about 1200 g. Pipette the supernatant serum into another tube and centrifuge for 10 min at about 1200 g. Transfer the serum to tubes for tests or for storage. For most tests, serum should be kept at 4°C, before use, but if testing is delayed, serum can be stored –20°C for up to 3 months and at –40°C or lower for long-term storage. Frozen specimens should be thawed on the bench or in a water-bath at room temperature, then inverted several times to ensure homogeneity before use for a test. Do not refreeze thawed specimens.

Defribrinating whole blood
When serum is required urgently or when both serum and cells are required, as in the investigation of certain types of haemolytic anaemia, the sample can be defibrinated. This can be simply performed by placing the blood in a receiver such as a conical flask containing a central glass rod on to which small pieces of glass capillary have been fused (Fig. 1.2). The blood is whisked around the central rod by moderately rapid rotation of the flask. Coagulation is usually complete within 5 min, most of the fibrin collecting upon the central rod. When fibrin formation seems complete, the defibrinated blood may be centrifuged and serum obtained quickly and in relatively large volumes. Blood defibrinated in this way should not undergo any visible degree of lysis. The morphology of the red cells and the leucocytes is well preserved.

Cold agglutinins
If cold agglutinins are to be titrated, the blood must be kept at 37°C until the serum has separated, and if cold agglutinins are known to be

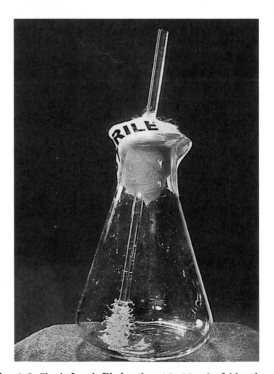

Fig. 1.2 Flask for defibrinating 10–50 ml of blood. The glass rod has had some small pieces of drawn-out glass capillary fused to its lower end.

---

* Room temperature is usually taken as 18–25°C.

present in high concentration, it is best to bring the patient to the laboratory and to collect blood into a previously warmed syringe and then to deliver the blood into containers which have been kept warm at 37°C. When filled, the containers should be promptly replaced in the 37°C water-bath. In this way, it is possible to obtain serum free from haemoglobin even when cold antibodies are present capable of causing agglutination at temperatures as high as 30°C. A practical way of warming the syringe is to place it in its container for 10 min in an oven at approximately 50°C or for 30 min or so in a 37°C incubator. When the clot has retracted in the sample and clear serum has been expressed, the serum is removed by a Pasteur pipette and transferred to a tube which has been warmed by being allowed to stand in a water-bath. It is then rapidly centrifuged so as to rid it of any suspended red cells.

ANTICOAGULANTS

For various purposes, a number of different anticoagulants are available. EDTA and sodium citrate remove calcium which is essential for coagulation. Calcium is either precipitated as insoluble oxalate (crystals of which may be seen in oxalated blood) or bound in a non-ionized form. Heparin works in a different way; it neutralizes thrombin by inhibiting the interaction of several clotting factors in the presence of a plasma co-factor, antithrombin III. Sodium citrate or heparin can be used to render blood incoagulable before transfusion. For better long-term preservation of red cells for certain tests and for transfusion purposes, citrate is used in combination with dextrose in the form of acid–citrate–dextrose (ACD), citrate–phosphate–dextrose (CPD) or Alsever's solution (see p. 603).

Ethylenediamine tetra-acetic acid

The sodium and potassium salts of EDTA are powerful anticoagulants and they are especially suitable for routine haematological work. EDTA acts by its chelating effect on the calcium molecules in blood. To achieve this requires a concentration of 1.2 mg of the anhydrous salt per ml of blood (c 4 μmol). The anticoagulant recommended by the International Council for Standardization in Haematology[12] is the dipotas-sium salt at a concentration of 1.50 ± 0.25 mg/ml of blood. At this concentration, the tripotassium salt produces some shrinkage of red cells which results in a 2–3% decrease in PCV and followed by a gradual increase in mean cell volume (MCV) on standing, whereas there are negligible changes when the dipotassium salt is used.[3]

Excess of EDTA, irrespective of which of its salts, affects both red cells and leucocytes, causing shrinkage and degenerative changes. EDTA in excess of 2 mg/ml of blood may result in a significant decrease in PCV by centrifugation and increase in mean cell haemoglobin concentration (MCHC).[3] The platelets are also affected; excess of EDTA causes them to swell and then disintegrate, causing an artifically high platelet count, as the fragments are large enough to be counted as normal platelets. Care must therefore be taken to ensure that the correct amount of blood is added, and that by repeated inversions of the container the anticoagulant is thoroughly mixed in the blood added to it. The dipotassium salt is very soluble (1650 g/l) and is to be preferred on this account to the disodium salt which is considerably less soluble (108 g/l).[13] Coating the inside surface of the container with a thin layer of EDTA improves the speed of its uptake by the blood.

The dilithium salt of EDTA is equally effective as an anticoagulant,[14] and its use has the advantage that the same sample of blood can be used for chemical investigation. However, it is less soluble than the dipotassium salt (160 g/l).

Blood films made from EDTA blood may fail to demonstrate basophilic stippling of the red cells in lead poisoning. Nor is it suitable for use in the investigation of coagulation problems and should not be used in samples for the prothrombin time test. It has been shown to cause leuco-agglutination affecting both neutrophils and lymphocytes,[15] and it is responsible for the activity of a naturally occurring antiplatelet auto-antibody[16] which may sometimes cause platelet adherence to neutrophils in blood films (see p. 98).

Trisodium citrate

100–120 mmol/l trisodium citrate (32 g/l $Na_3C_6H_5O_7.2H_2O$) is the anticoagulant of choice in coagulation studies. Nine volumes of blood are added to 1 volume of the sodium citrate solution and immediately well mixed with it. Sodium citrate is also the anticoagulant for the erythrocyte sedimentation rate (ESR); for this, 4 volumes of venous blood are diluted with 1 volume of the sodium citrate solution.

Heparin

This may be used at a concentration of 10–20 iu per ml of blood. Heparin is an effective anticoagulant and does not alter the size of the red cells; it is a good dry anticoagulant when it is important to reduce to a minimum the chance of lysis occurring after blood has been withdrawn. However, heparinized blood should not be used for making blood films as it gives a faint blue colouration to the background when the films are stained by Romanowsky dyes. This is especially marked in the presence of abnormal proteins. Heparin is the best anticoagulant to use for osmotic fragility tests and is suitable for immunophenotyping; otherwise, it is inferior to EDTA for general use and should not be used for leucocyte counts as it tends to cause the leucocytes to clump.

EFFECTS OF STORAGE ON BLOOD CELL MORPHOLOGY

If blood is allowed to stand in the laboratory before films are made, degenerative changes occur. The changes are not solely due to the presence of an anticoagulant for they also occur in defibrinated blood.

Irrespective of anticoagulant, films made from blood which has been standing for not more than 1 h at room temperature are not easily distinguished from films made immediately after collection of the blood. By 3 h, changes may be discernible and by 12–18 h these become striking. Some but not all neutrophils are affected; their nuclei may stain more homogeneously than in fresh blood, the nuclear lobes may become separated and the cytoplasmic margin may appear ragged or less well defined; small vacuoles appear in the cytoplasm (Fig. 1.3A,B). Some or many of the large monocytes develop marked changes; small vacuoles appear in the cytoplasm and the nucleus undergoes irregular lobulation which may almost amount to disintegration (Fig. 1.3C). Lymphocytes undergo similar changes: a few vacuoles may be seen in the cytoplasm, nuclei stain more homogeneously than usual and in some the

nucleus undergoes budding, giving rise to nuclei with two or three lobes (Fig. 1.3D–F). These artefactual changes must be distinguished from apoptosis which is natural cell degradation owing to programmed cell death.[17] It is characterized by shrinking of the cell with cytoplasmic condensation and nuclear fragmentation (Fig. 1.4). At least an occasional apoptotic cell may be seen in any blood film.[18]

Normal red cells are little affected by standing for up to 6 h at room temperature. Longer periods

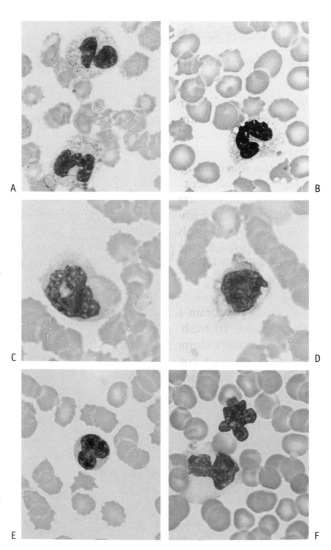

Fig. 1.3 Effect of storage on blood cell morphology. Photomicrographs from films made from EDTA-blood after 24 h at 20°C. (A) and (B): Polymorphonuclear neutrophils; (C): Monocytes; (D), (E) and (F): Lymphocytes. Red cell crenation is prominent in (B) and (E).

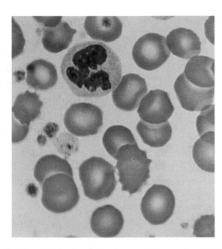

Fig. 1.4 Morphological features of apoptosis. See text.

lead to progressive crenation and sphering (Fig. 1.3 B, E and F). With an excess of EDTA (p. 5), a marked degree of creation occurs within a few hours.

All the above changes are retarded but not abolished in blood kept at 4°C. Their occurrence underlines the importance of making films as soon as possible after withdrawal. But delay of up to 1–3 h or so is certainly permissible.

Where possible, the practice of making films of blood before it is added to the anticoagulant is to be commended, especially when screening for lead toxicity, as the granules of punctuate basophilia may stain less obviously in anticoagulated blood. In fresh blood films, however, the platelets usually clump and it is less easy to estimate the platelet count from inspection of the films. Such films are nevertheless of particular value in investigating patients suffering from purpura, as in certain rare conditions the absence of platelet clumping is a useful pointer to the diagnosis (see p. 97).

QUANTITATIVE EFFECTS OF STORAGE ON BLOOD

In addition to the morphological changes described above, other changes take place when blood is allowed to stand in vitro at room temperature (18–25°C), and more rapidly at higher ambient temperatures. These occur regardless of the anticoagulant, although they are less marked in blood in ACD, CPD or Alsever's solution than in EDTA blood and, as described above, are greater in the tripotassium salt than in the dipotassium salt of EDTA. The red cells start to swell, with the result that the PCV and MCV increase, osmotic fragility and prothrombin time slowly increase and the sedimentation rate decreases; the leucocyte and platelet counts gradually fall.[3] If the blood is kept at 4°C, there is no significant change in PCV and MCV for up to 24 h. Other changes, too, take place more slowly at this temperature, so that for many purposes blood may safely be allowed to stand overnight in the refrigerator if precautions against freezing are taken. Nevertheless, it is best to count leucocytes and especially platelets within 2 h. The fall in leucocyte count, however, may become marked within 1–2 h if there is an excessive amount of EDTA (>4.5 mg/ml).[19] Degenerative changes in leucocyte morphology will especially affect automated differential counts, but can be largely prevented for up to 24 h if the blood is kept at 4°C. Reticulocyte counts are unchanged when the blood is kept in either EDTA or ACD anticoagulant for 24 h at 4°C, but at room temperature the count begins to fall within 6 h. Nucleated red cells disintegrate in the blood specimen within 1 to 2 days at room temperature. The advisability of making films as soon as possible has already been stressed.

Haemoglobin remains unchanged for days, provided that the blood does not become infected, as shown by turbidity or discolouration of the specimen. However, within 2 to 3 days, and especially at high ambient temperatures, the blood begins to lyse, resulting in a decrease in the red cell count and PCV, with an increase in MCH and MCHC.

SAMPLE HOMOGENEITY

In order to ensure homogeneity of blood, it is essential that specimens are effectively mixed immediately prior to taking a sample for testing. Place the specimen tube on a mechanical rotating mixer for at least 2 min or invert the tube 8 to 10 times by hand. If the specimen has been stored at 4°C, it will be viscid and the blood should be allowed to warm up to room temperature before mixing.

REFERENCES

1 National Committee for Clinical Laboratory Standards 1991 Procedures for the collection of diagnostic blood specimens by venipuncture. Document H3–A3 Vol 11. NCCLS, Villanova, PA.

2 International Committee for Standardization in Haematology 1982 Standardization of blood specimen collection procedures for reference values. Clinical and Laboratory Haematology 4:83–86.

3 Van Assendelft OW, Simmons A 1995 Specimen collection, handling, storage and variability. In: Lewis SM, Koepke JA (eds) Hematology laboratory management and practice. Butterworth Heinemann, Oxford, p 109–127.

4 Sutton CD, White SA, Edwards R 1999 A prospective controlled trial of the efficacy of isopropyl alcohol wipes before venesection in surgical patients. Annals of the Royal College of Surgeons 81:183–186.

5 Golder M, Chan CLH, O'Shea S, et al 2000 Potential risk of cross-infection during peripheral-venous access by contaminated tourniquets. Lancet 355:44.

6 Conway AM, Hinchliffe RF, Earland J, et al 1998 Measurement of haemoglobin using single drops of skin puncture blood: is precision acceptable? Journal of Clinical Pathology 51:248–250.

7 Meitis S 1988 Skin puncture and blood collecting techniques for infants: updates and problems. Clinical Chemistry 34:1890–1894.

8 Hicks JR, Rowland GL, Buffone GJ 1976 Evaluation of a new blood collection device ('Microtainer') that is suitable for pediatric use. Clinical Chemistry 22:2034–2036.

9 Freundlich MH, Gerarde HW 1963 A new, automatic, disposable system for blood counts and hemoglobin. Blood 21:648–655.

10 Daae LNW, Hallerud M, Halvorsen S 1988 A comparison between haematological parameters in 'capillary' and venous blood samples from hospitalized children aged 3 months to 14 years. Scandinavian Journal of Clinical and Laboratory Investigation 51:651–654.

11 Daae LNW, Halvorsen S, Mathison PM, et al 1988 A comparison between haematological parameters in 'capillary' and venous blood from healthy adults. Scandinavian Journal of Clinical and Laboratory Investigation 48:723–726.

12 International Council for Standardization in Haematology 1993 Recommendations for EDTA-anticoagulation of blood for hematology testing. American Journal of Clinical Pathology 100:371–372.

13 Hadley GG, Weiss SP 1955 Further notes on use of salts of ethylenediamine tetraacetic acid (EDTA) as anticoagulants. American Journal of Clinical Pathology 25:1090–1093.

14 Sacker LS, Saunders KE, Page B, et al 1959 Dilithium sequestrene as an anticoagulant. Journal of Clinical Pathology 12:254–257.

15 Deal I, Hernandez AM, Pierre RV 1995 Ethylenediamine tetraacetic acid-associated leukoagglutination. American Journal of Clinical Pathology 103:338–340.

16 Bizzaro N 1995 EDTA-dependent pseudothrombocytopenia: a clinical and epidemiological study of 112 cases with 10-year follow-up. American Journal of Cancer 26:239–257.

17 Kerr JF, Wylie AH, Currie AR 1972 Apoptosis: a basic biological phenomenon with wide-ranging implications in tissue kinetics. British Journal of Cancer 26:239–257.

18 Lach-Szyrma V, Brito-Babapulle F 1999 The clinical significance of apoptotic cells in peripheral blood smears. Clinical and Laboratory Haematology 21:277–280.

19 Goosens W, Van Duppen V, Verwilghen RL 1991 K_2 or K_3 EDTA: the anticoagulant of choice in routine haematology? Clinical and Laboratory Haematology 13:291–295.

2

Reference ranges and normal values

S. Mitchell Lewis

A number of factors affect haematological values in apparent health. The technique and timing of collection, transport and storage of specimens and differences in the subject's posture when the sample is taken and whether ambulant or confined to bed, may have an effect, as described in Chapter 1. Variation in the analytical methods used may also affect the measurements. These can all be standardized. More problematic are the inherent factors of sex, age, occupation, body build, genetic background as well as adaptation to diet and to environment, especially altitude.

These variables must be recognized when establishing physiologically normal values. Furthermore, it is difficult to be certain in any survey of a population for the purposes of obtaining data from which normal ranges may be constructed that the 'normal' subjects are completely healthy and do not have mild chronic infections, parasitic infestations or nutritional deficiencies, or have been affected by smoking.

Haematological values for the normal and abnormal will overlap, and a value within the recognized normal range may be definitely pathological in a particular subject. For these reasons the concept of 'normal values' and 'normal ranges' has been replaced by *reference values* and *reference limits* in which the variables are defined when establishing the values for the *reference population* in a particular test, and the range between the reference limits is termed the *reference interval*.[1,2] Ideally, each laboratory should establish a data bank of reference values which take account of the physiological variables mentioned above, so that an individual's result can be expressed and interpreted relative to a comparable normal.

REFERENCE RANGES

A reference range for a population can be established from measurements on a relatively small number of subjects (see below) if they are assumed to be representative of the population as a whole.[1,3] The conditions for obtaining samples from the individuals must be standardized and data should be analysed separately for different variables such as individuals in bed or ambulant, smokers or non-smokers. The samples should be collected at about the same time of day, preferably in the morning before breakfast; the last meal should have been eaten not later than 9 p.m. on the previous evening and at that time alcohol should have been restricted to one bottle of beer or an equivalent amount of other alcoholic drink.[4]

STATISTICAL PROCEDURE[5]

It is usually assumed that the data will fit a specified type of pattern, either symmetric (Gaussian) or asymmetric with a skewed distribution (non-Gaussian) (p. 612). If the data fit a Gaussian distribution, the arithmetic mean ($\bar{x}$) and SD may be calculated as described on page 613.

Alternatively, a frequency histogram is plotted (Fig. 2.1). Taking the modal value (mode) and the

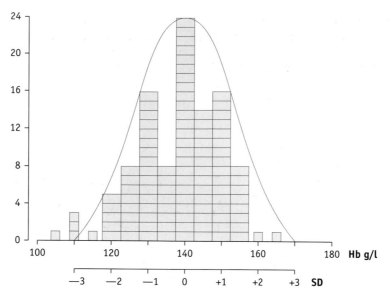

Fig. 2.1 Example of establishing a reference range. Histogram of data of haemoglobin measurements in a population, with Gaussian curve superimposed. The ordinate shows the number which occurred at each reference point.

calculated standard deviation (SD) as reference points, a Gaussian curve is superimposed. From this curve, practical reference limits can be determined even if the original histogram included outlying results from some subjects not belonging to the normal population. Limits representing the 95% range (reference interval) are calculated from arithmetic mean ±2SD (or more accurately ± 1.96SD). When there is a log normal (skew) distribution of measurements, the range to −2SD may extend below zero (Fig. 2.2). To avoid this anomaly, the data should be converted to their logarithms by means of log-tables or a calculator with the appropriate facility. The mean and SD are calculated in

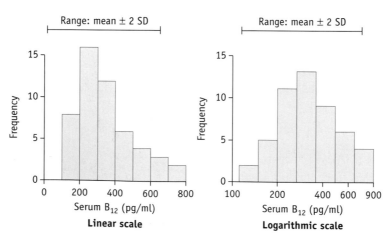

Fig. 2.2 Example of log normal distribution. Data of vitamin B_{12} measurements in a population. Left: arithmetic scale. Right: geometric scale. Arithmetic mean 343 pg/ml and SD 161 pg/ml; 2SD range would thus be 21–665 pg/ml. When the data are converted to their logarithms as described on page 612, the geometric mean is 308 pg/ml, and a 2SD range is 121–783 pg/ml. (Reproduced with permission from England JM 1975 Medical Research: A Statistical and Epidemiological Approach. Churchill Livingstone, Edinburgh, p. 20.)

the usual way (p. 613); the figures are then converted to their antilogs in order to express the data in the original scale.

When it is not possible to make an assumption about the type of distribution, a non-parametric procedure may be used instead. For this, the data are sorted out and ranked according to increasing numerical values. The total number of results = n; subsequent calculations are based on n + 1. The lower reference limit will correspond to the rank number at which 2.5% of n + 1 results occur; the upper reference limit is similarly taken as the rank number at which 97.5% of n + 1 results have accumulated. If these numbers are not integers, it may be necessary to interpolate between two adjacent rank values.

In any of the methods of analysis, a reasonably reliable estimate can be obtained with 40 values, although a larger number (120 or more) is preferable (Fig. 2.3).[5,6] When a large set of reference values is unattainable and precise estimation impossible, a smaller number of values may still serve as a useful clinical guide.

The data given in Tables 2.1 and 2.2 provide a guide to normal reference values which are applic-able to most healthy adults and children, respectively, in industrialized countries. The data have been based on personal observations as well as various published reports.[7-11] The reference interval, which comprises a range of ±2SD from the mean, indicates the limits which should cover 95% of normal subjects; 99% of normal subjects will be included in a range of ±3SD. Age and sex differences have been taken into account for some values. Even so, the wide ranges which are shown for some tests reflect the influence of various factors as described on p. 13. Narrower ranges would be expected under standardized conditions.

It should be noted that in Table 2.1 the differential white cell count is shown as percentages as well as in absolute numbers. However, automated analysers provide absolute counts for each type of leucocyte, and because proportional (percentage) counting is less likely to interpret correctly their absolute increase or decrease, the International Council (formerly Committee) for Standardization in Haematology has recommended that the differential leucocyte count should always be expressed as the absolute number of each cell type per unit volume of blood.[12]

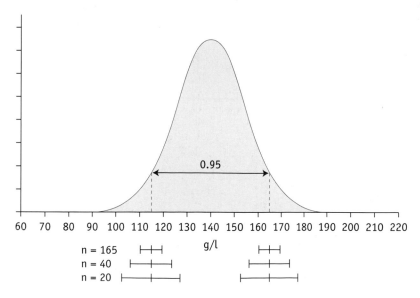

Fig. 2.3 Effect of sample size on reference values. A smoothed distribution graph was obtained for haemoglobin measurement from a group of normal women: the ordinate shows the frequency distribution. The 95% reference interval is defined by the lower and upper reference limits which were calculated as 115 and 165 g/l respectively. The confidence levels for the precision of these reference limits are shown for three sample sizes of 20, 40 and 165 values, respectively.

Table 2.1 Haematological values for normal adults expressed as a mean ±2SD (95% range)

Red blood cell count			*Protein S*	
Men	$5.0 \pm 0.5 \times 10^{12}/l$		Total	0.78–1.37 u/ml
Women	$4.3 \pm 0.5 \times 10^{12}/l$		Free	0.68–1.52 u/ml
			Activity	
Haemoglobin			Men	0.60–1.35 u/ml
Men	150 ± 20 g/l		Women	0.55–1.35 u/ml
Women	135 ± 15 g/l			
			Heparin co-factor II	0.55–1.45 u/ml
Packed cell volume (PCV) or haematocrit (Hct) value				
Men	0.45 ± 0.05 (l/l)		*Median red cell fragility (MCF) (g/l NaCl)*	
Women	0.41 ± 0.05 (l/l)		Fresh blood	4.0–4.45 g/l NaCl
			24 h at 37°C	4.65–5.9 g/l NaCl
Mean cell volume (MCV)				
Men and women	92 ± 9 fl		*Cold agglutinin titre (4°C)*	<64
Mean cell haemoglobin (MCH)			*Blood volume (normalized to "ideal weight")*	
Men and women	29.5 ± 2.5 pg		Red cell volume: men	30 ± 5 ml/kg
			women	25 ± 5 ml/kg
Mean cell haemoglobin concentration (MCHC)			Plasma volume	45 ± 5 ml/kg
Men and women	330 ± 15 g/l		Total blood volume	70 ± 10 ml/kg
Red cell distribution width (RDW)			*Red cell life-span*	120 ± 30 days
As coefficient of variation (CV)	$12.8 \pm 1.2\%$			
As standard deviation (SD)	42.5 ± 3.5 fl		*Serum iron*	
			Men	12–24 μmol/l (0.6–1.3 mg/l)
Red cell diameter (mean values)			Women	9–23 μmol/l (0.5–1.3 mg/l)
Dry films	6.7–7.7 μm			
			Total iron-binding capacity	
Red cell density	1092–1100 g/l		Men	54–72 μmol/l (3.0–4.0 mg/l)
			Women	55–81 μmol/l (3.1–4.5 mg/l)
Reticulocyte count	$50–100 \times 10^9/l$ (0.5–2.5%)			
			Transferrin saturation	
White blood cell count	$7.0 \pm 3.0 \times 10^9/l$		Men	18–40%
			Women	13–37%
Differential white cell count				
Neutrophils	$2.0–7.0 \times 10^9/l$ (40–80%)		*Ferritin*	
Lymphocytes	$1.0–3.0 \times 10^9/l$ (20–40%)		Men	15–300 μgl/l (median 100 μg/l)
Monocytes	$0.2–1.0 \times 10^9/l$ (2–10%)		Women	15–200 μg/l (median 30 μg/l)
Eosinophils	$0.02–0.5 \times 10^9/l$ (1–6%)			
Basophils	$0.02–0.1 \times 10^9/l$ (<1–2%)		*Serum vitamin B_{12}*	160–760 ng/l
Platelet count	$150–400 \times 10^9/l$		*Serum folate*	3–20 μg/l
Bleeding time			*Red cell folate*	160–640 μg/l
Ivy's method	2–7 min			
Template method	2.5–9.5 min		*Plasma haemoglobin*	10–40 mg/l
Prothrombin time	11–16 s		*Serum haptoglobin*	
Recombinant thromboplastin	10–12 s		Radial immunodiffusion	0.8–2.7 g/l
			Haemoglobin binding capacity	0.3–2.0 g/l
Activated partial thromboplastin time (APTT)	30–40 s			
			Hb A_2	2.2–3.5%
Thrombin time	15–19 s			
			Hb F	<1.0%
Plasma fibrinogen				
Clauss	2.0–4.0 g/l		*Methaemoglobin*	<2.0%
Dry clot	1.5–4.0 g/l			
			Sedimentation rate (mm in 1 h at 20 ± 3°C)	
Fibrinogen titre	≥128		Men 17–50 yr	10 or <
			51–60 yr	12 or <
Plasminogen	0.75–1.60 u/ml		61–70 yr	14 or <
			>70 yr	30 or <
Euglobulin lysis time	90–240 min		Women 17–50 yr	12 or <
			51–60 yr	19 or <
Antithrombin III			61–70 yr	20 or <
Function	0.86–1.32 u/ml		>70 yr	35 or <
Antigen	0.79–1.11 u/ml			
			Plasma viscosity	
β-Thromboglobulin	<50 ng/ml		25°C	1.50–1.72 mPa/s
			37°C	1.16–1.33 mPa/s
Platelet factor 4	<10 ng/ml			
			Heterophile (anti-sheep red cell) agglutinin titre	<80
Protein C			After absorption with guinea-pig kidney	<10
Function	0.70–1.40 u/ml			
Antigen	0.61–1.32 u/ml			

Table 2.2 **Haematological values for normal infants and children.** Amalgamation of data derived from various sources; expressed as mean ± 2SD or 95% range.

	Birth	Day 3	1 month	2 months	3–6 months	1 year	2–6 years	6–12 years
Red cell count ×10^{12}/l	6.0 ± 1.0	5.3 ± 1.3	4.2 ± 1.2	3.7 ± 0.6	4.7 ± 0.6	4.5 ± 0.6	4.6 ± 0.6	4.6 ± 0.6
Haemoglobin g/l	180 ± 40	180 ± 30	140 ± 25	112 ± 18	126 ± 15	126 ± 15	125 ± 15	135 ± 20
Packed cell volume (PCV) l/l	0.60 ± 0.15	0.56 ± 0.11	0.43 ± 0.10	0.35 ± 0.07	0.35 ± 0.05	0.34 ± 0.04	0.37 ± 0.03	0.40 ± 0.05
Mean cell volume (MCV) fl	110 ± 10	105 ± 13	104 ± 12	95 ± 8	76 ± 8	78 ± 6	81 ± 6	86 ± 9
Mean cell Hb (MCH) pg	34 ± 3	34 ± 3	33 ± 3	30 ± 3	27 ± 3	27 ± 2	27 ± 3	29 ± 4
Mean cell Hb conc (MCHC) g/l	330 ± 30	330 ± 40	330 ± 40	320 ± 35	330 ± 30	340 ± 20	340 ± 30	340 ± 30
Reticulocytes ×10^9/l	120–400	50–350	20–60	30–50	40–100	30–100	30–100	30–100
White cell count ×10^9/l	18 ± 8	15 ± 8	12 ± 7	10 ± 5	12 ± 6	11 ± 5	10 ± 5	9 ± 4
Neutrophils ×10^9/l	4–14	3–5	3–9	1–5	1–6	1–7	1.5–8	2–8
Lymphocytes ×10^9/l	3–8	2–8	3–16	4–10	4–12	3.5–11	6–9	1–5
Monocytes ×10^9/l	0.5–2.0	0.5–1.0	0.3–1.0	0.4–1.2	0.2–1.2	0.2–1.0	0.2–1.0	0.2–1.0
Eosinophils ×10^9/l	0.1–1.0	0.1–2.0	0.2–1.0	0.1–1.0	0.1–1.0	0.1–1.0	0.1–1.0	0.1–1.0
Platelets ×10^9/l	150–450	210–500		210–650	200–550	200–550	200–450	180–400

PHYSIOLOGICAL VARIATION

PHYSIOLOGICAL VARIATION IN Hb, PCV AND RED CELL COUNTS

Some of the earlier studies should, perhaps, be interpreted cautiously as techniques for the blood count were less precise than those now available. But there is no doubt that there is considerable variation in the red cell count and Hb content at different periods of life. At birth the Hb is higher than at any period subsequently (Table 2.2). The red cell count is high immediately after birth[9,13,14] and values for Hb greater than 200 g/l, red cell count higher than 6.0 × 10^{12}/l and a packed cell volume (PCV) of 0.65 are encountered frequently when the cord is tied late after delivery. Probably it is the cessation of pulsation of the umbilical artery in the cord as well as the uterine contractions which result in much of the blood contained in the placenta re-entering the infant's circulation. After the immediate postnatal period, the Hb falls fairly steeply to a minimum by about the 2nd month (Fig. 2.4). The red cell count and PCV also fall, though less steeply, and the cells may become microcytic with the development of 'physiological' iron deficiency.[15]

In the neonate and until about the 2nd month, the average mean cell haemoglobin (MCH) is 34 pg; the mean cell haemoglobin concentration

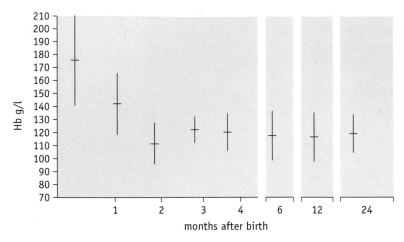

Fig. 2.4   Changes in haemoglobin values in the first 2 years after birth. The perpendicular lines show means and 2SD ranges.

(MCHC) is about 330 g/l and does not alter significantly during the first 3 years. The mean MCV is 110 fl in the neonate, 95 fl at 2 months, and within the adult range by 3 years.

The Hb content and red cell count normally rise gradually to almost adult levels by the time of puberty,[10] the levels in women tend to be significantly lower than those of men.[7,16] Factors influencing the difference between men and women include a hormonal influence on haemopoiesis and conversely menstrual blood loss; the extent to which the latter is a significant factor is not clear, as a loss of up to 100 ml of blood with each period does not appear to cause a fall in Hb although it results in lower levels of serum iron.[17,18] Moreover, arrest of menstruation by oral contraceptives causes an increase in serum iron without affecting the haemoglobin level.[19]

In normal pregnancy, there is an increase in erythropoietic activity. However, at the same time, an increase in plasma volume occurs and this results in a progressive fall in Hb, PCV and red cell count.[20,21] The level returns to normal about a week after delivery. There is a slight increase in MCV during the 2nd trimester.[22] Serum ferritin falls in early pregnancy and usually remains low throughout pregnancy, even when supplementary iron is given.[23]

In old age Hb is reported to fall progressively in men; in one study, this was found to be to a mean level of 134 g/l at 65, 129 g/l at 75, and 122 g/l at over the age of 85.[24] Lesser differences have

been recorded by others.[7,8,16] By contrast, in older women the level tends to rise, so that a difference of 20 g/l in younger age groups is reduced to 10 g/l or less in old age. In women a progressive fall with time, on average 0.35 g/l per year has also been reported.[17,25,26] There is a concomitant increase in serum iron although serum ferritin levels remain higher in men than in women. In healthy men and women, Hb, red cell count, PCV and related parameters remain remarkably constant until the 6th decade.[27]

In addition to the permanent effects of age and sex, there seem to be transient fluctuations, the significance of which is often difficult to assess. Strenuous muscular activity, in the short term, raises the red cell count and Hb, largely because of reduction in plasma volume and to a lesser extent to the re-entry into the circulation of cells previously sequestered in the spleen,[28,29] the red cell count increases by $0.5 \times 10^{12}/l$ and Hb by 15 g/l. Posture, too, appears to cause transient alterations in the plasma volume, and thus in Hb and PCV. There is a small but significant increase as the posture changes from lying to sitting, especially in women[30] and, conversely, change from walking about to lying down results in a 5–10% fall in the Hb and PCV. This occurs within 20 min, after which time the PCV is stabilized at the lower level.[31,32] Consistently similar findings have also been reported by Eisenberg in a study of 25 subjects.[33] He also showed that the position of the arm during venous sampling affected the magnitude of the increase in

PCV; it was 2–4% lower when the arm was held at the atrial level instead of being dependent.

It is not clear whether emotion or light exercise raises the red cell count or Hb significantly above the baseline observed with the subject at rest; the effects may be small enough to be submerged in the technical errors of estimation.[34] More significant changes occur in athletes, resulting in so-called 'sports anaemia' with a slightly lower Hb and red cell count[35] probably owing to increased plasma volume;[36] endurance training leads to a higher total red cell volume with a concomitant further rise in plasma volume.[37]

Diurnal variation in Hb and red cell count is usually slight, about 3%, but variation of 20% occurs with reticulocytes.[11] Pronounced diurnal variations are seen in serum iron and ferritin in healthy as well as in anaemic subjects.[38–40] Decreased levels occur during endurance training, possibly associated with loss of iron in sweat.[41]

It has been suggested that minor seasonal variations also occur, but the evidence for this is conflicting.[42–45] One study demonstrated a lower Hb and PCV in summer than in winter, with a concomitant 5% increase in plasma volume.[46] There may be an ethnic difference in red cell indices; lower levels of Hb and MCV have been reported in healthy Africans and West Indians living in Britain not related to nutritional status and probably due to α thalassaemia trait.[47]

The effect of altitude is to raise the Hb and PCV and increase the number of circulating red cells with a lower MCV.[48,49] The magnitude of the polycythaemia depends on the degree of anoxaemia.[48] At an altitude of 2 km (c 6500 ft), the Hb is c 10 g/l higher than at sea level; at 3 km (c 10 000 ft), it is c 20 g/l higher. Corresponding increases occur at intermediate altitudes.[49,69] These increases appear to be due both to increased erythropoiesis as a result of the anoxic stimulus and to the decrease in plasma volume which occurs at high altitudes.[50,51] Smoking ten or more cigarettes a day results in slightly higher Hb, PCV and MCV.[52,53] This is probably in consequence of the accumulation of carboxyhaemoglobin in the blood together with a decrease in plasma volume. After a single cigarette, the carboxyhaemoglobin level increases by about 1%,[54] and in heavy smokers the carboxyhaemoglobin may constitute c 4–5% of the total haemoglobin. There may be polycythaemia.[55]

PHYSIOLOGICAL VARIATION IN THE TOTAL LEUCOCYTE COUNT

The effect of age is indicated in Tables 2.1 and 2.2; at birth, the total leucocyte count is high; neutrophils predominate, reaching a peak of c 13.0 × 10^9/l at 12 h and then falling to c 4.0 × 10^9/l over the next few weeks, and then to a level at which the count remains steady. The lymphocytes fall during the first 3 days of life to a low level of c 2.0–2.5 × 10^9/l and then rise up to the 10th day; after this time, they are the predominant cell (up to about 60%) until the 5th to 7th year when they give way to the neutrophils. From that age onwards, the levels are the same as for adults.[10] There are slight sex differences; the total leucocyte count and the neutrophil count may be slightly higher in girls than in boys,[10] and in women than men.[56] After the menopause, the counts fall in women so that they tend to become lower than in men of similar age.[17,56,57]

People differ considerably in their leucocyte counts. Some tend to maintain a relatively constant level over long periods of time;[57] others have counts which may vary by as much as 100% at different times. In some subjects, there appears to be a rhythm, occurring in cycles of 14 to 23 days, and in women this may be related to some extent to the menstrual cycle.[58] Some forms of oral contraception have been reported to raise the leucocyte count.[56] There is also diurnal variation with differences of 14% for the total leucocyte count, 10% for neutrophils, 14% for lymphocytes and 20% for eosinophils;[11] it affects the total leucocyte count as well as all the individual cell types. The minimum counts are found in the morning with the subject at rest.[34] Random activity may raise the count slightly; strenuous exercise causes rises of up to 30 × 10^9/l, chiefly because of decreased splenic blood flow resulting in reduced pooling of neutrophils in the spleen, and to some extent because of liberation into the bloodstream of neutrophils formerly sequestered in shut-down capillaries and in the spleen.[29] Large numbers of lymphocytes and monocytes also enter the bloodstream during strenuous exercise.

Adrenaline (epinephrine) injection causes an increase in the leucocyte count; here, too, increases in the numbers of all major types of leucocytes (and platelets) occur.[59] The rise has been thought to be a reflection of the extent of the reservoir of mature blood cells present not only in the bone marrow and spleen but also in other tissues and organs of the body. Emotion may possibly cause an increase in the leucocyte count in a similar way. The effect of ingestion of food is uncertain. Cigarette smoking causes a significant increase in the leucocyte count;[16,53,60] all types of cells are affected proportionately.[61]

A moderate leucocytosis of up to $15 \times 10^9/l$ is common during pregnancy, owing to a neutrophilia, with the peak in the 2nd trimester.[22] The count returns to normal levels a week or so after delivery.[62]

The environment may influence the leucocyte count. Thus, in tropical Africa, there is a tendency for a reversal of the neutrophil:lymphocyte ratio in individuals with a low total leucocyte count.[63] This may be partly due to endemic parasitic and proto-zoal disease; however, genetics are also likely to play a part as significantly lower leucocyte counts, especially neutrophil counts, have been observed in Africans living in Britain.[64] In some tropical areas, reactive eosinophilia or monocytosis is suf-ficiently common to be regarded as a reference value for that population. Elderly people receiving influenza vaccination show a lower total leucocyte count owing to a decrease in lymphocytes.[65]

PHYSIOLOGICAL VARIATION IN THE PLATELET COUNT

There may be a sex difference; thus, in women, the count has been reported to be about 20% higher than in men.[66] A fall in the platelet count may occur in women at about the time of menstruation and there is some evidence of a cycle with a 21 to 35 day rhythm.[67] There is no evidence that oral contraceptives affect the platelet count. There is a slight diurnal variation of about 5%;[11] this occurs during the course of a day as well as from day to day.[34] Within the wide normal reference range, there are some ethnic differences, and in healthy West Indians and Africans platelet counts may on average be 10–20% lower than those in Europeans living in the same environment.[68] There are no obvious age differences; however, in the first year after birth the platelet count tends to be at the higher level of the adult normal reference range. Strenuous exercise causes a 30–40% increase in platelet count;[29] the mechanism is similar to that which occurs with leucocytes.

Modern blood counting systems provide a high level of precision, so that even small differences in successive measurements may be significant. It is thus most important to establish and understand the limits of physiological variation etc. for the various tests. With this proviso, present-day blood count data can now provide sensitive indications of minor abnormalities which may be important in clinical interpretation and health screening.

REFERENCES

1 International Committee for Standardization in Haematology 1981 The theory of reference values. Clinical and Laboratory Haematology 3:369–373.

2 International Federation of Clinical Chemistry and International Council for Standardization in Haematology 1987 The theory of reference values Part 6: Presentation of observed values related to reference values. Journal of Clinical Biochemistry 25:657–662.

3 Viteri FE, DeTuna V, Guzman MA 1972 Normal haematological values in the Central American population. British Journal of Haematology 23:189.

4 International Committee for Standardization in Haematology 1982 Standardization of blood specimen collection procedures for reference values. Clinical and Laboratory Haematology 4:83–86.

5 International Federation of Clinical Chemistry and International Council for Standardization in Haematology 1987 The theory of reference values Part 5: Statistical treatment of collected reference values. Determination of reference limits. Journal of Clinical Chemistry and Clinical Biochemistry 25:645–656.

6 Reed AH, Henry RJ, Mason WB 1971 Influence of statistical method used on the resulting estimate of normal range. Clinical Chemistry 17:275.

7 Kelly A, Munan L 1977 Haematologic profile of natural populations: red cell parameters. British Journal of Haematology 35:153.

8 Nillson-Ehle H, Jagenburg R, Landahl S, et al 1989 Decline of blood haemoglobin in the aged: a longitudinal study of an urban Swedish population from age 70 to 81. British Journal of Haematology 71:437.

9 Lilleyman JS, Hann IM, Blanchette VS 1999 Pediatric hematology, 2nd edn. Churchill Livingstone, London.

10 Taylor MRH, Holland CV, Spencer R, et al 1997 Haematological reference ranges for school children. Clinical and Laboratory Haematology 19:1–15.

11 Richardson Jones A, Twedt D, Swaim W, et al 1996 Diurnal change of blood count analytes in

normal subjects. American Journal of Clinical Pathology 106:723–727.

12 International Council for Standardization in Haematology: Expert Panel on Cytometry 1995 Recommendation of the International Council for Standardization in Haematology on reporting differential leucocyte counts. Clinical and Laboratory Haematology 17:113.

13 DeMarsh QB, Alt HL, Windle WF, et al 1941 The effect of depriving the infant of its placental blood. Journal of the American Medical Association 116:2568.

14 Matoth Y, Zaizon R, Varsano I 1971 Post-natal changes in some red cell parameters. Acta Paediatrica Scandinavica 60:317.

15 Burman D 1972 Haemoglobin levels in normal infants aged 3 to 24 months and the effect of iron. Archives of Diseases in Childhood 47:261.

16 Helman N, Rubenstein LS 1975 The effects of age, sex and smoking on erythrocytes and leukocytes. American Journal of Clinical Pathology 63:35.

17 Cruickshank JM, Alexander MK 1970 The effect of age, parity, haemoglobin level and oral contraceptive preparations on the normal leucocyte count. British Journal of Haematology 18:541.

18 Hallberg L, Hogdahl AM, Nilsson L, et al 1966 Menstrual blood loss and iron deficiency. Acta Medica Scandinavica 180:639.

19 Burton JL 1967 Effect of oral contraceptives on haemoglobin, packed cell volume, serum-iron and total iron-binding capacity in healthy women. Lancet i:978.

20 Chesley LC 1972 Plasma and red cell volumes during pregnancy. American Journal of Obstetrics and Gynecology 112:440.

21 Large RD, Dynesius R 1973 Blood volume changes during normal pregnancy. Clinics in Haematology 2:433.

22 Balloch AJ, Cauchi MN 1993 Reference ranges for haematology parameters in pregnancy derived from patient populations. Clinical and Laboratory Haematology 15:7–14.

23 Howells MR, Jones SE, Napier JAF, et al 1986 Erythropoiesis in pregnancy. British Journal of Haematology 64:595.

24 Smith JS, Whitelaw DM 1971 Hemoglobin values in aged men. Canadian Medical Association Journal 105:816.

25 Mattila KS, Kuusela V, Pelliniemi TT, et al 1986 Haematological laboratory findings in the elderly; influence of age and sex. Scandinavian Journal of Clinical and Laboratory Investigation 46:411.

26 Myers AM, Saunders CRG, Chalmers DG 1968 The haemoglobin level of fit elderly people. Lancet ii:261.

27 Ross DM, Ayscue LH, Watson J, et al 1988 Stability of hematologic parameters in healthy subjects: intra-individual versus inter-individual variation. American Journal of Clinical Pathology 90:262.

28 Allsop P, Peters AM, Arnot RN, et al 1992 Intrasplenic blood cell kinetics in man before and after brief maximal exercise. Clinical Science 83:47.

29 Allsop P, Arnot R, Gwilliam M, et al 1988 Does splenic autotransfusion occur during high intensity cycle exercise in man? Journal of Physiology (London) 407:24P.

30 Felding P, Tryding N, Hyltoft Petersen P, et al 1980 Effects of posture on concentration of blood constituents in healthy adults: practical application of blood specimen collection procedures recommended by the Scandinavian Committee on Reference Values. Scandinavian Journal of Clinical and Laboratory Investigation 40:615.

31 Ekelund LG, Eklund B, Kaijser L 1971 Time course for the change in hemoglobin concentration with change in posture. Acta Medica Scandinavica 190:335.

32 Mollison PL 1983 Blood transfusion in clinical medicine, 7th edn. Blackwell Scientific, Oxford, p 77.

33 Eisenberg S 1963 The effect of posture and position of the venous sampling site on the hematocrit and serum protein concentration. Journal of Laboratory and Clinical Medicine 51:755.

34 Statland BE, Winkel P, Harris SC, et al 1978 Evaluation of biologic sources of variation of leukocyte counts and other hematologic quantities using very precise automated analyzers. American Journal of Clinical Pathology 69:48.

35 Smith JA 1995 Exercise, training and red blood cell turnover. Sports Medicine 19:9–31.

36 Brotherhood J, Brozovic B, Pugh LGC 1975 Haematological status of middle and long distance runners. Clinical Science and Molecular Medicine 48:139.

37 Green HJ, Sutton JR, Coates G, et al 1991 Response of red cell and plasma volume to prolonged training in humans. Journal of Applied Physiology 70:1810–1815.

38 Piton VA, Howanitz PJ, Howanitz JH, et al 1981 Day-to-day variation in serum ferritin concentration in healthy subjects. Clinical Chemistry 27:78.

39 Romslo I, Talstad I 1988 Day-to-day variations in serum iron, serum iron binding capacity, serum ferritin and erythrocyte protoporphyrin concentration in anaemic subjects. European Journal of Haematology 40:79.

40 Statland EE, Winkel P 1976 Variation in serum iron concentration in young healthy men: within-day and day-to-day changes. Clinical Biochemistry 9:26.

41 Cook JD 1994 The effect of endurance training on iron metabolism. Seminars in Hematology 31:146–154.

42 Natvig H, Bierkedal T, Jonassen O 1963 Studies on hemoglobin values in Norway. III. Seasonal variations. Acta Medica Scandinavica 174:351.

43 Rocker L, Feddersen HM, Hoffmeister H, et al 1980 Seasonal variation of blood components important for diagnosis. Klinische Wochenschrift 58:769–778.

44 Costongs GMPJ, Janson PCW, Bas BM, et al 1985 Short-term and long-term intra-individual variations and critical differences of haematological laboratory parameters. Journal of Clinical Chemistry and Biochemistry 23:69–76.

45 Ross DW, Ayscue LH, Watson J, et al 1988 Stability of hematologic parameters in healthy subjects: intraindividual versus interindividual variation. American Journal of Clinical Pathology 90:262–267.

46 Kristal-Boneh E, Froom P, Harari G, et al 1997 Seasonal differences in blood cell parameters and the association with cigarette smoking. Clinical and Laboratory Haematology 19:177–181

47 Godsland IF, Seed M, Simpson R, et al 1983 Comparison of haematological indices between women of four ethnic groups and the effect of oral contraceptives. Journal of Clinical Pathology 36:184.

48 Hurtado A, Merino C, Delgado E 1945 Influence of anoxemia on the hemopoietic activity. Archives of Internal Medicine 75:284.

49 Ruiz-Arguelles GJ, Sanchez-Medal L, Loria A, et al 1980 Red cell indices in normal adults residing at altitudes from sea level to 2670 meters. American Journal of Hematology 8:265–271.

50 Levin NW, Metz J, Hart D, et al 1960 The blood volume of healthy adult males resident in Johannesburg (altitude 5740 feet). South African Journal of Medical Sciences 28:132.

51 Myhre LD, Dill DB, Hall FG, et al 1970 Blood volume changes during three week residence at high altitude. Clinical Chemistry 16:7.

52 Isager H, Hagerup L 1971 Relationship between cigarette smoking and high packed cell volume and haemoglobin levels. Scandinavian Journal of Haematology 8:241.

53 Whitehead TP, Robinson D, Allaway SL, et al 1995 The effects of cigarette smoking and alcohol consumption on blood haemoglobin, erythrocytes and leucocytes: a dose related study on male subjects. Clinical and Laboratory Haematology 17:131–138.

54 Russel MAH, Wilson C, Cole PV, et al 1973 Comparison of increases in carboxyhaemoglobin after smoking 'extramild' and 'non mild' cigarettes. Lancet ii:687.

55 Smith JR, Landow SA 1978 Smoker's polycythemia. New England Journal of Medicine 298:6.

56 England JM, Bain BJ 1976 Total and differential leucocyte count. British Journal of Haematology 33:1.

57 Booth K, Hancock RET 1961 A study of the total and differential leucocyte counts and haemoglobin levels in a group of normal adults over a period of two years. British Journal of Haematology 7:9.

58 Morley A 1973 Correspondence. Blood 41:329.

59 Chatterjea JB, Dameshek W, Stefanini M 1953 The adrenalin (epinephrin) test as applied to hematologic disorders. Blood 8:211.

60 Corre F, Lellouch J, Schwartz D 1971 Smoking and leucocyte counts; results of an epidemiological survey. Lancet ii:632.

61 Parry H, Cohen S, Schlarb J 1997 Smoking, alcohol consumption and leukocyte counts. American Journal of Clinical Pathology 107:64–67.

62 Cruickshank JM 1970 The effects of parity on the leucocyte count in pregnant and non-pregnant women. British Journal of Haematology 18:531.

63 Woodliff HJ, Kataaha PK, Tibaleka AK, et al 1972 Total leucocyte count in Africans. Lancet ii:875.

64 Bain BJ, Seed M, Godsland I 1984 Normal values for peripheral blood white cell counts in women of four different ethnic origins. Journal of Clinical Pathology 37:188.

65 Cummins D, Wilson ME, Foulger KJ, et al 1998 Haematological changes associated with influenza vaccination in people aged over 65: case report and prospective study. Clinical and Laboratory Haematology 20:285–287.

66 Stevens RF, Alexander MK 1977 A sex difference in the platelet count. British Journal of Haematology 37:295.

67 Morley A 1969 A platelet cycle in normal individuals. Australasian Annals of Medicine 18:127.

68 Bain BJ, Seed M 1986 Platelet count and platelet size in healthy Africans and West Indians. Clinical and Laboratory Haematology 8:43.

69 Narayanan S 2000 The preanalytic phase: an important component of laboratory medicine. American Journal of Clinical Pathology 113: 429–452

3

Basic haematological techniques

Barbara J. Bain & Imelda Bates

It is possible to use manual, semi-automated or automated techniques to determine the various components of the full blood count (FBC). Manual techniques are generally low cost with regard to equipment and reagents but are labour intensive; automated techniques entail high capital costs but permit rapid performance of a large number of blood counts by a smaller number of laboratory workers. Automated techniques are more precise and, if instruments are correctly calibrated, can be as accurate as manual techniques. Many laboratories now use automated techniques almost exclusively, but manual techniques are the basis of laboratory practice and are essential for standardization of laboratory methods.

All the tests discussed in this chapter can be performed on venous or free-flowing capillary blood which has been anticoagulated with EDTA (p. 5). Thorough mixing of the blood specimen before sampling is essential for accurate test results. Ideally, tests should be performed within 6 h of obtaining the blood specimen, since some test results are altered by longer periods of storage. However, results of acceptable accuracy for clinical purposes, can be obtained on blood stored for up to 24 h at 4°C (see Ch. 1).

MANUAL TECHNIQUES

ESTIMATION OF HAEMOGLOBIN CONCENTRATION

The haemoglobin concentration (Hb) of a solution may be estimated by several methods: by measurement of its colour, by its power of combining with oxygen or carbon monoxide or by its iron content. The methods to be described are all colour or light-intensity matching techniques, which also measure, with different degrees of efficiency, any inert pigments, i.e. methaemoglobin (Hi) or sulphaemoglobin (SHb), that may be present. The oxygen-combining capacity of blood is 1.34 ml O_2 per g haemoglobin. Ideally, for assessing *clinical* anaemia a functional estimation of Hb should be carried out by measurement of oxygen capacity, but this is hardly practicable in the routine haematology laboratory. It gives results at least 2% lower than the other methods probably because a small proportion of inert pigment is always present. The iron content of haemoglobin can be estimated accurately,[1] but again the method is impracticable for routine purposes. Estimations based on iron content are generally taken as authentic, but iron bound to inactive pigment is included. Iron content is converted into Hb by assuming the following relationship: 0.347 g iron = 100 g haemoglobin.[2]

MEASUREMENT OF HAEMOGLOBIN CONCENTRATION USING A SPECTROMETER* OR PHOTOELECTRIC COLORIMETER

Two methods are in common use: (a) haemiglobin-cyanide (HiCN; cyanmethaemoglobin) method, and (b) oxyhaemoglobin (HbO_2) method.

There is little to choose in accuracy between these methods, although a major advantage of the HiCN method is the availability of a stable and reliable reference preparation.

Other methods which have been used include Sahli's acid-haematin method which is less accurate as the colour develops slowly, is unstable and begins to fade almost immediately after it reaches its peak. The alkaline-haematin method[3,4] may occasionally be useful as it gives a true estimate of total Hb even if HbCO, Hi or SHb is present, and plasma proteins and lipids have little effect on the development of colour, although they cause turbidity. But the method is more cumbersome and less accurate than the HiCN or HbO_2 methods, and is thus unsuitable for routine use.

Although Drabkin's solution contains only 50 mg of potassium cyanide per litre and 600–1000 ml would have to be swallowed to produce serious effects, the use of potassium cyanide has been viewed as a potential hazard; alternative reagents which have been proposed as non-hazardous substitutes are sodium azide[5,6] and sodium lauryl sulphate[7] which convert haemoglobin to haemiglobinazide and haemiglobinsulphate, respectively. They are used in some automated systems, but they, too, must be handled with care, and no stable standards are available.

HAEMIGLOBINCYANIDE (CYANMETHAEMOGLOBIN) METHOD

This is the World Health Organization's recommended method for determining the haemoglobin concentration of blood.[8] The basis of the method is dilution of blood in a solution containing potassium cyanide and potassium ferricyanide.[9] Haemoglobin, methaemoglobin (Hi) and carboxyhaemoglobin (HbCO), but not sulphaemoglobin (SHb), are converted to HiCN. The absorbance of the solution is then measured in a spectrometer at a wavelength of 540 nm or a photoelectric colorimeter with a yellow-green filter.[†]

Diluent

This is based on Drabkin's cyanide-ferricyanide solution.[9] The original Drabkin reagent had a pH of 8.6. The following modified solution, Drabkin-type reagent, as recommended by the International Committee for Standardization in Haematology,[2] has a pH of 7.0–7.4. It is less likely to cause turbidity from precipitation of plasma proteins and requires a shorter conversion time (3–5 min) than the original Drabkin's solution, but it has the disadvantage that the detergent causes some frothing:

Potassium ferricyanide (0.607 mmol/l)	200 mg
Potassium cyanide (0.768 mmol/l)	50 mg
Potassium dihydrogen phosphate (1.029 mmol/l)	140 mg
Non-ionic detergent	1 ml
Distilled or deionized water	to 1 litre

Suitable non-ionic detergents include Nonidet P40 (Sigma), Saponic 218 (Alcoac Inc.) and Triton X-100 (Rohm and Haas).

The pH should be 7.0–7.4 and must be checked with a pH meter at least once a month. The diluent should be clear and pale yellow in colour. When measured against water as blank in a spectrometer at a wavelength of 540 nm, absorbance must be zero. If stored at room temperature in a brown borosilicate glass bottle, the solution keeps for several months. If the ambient temperature is more than 30°C, the solution should be stored in the refrigerator, but brought to room temperature before use. It must not be allowed to freeze, as this can result in its

---

†(e.g. Ilford 625, Wratten 74, Chance 0 Grl)

decomposition.[10] The reagent must be discarded if it becomes turbid, if the pH is found to be outside the 7.0–7.4 range or if it has an absorbance other than zero at 540 nm against a water blank.

Haemiglobincyanide reference preparation

With the advent of HiCN solution, which is stable for many years, other standards have become outmoded.[11] The International Committee for Standardization in Haematology has defined specifications on the basis of a relative molecular mass (molecular weight) of human haemoglobin of 64 458 and a millimolar coefficient extinction ('molar area absorbance') of 44.0.[*2] Some standards are prepared from ox blood which has the same coefficient extinction but a molecular weight of 64 532. These specifications have been widely adopted; a WHO International Standard has been established, and a comparable reference material is also available from the European Community Bureau of Reference (BCR) (see p. 608). Reference solutions that conform to these international specifications are available commercially. They contain 550–850 mg of haemoglobin per litre and the exact concentration is indicated on the label.

The HiCN solution is dispensed in 10 ml sealed ampoules and is regarded as a dilution of whole blood. The original Hb that it represents is obtained by multiplying the figure stated on the label by the dilution to be applied to the blood sample. Thus, if the standard solution contains 800 mg of haemoglobin per litre, it will have the same optical density as a blood sample containing 160 g haemoglobin per litre diluted 1 to 200, or as one containing 200 g haemoglobin per litre diluted 1 to 250.[†]

The HiCN reference preparation is intended primarily for direct comparison with blood which is also converted to HiCN. It can also be used for the standardization of a whole-blood standard in the HbO_2 method (see below).

Method

Make a 1 in 201 dilution of blood by adding 20 µl of blood to 4 ml of diluent. Stopper the tube containing the solution and invert it several times. After being allowed to stand at room temperature for at least 5 min (to ensure the complete conversion of haemoglobin to haemiglobinocyanide), pour the test sample into a cuvette and read the absorbance in a spectrometer at 540 nm or in a photoelectric colorimeter with a suitable filter,[‡] against a reagent blank. The absorbance of the test sample must be measured within 6 h of its initial dilution. The absorbance of a commercially available HiCN standard (brought to room temperature if previously stored in a refrigerator) should also be compared to a reagent blank in the same spectrometer or photoelectric colorimeter as the patient sample. The standard should be kept in the dark and, to ensure that contamination is avoided, any unused solution should be discarded at the end of the day on which the ampoule is opened.

Calculation of haemoglobin concentration

$$\frac{Hb}{(g/l)} = \frac{{}^\S A^{540} \text{ of test sample}}{A^{540} \text{ of standard}} \times \frac{\text{Conc.}}{\text{of standard}} \times \frac{\text{Dilution factor (201}^\P\text{)}}{1000}$$

Preparation of standard graph and standard table

When many blood samples are to be tested, it is convenient to read the results from a standard graph or table relating absorbance readings to Hb in g/l for the individual instrument. This graph should be prepared each time a new photometer is put into use and can be prepared as follows.

Prepare five dilutions of the HiCN reference solution (brought to room temperature) with the Drabkin-type reagent according to Table 3.1. As the graph will be used to determine the haemoglobin

---

[*]i.e. the absorbance of a solution containing 4×55.8 mg of haemoglobin iron per litre at 540 nm.

[†]Within the SI system, many measurements are now expressed in terms of substance concentration, using the mole as unit. For clinical purposes, there are practical advantages in continuing to express Hb in mass concentration, as g/l or g/dl.

[‡]e.g. Ilford 625, Wratten 74 or Chance 0 Gr1.

[§]i.e. absorbance; formerly called optical density. In some instruments, measurements are read as percentage transmittance.

[¶]It is also acceptable to use an initial dilution of 1 to 251 instead of 1 to 201 by adding 20 µl blood to 5 ml Drabkin-type reagent; in this case, the dilution factor will be 251 instead of 201.

Table 3.1 Dilutions of HiCN reference solution for preparation of standard graph

Tube	Hb*	HiCN volume	Reagent volume
1	100% (full strength)	4 ml (neat)	none
2	75%	3.0 ml	1.0 ml
3	50%	2.0 ml	2.0 ml
4	25%	1.0 ml	3.0 ml
5	0	none	4 ml (neat)

* As percent of Hb on reference solution label.

measurements, it is essential that the dilutions are performed accurately.

The haemoglobin concentration of the reference solution in each tube should be plotted against the absorbance measurement. For example, if the label on the HiCN reference solution states that it contains 800 mg/l and the method for haemoglobin measurement uses a dilution of 1:201, the respective haemoglobin concentrations of tubes 1–5 would be 160 g/l, 120 g/l, 80 g/l, 40 g/l and zero.

Using linear graph paper, plot the absorbance values on the vertical axis and the haemoglobin values on the horizontal axis. (If the readings are in percentage transmittance, use semi-logarithmic paper with the transmittance recorded on the vertical (log) scale.) The points should fit a straight line that passes through the origin. Providing that the standard has been correctly diluted, this provides a check that the calibration of the photometer is linear. From the graph, it is possible to construct a table of readings and corresponding haemoglobin values. This is more convenient than reading values from a graph when large numbers of measurements are made. It is important that the performance of the instrument should not vary and that its calibration remains constant in relation to Hb measurements. To ensure this, the reference preparation should be measured at frequent intervals, preferably with each batch of blood samples.

The main advantages of the HiCN method for Hb determination are that it allows direct comparison with the HiCN standard and that the readings need not be made immediately after dilution so batching of samples is possible. It also has the advantage that all forms of haemoglobin, except SHb, are readily converted to HiCN.

The rate of conversion of blood containing HbCO is markedly slow. This difficulty can be overcome by prolonging the reaction time to 30 min before reading.[12] The difference between the 5 and 30 min readings can be used as a semi-quantitative method for estimating the percentage of HbCO in the blood.

As referred to above, lauryl sulphate can be used as a non-hazardous substitute for potassium cyanide.[13] However, no stable standard is available for this method so a sample of blood which has first had a haemoglobin value assigned by the HiCN method needs to be used as a secondary standard.

Abnormal plasma proteins or a high leucocyte count may result in turbidity when the blood is diluted in the Drabkin-type reagent. The turbidity can be avoided by centrifuging the diluted sample or by increasing the concentration of potassium dihydrogen phosphate to 33 mmol/l (4.0 g/l).[14]

OXYHAEMOGLOBIN METHOD

This method is the simplest and quickest method for general use with a photometer. Its disadvantage is that it is not possible to prepare a stable HbO_2 standard so the calibration of these instruments should be checked regularly using HiCN reference solutions or a secondary standard of preserved blood or lysate (p. 568). The reliability of the method is not affected by a moderate rise in plasma bilirubin but it is not satisfactory in the presence of HbCO, Hi or SHb.

Method

Wash 20 µl of blood into a tube containing 4 ml of 0.4 ml/l ammonia (specific gravity 0.88) to give a 1:200 dilution.* Use a tightly fitting stopper and mix by inverting the tube several times. The solution of HbO_2 is then ready for matching against a standard in a spectrometer at 540 nm or a photometer with a yellow-green filter (e.g. Ilford 625) against a water blank. If the absorbance of the haemoglobin solution exceeds 0.7, dilute the blood further with an equal volume of water and read again. Fresh ammonia solution must be made up each week. Once diluted, the blood sample is stable at 20°C for about 2 days.

---

*i.e., 1 in 201

Standard

A standard should be prepared from a specimen of normal anticoagulated whole blood. Its Hb is first determined by the HiCN method (p. 20). The blood is then diluted 1 in 201 by pipetting 20 μl of the well-mixed blood into 4 ml of ammonia; sequential dilutions are made in ammonia and absorbance is read in a spectrometer at 540 nm or photometer using a yellow-green filter (Ilford 625, Wratten 74 or Chance 0 Gr 1). The readings are plotted on arithmetic graph paper. Linearity of response is checked and absorbance is related to Hb from the measurement obtained in the original sample by the HiCN method.

Colorimeters and light filters unfortunately differ sufficiently one from the other to make it essential to check the chosen standard at frequent intervals against a HiCN reference preparation in the photometer in which it is going to be used. It is probably preferable to use a new fresh whole-blood sample each day as a secondary standard after measuring its Hb by the HiCN method. Preserved blood or lysate (p. 568) can be used instead.

Direct calculation from a standard:

$$\text{Hb (g/l)} = \frac{A^{540} \text{ test sample}}{A^{540} \text{ standard}} \times \frac{\text{Conc. of}}{\text{standard}} \times \frac{\text{Dilution}}{\text{factor}}$$

If the HiCN method is not available, a neutral grey filter of 0.475 density (Ilford or Chance) can be used as a calibration standard. This corresponds to a 1:200 dilution of blood with 146 g/l haemoglobin in a 1 cm cuvette at a wavelength of 540 nm.

DIRECT READING HAEMOGLOBINOMETRY
Colour comparators

These are simple clinical devices which compare the colour of blood, without conversion to a derivative, against a range of colours which represent haemoglobin concentrations. They include the *Lovibond Comparator*, which requires the blood to be diluted, and the *BMS Grey Wedge Photometer* which does not.

The *WHO Hb Colour Scale* provides an estimate of Hb within 1 g/dl (10 g/l) by comparing the colour of a drop of blood on a special test strip with a printed colour scale (see p. 594).

Portable haemoglobinometers

These instruments have a built-in filter and a scale calibrated for direct reading of Hb in g/dl or g/l. They are generally based on the oxyhaemoglobin method. A number of instruments are now available which utilize a light-emitting diode of appropriate wavelength and are standardized to give the same results as with the haemiglobincyanide method. The HemoCue system consists of a pre-calibrated, portable, battery-operated photometer and no dilution is necessary as blood is run by capillary action directly into a cuvette containing sodium nitrite and sodium azide which convert the haemoglobin to azidemethaemoglobin. The absorbance is measured at wavelengths of 565 and 880 nm. It is reliable, easy for non-technical personnel to operate and measurements are not affected by high levels of bilirubin, lipids or white cells.

Spectrometry

The Hb of a diluted blood sample can be determined accurately by spectrometry. The blood is diluted 1:201 (or 1:251) with cyanide-ferricyanide reagent (p. 20) and the absorbance is measured at 540 nm. Hb is calculated as follows:

$$\text{Hb (g/dl)} = \frac{A^{540} \text{ HiCN} \times 64\,500 \times \text{Dilution factor}}{44.0 \times d \times 1000}$$

where A^{540} = absorbance of solution at 540 nm; 64 500 = molecular weight of haemoglobin (derived from 64 458*); dilution = 201 when 20 μl of blood are diluted in 4 ml of reagent; 44.0 = millimolar coefficient extinction; d = layer thickness in cm; and 1000 = conversion of mg to g.

Calibration of the spectrophotometer should be checked regularly by verifying that it gives an accurate value for the HiCN standard. Slight deviations from the expected A^{540} HiCN value for the standard may be used to correct the results of test samples for a bias in measurement.[2]

Range of Hb in health

See pages 12 and 13.

Slightly lower mean values for men (145 g/l) and women (128 g/l) have been reported in a Health survey in England.[89]

DETERMINATION OF PACKED CELL VOLUME OR HAEMATOCRIT VALUE

The packed cell volume (PCV) can be used as a simple screening test for anaemia and as a reference

---

*or 64532 for OX blood

method for calibrating automated blood count systems.[15] It can also be used as a rough guide to the accuracy of haemoglobin measurements as the PCV as a percentage should be about three times the haemoglobin value. In conjunction with estimations of Hb and red cell count, it is used in the calculation of red cell indices. However, its use in under-resourced laboratories may be limited by the need for a specialized centrifuge and a reliable supply of capillary tubes. The macro-method of Wintrobe for PCV measurement is no longer in routine use, having been replaced by the micro-haematocrit method.

MICRO-HAEMATOCRIT

The centrifuge used for capillary tubes provides a centrifugal force of c 12 000 g and 5 min centrifugation results in a constant PCV. When the PCV is greater than 0.5, it may be necessary to centrifuge for a further 5 min.

Method

Capillary tubes 75 mm in length and having an internal diameter of about 1 mm are required. They can be obtained plain or coated inside with 2 iu of heparin. The latter type is suitable for the direct collection of capillary blood. Plain tubes are used for anticoagulated venous blood which must be well mixed before use.

Allow the blood to enter the tube by capillarity, leaving at least 15 mm unfilled. Then seal the tube by a plastic seal, e.g. Cristaseal (Hawksley, Lancing, Sussex) or by heating the dry end of the tube rapidly in a fine flame, e.g. the pilot light of a Bunsen burner, combined with rotation. After centrifugation for 5 min, measure the proportion of cells to the whole column (i.e. the PCV) using a reading device.

Accuracy of micro-haematocrit

Failure to mix the blood sample adequately will produce an inaccurate result. EDTA anticoagulant in excess of 1.5 mg/ml may cause a falsely low PCV as it causes cell shrinkage. The degree of oxygenation of the blood also affects the result, as the PCV of venous blood is ~2% higher than that of fully aerated blood (which has lost CO_2 and taken up O_2)[90]. Variation of the bore of the tubes may also cause serious errors if they are not manufactured within the narrow limits of precision that

conform to defined standards, e.g. British Standard for Apparatus for Measurement of Packed Red Cell Volume (BS 4316: 1968).

Other errors are caused by difficulty in heat-sealing the lower end of the tube so as to obtain a flat base and difficulties in reading. To avoid errors in reading with the special reading device, a magnifying glass should be used. If a special reading device is not available, the ratio of red cell column to whole column (i.e. red cells, buffy layer and plasma) can be calculated from measurements obtained by placing the tube against arithmetic graph paper or against a ruler.

Plasma trapping, especially in the lower end of the red cell column, and red cell dehydration during centrifugation generally counterbalance each other and the error caused by trapped plasma is usually not more than 0.01 PCV units. Thus, in routine practice, it is unnecessary to correct for trapped plasma, but when the PCV is required for calibrating a blood cell analyser or for calculating blood volume, the observed PCV should be reduced by a 2% correction factor after centrifuging for 5 min.[16] When the PCV is more than 0.5, centrifugation should be continued for a further 5 min and 2% should be deducted from the observed reading. Plasma trapping is increased in macrocytic anaemias,[17] spherocytosis, thalassaemia, hypochromic anaemias and sickle-cell anaemia;[18] it may be as high as 20% in sickle-cell anaemia if all the cells are sickled.[17]

Range of packed cell volume in health
See pages 12 and 13.

MANUAL CELL COUNTS AND RED CELL INDICES

The principles of manual cell counts, methods for manually counting white cells and platelets, and the limitations of these measurements are described in Chapter 26.

TOTAL RED BLOOD CELL COUNT (RBC) AND RED CELL INDICES

In addition to being intrinsically useful, an accurate red blood cell count (RBC) enables the mean cell volume (MCV) and mean cell haemoglobin (MCH) to be calculated. In well-equipped laboratories, where these indices are provided by an automated system (p. 35), they are of considerable clinical importance and are widely used in the classification of anaemia. Where automated analysers are not used, manual red cell counts (and consequently, calculations of these red cell indices) are so inaccurate and time-consuming that they have become obsolete.

The only measurement which can be obtained with reasonable accuracy by manual methods is mean cell haemoglobin concentration (MCHC), as this is derived from Hb and PCV from the formula:

$$MCHC \ (g/l) = Hb \ (g/l) \div PCV \ (l/l).$$

Range of MCHC in health
See pages 12 and 13.

BASOPHIL AND EOSINOPHIL COUNTS
Counting chamber methods for eosinophil and basophil counts were described in previous editions. They are similar to the method for total leucocyte count (p. 595): the blood is diluted with a dye solution which stains, respectively, the eosinophils (eosin or phloxine)[19,20] or the basophils (alcian blue)[21] whilst lysing the red cells. A preferred method is to count the percentage of eosinophils or basophils in a manual differential leucocyte count of 500 cells on a stained blood film, and then calculate the eosinophil or basophil count per litre from the total leucocyte count.

Range of eosinophil count in health
See pp. 12 and 13
There is normally considerable diurnal variation in the eosinophil count, and differences amounting to as much as 100% have been recorded. The lowest counts are found in the morning (10 a.m. to noon) and the highest at night (midnight to 4 a.m.)[22-24] Muehrcke et al.[25] found that the counts of 42 healthy but fasting young males conformed to a log-normal distribution.

Range of basophil count in health[26]
See p. 12
Gilbert & Ornstein[21] reported a 95% distribution in normal subjects of $0.01-0.08 \times 10^9/l$. There are no age or sex differences although serial counts have shown lower levels during ovulation.[27]

MANUAL DIFFERENTIAL LEUCOCYTE COUNT
Differential leucocyte counts are usually performed by visual examination of blood films which are prepared on slides by the spread or 'wedge' technique (p. 47). Unfortunately, even in well-spread films, the distribution of the various cell types is not totally random (see below).

For a reliable, differential count on films spread on slides, the film must not be too thin and the tail of the film should be smooth. To achieve this, the film should be made with a rapid movement using a smooth glass spreader. This should result in a film in which there is some overlap of the red cells, diminishing to separation near the tail, and in which the white cells in the body of the film are not too badly shrunken. If the film is too thin, or if a rough-edged spreader is used, many of the white cells, perhaps even 50% of them, accumulate at the edges and in the tail (Fig. 3.1). Moreover, a gross qualitative irregularity in distribution is the rule: polymorphonuclear neutrophils and monocytes predominate at the margins and the tail; lymphocytes in the middle of the film (Fig. 3.2). This separation probably depends upon differences in stickiness, size and specific gravity of the different types of cells.

Differences in distribution of the various types of cells are probably always present to a small extent even in well-made films. Various systems for performing the differential count have been advocated but none can compensate for the gross irregularities in distribution in a badly made film. On well-made films, the following technique of counting is recommended.

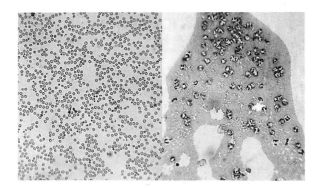

Fig. 3.1 Centre (left) and tail (right) of a badly made blood film. The centre of the film is almost devoid of white cells; in the tail, neutrophils, particularly, are present in large numbers. ×100.

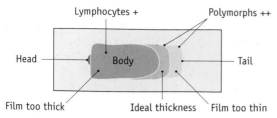

Fig. 3.2 Schematic drawing of a blood film made on a slide. The film has been spread from left to right. An indication is given of the way the white blood cells are distributed (see text).

Method

Count the cells using a ×40 dry lens in a strip running the whole length of the film. Avoid the lateral edges of the film. Inspect the film from the head to the tail, and if fewer than 100 cells are encountered in a single narrow strip, examine one or more additional strips until at least 100 cells have been counted. Each longitudinal strip represents the blood drawn out from a small part of the original drop of blood when it has spread out between the slide and spreader (Fig. 3.3). If all the cells are counted in such a strip, the differential totals will approximate closely to the true differential count. This technique is liable to error if cells in the thick part of the film cannot be identified; also, it does not allow for any excess of neutrophils and monocytes at the edges of the film, but this preponderance is slight in a well-made film and in practice makes little difference to the result.

The above technique is easy to carry out; with high counts (10–30 × 10⁹ cells per litre) a short,

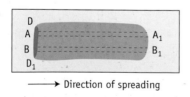

Fig. 3.3 Schematic drawing illustrating the longitudinal method of performing differential leucocyte counts. The original drop of blood spreads out between spreader and slide (D–D₁). The film is made in such a way that representative strips of films, such as A–A₁ and B–B₁ are formed from blood originally at A and B, respectively. In order to perform an accurate differential count, all the leucocytes in one or more strips, such as A–A₁ and B–B₁, should be inspected and classified.

2–3 cm, film is desirable. In patients with very high counts (as in leukaemia), the method has to be abandoned and the cells should be counted in any well-spread area where the cell types are easy to identify. Other systems of counting, such as the 'battlement' count, are more elaborate but may minimize error owing to variation of distribution of cells between the centre and the edge of the film. The results of the differential count can be recorded using a multiple manual register or directly entered onto a computer.

The variance differential count depends not only on artefactual differences in distribution owing to the process of spreading, but also on 'random' distribution; together they are by far the most important cause of unreliable differential counts.[28] The random distribution means that, if a total of 100 cells are counted, with a true neutrophil proportion of 50%, the range (± 2SD) within which 95% of the counts will fall, is of the order of ± 14%, i.e. 36–64% neutrophils. A 200-cell count can provide a more accurate estimate; in the above example, the ± 2SD range will be about 40–60%. In a 500-cell count, the range would be reduced to 44–56% neutrophils. In practice, a 100- or 200-cell count is recommended as a routine procedure. However, if abnormal cells are present in small numbers, they are more likely to be detected when 200–500 cell counts are performed than with a 100-cell count.

Reporting the differential leucocyte count

The differential count, expressed as the percentage of each type of cell, should be related to the total leucocyte count and the results reported in absolute numbers (× 10⁹/l). Myelocytes and metamyelocytes, if present, are recorded separately from neutrophils. Band (stab) cells are generally counted as neutrophils but it may be useful to record them separately. They normally constitute less than 6% of the neutrophils; an increase may point to an inflammatory process even in the absence of an absolute leucocytosis.[29] However, the band cell count is very imprecise and is not helpful in predicting occult bacteraemia in infants.[30]

Correcting the count for nucleated red blood cells

When nucleated red blood cells (NRBC) are present, they will be included in the total white blood cell count (WBC), which is really a 'total nucleated cell count' (TNCC). They should also be included in the differential count, as a percentage of the TNCC, and reported in absolute numbers ($\times 10^9$/l) in the same way as the different types of leucocytes. If they are present in significant numbers, the TNCC should be corrected to obtain the true total WBC. Thus, for example, if total WBC is 8.0×10^9/l and the percentage of NRBCs on the differential count is 25%, then

Corrected WBC = $8 - (8 \times 25/100) = 6 \times 10^9$/l.

Care should be taken to differentiate small lymphocytes from nucleated red blood cells (e.g. p. 86 Fig. 5.64).

Range of differential white cell counts in health

See pages 12 and 13.

PLATELET COUNT

The method for manual counting of platelets using a counting chamber is described on page 596. If a red cell count by a semi-automated counter is available, it is possible to obtain an approximation of the platelet count by counting the proportion of platelets to red cells in a thin part of a film made from an EDTA blood sample, using the $\times 100$ oil-immersion objective and if possible eyepieces provided with an adjustable diaphragm, as for a reticulocyte count (p. 29).

RETICULOCYTE COUNT

Reticulocytes are juvenile red cells; they contain remnants of the ribosomal ribonucleic acid which was present in larger amounts in the cytoplasm of the nucleated precursors from which they were derived. Ribosomes have the property of reacting with certain basic dyes such as azure B, brilliant cresyl blue or New methylene blue* to form a blue or purple precipitate of granules or filaments.

This reaction takes place only in vitally stained unfixed preparations. Stages of maturation can be identified by their morphological features.[31,32] The most immature reticulocytes are those with the largest amount of precipitable material; in the least immature, only a few dots or short strands are

seen. Reticulocytes can be classified into four groups ranging from the most immature reticulocytes, with a large clump of reticulin (group I), to the most mature, with a few granules of reticulin (group IV) (Fig. 3.4).

If a blood film is allowed to dry and is afterwards fixed with methanol, reticulocytes appear as red cells staining diffusely basophilic if the film is stained with one of the basic dyes.

Complete loss of basophilic material probably occurs in the bloodstream and, particularly, in the spleen[33] after the cells have left the bone marrow.[34] The ripening process is thought to take 2 to 3 days, of which about 24 h are spent in the circulation.

The number of reticulocytes in the peripheral blood is a fairly accurate reflection of erythropoietic activity, assuming that the reticulocytes are released normally from the bone marrow, and that they remain in circulation for the normal period of time. These assumptions are not always valid as an increased erythropoietic stimulus leads to premature release into the circulation. The maturation time of these so-called 'stress' or stimulated reticulocytes may be as long as 3 days. In such cases, it is possible to deduce the reticulocyte maturation time and calculate a 'corrected' reticulocyte count by using plasma-iron turnover data.[35,36] Nevertheless, adequate information is usually obtained from a simple reticulocyte count recorded as a percentage of the red cells or preferably, if the red cell count is known, expressed as absolute numbers.

Stains

Better and more reliable results are obtained with New methylene blue than with brilliant cresyl blue. New methylene blue stains the reticulofilamentous material in reticulocytes more deeply and more uniformly than does brilliant cresyl blue, which varies from sample to sample in its staining ability. Purified azure B is a satisfactory substitute for New methylene blue; it has the advantage that the dye does not precipitate[37] and it is available in pure form.[38] It is used in the same concentration and the staining procedure is the same as with New methylene blue.

Staining solution

Dissolve 1.0 g of New methylene blue (CI 52030)* or azure B (CI 52010) in 100 ml of iso-osmotic phosphate buffer pH 6.5 (p. 605).

---

*New methylene blue is chemically different from methylene blue which is a poor reticulocyte stain.

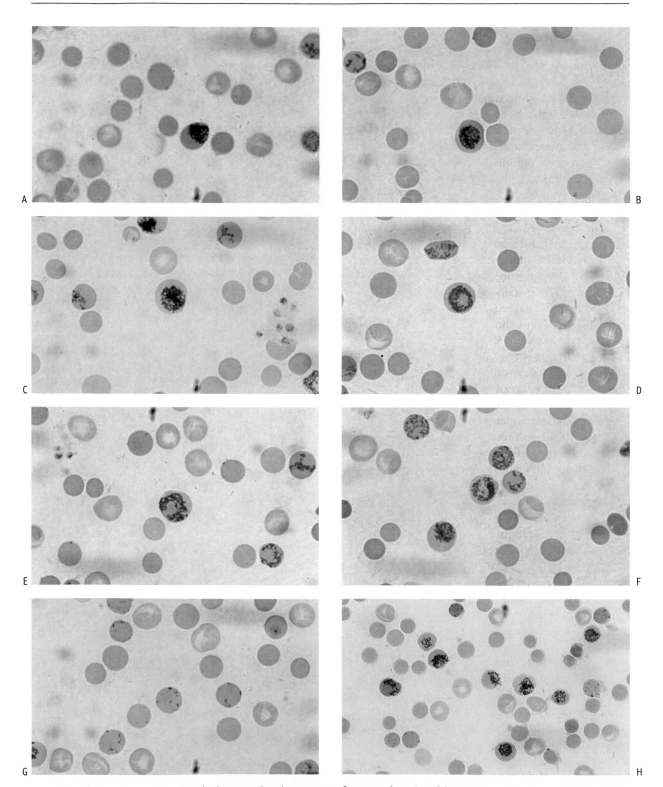

Fig. 3.4 Photomicrographs of reticulocytes showing stages of maturation. A and B, most immature (group I); C and D, intermediate (group II); E and F, later stage itermediate (group III); G, most mature (group IV); H, haemolytic anaemia, stained supravitally by new methylene blue.

Method

Deliver 2 or 3 drops of the dye solution into a 75 × 10 mm glass or plastic tube by means of a plastic Pasteur pipette. Add 2–4 volumes of the patient's EDTA-anticoagulated blood to the dye solution and mix. Keep the mixture at 37°C for 15–20 min. Re-suspend the red cells by gentle mixing and make films on glass slides in the usual way. When dry, examine the films without fixing or counterstaining.

The exact volume of blood to be added to the dye solution for optimal staining depends upon the red cell count. A larger proportion of anaemic blood, and a smaller proportion of polycythaemic blood, should be added than of normal blood. In a successful preparation, the reticulofilamentous material should be stained deep blue and the non-reticulated cells stained diffusely shades of pale greenish blue. Films should not be counterstained. The reticulofilamentous material is not better defined after counterstaining and precipitated stain overlying cells may cause confusion. Moreover, Heinz bodies will not be visible in fixed and counterstained preparations. If the stained preparation is examined under phase contrast, both the mature red cells and reticulocytes are well defined. By this technique, late reticulocytes characterized by the presence of remnants of filaments or threads are readily distinguished from cells containing inclusion bodies. Satisfactory counts may be made on blood that has been allowed to stand (unstained) for as long as 24 h, although the count will tend to fall slightly after 6–8 h unless the blood is kept at 4°C.

Counting reticulocytes

An area of film should be chosen for the count where the cells are undistorted and where the staining is good. A common fault is to make the film too thin; however, the cells should not overlap. To count the cells, use the × 100 oil-immersion objective and, if possible, eyepieces provided with an adjustable diaphragm. If eyepieces with an adjustable diaphragm are not available, a paper or cardboard diaphragm, in the centre of which has been cut a small square with sides about 4 mm in length, can be inserted into an eyepiece and used as a less convenient substitute.

The counting procedure should be appropriate to the number of reticulocytes present. Very large numbers of cells have to be surveyed if a reason-ably accurate count is to be obtained when only small numbers of reticulocytes are present.[34] When the count is less than 10%, a convenient method is to survey successive fields until at least 100 reticulocytes have been counted and to count the total red cells in at least ten fields in order to determine the average number of red cells per field.

Calculation

Number of reticulocytes in n fields = x
Average number of red cells per field = y
Total number of red cells in n fields = n × y
Reticulocyte percentage = [x ÷ (n × y)] × 100%
Absolute reticulocyte count = % × RBC

Thus, when the reticulocyte percentage is 3.3 and the RBC is $5 \times 10^{12}/l$, the absolute reticulocyte count per litre is: $[3.3/100] \times 5 \times 10^{12} = 165 \times 10^9$

It is essential that the reticulocyte preparation be well spread to ensure an even distribution of cells in successive fields.

When the reticulocyte count exceeds 10%, only a relatively small number of cells will have to be surveyed to obtain a standard error of 10%.

An alternative method is based on the principle of 'balanced sampling', using a Miller ocular.* This is an eyepiece giving a square field, in the corner of which is a smaller ruled square, one-ninth the area of the total square (Fig. 3.5). Reticulocytes are counted in the large square and the total number of red cells in the small square.

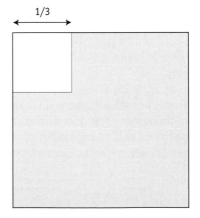

Fig. 3.5 Miller ocular.

*e.g. Graticules Ltd, Morley Road, Tonbridge, UK.

Table 3.2 Accuracy of reticulocyte counts with Miller ocular

Reticulocytes		Standard error (σ)		
%	Proportion (p)	2%	5%	10%
1	0.01	27500	4400	1100
2	0.02	13600	2180	550
5	0.05	5280	845	210
10	0.10	2500	400	100
25	0.25	835	135	35

Columns 3–5 indicate the total number of red cells to be counted *in the small squares* so as to give the required standard error at different reticulocyte levels. It is derived from:
$\sigma = \sqrt{p(1 - p)/\lambda}$, where p = Number of reticulocytes in n large squares ÷ (Number of red cells in n small squares × f)
f = ratio of large to small squares (i.e. 9), and λ = approximate total number of cells in n large squares.

The number of fields which should be surveyed to obtain a desired degree of precision depends on the proportion of reticulocytes (Table 3.2).

It is essential that the reticulocyte preparation be well spread and well stained. Other important factors which affect the accuracy of the count are the visual acuity and patience of the observer and the quality and resolving power of the microscope. The most accurate counts are carried out by a conscientious observer who has no knowledge of the supposed reticulocyte level, thus eliminating the effect of conscious or unconscious bias.

Differentiating between reticulocytes and other red cell inclusions

The decision as to what is and what is not a reticulocyte may be difficult, as the most mature reticulocytes contain only a few dots or threads of reticulofilamentous material. Fortunately, in well-stained preparations, viewed under the light microscope, the Pappenheimer (iron-containing) type of granular material – usually present as a single small dot, less commonly as multiple dots – stains a darker shade of blue than does the reticulofilamentous material of the reticulocyte. As described above, phase contrast will help to distinguish them. If there is any doubt, Pappenheimer bodies can be identified by overstaining the film for iron by Perls' reaction (see p. 270).

HbH undergoes denaturation in the presence of brilliant cresyl blue or New methylene blue, resulting in round inclusion bodies which stain greenish-blue (Figs 13.7 and 13.8, p. 274). These can be easily differentiated from reticulofilamentous material (Fig. 13.9).

Heinz bodies are also stained by New methylene blue, but they stain a lighter shade of blue than the reticulofilamentous material of reticulocytes and stain well with methyl violet (Figs 13.5 and 13.6, p. 273).

Fluorescence methods for performing a reticulocyte count

Reticulocytes can be counted by fluorescence microscopy.[39,40] Add 1 volume of acridine orange solution (50 mg/100 ml of 9 g/l NaCl) to 1 volume of blood. Mix gently for 2 min; make films on glass slides, dry rapidly and examine by a fluorescent microscope. RNA gives an orange-red fluorescence whilst nuclear material (DNA) fluoresces yellow. However, the method is not suitable for routine use for reticulocyte counting. Although the amount of fluorescence is proportional to the amount of RNA, the brightness and colour of the fluorescence fluctuates and the preparation quickly fades when exposed to light; also, it requires a special fluorescence microscope.

Fluorescent staining combined with flow cytometry has been developed as a method for automated reticulocyte counting (see p. 41).[41–43]

Range of reticulocyte count in health

Adults and children 50–100 × 10^9/l. (0.5–2.5%). Infants (full term, cord blood) 2–5% (see p. 13).

AUTOMATED TECHNIQUES

A variety of automated instruments for performing blood counts have been developed and are now in widespread use. Semi-automated instruments require some steps, e.g. dilution of a blood sample, to be carried out by the operator. Fully automated instruments require only that an appropriate blood sample is presented to the instrument. Semi-automated instruments often measure a small number of components, e.g. WBC and Hb. Fully automated multi-channel instruments usually measure from 8 to 20 components, including some new variables which have no equivalent in manual techniques. Automated instruments usually have a high level of precision which, for cell counting and cell-sizing techniques, is greatly superior to that which can be achieved with manual techniques. If instruments are carefully calibrated and their correct operation is assured by quality control procedures, they produce test results that are generally accurate. When blood has abnormal characteristics, the results for one or more parameters may be aberrant; instruments are designed so that such inconsistent results are 'flagged' for subsequent review. The abnormal characteristics which lead to inaccurate counts vary between instruments, so that it is important for instrument operators to be familiar with the types of factitious results to which their instruments are prone. The most recently developed blood cell counters have automated procedures for sample recognition (e.g. by bar-coding), for ensuring that adequate sample mixing occurs, for taking up the test sample automatically and for detection of clots or inadequately sized samples. Ideally, blood sampling is carried out by piercing the cap of a closed tube so that samples which carry an infection hazard can be handled with maximum safety.

Laboratories performing large numbers of blood counts each day require fully automated blood counters capable of the rapid production of accurate and precise blood counts, including platelet counts and differential counts, either three-part or five-part. The sample throughput required varies with the workload and the timing of arrival of blood specimens in the laboratory, but for most large laboratories a throughput of 80–100 samples per hour is required. Sample size and the availability of a 'pre-dilute' mode are particularly relevant if the laboratory receives many paediatric specimens. Choice of an instrument for an individual laboratory should take account of capital expenditure and running costs, including maintenance and reagents; size of instrument, requirements of services such as water, compressed air, drainage and an electricity supply with stable voltage; environmental disturbance by generation of heat, vibration and noise; any influence on performance by the ambient temperature and humidity; storage requirements for the often bulky reagents; ease of operation; the likely level of support which can be expected from the manufacturer. A practical guide on the principles of the various systems has been published,[44] and there are guidelines to help in the choice of an instrument suitable for the needs of an individual laboratory and also to assess its performance, as compared with the claims of the manufacturer, when it has been installed and is being used in routine practice.[45] Choice of instrument may be aided by reference to published reports of instrument evaluations, of which there are many, and to reports from the UK National Health Service Medical Devices Agency. A number of monographs are available.[31,44,46] Some semi-automated instruments aspirate a sample of accurately determined volume and so can perform absolute cell counts and accurate estimations of Hb. Most automated instruments, however, count for a specified period of time rather than on an exact volume of blood; they therefore require calibration by means of the direct counts derived from instruments counting cells in a defined volume of diluted blood. For some variables, instruments are calibrated by the manufacturer, but others require calibration in the laboratory (see p. 33). Performance characteristics of an instrument vary over time so that periodic recalibration is needed, both when quality control procedures indicate the necessity and when certain components are replaced.

HAEMOGLOBIN CONCENTRATION

Most automated counters measure Hb by a modification of the manual HiCN method. Modifications include alterations in the concentration of reagents and in the temperature and pH of the reaction. A non-ionic detergent is included to ensure rapid cell lysis and to reduce turbidity caused by cell membranes and plasma lipids. Measurements of absorbance are made at a set time interval after mixing of blood and the active reagents but before the reaction is completed.

In some Sysmex instruments, HiCN has been replaced with a method using a non-toxic chemical, sodium lauryl sulphate, in order to reduce possible environmental hazards from disposal of large volumes of cyanide-containing waste. This has been found to be a reliable routine method with estimations of Hb being generally equivalent to those produced by the HiCN method.[13]

RED BLOOD CELL COUNT

Red cells and other blood cells can be counted in systems based on either aperture impedance or light-scattering technology. As large numbers of cells can be counted rapidly, there is a high level of precision. Consequently, electronic counts have rendered the RBC and the red cell indices derived from it (the MCV and the MCH) of much greater clinical relevance than was possible when only a slow and imprecise manual RBC was available.

Impedance counting

Impedance counting, first described by Wallace Coulter in 1956,[47] depends on the fact that red cells are poor conductors of electricity whereas certain diluents are good conductors; this difference forms the basis of the counting systems used in Beckman–Coulter, Sysmex, Abbott, Roche and a number of other instruments.

For a cell count, blood is highly diluted in a buffered electrolyte solution. The flow rate of this diluted sample is controlled by a mercury siphon (as in the original Coulter system) or by displacement of a tightly fitting piston. This result is a measured volume of the sample passing through an aperture tube of specific dimensions, e.g. 100 μm in diameter and 70 μm in length. By means of a constant source of electricity, a direct

current is maintained between two electrodes, one in the sample beaker or the chamber surrounding the aperture tube and another inside the aperture tube. As a blood cell is carried through the aperture, it displaces some of the conducting fluid and increases the electrical resistance. This produces a corresponding change in potential between the electrodes which lasts as long as the red cell takes to pass though the aperture; the height of the pulses produced indicates the volume of the cells passing through. The pulses can be displayed on an oscillograph screen. The pulses are led to a threshold circuit provided with an amplitude discriminator for selecting the minimal pulse height which will be counted (Fig. 3.6). The height of the pulses is used to determine the volume of the red cells (see p. 35).

Light scattering

Red cells and other blood cells may be counted by means of electro-optical detectors.[48] A diluted cell suspension flows through an aperture so that the cells pass, in single file, in front of a light source; light is scattered by the cells passing through the light beam. Scattered light is detected by a photomultiplier or photodiode which converts it into electrical impulses which are accumulated and counted. The amount of light scattered is proportional to the surface area and therefore the volume of the cell so that the height of the electrical pulses can be used to estimate the cell volume. The high intensity coherent laser beams used in current instruments have superior optical qualities to the non-coherent tungsten light of earlier instru-

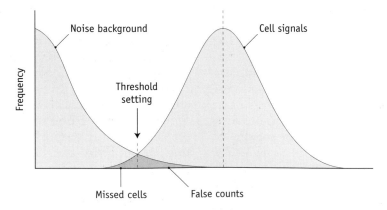

Fig. 3.6 Effect of threshold discrimination (horizontal axis) in separating cell signals from background noise.

ments. Sheathed flow allows cells to flow in an axial stream with a diameter not much greater than that of a red cell; light can be very precisely focused on this stream of cells. Electro-optical detectors are employed for red cell sizing and counting in Bayer–Technicon systems, and for white cell differential counting in a number of other instruments.

RELIABILITY OF ELECTRONIC COUNTERS

Electronic counts are precise but care needs to be taken so that they are also accurate. The recorded count on the same sample may vary from instrument to instrument and even between different models of the same instrument. Inaccuracy may be introduced by coincidence (i.e. by two cells passing through an orifice simultaneously and being counted as one cell, or by a pulse being generated during the electronic dead time of the circuit), by recirculation of cells which have already been counted, by red cell agglutination (which causes a clump of cells to be counted as one cell) and by the counting of bubbles, lipid droplets, microorganisms or extraneous particles as cells. Faulty maintenance may lead to variation in the volume aspirated or the flow rate. Single-channel instruments may have their thresholds set incorrectly and multi-channel instruments may be incorrectly calibrated.

A statistical correction may be applied for coincidence (coincidence correction); in some instruments, this is done automatically by electronic editing. Errors of coincidence can be detected by carrying out a series of measurements at various dilutions of the same specimen, plotting the data on graph paper and then extrapolating the graph to the baseline for the true value. Alternatively, the need for coincidence correction can be avoided by having the dimensions and flow characteristics of the aperture through which the cells pass such that cells can only pass in single file; this may be achieved by sheath flow or hydrodynamic focusing in which diluted blood is injected into a sheath of fluid as it flows into the sensing zone. This induces the cells to pass through the centre of the sensing zone in single file and free of distortion. Coincidence can be more effectively reduced with sheathed flow and precisely focused light in an electro-optical detector than in an impedance counter so that less dilution of the blood sample is

needed.[48] Electrical impulses generated by recirculation of cells can be eliminated by electronic editing or, alternatively, recirculation of cells in the region of the aperture can be prevented by 'sweep flow' in which a directed stream of diluent sweeps cells and debris away from the aperture, thus preventing cells from being recounted and debris from being counted as cells.

Inaccurate counts consequent on red cell agglutination are usually due to cold agglutinins. They are recognized as erroneous because of an associated marked factitious elevation of the MCV. A correct count can be achieved by pre-warming the blood sample and, if necessary, also pre-warming the diluent.

A correct red cell count and, particularly, a correct measurement of the MCV is dependent on the use of an appropriate diluent. For impedance counters, pH, temperature and rate of ionization have to be standardized and remain constant, since changes alter the electrical field and may lead to artefactual alterations in the size, shape and stability of the blood cells in the diluent. Diluents must be free of particles and give a background count of less than 50 particles in the measured volume. The correct diluent for each individual instrument must be used; other diluents, even those made by the same manufacturer, may not be interchangeable. Any laboratories using diluents other than those recommended by the manufacturer of the instrument must satisfy themselves that no error is being introduced.

For red cell counting in simple single-channel counters a suitable diluent requires a pH of 7.0–7.5 and osmolality of 340 ± 10 mmol. Physiological saline (9 g/l NaCl) or phosphate buffered saline (p. 606), which have the advantages of simplicity and ready availability, can be used as a red cell diluent, provided that the counts are performed immediately after dilution in order to avoid errors owing to sphering. Commercial solutions of saline (for intravenous use) are usually particle-free. Other solutions may require filtration through a 0.22 or 0.45 μm micropore filter to remove dust.

Setting discrimination thresholds
An accurate RBC requires that thresholds be set so that all red cells, but a minimum of other cells, are included in the count. Some counters have a lower threshold but no upper threshold so that white

cells are included in the 'red cell count'. Since the WBC is usually very low in relation to the RBC, this is not usually of practical importance; however, an appreciable error can be introduced if the WBC is greatly elevated, particularly if the patient is also anaemic. The setting of the lower threshold is of considerable importance since it is necessary to ensure that microcytic red cells are included in the count without also counting large platelets.

Current multi-channel instruments, both impedance counters and counters employing light-scattering technology, have thresholds which are either pre-calibrated by the manufacturer or are automatically adjusted, depending on the characteristics of individual blood samples. Single-channel impedance instruments capable of performing a direct RBC require setting of thresholds so as to separate pulses generated by red cells from background noise and from pulses generated by platelets. This is done by adjusting the aperture current and the pulse amplification. A simple method is to dilute a fresh blood sample and carry out successive counts on the suspension, whilst the lower threshold control is moved incrementally from its maximum to its minimum position. At the maximum position, the count should be zero or close to zero, and the counts will rise as the amplitude is reduced. The counts at each setting are plotted on arithmetic graph paper (Fig. 3.7). The correct threshold setting is at the left of the horizontal part of the graph before the line begins to slope. It is important to check that the setting selected is valid for microcytic cells. The threshold can be defined more precisely for an individual sample by means of a pulse height analyser linked to the counting system. The lower threshold is correctly set if beyond this point there are fewer than 0.5% of the counts at the peak (mode) of the pulse size distribution curve (Fig. 3.6).

PACKED CELL VOLUME AND MEAN CELL VOLUME

Modern automated blood cell counters estimate PCV by technology which has little connection with packing red cells by centrifugation. It is sometimes convenient to use different terms to distinguish the manual and automated tests, and for this reason the International Council for Standardization in Haematology has suggested that the term 'haematocrit' (Hct) rather than PCV should be used for the automated measurement. However, it should be noted that, in the past, the terms 'packed cell volume' and 'haematocrit' have been used interchangeably for the manual procedure.

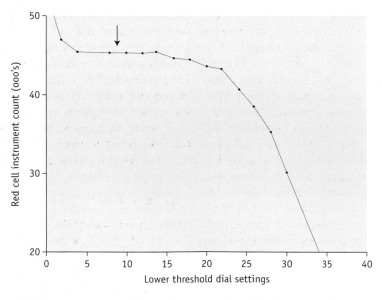

Fig. 3.7 Method to establish working conditions of cell counters. The correct setting of the threshold (at arrow) is intended to exclude noise pulses without loss of the signal pulses produced by the blood cells.

With automated instruments, the derivation of the RBC, PCV and MCV are closely interrelated. The passage of a cell through the aperture of an impedance counter or through the beam of light of a light-scattering instrument leads to the generation of an electrical pulse the height of which is proportional to cell volume. The number of pulses generated allows the RBC to be determined, as discussed above. Pulse height analysis allows either the MCV or the PCV to be determined. If the average pulse height is computed, this is indicative of the MCV, and the PCV can be derived by multiplying the estimated MCV by the RBC. Similarly, if the pulse heights are summated, this figure is indicative of the PCV, and the MCV can, in turn, be derived by dividing the PCV by the RBC.

Automated instruments require calibration before the PCV or MCV can be determined. Calibration of the PCV can be based on manual PCV determinations. Alternatively, the MCV can be calibrated by means of the pulse heights generated by latex beads,* stabilized cells or some other calibrant containing particles of known size; however, unfixed human red cells which are biconcave and flexible will not necessarily show the same characteristics in a cell counter as latex particles or some other artificial calibrant. Aperture-impedance systems measure an apparent volume which is greater than the true volume, being influenced by a 'shape factor';[49] this factor is less than 1.1 for young, flexible red cells; is between 1.1 and 1.2 for fixed biconcave cells; and is about 1.5 for spheres, whether they be fixed cells or latex spheres.[48,49]

The MCV and therefore the PCV, as determined by an automated counter, will vary with certain cell characteristics other than volume. As indicated above, such characteristics include shape which in turn is partly determined by flexibility. With impedance counters, the normal disc-shaped red cell becomes elongated into a cigar shape as it passes through the aperture; this is caused by deformation in response to shear force which occurs in cells of normal flexibility. Cells with a reduced haemoglobin concentration undergo more elongation than normal cells; this leads to a reduced 'shape factor', a reduced pulse height in relation to the true size of the cell and under-

estimation of the MCV. Conversely, cells with abnormally rigid membranes and cells such as spherocytes with a high haemoglobin concentration will undergo less deformation than normal and the MCV will be overestimated. Earlier light-scattering instruments also underestimated the volume of red cells with a reduced haemoglobin concentration since light scattering was affected by the haemoglobin concentration.[50] These artefacts are seen even with normal red cells of varying haemoglobin concentration but are more apparent with red cells from patients with defects in haemoglobin synthesis such as those from patients with iron deficiency. Several light-scattering instruments from Bayer–Technicon (H1, H2, H3 and Advia) have recently been developed to avoid artefacts of this type. Cells are isovolumetrically sphered so that their light-scattering characteristics are uniform and should follow the laws of physics. Light scattering by each individual cell is measured at two angles, which permits computation of both its volume and its haemoglobin concentration;[50,51] the latter measurement is designated the cellular haemoglobin concentration mean (CHCM) to distinguish it from the traditional MCHC derived from the Hb and the PCV. If all measurements are accurate, the CHCM and the MCHC should give the same results, thus providing an internal quality control mechanism.

The automated MCV and PCV are prone to certain errors which do not occur or are less of a problem with manual methods. Alterations in plasma osmolarity occurring, for example, in severe hyperglycaemia cause factitious elevation of the MCV and PCV.[52,53] Cold agglutinins are a relatively common cause of factitious elevation of the MCV since clumps of cells are sized as if they were single cells. Since the RBC is underestimated, the PCV is less affected, although it is also inaccurate. It is rare for warm agglutinins to cause a similar problem.

RED CELL INDICES

These have traditionally been the derived parameters of MCV, MCH and MCHC; more recently, red cell distribution width (RDW) has also been included. These indices are the basis for classifying anaemias and in various combinations they have been used to distinguish between iron deficiency and thalassaemias[54,55] (p. 256).

---

*Available as certified reference materials from the Commission of the European Union (see p. 608).

Mean cell volume

As described above, in automated systems, MCV is measured directly, but in semi-automated counters MCV is calculated by dividing the PCV by RBC.

Thus, e.g. if the PCV is 0.45 (i.e. 0.45 litres of red cells per litre of blood), and the RBC is 5×10^{12} per litre,

Volume of 1 cell = $0.45 \div 5 \times 10^{12}$ = 90 femtolitres (fl).

Mean cell haemoglobin and mean cell haemoglobin concentration

MCH is derived from the Hb divided by RBC.

Thus, e.g. if there are 150 g of Hb and 5×10^{12} red cells per litre,

MCH = $150 \div 5 \times 10^{12}$ = $3 \div 10^{11}$ g = 30 picograms (pg).

The MCHC is derived in the traditional manner (p. 25) from the Hb and the PCV with instruments that measure the PCV and calculate the MCV, whereas when the MCV is measured directly and the PCV is calculated, the MCHC is derived from the Hb, MCV and RBC according to the formula:

$$\text{MCHC (g/l)} = \frac{\text{Hb (g/l)} \times 1000}{\text{MCV (fl)} \times \text{RBC} \times 10^{-12}/\text{l}}$$

e.g. if Hb is 150 g/l, MCV is 90 fl and RBC is 5×10^{12}/l,

$$\text{MCHC} = 150 \times \frac{1000}{90 \times 5}$$
$$= 333 \text{ g/l}.$$

As mentioned above, the CHCM, which is determined in the Bayer–Technicon instruments, is a more directly measured equivalent of the MCHC.

As automated counters were developed and introduced, it was noted that the lowered MCHC which, with manual methods, had been a useful indicator of hypochromia in early iron deficiency was a less sensitive indicator of developing iron deficiency. The explanation of this is complex. In iron deficiency, there is not only true hypochromia but also increased plasma trapping within the column of red cells in a micro-haematocrit tube which increases the PCV and exaggerates the fall in the MCHC. The lowered MCHC is thus partly a true reflection of hypochromia and partly an artefact. When the MCHC is derived by auto-mated counters, the artefact of increased plasma trapping is no longer present but the instruments are also less sensitive to a true reduction of the MCHC because of the underestimation of the size of hypochromic red cells described above. Since the MCHC is calculated from the formula given above, the underestimation of the MCV leads to an overestimation of the MCHC. The MCHC thus shows little alteration as cells become hypochromic. In the newer Bayer–Technicon instruments, sensitivity to iron deficiency has improved and the MCHC and the CHCM fall as hypochromia develops.[51]

DISTRIBUTION OF RED CELL VOLUMES – RED CELL DISTRIBUTION WIDTH

Automated instruments produce volume distribution histograms which allow the presence of more than one population of cells to be appreciated. Instruments may also assess the percentage of cells falling above and below given MCV thresholds and 'flag' the presence of an increased number of microcytes or macrocytes. Such measurements may indicate the presence of a small but significant increase in the percentage of either microcytes or macrocytes before there has been any change in the MCV.

Most instruments also produce a quantitative measurement of the variation in cell volume, an equivalent of the microscopic assessment of the degree of anisocytosis. This new parameter has been named the 'red cell distribution width'. The RDW is derived from pulse height analysis and can be expressed either as the standard deviation (in fl) or as the coefficient of variation (CV) (%) of the measurements of the red cell volume. Current Beckman–Coulter and Bayer–Technicon instruments express the RDW as the SD, and Sysmex instruments express it as either the SD or the CV. Widely different reference ranges have been reported for the RDW with the CV varying between 7.4 and 13.4.[45,56–58] It is therefore important for laboratories to determine their own reference ranges. The RDW expressed as the CV has been found of some value in distinguishing between iron deficiency (RDW usually increased) and thalassaemia trait (RDW usually normal) and between megaloblastic anaemia (RDW often increased) and other causes of macrocytosis (RDW more often normal).

Range of RDW values in health

See page 12.

DISTRIBUTION OF RED CELL HAEMOGLOBINIZATION – HAEMOGLOBIN DISTRIBUTION WIDTH

Instruments such as the Bayer–Technicon system which determine the haemoglobin concentration of individual red cells provide distribution curves of the haemoglobin concentration and are able to 'flag' the presence of increased numbers of hypochromic cells and hyperchromic cells. Since the volume of individual red cells is also determined, it is possible to distinguish between hypochromic microcytes, which are indicative of a defect in haemoglobin synthesis, and hypochromic macrocytes, which often represent reticulocytes.[59] The identification of an increased percentage of hyperchromic cells may be caused by the presence of spherocytes, 'irregularly contracted cells' or sickled cells. The degree of variation in red cell haemoglobinization is quantified as the haemoglobin distribution width or HDW; this is the CV of the measurements of haemoglobin concentration of individual cells. The normal 95% range is 1.82–2.64.

TOTAL WHITE BLOOD CELL COUNT

The total WBC is determined in whole blood in which red cells have been lysed. The lytic agent is required to destroy the red cells and reduce the red cell stroma to a residue which causes no detectable response in the counting system without affecting leucocytes in such a manner that the ability of the system to count them is altered. Various manufacturers recommend specific reagents and for multi-channel instruments which also perform an automated differential count use of the recommended reagent is essential. For a simple single-channel impedance counter, the following fluid is satisfactory:

Cetrimide 20 g
10% formaldhyde (in 9 g/l NaCl) 2 ml
Glacial acetic acid 16 ml
NaCl 6 g
Water to 1 litre.

Relatively simple instruments are also available which determine the Hb and the WBC by consecutive measurements on the one blood sample. The diluent contains a reagent to lyse the red cells and another to convert haemoglobin to haemiglobin cyanide. Hb is measured by a modified HiCN method and white cells are counted by impedance technology. Apart from the reagents specified by the manufacturers, a diluent containing potassium cyanide and potassium ferricyanide together with ethylhexadecyldimethyl-ammonium bromide can be used.[60,61]

Fully automated multi-channel instruments perform WBCs by either impedance or light-scattering technology or both. Residual particles in a diluted blood sample are counted after red cell lysis or, in the case of some light-scattering instruments, after the red cells have been rendered transparent. Thresholds are set to exclude normal platelets from the count, although giant platelets are included. Some or all of any nucleated red cells present are usually included, so that when nucleated red cells are present the count approximates more to the TNCC than to the WBC.

Factitiously low automated WBCs occasionally occur as a consequence of white cell agglutination. Factitiously high counts are more common and usually result from failure of lysis of red cells; with certain instruments this may occur with the cells of neonates or be consequent on uraemia or on the presence of an abnormal haemoglobin such as haemoglobin S or haemoglobin C.

AUTOMATED DIFFERENTIAL COUNT

Automated differential counters which are now available use flow cytometry incorporated into a full blood counter rather than being stand-alone differential counters. Differential counters based on pattern recognition in stained blood films were initially preferred by many haematologists but they were relatively slow, and since they could count only a small number of cells in a reasonable time, the precision of the automated count was no better than that of a manual count.

Increasingly, automated blood cell counters have a differential counting capacity, providing either a three-part or a five- to seven-part differential count. Counts are performed on diluted whole blood in which red cells are either lysed or are rendered transparent. A three-part differential count assigns cells to categories usually designated: (i) 'granulocytes' or 'large cells'; (ii) 'lymphocytes' or small cells; and (iii) 'monocytes', 'mononuclear cells' or 'middle cells'. In theory, the granulocyte category includes eosinophils and basophils, but in practice it is common for an appreciable proportion of cells of these types to be excluded from the granulocyte category and to be counted instead in the monocyte category.[62,63] Five- to seven-part differential counts classify cells, as neutrophils, eosinophils, basophils, lymphocytes and monocytes,[46,51,64,65] and may also include large immature cells (composed of blasts and immature granulocytes) and atypical lymphocytes (including small blasts). Automated instruments performing three-part or five-to seven-part differential counts are able to 'flag' or reject counts from the majority of samples with nucleated red cells, myelocytes, promyelocytes, blasts and atypical lymphocytes.[64,65,66] To a lesser extent, instruments incorporating a three-part differential count, although not capable of enumerating eosinophils or basophils, are able to flag a significant proportion of samples which have an increased number of one of these cell types.[21]

Both impedance counters and light-scattering instruments are capable of producing three-part differential counts from a single channel; the categorization is based on the different volume of various types of cell following partial lysis and cytoplasmic shrinkage. Most five- to seven-part differential counts require two or more channels in which cell volume and other characteristics are analysed by various modalities (Table 3.3). Analysis may be dependent only on volume and other physical characteristics of the cell or also on activity of cellular enzymes such as peroxidase. Technologies employed to study cell characteristics include light scattering and absorbance and impedance measurements with low- and high-frequency electromagnetic current or radio-frequency current. Cells may have been exposed to lytic agents or a cytochemical reaction may have occurred before cell characteristics are studied. Two-parameter analysis or more complex discriminant functions divide cells into clusters which can be matched with the position of the various white cell clusters in normal blood. Thresholds, some fixed and some variable, divide clusters from one another, permitting cells in each cluster to be counted.

Automated differential counters employing flow cytometry classify far more cells than is possible with a manual differential count. Automated counts are consequently much more precise than manual counts; however, with certain cell categories – specifically monocytes and basophils – the degree of precision is sometimes less than would be expected for the number of cells counted, indi-

Table 3.3 Automated full blood counters with a five-part or more differential counting capacity

Instrument and manufacturer	Technology employed for differential count
Coulter STKS (Beckman–Coulter Electronics Ltd)	Impedance with low-frequency electromagnetic current Impedance with high-frequency electromagnetic current Laser light scattering
Sysmex NE-8000 (Sysmex Corporation)	Impedance with low-frequency direct current Impedance with radiofrequency current
H1, H2 and H3, Advia (Technicon Division of Bayer)	Light scattering and absorbance following peroxidase reaction Two-angle light scatter following differential cytoplasmic stripping
Cell-Dyn 3500 (Abbott Diagnostics Division)	Four light-scattering parameters: forward light scatter, orthogonal light scatter, narrow-angle light scatter, depolarized orthogonal light scatter
Cobas Argos 5 Diff (Roche Diagnostics Systems)	Electrical impedance with intact cells and following differential cytoplasmic stripping Light absorbance

cating that such cells are not always classified in a consistent manner. The accuracy of automated counters is less impressive than their precision. With all types of counter, unusual cell characteristics or ageing of a blood specimen can lead to misclassification of cells. Although the majority of samples containing abnormal cells are 'flagged', this is not invariably so; the presence of nucleated red cells, immature granulocytes, atypical lymphocytes and blasts (even occasionally quite large numbers of blasts) may not give rise to a 'flag'. However, human observers performing a 100-cell manual differential count also miss significant abnormalities. In general, automated counts have compared reasonably favourably with routine manual counts if the instruments are assigned only two functions – performing differential counts on normal samples, and 'flagging' abnormal samples. If a differential count shows other than distributional abnormalities, there is, as yet, no substitute for the human observer for the recognition and enumeration of abnormal cells.

The instrument–reagent systems which have been developed to permit automated differential counts often include some but not all NRBC in the total 'white cell count'. Thus, in the presence of a significant number of NRBC, the total count is neither a true 'white cell count' nor a true 'total nucleated cell count' and the absolute WBC counts calculated from the total will necessarily be somewhat erroneous. This differs from the situation with earlier instruments which included any nucleated red cells in the 'white cell count'. It may be possible to make some assessment of the proportion of the nucleated red cells included in the total count by studying the graphical output of the instrument, but if accurate absolute counts of different leucocyte types are needed, it is necessary to revert to earlier instruments to provide the TNCC.

New white cell parameters

Automated white cell counters analyse cell characteristics by novel technologies and identify cell types by features which differ greatly from those used when a blood film is examined visually. It is possible, for example, to identify eosinophils by the ability of their granules to polarize light[64] or to detect a left shift or the presence of blasts by the reduced light-scattering of the nuclei of more immature granulocytes. There is also the potential

to produce information which is not directly analogous with that available from a manual differential count. Instruments that incorporate a cytochemical reaction give information on enzyme activity expressed as the mean peroxidase activity index (MPXI). An increased MPXI has been observed in infections, in some myelodysplasias and leukaemias, in the acquired immune deficiency syndrome (AIDS) and in megaloblastic anaemia, whereas a reduced MPXI occurs in inherited and acquired neutrophil peroxidase deficiency.[46,51,67,68] Such measurements may prove to be clinically useful.

AUTOMATED INSTRUMENT GRAPHICAL REPRESENTATIONS

Current fully automated instruments produce a graphical display of much of the data produced. This is displayed on a colour monitor and can be printed, either in black and white or in colour. Inspection of the graphical display can give further information beyond that which is available from assessment of the numerical data. Displays usually include histograms of red cell, white cell and platelet size and sometimes histograms of red cell haemoglobin concentration and scatter plots of size versus haemoglobin concentration. Differential counts are graphically represented as scatter plots of two variables or scatterplots of discriminant functions derived from more than two variables.

Typical printouts of histograms or scatter-plots of current automated instruments are shown in Figure 3.8.

PLATELET COUNT

Platelets can be counted in whole blood using the same techniques of electrical or electro-optical detection as are employed for counting red cells. An upper threshold is needed to separate platelets from red cells and a lower threshold to separate platelets from debris and electronic noise. Recirculation of red cells near the aperture should be prevented or pulses produced may simulate those generated by platelets. Three techniques for setting thresholds have been used: (i) platelets can be counted between two fixed thresholds, e.g. between 2 and 20 fl; (ii) pulses between fixed thresholds can be counted with subsequent fitting of a curve and

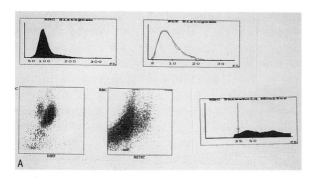

A

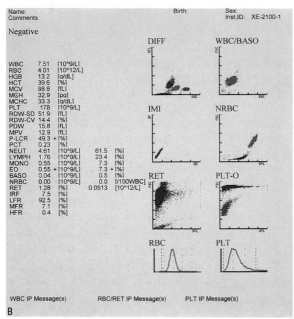

B

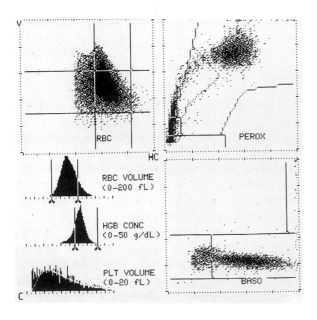

C

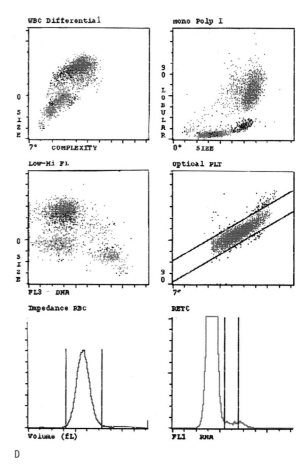

D

Fig. 3.8 Patterns of blood count print out of some automated systems. A, Beckman Coulter Gen S; B, Sysmex XE 2100; C, Bayer H1; D, Abbot Cell-Dyne 4000.

extrapolation so that platelets falling outside the fixed thresholds are included in the computed count; and (iii) thresholds can vary automatically, depending on the characteristics of individual blood samples, to make allowance for microcytic or fragmented red cells or for giant platelets. A reference method for platelet counting is based on establishing the platelet: red cell ratio by flow cytometry in which the platelets are identified by labelling them with specific antibodies (CD 61 and CD 41).[69]

Platelet count in health

In health, there are approximately $150–400 \times 10^9$ platelets per litre of blood. The counts are somewhat higher in women than in men,[70] and there is a cycling, with slightly lower count at about the time of menstruation.[71] Lower platelet counts have been observed in apparently healthy West Indians and Africans than in Caucasians[72] (see also p. 16).

Mean platelet volume and other platelet parameters

The same techniques which are used to size red cells can be applied to platelets. The calculated mean platelet volume (MPV) is very dependent on the technique of measurement and on length and conditions of storage prior to testing the blood. When MPV is measured by impedance technology, it has been found to vary inversely with the platelet count in normal subjects. If this curve is extrapolated, it has been found that data fit the extrapolated curve when thrombocytopenia is caused by peripheral platelet destruction; however, the MPV is lower than predicted when thrombocytopenia is caused by megaloblastic anaemia or bone marrow failure.[73] The MPV is generally greater than predicted in myeloproliferative disorders, but differentiating essential thrombocythaemia from reactive thrombocytosis on this basis has not been very successful.

Other platelet parameters which can be computed by automated counters include the platelet distribution width (PDW) which is a measure of platelet anisocytosis and the 'plateletcrit' which is the product of the MPV and platelet count and, by analogy with the haematocrit, may be seen as indicative of the volume of circulating platelets in a unit volume of blood. The PDW has been found to be of some use in distinguishing essential thrombocythaemia (PDW increased) from reactive thrombocytosis (PDW normal). The plateletcrit does not appear to provide any information of clinical value.

With some automated blood counting systems and flow cytometers, it is possible to identify young platelets with a higher RNA content; by analogy with the reticulocyte count, these have been called 'reticulated platelets'.[74] However, as there is a constant exchange of platelets between the circulation and the spleen, it is not clear whether their presence in the blood has the same significance as reticulocytes.

RETICULOCYTE COUNT

An automated reticulocyte count can be performed utilizing the fact that various dyes and fluorochromes combine with the RNA of reticulocytes; however, they also combine with the DNA of nucleated cells. Following binding of the dye, fluorescent cells can be enumerated using a flow cytometer, either a general purpose flow cytometer or a committed automated reticulocyte and many fully automated blood counters also now incorporate a reticulocyte counting capacity. The dyes used in these systems include auramine O (Sysmex), thiazole orange (ABX), CD4K 530 (Abbott) as well as non-fluorescent dyes such as oxazine 750 (Bayer–Technicon) and the traditional New methylene blue (Beckman–Coulter, Abbott).

Automated reticulocyte counts correlate well with manual reticulocyte counts, although absolute counts may differ since automated counts are dependent on the conditions of incubation and the method of calibrating the instrument. Precision is much superior to that of the manual count since many more cells are counted and the subjective element inherent in recognizing late reticulocytes is eliminated. Potential sources of inaccuracy are the inclusion of some leucocytes and platelets and, less often, Howell–Jolly bodies or malarial parasites, in the 'reticulocyte' count.

An automated reticulocyte counter also permits assessment of reticulocyte maturity since the most immature reticulocytes, produced when erythropoietin levels are high, have more RNA and fluoresce more strongly than the mature reticulocytes normally present in the peripheral blood.

Parameters indicating reticulocyte immaturity have potential clinical relevance. For example, an increase in mean fluorescence intensity has been noted as an early sign of engraftment following bone marrow transplantation.[75] The appearance of reticulocytes with high fluorescence heralds response when severe aplastic anaemia is being treated with immunosuppressive therapy,[76] and is a reliable indication of haemopoietic regeneration after marrow ablative chemotherapy. The immature reticulocyte percentage has also been found to be useful in predicting the optimal time for stem cell harvests in some but not all studies.[77]

Automated reticulocyte counts are fairly stable in blood which has been stored for 1 to 2 days at room temperature or up to 3 to 5 days at 4°C.

Fully automated instruments provide a graphical output representing reticulocytes of various degrees of maturity.

Reticulocyte counts in health

Reference ranges reported for automated reticulocyte counts have varied considerably between methods. Ranges of $19–59 \times 10^9/l$ $(0.2–1.6\%)$[78] and $40–140 \times 10^9/l$ $(1–3\%)$[75] have been reported for thiazole orange with a Coulter Epic Flow Cytometer. With the Sysmex R-1000, absolute ranges have been reported as $19–98$,[79] $20–70$,[80] and $10–90 \times 10^9/l$,[80] and percentage ranges as $0.4–2.1$[79] and $0.27–2.11$.[81]

CALIBRATION OF AUTOMATED BLOOD CELL COUNTERS

There are three satisfactory methods for calibrating an automated blood cell counter:[82–84]

1. using fresh normal blood specimens to which values have been assigned for Hb, PCV, RBC, WBC and platelet count by standardized reference methods
2. using a stable calibrant (either preserved blood or a substitute) to which values appropriate for the instrument in question have been assigned by comparison with fresh normal blood
3. by use of a commercial calibrant with assigned values suitable for the instrument in question.

For reasons of convenience and economy, control materials are commonly used as calibrants; but this practice is not recommended. Such materials are not

sufficiently stable to serve as calibrants and their stated values are often approximations which are not assigned by reference methods. They are designed to give test results within a stated range over a stated period of time rather than a specific result.

The procedure for assigning values to fresh blood samples and indirectly to a stable calibrant is as follows:

1. 4 ml blood specimens are obtained from three haematologically normal volunteers and are anticoagulated with K_2 EDTA.
2. The Hb value is assigned by using the haemiglobincyanide method (see p. 20) and the mean of two measurements.
3. The PCV is assigned by the micro-haematocrit method (see p. 23), taking the mean of measurements in four micro-haematocrit tubes.
4. The RBC is assigned by performing counts on a single-channel aperture-impedance counter capable of performing a direct cell count; the mean of two dilutions, each counted twice, is used.
5. The MCV is assigned by calculation from the RBC and PCV.
6. The WBC is assigned by performing counts on a single-channel aperture-impedance instrument capable of performing direct cell counts; the mean of two dilutions, each counted twice, is used.
7. The platelet count is assigned by using a counter capable of measuring the ratio of platelets to red cells, the platelet count being calculated from the ratio and an independently measured RBC.

Methods have recently been described in which the platelets are labelled with a specific fluorescent monoclonal antibody (e.g. CD41, CD42a or b, CD61) and the sample is then counted in a multiparameter flow cytometer to obtain the ratio of platelets to red cells and thereby the absolute platelet count.[85–87]

To calibrate the automated counter directly from the three fresh blood samples, perform two counts with each sample and take the means. If the measured counts differ from those assigned, recalibrate the counter appropriately.

To calibrate a stable calibrant, perform two counts on the calibrant and on each fresh sample using the automated instrument, A, and take the means. From the ratio of the test results on fresh blood to those on the calibrator, assign corrected values to the calibrator by using the following calculations.

Corrected calibrator value =

$$A_C \times \sqrt[3]{\frac{D_{F1}}{A_{F1}} \times \frac{D_{F2}}{A_{F2}} \times \frac{D_{F3}}{A_{F3}}}$$

where:
A_C = measurement of calibrator by automated counter
A_F = measurement of the fresh bloods (1, 2 and 3) by automated counter
D_F = direct measurement of the fresh bloods (1, 2 and 3).

Considerable care is required to ensure that the initial measurements on the fresh blood are as accurate as possible. Dilutions should be made with individually calibrated pipettes and grade A volumetric flasks. The cell counter should be calibrated as described on page 33, with a signal to noise ratio of greater than 100:1, and the count corrected for coincidence. Details of procedures to be used are described by the International Committee for Standardization in Haematology.[81] Procedures for verification of the performance of multi-channel analysers by the users have also been published in the USA by the National Committee for Clinical Laboratory Standards.[88]

REFERENCES

1 Zijlstra WG, van Kampen EJ 1960 Standardization of hemoglobinometry. I. The extinction coefficient of hemiglobincyanide at λ = 540 mμ: ε^{540}HiCN. Clinica Chimica Acta 91:339.

2 International Committee for Standardization in Haematology 1978 Recommendations for reference method for haemoglobinometry in human blood and specifications for international haemiglobincyanide reference preparation. Journal of Clinical Pathology 31:139.

3 Clegg JW, King EJ 1942 Estimation of haemoglobin by the alkaline haematin method. British Medical Journal ii:329.

4 Gibson QH, Harrison DC 1945 An artificial standard for use in the estimation of haemoglobin. Biochemical Journal 39:490.

5 Vanzetti G 1966 An azide-methemoglobin method for hemoglobin determination in blood. Journal of Laboratory and Clinical Medicine 67:116–126.

6 Bridges N, Parvin RM, van Assendelft OW 1987 Evaluation of a new system for hemoglobin measurement. American Clinical Products Review 6:22–25.

7 Oshiro I, Takenaka T, Maeda J 1982 New method for hemoglobin determination by using sodium lauryl sulphate (SLS). Clinical Biochemistry 15:83–88.

8 Van Assendelft OW, Lewis SM 1991 Recommended method for the determination of the haemoglobin concentration of blood. World Health Organization Document LAB/84.10, Rev 1.

9 Drabkin DL, Austin JH 1932 Spectrophotometric studies: spectrometric constants for common haemoglobin derivatives in human, dog and rabbit blood. Journal of Biological Chemistry 98:719.

10 Zweens J, Frankena H, Zijlstra WG 1979 Decomposition on freezing of reagents used in the ICSH recommended method for the determination of total haemoglobin in blood; its nature, cause and prevention. Clinica Chimica Acta 91:339.

11 Van Assendelft OW, Buursma A, Zijlstra WG 1996 Stability of haemiglobincyanide standards. Journal of Clinical Pathology 49:275–277.

12 Van Kampen EJ, Zijlstra WG 1983 Spectrophotometry of hemoglobin and hemoglobin derivatives. Advances in Clinical Chemistry 23:199.

13 Lewis SM, Garvey B, Manning R, et al 1991 Lauryl sulphate haemoglobin: a non-hazardous substitute for HiCN in haemoglobinometry. Clinical and Laboratory Haematology 13:279.

14 Matsubara T, Okuzono H, Senba U 1979 Modification of Van Kampen–Zijlstra's reagent for the hemiglobincyanide method. Clinica Chimica Acta 93:163.

15 International Committee for Standardization in Haematology 1980 Recommendations for reference method for determination by centrifugation of packed cell volume of blood. Journal of Clinical Pathology 33:1.

16 International Committee for Standardization in Haematology 1980 Recommended methods for measurement of red-cell and plasma volume. Journal of Nuclear Medicine 21:793–800.

17 England JM, Walford DM, Waters DAW 1972 Reassessment of the reliability of the haematocrit. British Journal of Haematology 23:247.

18 Pearson TC, Guthrie DL 1982 Trapped plasma in microhematocrit. American Journal of Clinical Pathology 78:770.

19 Dungar R 1910 Eine einfache Methode der Zählung der eosinophilen Leukozyten und der praktische Wert dieser Untersuchung. Münchener Medizinische Wochenschrift 57:1942.

20 Spiers RS The principles of eosinophil diluents. Blood 7:550.

21 Gilbert HS, Ornstein L 1975 Basophil counting with a new staining method using Alcian blue. Blood 46:279.

22 Best WR, Samster M 1951 Variation and error in eosinophil counts of blood and bone marrow. Blood 6:61.

23 Rud F 1947 The eosinophil count in health and mental disease. Acta Psychiatrica et Neurologica (København) 40 (Suppl.).

24 Uhrbrand H 1958 The number of circulating eosinophils: normal figures and spontaneous variations. Acta Medica Scandinavica 160:99.

25 Muehrcke RC, Eckert EL, Kark RM 1952 A statistical study of absolute eosinophil cell counts in healthy young adults using logarithmic analysis. Journal of Laboratory and Clinical Medicine 40:161.

26 Shelley WB, Parnes HM 1965 The absolute basophil count. Technique and significance. Journal of the American Medical Association 192:368.

27 Mettler L, Shirwani D 1974 Direct basophil count for timing ovulation. Fertility and Sterility 25:718.

28 England JM 1979 Prospect for automated differential leucocyte counting in the routine laboratory. Clinical and Laboratory Haematology 1:263.

29 Mathy KA, Koepke JA 1974 The clinical usefulness of segmented vs stab neutrophil criteria for differential leucocyte counts. American Journal of Clinical Pathology 61:947.

30 Gombos M, Bienkowski R, Gochman R, et al 1998 The absolute neutrophil count: Is it the best indicator for occult bacteraemia in infants? American Journal of Clinical Pathology 109:221–225.

31 Bain BJ 2000 Blood cells: a practical guide, 3rd edn. Blackwell Science Oxford.

32 Gilmer PR, Koepke JA 1976 The reticulocyte: an approach to definition. American Journal of Clinical Pathology 66:262.

33 Berendes M 1973 The proportion of reticulocytes in the erythrocytes of the spleen as compared with those of circulating blood, with special reference to hemolytic states. Blood 14:558.

34 Seip M 1953 Reticulocyte studies: the liberation of red blood corpuscles from the bone marrow into the peripheral blood and the production of erythrocytes elucidated by reticulocyte investigations. Acta Medica Scandinavica (Suppl. 282).

35 Hillman RS 1969 Characteristics of marrow production and reticulocyte maturation in normal man in response to anemia. Journal of Clinical Investigation 48:443.

36 Hillman RS, Finch CA 1969 The misused reticulocyte. British Journal of Haematology 17:313.

37 Marshall PN, Bentley SA, Lewis SM 1976 Purified azure B as a reticulocyte stain. Journal of Clinical Pathology 29:1060.

38 Wittekind D, Schulte E 1987 Standardized azure B as a reticulocyte stain. Clinical and Laboratory Haematology 9:395.

39 Jahanmehr SAH, Hyde K, Geary CG, et al 1987 Simple technique for fluorescence staining of blood cells with acridine orange. Journal of Clinical Pathology 40:926.

40 Vander JB, Harris CA, Ellis SR 1963 Reticulocyte counts by means of fluorescence microscopy. Journal of Laboratory and Clinical Medicine 62:132.

41 Sage BH, O'Connell JP, Mercolino TJ 1983 A rapid, vital staining procedure for flow cytometric analysis of human reticulocytes. Cytometry 4:222.

42 Tanke HJ, Rothbarth PH, Vossen JMJJ, et al 1983 Flow cytometry of reticulocytes applied to clinical hematology. Blood 61:1091.

43 Vaughan WP, Hall J, Johnson K, et al 1985 Simultaneous reticulocyte and platelet counting on a clinical flow cytometer. American Journal of Haematology 18:385.

44 Groner W, Simson E 1995 Practical guide to modern haematology analyzers. Wiley, Chichester.

45 International Council for Standardization in Haematology 1994 Guidelines for the evaluation of blood cell analysers including those used for differential leucocyte and reticulocyte counting and cell marker applications. Clinical and Laboratory Haematology 16:157.

46 Simson E, Ross DW, Kocher WD 1988 Atlas of automated cytochemical hematology. Technicon, Tarrytown, NY.

47 Coulter WH 1956 High speed automatic blood cell counter and cell size analyser. Proceedings of National Electronics Conference 12:1034.

48 Thom R 1990 Automated red cell analysis. Baillière's Clinical Haematology 3:837.

49 England JM, van Assendelft OW 1986 Automated blood counters and their evaluation. In: Rowan RM, England JM (eds) Automation and quality assurance in haematology. Blackwell Scientific, Oxford.

50 Mohandas N, Kim YR, Tycko DH, et al 1986 Accurate and independent measurement of volume and hemoglobin concentration of individual red cells by laser scattering. Blood 68:506.

51 Ross DW, Bentley SA 1986 Evaluation of an automated hematology system (Technicon H-1).

Archives of Pathology and Laboratory Medicine 110:803.

52 Evan-Wong L, Davidson RJ 1983 Raised Coulter mean corpuscular volume in diabetic ketoacidosis, and its underlying association with marked plasma hyperosmolarity. Journal of Clinical Pathology 36:334.

53 Holt JT, DeWandler MJ, Arvan DA 1982 Spurious elevation of the electronically determined mean corpuscular volume and hematocrit caused by hyperglycemia. American Journal of Clinical Pathology 77:568.

54 Bentley SA, Ayscue LH, Watson JM, et al 1989 The clinical utility of discriminant functions in the differential diagnosis of microcytic anemias. Blood Cells 15:575–582.

55 Lafferty JD, Crowther MA, Ali MA, et al 1996 The evaluation of various mathematical RBC indices and their efficacy in discriminating between thalassemic and non-thalassemic microcytosis. American Journal of Clinical Pathology 106:201–295.

56 Bessman JD, Gilmer PR, Gardner FH 1983 Improved classification of anemias by MCV and RDW. American Journal of Clinical Pathology 80:322.

57 Roberts GT, El Badawi SB 1985 Red blood cell distribution width index in some hematologic diseases. American Journal of Clinical Pathology 83:222.

58 Rowan RM 1983 Blood cell volume analysis – a new screening technology for the haematologist. Albert Clark, London.

59 Bain BJ, Cavill I 1993 Hypochromic macrocytes – are they reticulocytes? Journal of Clinical Pathology 46:963.

60 Ballard BCD 1972 Lysing agent for the Coulter S. Journal of Clinical Pathology 25:460.

61 Skinnider LF, Musglow E 1972 A stromatolysing and cyanide reagent for use with the Coulter Counter Model S. American Journal of Clinical Pathology 57:537.

62 Bain BJ 1986 An assessment of the three population differential count on the Coulter Model S Plus IV. Clinical and Laboratory Haematology 8:347.

63 Clark PT, Henthorn SJ, England JM 1985 Differential white cell counting on the Coulter Counter Model S Plus IV (three population) and the Technicon H6000: a comparison by simple and multiple regression. Clinical and Laboratory Haematology 7:335.

64 Cornbleet PJ, Myrick D, Judkins S, et al 1992 Evaluation of the CELL-DYN 3000 differential. American Journal of Clinical Pathology 98:603.

65 Mansberg HP, Saunders AM, Groner W 1974 The Hemalog D white cell differential system. Journal of Histochemistry and Cytochemistry 22:711.

66 Robertson EP, Lai HW, Wei DCC 1992 An evaluation of leucocyte analysis on the Coulter STKS. Clinical and Laboratory Haematology 14:53.

67 D'Onofrio G, Zini G, Tommasi M, et al 1992 Anomalie ultramorpholigiche dei granulociti neutrofili nelle infezioni da virus HIV. Atti del V Incontro del Club Utilizzatori Sistemi Ematologici Bayer–Technicon, Montecatini Terme, 1991.

68 Taylor C, Bain BJ 1991 Technicon H1 automated white cell parameters in the diagnosis of megaloblastic erythropoiesis. European Journal of Haematology 46:248.

69 ICSH (Expert Panel on Cytometry) and International Society of Laboratory Hematology (ISLH) Task-force on Platelet counting 2001 Platelet counting by the PLT/RBC ratio – a reference method. American Journal of Clinical Pathology. 115: 460–464.

70 Bain BJ 1985 Platelet count and platelet size in males and females. Scandinavian Journal of Haematology 35:77.

71 Morley A 1969 A platelet cycle in normal individuals. Australasian Annals of Medicine 18:127.

72 Bain BJ, Seed M 1986 Platelet count and platelet size in Africans and West Indians. Clinical and Laboratory Haematology 8:43.

73 Bessman JD, Williams LJ, Gilmer PR 1982 Platelet size in health and hematologic disease. American Journal of Clinical Pathology 78:150.

74 Takubo T, Yamane T, Hino M, et al 1998 Usefulness of determining reticulated and large platelets in idiopathic thrombocytopenic purpura. Acta Haematologica 99:109–110.

75 Sica S, Sora F, Laurenti L, et al 1999 Highly fluorescent reticulocyte count predicts haemopoietic recovery after immunosuppression for severe aplastic anaemia. Clinical and Laboratory Haematology 21:387.

76 Davies SV, Cavill I, Bentley N, et al 1992 Evaluation of erythropoiesis after bone marrow transplantation: quantitative reticulocyte counting. British Journal of Haematology 81:12.

77 Gowans ID, Hepburn MD, Clark DM, et al 1999 The role of the Sysmex SE9000 immature myeloid index and Sysmex R2000 reticulocyte parameters in optimizing the timing of peripheral blood cell harvesting in patients with lymphoma and myeloma. Clinical and Laboratory Haematology 21:331–336.

78 Nobes PR, Carter AB 1990 Reticulocyte counting using flow cytometry. Journal of Clinical Pathology 43:675.

79 Chin-Yee I, Keeney M, Lohmann C 1991 Flow cytometric reticulocyte analysis using thiazole orange; clinical experience and technical limitations. Clinical and Laboratory Haematology 13:177.

80 Hoy TG 1990 Flow cytometry: clinical applications in haematology. Baillière's Clinical Haematology 3:977.

81 Tatsumi N, Niri M, Tsuda IO 1992 No correlation between reticulocyte count and erythrocyte count. Clinical and Laboratory Haematology 14:92.

82 International Committee for Standardization in Haematology; Expert Panel on Cytometry 1988 The assignment of values to fresh blood used for calibrating automated blood cell counters. Clinical and Laboratory Haematology 10:203.

83 Lewis SM, Wardle J, Cousins S, et al 1979 Platelet counting – development of a reference method and a reference preparation. Clinical and Laboratory Haematology 1:227.

84 Lewis SM, England JM, Rowan RM 1991 Current concerns in haematology 3: Blood count calibration. Journal of Clinical Pathology 44:881.

85 Dickerhoff R, von Ruecker A 1995 Enumeration of platelets by multiparameter flow cytometry using platelet specific antibodies and fluorescent reference particles. Clinical and Laboratory Haematology 17:163–172.

86 Tanaka C, Isii T, Fujimoto D 1996 Flow cytometric platelet enumeration utilizing monoclonal antibody CD42a. Clinical and Laboratory Haematology 18:265–269.

87 Harrison P, Horton A, Grant D, et al 2000 Immunoplatelet counting: a proposed new reference procedure. British Journal of Haematology 108:228–235.

88 National Committee for Clinical Laboratory Standards 1996 Performance goals for the internal quality control of multichannel hematology analyzers; approved standard. NCCLS, Wayne, PA.

89 White A, Nicolaas G, Foster K et al 1991 Health survey for England: Office of population censuses and surveys, Social Survey Division. Stationery Office, Norwich, NR3 IPD.

90 Bryner MA, Houwen B, Westengard J, Klein O 1997 The spun haematocrit and mean red cell volume are affected by changes in the oxygenation state of red blood cells. Clinical and Laboratory Haematology 19:99–103.

4

Preparation and staining methods for blood and bone marrow films

Barbara J. Bain   S. Mitchell Lewis

PREPARATION OF BLOOD FILMS ON SLIDES

Blood films should be made on clean glass slides. Films made on cover-glasses have negligible advantages and are unsuitable for modern laboratory practice. Films may be spread by hand or by means of an automated slide-spreader, the latter being either a stand-alone instrument or a component of an automated blood cell counter.

Manual method

Blood films can be prepared from fresh blood with no anticoagulant added or from EDTA-anticoagulated blood. Heparinized blood should not generally be used since its staining characteristics differ from those of EDTA-anticoagulated blood. Good films can be made in the following manner, using clean slides (p. 609), if necessary wiped free from dust immediately before use. Ideally, slides should be frosted at one end to facilitate labelling but these are more expensive.

First, make a spreader from a glass slide which has a smooth end. Using a glass cutter, break off one corner of the slide, leaving a width of about 18 mm as the spreader. A spreader can be used repeatedly unless the edge becomes chipped, but it must be cleaned carefully between films.

Place a small drop of blood in the centre line of a slide about 1 cm from one end. Then, without delay, place a spreader in front of the drop at an angle of about 30° to the slide and move it back to make contact with the drop. The drop should spread out quickly along the line of contact. With a steady movement of the hand, spread the drop of blood along the slide. The spreader must not be lifted off until the last trace of blood has been

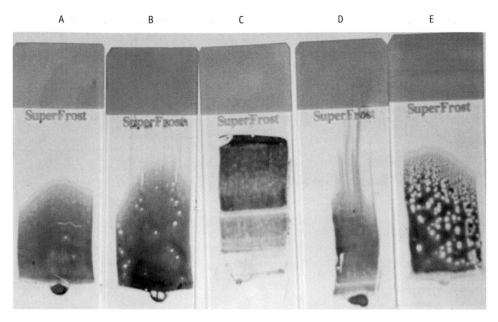

A   B   C   D   E

Fig. 4.1 Blood films made on slides. (A) A well-made film. (B) An irregular patchy film on a dusty slide. (C) A film which is too thick. (D) A film which has been spread with inconsistent pressure and using an irregularly-edged spreader, resulting in long tails. (E) A film made on a very greasy slide.

spread out; with a correctly sized drop, the film should be about 3 cm in length. It is important that the film of blood finishes at least 1 cm before the end of the slide (Fig. 4.1).

The thickness of the film can be regulated by varying the pressure and speed of spreading, and by changing the angle at which the spreader is held. With anaemic blood, the correct thickness is achieved by using a wider angle and, conversely, with polycythaemic blood, the angle should be narrower. The ideal thickness is such that there is some overlap of red cells throughout much of the film's length (see p. 25). The leucocytes should be easily recognizable throughout most of the film. An irregular streaky film will occur if the slide is greasy and dust on the surface will cause patchy spots (Fig. 4.1).

Automated methods

The instructions of the manufacturer should be followed unless local experience has demonstrated that variation of the recommended technique achieves better results.

Labelling blood films

The film should be labelled immediately after spreading. Write either a laboratory reference number or the name of the patient and the date in pencil on the frosted end of the slide or on the film itself (writing on the thickest part, which is least suitable for microscopic examination). A label written in pencil will not be removed by staining. A paper label should be affixed to the slide later. If blood films are to be stored for future reference, the paper label should be applied in such a manner that it is easily read when the slides are filed.

Bar-coded specimen identification labels are convenient, when available, in a computerized laboratory.

Fixing blood films

To preserve the morphology of the cells, films must be fixed without delay, and they should never be left unfixed for more than a few hours. If the films are left unfixed at room temperature for several days, it may be found that the background of dried plasma stains a pale blue which is impossible to remove without spoiling the staining of the blood cells. If films are sent to the laboratory by post, it is preferable that, when possible, they are thoroughly dried and fixed before despatch.

It is important to prevent any contact with water before fixation is complete. Methyl alcohol (methanol) is the fixative of choice although ethyl alcohol ('absolute alcohol') can also be used. To prevent the alcohol from becoming contaminated with absorbed water, it must be stored in a bottle with a tightly fitting stopper and not left exposed to the atmosphere, especially in humid climates. Methylated spirits must not be used as it contains water.

BONE MARROW FILMS

The method for preparation of films from aspirated bone marrow is described on page 105. They should be made without delay. At least one film should be fixed for a Perls' stain and, if necessary, films should be fixed in the appropriate fixatives for special staining (Ch. 13); others should be fixed and stained with a Romanowsky stain as described below. Crushed bone marrow particles and touch preparations from trephine biopsy specimens can be stained in the same manner.

STAINING BLOOD AND BONE MARROW FILMS

Romanowsky stains are universally employed for routine staining of blood films, and very satisfactory results can be obtained. The remarkable property of the Romanowsky dyes of making subtle distinctions in shades of staining, and of staining granules differentially, depends on two components, namely, azure B (trimethylthionin) and eosin Y (tetrabromo-fluorescein).[1,2]

The original Romanowsky combination was polychrome methylene blue and eosin. Several of the stains now used routinely which are based on azure B also include methylene blue, but the need for this is debatable. Its presence in the stain is thought by some to enhance the staining of nucleoli and polychromatic red cells; in its absence, normal neutrophil granules tend to stain heavily and may resemble 'toxic granules' in conventionally stained films.[3]

There are a number of causes for variation in staining. One of the main factors is the presence of contaminants in the commercial dyes and a simple combination of pure azure B and eosin Y is preferable to the more complex stains, as this ensures consistent results from batch to batch.[1,4,5] However, in practice, absolutely pure dyes are expensive, and it is sufficient to ensure that the stains contain at least 80% of the appropriate dye.[6] Amongst the Romanowsky stains now in use, Jenner's is the simplest and Giemsa's the most complex. Leishman's stain, which occupies an intermediate position, is still widely used in the routine staining of blood films, although the results are inferior to those obtained by the combined May–Grünwald–Giemsa, Jenner–Giemsa and azure B–eosin Y methods. Wright's stain, which is widely used in North America, gives results that are similar to those obtained with Leishman's stain.

A pH to the alkaline side of neutrality accentuates the azure component at the expense of the eosin and vice versa. A pH of 6.8 is usually recommended for general use, but to some extent this depends on personal preference. (When looking for malaria parasites, a pH of 7.2 is recommended in order to see Schüffner's dots.) To achieve a uniform pH, 50 ml of 66 mmol/l Sörensen's phosphate buffer (p. 606) may be added to each 1 litre of the water used in diluting the stains and washing the films.

The mechanism by which certain components of a cell's structure stain with particular dyes and other components fail to do so, although staining with other dyes, depends on complex differences in binding of the dyes to chemical structures and interactions between the dye molecules.[7] Azure B is bound to anionic molecules, and eosin Y is bound to cationic sites on proteins.

Thus, the acidic groupings of the nucleic acids and proteins of the cell nuclei and primitive cytoplasm determine their uptake of the basic dye azure B and, conversely, the presence of basic groupings on the haemoglobin molecule results in its affinity for acidic dyes and its staining by eosin. The granules in the cytoplasm of neutrophil leucocytes are weakly stained by the azure complexes. Eosinophilic granules contain a spermine derivative with an alkaline grouping which stains strongly with the acidic component of the dye, whereas basophilic granules contain heparin which has an affinity for the basic component of the dye. These effects depend on molar equilibrium between the two dyes in time-dependent reactions.[2] DNA binds rapidly, RNA slower and haemoglobin slower still; hence the need to have the correct azure B:eosin ratio, to avoid contamination of the dyes and to stain for the right time. Standardized stains and staining method have been proposed (p. 51).

The colour reactions of the Romanowsky effect are shown in Table 4.1; causes of variation in staining are given in Table 4.2.

Table 4.1 Colour responses of blood cells to Romanowsky staining

Cellular component	Colour
Nuclei	
Chromatin	Purple
Nucleoli	Light blue
Cytoplasm	
Erythroblast	Dark blue
Erythrocyte	Dark pink
Reticulocyte	Grey-blue
Lymphocyte	Blue
Metamyelocyte	Pink
Monocyte	Grey-blue
Myelocyte	Pink
Neutrophil	Pink/orange
Promyelocyte	Blue
Basophil	Blue
Granules	
Promyelocyte (primary granules)	Red or purple
Basophil	Purple black
Eosinophil	Red-orange
Neutrophil	Purple
Toxic granules	Dark Blue
Platelet	Purple
Other inclusions	
Auer body	Purple
Cabot ring	Purple
Howell–Jolly body	Purple
Döhle body	Light blue

Table 4.2 Factors giving rise to faulty staining

Appearances	Causes
Too blue, nuclei blue to black	Eosin concentration too low. Incorrect preparation of stock. Stock stain exposed to bright daylight. Batch of stain solution overused. Impure dyes. Staining time too short. Staining solution too acid. Smear too thick. Inadequate time in buffer solution
Too pink	Incorrect proportion of azure B–eosin Y. Impure dyes. Buffer pH too low. Excessive washing in buffer solution
Pale staining	Old staining solution. Overused staining solution. Incorrect preparation of stock. Impure dyes, especially azure A and/or C. High ambient temperature
Neutrophil granules not stained	Insufficient azure B
Neutrophil granules dark blue/black (pseudo-toxic)	Excess azure B
Other stain anomalies	Various contaminating dyes and metal salts
Stain deposit on film	Stain solution left in uncovered jar. Stain solution not filtered
Blue background	Inadequate fixation or prolonged storage before fixation. Blood collected into heparin as anticoagulant

PREPARATION OF SOLUTIONS OF ROMANOWSKY DYES

May–Grünwald stain. Weigh out 0.3 g of the powdered dye and transfer to a conical flask of 200–250 ml capacity. Add 100 ml of methanol and warm the mixture to 50°C. Allow the flask to cool to *c* 20°C and shake several times during the day. After standing for 24 h, filter the solution. It is then ready for use, no ripening being required.

Jenner's stain.   Prepare a 5 g/l solution in methanol in exactly the same way as described above for the May–Grünwald stain.

Giemsa's stain.   Weigh 1 g of the powdered dye and transfer to a conical flask of 200–250 ml capacity. Add 100 ml of methanol and warm the mixture to 50°C; keep at this temperature for 15 min with occasional shaking, then filter the solution. It is then ready for use, but will improve on standing.

Azure B–eosin Y stock solution.   Azure B, tetra-fluoroborate or thiocyanate (CI 52010), >80% pure. Eosin Y (CI 45380), >80% pure.

   Dissolve 0.6 g of azure B in 60 ml dimethyl sulphoxide (DMSO) and 0.2 g of eosin Y in 50 ml DMSO; preheat the DMSO at 37°C before adding the dyes. Stand at 37°C, shaking vigorously for 30 s at 5 min intervals until both dyes are completely dissolved. Add the eosin Y solution to the azure B solution and stir well. This stock solution should remain stable for several months if kept at room temperature in the dark. DMSO will crystallize below 18°C; if necessary allow it to redissolve before use.

Buffered water.   Make up 50 ml of 66 mmol/l Sörensen's phosphate buffer of the required pH to 1 litre with water at a pH of 6.8 (see p. 606). An alternative buffer may be prepared from buffer tablets which are available commercially. Solutions of the required pH are obtained by dissolving the tablets in water.

STAINING METHODS

May–Grünwald–Giemsa stain

Dry the films in the air, then fix by immersing in a jar of methanol for 5–10 min. For bone marrow films, allow longer time to ensure thorough drying and then leave for 15–20 min in the methanol. Transfer to a staining jar containing May–Grünwald stain freshly diluted with an equal volume of buffered water. After the films have been allowed to stain for *c* 15 min, transfer them without washing to a jar containing Giemsa's stain

freshly diluted with 9 volumes of buffered water, pH 6.8. After staining for 10–15 min, transfer the slides to a jar containing buffered water, pH 6.8, rapidly wash in three or four changes of water and finally allow to stand undisturbed in water for a short time (usually 2–5 min) for differentiation to take place. This may be controlled by inspection of the wet slide under the low power of the microscope; with experience, the naked-eye colour of the film is often a good guide. The slides should be transferred from one staining solution to the other without being allowed to dry. As the intensity of the staining is affected by any variation in the thickness of a film, it is not easy to obtain uniform staining throughout a film's length.

   When differentiation is complete, stand the slides upright to dry.

   The May-Grünwald-Giemsa staining method described above is designed for staining a number of films at the same time. Single slides may be stained by flooding the slide with a combined fixative and staining solution (e.g. Leishman's stain).

   A relatively prolonged fixation, at least 10 min, is required for good staining, particularly when staining films of bone marrow. It is important to ensure that the methanol used as fixative is completely water-free. As little as 1% water may affect the appearance of the films and a higher water content causes gross changes (Fig. 4.2). The red cells will also be affected by traces of detergent on inadequately washed slides (Fig. 4.3).

   The diluted stains usually retain their staining powers sufficiently well for several batches of slides to be stained in them. They must be made up freshly each day, and it is probably best to stain the day's films in two batches, morning and afternoon. There is no need to filter the stains before use unless a deposit is present.

Standardized Romanowsky stain[2,5]

This is based on a method with pure dyes proposed by the International Committee for Standardization in Haematology. Its advantage is that it ensures consistent results from batch to batch so that it can be used for checking the performance of other stains and for automated pattern recognition methods. Its disadvantage in a routine laboratory is that it requires the use of DMSO which is a potentially toxic solvent with an unpleasant smell. The stained films tend to fade after a few months.

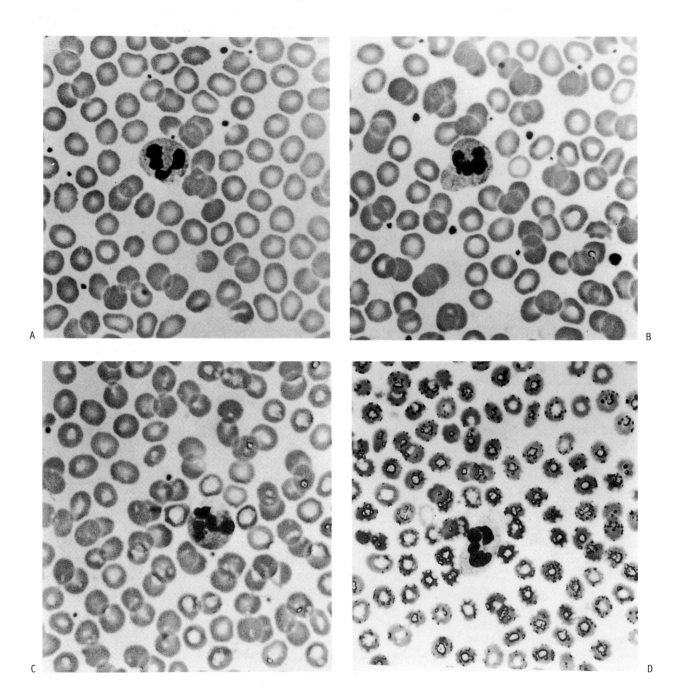

Fig. 4.2 Blood film appearances following methanol fixation. Photomicrographs of Romanowsky-stained blood films that have been fixed in methanol containing: (A) 1% water; (B) 3% water; (C) 4% water; (D) 10% water. The red cells and leucocytes are well fixed in A and B, but badly fixed in C and D.

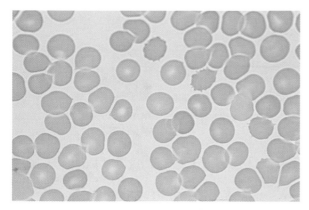

Fig. 4.3 Effect of traces of detergent on the slide. Photomicrograph of a Romanowsky-stained blood film on an inadequately washed slide with residual traces of detergent.

Fixative. Mix 1 volume of stock solution of azure B–eosin Y with 14 volumes of methanol.

Staining solution. Immediately before use, dilute 1 volume of the stock solution (see above) with 14 volumes of HEPES buffer, pH 6.6 (p. 605). This solution is stable for about 8 h.[8]

Method. Dry the films in the air. Leave for 3 min in the fixative. Leave the slides in the diluted staining solution for 15 min. Rinse in phosphate buffer solution, pH 6.8, for 1 min. Then rinse with water, air dry and mount. For bone marrow films, fix for 5 min and leave the slides to stain for 25–30 min.

When several batches of films are being stained in succession, the staining solution should be renewed at intervals (e.g. after each 50 slides). Loss of staining power is usually due to precipitation of the eosin Y and this will result in the nuclei staining blue instead of purple (see Table 4.2).

Jenner–Giemsa stain

Jenner's stain may be substituted for May–Grünwald stain in the technique described on p. 51. The results are a little less satisfactory. The stain is used with 4 volumes of buffered water and the films, after being fixed in methanol, are immersed in it for approximately 4 min before being transferred to the Giemsa's stain. They should be allowed to stain in the latter solution for 7–10 min. Differentiation is carried out as described above.

Leishman's stain

Dry the film in the air and flood the slide with the stain. After 2 min, add double the volume of water and stain the film for 5–7 min. Then wash it in a stream of buffered water until it has acquired a pinkish tinge (up to 2 min). After the back of the slide has been wiped clean, set it upright to dry.

AUTOMATED STAINING

Automatic staining machines are available which enable large batches of slides to be handled. Some apply staining solutions to slides lying horizontally (flat-bed staining) while others either immerse a slide or slides in a bath of staining solution ('dip-and dunk' technique) or spray stain onto slides in a cytocentrifuge. Problems include increased background staining, inadequate staining of neutrophil granules, degranulation of basophils and blue or green rather than pink staining of erythrocytes. These problems are usually related to the specific stains and staining protocols employed than to the type of instrument, although flat-bed stainers are more likely to cause problems with stain deposit. However, as a rule, staining is satisfactory provided that reliable stains are used and there is careful control of the cycle time and other variables.[9]

RAPID STAINING METHOD

Field's method[10,11] was introduced to provide a quick method for staining thick films for malaria parasites (see below). With some modifications, it can be used fairly satisfactorily for the rapid staining of thin films. The stains are available commercially ready for use or they can be prepared as described below.

Stains
Stain A (polychromed methylene blue)
Methylene blue 1.3 g
Disodium hydrogen phosphate (Na_2HPO_4. $12H_2O$) 12.6 g
Potassium dihydrogen phosphate (KH_2PO_4) 6.25 g
Water 500 ml.
Dissolve the methylene blue and the disodium hydrogen phosphate in 50 ml of water. Then boil the solution in a water-bath almost to dryness in order to 'polychrome' the dye. Add the potassium

dihydrogen phosphate and 500 ml of freshly boiled water. After stirring to dissolve the stain, set aside the solution for 24 h before filtering. Filter again before use. The pH is 6.6–6.8.

Alternatively, azure B may be added to the methylene blue in the proportion of 0.5 g of azure B to 0.8 g of methylene blue. In this case, the dyes can be dissolved directly in the phosphate buffer solution.

Stain B (eosin)
Eosin 1.3 g
Disodium hydrogen phosphate $(Na_2HPO_4. 12H_2O)$ 12.6 g
Potassium dihydrogen phosphate (KH_2PO_4) 6.25 g
Water 500 ml.

Dissolve the phosphates in warm freshly boiled water, and then add the dye. Filter the solution after standing for 24 h.

METHOD OF STAINING
Fix the film for 10–15 s in methanol. Pour off the methanol and drop on the slide 12 drops of diluted Stain B (1 volume of stain to 4 volumes of water). Immediately, add 12 drops of Stain A. Agitate the slide to mix the stains. After 1 min, rinse the slide in water, then differentiate the film for 5 s in phosphate buffer at pH 6.6, wash the slide in water and then place it on end to drain and dry. Two-stage stains of this type are also available commercially.

MOUNTING OF COVER-GLASS

When thoroughly dry, cover the blood film with a rectangular No. 1 cover-glass, using for this purpose a mountant, which is miscible with xylol (e.g. DPX Mountant, Merck). For a temporary mount, cedarwood oil may be used.

The cover-glass should be sufficiently large to overlie the whole film, so that the edges and the tail of the film can be examined. If a neutral mounting medium is used, the staining should be preserved for many years if kept in the dark. Although it is probable that stained films keep best unmounted, there are objections to this course: it is almost impossible to keep the slides free from dust and from being scratched, and in the absence of a cover-glass the observer is tempted to examine the film solely with the oil-immersion objective, a practice which is to be deprecated.

EXAMINATION OF BLOOD FILMS FOR PARASITES

A number of screening tests based on immunological methods have been developed for the detection of malarial antigens (see Ch. 22, p. 538). But the essential method for a definitive diagnosis remains the finding of parasites in a blood film and the identification of the species by morphology.[12,13]

In addition to standard thin films, thick films are extremely useful when parasites are scanty, and these should be prepared and examined as a routine, although identification of the species is less easy than in thin films and mixed infections may be missed. However, an experienced observer should be able to find and recognize parasites with certainty even in badly stained thick films, whilst in a well-stained film, parasites should be easily recognized even by beginners. If 5 minutes are spent examining a thick film this is equivalent to about 1 h spent in traversing a thin film. Once the presence of parasites has been confirmed, a thin film should be used for determining the species and, in the case of *Plasmodium falciparum*, for assessing the severity of the infection by counting the percentage of positive cells. Seldom, if ever, should there be any doubt as to whether or not an object is a malaria parasite when a film has been well stained.

Rapid screening for malaria can also be carried out on films by fluorescence microscopy at low magnification, as malaria parasites fluoresce intensely with acridine orange.[14,15]

Thick blood films are also useful for the detection of microfilaria. When they are used for this purpose, it is important to scan the entire film using a low-power objective or parasites may be missed. Examination of fresh liquid blood (see below) can also be used for the identification of microfilariae and has the advantage that as the parasites are moving they are easily detected. A stained film is necessary for confirmation of species.

MAKING THICK FILMS

Make a thick film by placing a small drop of blood in the centre of a slide and spreading it out with a corner of another slide to cover an area about four times its original area. The correct thickness for a satisfactory film will have been achieved if, with the slide placed on a piece of newspaper, small print is just visible.

Allow the film to dry thoroughly for at least 30 min at 37°C before attempting to stain it. If it is necessary to hurry the procedure, the slide can be left near a light bulb where the temperature is 50–60°C, but not touching it, for *c* 7 min; the quality of the film may deteriorate if overheated. Absolutely fresh films, although apparently dry, often wash off in the stain.

STAINING THICK FILMS

Field's method of staining[10,11] is quick and usually satisfactory for thick films, but the method is not practical for staining large numbers of films; for this purpose the Giemsa, Leishman or azure B–eosin Y methods are more suitable. Careful attention to pH is critical.

Field's stain[10,11]

The preparation of the stains is described on page 53.

1. Dip the slide with the dried but otherwise unfixed film on it into Stain A for 3 s.
2. Dip into a jar of tap water for 3 s with gentle agitation.
3. Dip into Stain B for 3 s.
4. Wash gently in tap water for a few seconds until all excess stain is removed.
5. Drain the slide vertically and leave to dry. Do not blot.

Giemsa's stain

1. Dry the films thoroughly as above.
2. Without fixing, immerse the slides for 20–30 min in a staining jar containing Giemsa's stain freshly diluted with 20 volumes of buffered water (pH 7.2).
3. Wash in buffered water pH 7.2 for 3 min.
4. Stand the slides upright to dry. Do not blot.

Azure B–eosin Y stain

1. Prepare a staining solution from the stock stain, as described on page 51, but using HEPES buffer at pH 7.2.
2. After the films have been dried as described above, stain for 10 min in the staining solution.
3. Rinse for 1 min in buffered water, pH 7.2.
4. Stand the slides upright to dry. Do not blot.

Sometimes when thick films are stained, they become overlaid by a residue of stain or spoilt by the envelopes of the lysed red cells. These defects can be minimized by adding 0.1% Triton X-100 to the buffer before diluting the stock stain.[16] An alternative, but more laborious, method is to lyse 1 volume of blood with 3 volumes of 1% saponin in saline for 10 min, then centrifuge for 5 min, decant the supernatant and make films from the residual pellet.[17]

STAINING THIN FILMS

Thin films should be stained with Giemsa's stain or Leishman's stain at pH 7.2, not with a standard May–Grünwald–Giemsa stain.

Leishman's stain[12]
Stain
Use commercially available stain or prepare stain as follows:

1. Add glass beads to 500 ml of methanol.
2. Add 1.5 g of Leishman's powder.
3. Shake well, leave on a rotary shaker during the day, then incubate at 37°C overnight.

There is no need to filter.

Method

1. Make a thin film and air-dry rapidly

2. Place the film on a staining rack, flood with Leishman's stain and leave for 30 s to 1 min to fix.
3. Add twice as much buffered distilled water (preferably from a plastic wash bottle as this permits better mixing of the solution), pH 7.2.
4. Leave to stain for 10 min.
5. Wash off stain with tap water.

EXAMINATION OF WET BLOOD FILM PREPARATIONS

The examination of a drop of blood sealed between a slide and cover-glass is sometimes of considerable value.

The preparation may be examined in several ways; by ordinary illumination, by dark-ground or by Nomarski (interference) illumination. Chemically clean slides and cover-glasses (p. 609) must be used and the blood allowed to spread out thinly between them. If the glass surfaces are free from dust, the blood will spread out spontaneously, and pressure, which is undesirable, should not be necessary. The edges of the preparation may be sealed with a melted mixture of equal parts of petroleum jelly and paraffin wax or with nail varnish.

Red cells

Rouleaux formation is usually seen in varying degrees in 'wet' preparations of whole blood and has to be distinguished from auto-agglutination.

Rouleaux formation versus auto-agglutination
The distinction between rouleaux formation and auto-agglutination is sometimes a matter of considerable difficulty, particularly when, as not infrequently happens, rouleaux formation is superimposed on agglutination. The rouleaux, too, may be notably irregular in haemolytic anaemias characterized by spherocytosis, while the clumping caused by massive rouleaux formation of normal type may closely simulate true agglutination. This 'pseudo-agglutination' owing to massive rouleaux formation may be distinguished from true agglutination in two ways:

1. By noting that the red cells, although forming parts of larger clumps, are mostly arranged side by side as in typical rouleaux.
2. By adding 3–4 volumes of 9 g/l NaCl to the preparation. Pseudo-agglutination owing to massive rouleaux formation should either disperse completely or transform itself into typical rouleaux. The addition of saline to blood that has undergone true agglutination may cause the agglutinates to break up somewhat, but a major degree of it is likely to persist and typical rouleaux will not be seen.

Anisocytosis and poikilocytosis can be recognized in 'wet' preparations of blood, but the tendency to crenation and the formation of rouleaux tend to make observations on shape changes rather difficult. Such changes can best be studied in a wet preparation after fixation. For this, freshly collected heparinized or EDTA-blood is diluted in 10 volumes of iso-osmotic phosphate buffer, pH 7.4 (see p. 605) and immediately fixed with an equal volume of 0.3% glutaraldehyde in iso-osmotic phosphate buffer, pH 7.4. After standing for 5 min, one drop of this suspension is added to 4 drops of glycerol and 1–2 drops are placed on a glass slide which is then sealed.[18]

Normally, less than 2% of the circulating red cells show pitting; an increase above 4% is an indication of splenic dysfunction. The pits are readily identified by Nomarski illumination, when they have the appearance of small crater-like identations on the cell surface.[19]

The sickling of red cells in 'wet' preparations of blood is described on page 251.

Parasites

Wet preparations of blood are suitable for the detection of microfilariae, trypanosomes and the spirochaetes of relapsing fever. The presence of small numbers of trypanosomes or spirochaetes is revealed by occasional slight agitation of groups of red cells. Examination of a Romanowsky-stained film confirms their nature.

Leucocytes

The motility of leucocytes can be readily studied in heparinized blood if the microscope stage can be warmed to c 37°C. Usually, only the granulocytes show significant progressive movements. However, the examination of living neutrophils in plasma is not useful in day-to-day routine haematological practice. Specialized microscopy techniques applicable to leucocytes are discussed in the eighth edition of this book.

SEPARATION AND CONCENTRATION OF BLOOD CELLS

A number of methods are available for the concentration of leucocytes or abnormal cells when they are present in only small numbers in the peripheral blood. Concentrates are most simply prepared from the buffy coat of centrifuged blood.

Making a buffy-coat preparation

Defibrinate venous blood in a flask and then centrifuge a sample for 15 min in a Wintrobe haematocrit tube at 3000 rpm (1500 g). If a Wintrobe haematocrit tube is not available, a narrow test tube or capillary tube can be used. After centrifugation, remove the supernatant serum carefully with a fine pipette, and with the same pipette deposit the platelet and underlying leucocyte layers on to one or two slides. Emulsify the buffy coat in a drop of the patient's plasma and then spread the films. Allow them to dry in the air and then fix and stain in the usual way.

When leucocytes are scanty or if many slides are to be made, it is worth while centrifuging the blood twice; first, c 5 ml are centrifuged and a haematocrit tube is then filled from the upper cell layers of this sample.

As an alternative to centrifugation, the blood may be allowed to sediment, with the help of sedimentation-enhancing agents such as fibrinogen, dextran, gum acacia, Ficoll (Pharmacia) or methylcellulose.[20,21] Bøyum's reagent[22,23] (methylcellulose and sodium metrizoate) is particularly suitable for obtaining leucocyte preparations with minimal red cell contamination.

Most methods of separation affect to some extent subsequent staining properties, chemical reactions and the viability of the separated cells.

The buffy coat

It is well known that atypical or primitive blood cells circulate in small numbers in the peripheral blood in health. Thus, atypical mononuclear cells, metamyelocytes and megakaryocytes may be found. Even promyelocytes, blasts and nucleated red cells may occasionally be seen, but only in very small numbers. Efrati & Rozenszajn[24] described a method for the quantitative assessment of the numbers of atypical cells in normal blood and gave figures for the incidence of megakaryocyte fragments (e.g. mean 21.8 per 1 ml of blood) and of atypical mononuclears and metamyelocytes and myelocytes. In cord blood, the incidence of all types of primitive cells is considerably greater.[25]

In disease, leaving the leukaemias and allied disorders out of consideration, abnormal cells may be seen in buffy-coat preparations in much larger numbers than in films of whole blood. For instance, megakaryocytes and immature cells of the granulocyte series are found in relatively large numbers in disseminated carcinoma.[26] Megaloblasts, if present, may help in the diagnosis of a megaloblastic anaemia. Haemophagocytosis, which is more often observed in the bone marrow, may also sometimes be demonstrated in buffy-coat preparations in lymphomas.[27] Erythrophagocytosis may be conspicuous in cases of auto-immune haemolytic anaemia (Fig. 4.4), whilst in systemic lupus erythematosus

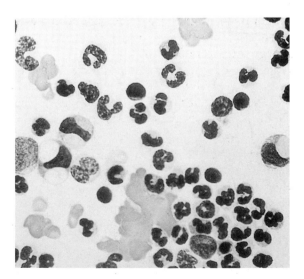

Fig. 4.4 Film of a buffy coat. Erythrophagocytosis in auto-immune haemolytic anaemia.

(SLE) a few LE cells may be found – this is not, however, the best way to demonstrate LE cells and in any event the detection of LE cells for the diagnosis of SLE has now largely been supplanted by immunological tests for the detection of antinuclear or anti-DNA antibodies.

Buffy-coat films can be useful for the detection of bacteria, fungi or parasites within neutrophils, monocytes or circulating macrophages.

With the availability of automated differential leucocyte counts, the use of buffy-coat films for differential counting of leucopenic samples is usually unnecessary.

Separation of specific cell populations

Differences in density of cells can be used to separate individual cell types, using gradient solutions of selected specific gravity.[21,23,28] These include an erythrocyte-aggregating polysaccharide (Ficoll, Pharmacia), polyvinyl pyrrolidone (PVP)-coated silica gel (Percoll, Pharmacia), and sodium metrizoate (e.g. Isopaque, Nycomed). Mixtures of Ficoll with sodium metrizoate (Lymphoprep, Nycomed), sodium metrizoate with methyl-cellulose and aqueous buffered solutions of sodium metrizoate (e.g. Nycodenz, Nycomed) will provide media of selected densities. In this way, it is possible to separate cell populations with reasonable purity. A simple convenient technique has been described for layering the blood or bone marrow over the density preparations.[29]

The median values for the main haemopoietic cells are given below. There is, however, considerable overlap in the density ranges between adjacent types of cells.[21,23,30]

Erythrocytes	1100
Eosinophils	1090
Neutrophils	1085
Myelocytes	1075
Lymphocytes	1070
Monocytes	1064
Myeloblasts	1062
Platelets	1035.

It is also possible to separate and harvest specific B cells, T cells and various haemopoietic progenitor cells by means of magnetic latex polymer particles coated with specific antibody (Dynabeads, Dynal Ltd).[31–33]

Isolation of tumour cells from blood

The methods used for demonstrating tumour cells in circulating blood involve elimination of the red cells and differential sedimentation or filtration of the leucocytes. Fleming & Stewart[34] assessed several methods critically and concluded that differential separation was to be preferred for routine use. They recommended a slight modification of the silicone flotation method of Seal.[35] Positive identifications are seldom made except in advanced cancer when the diagnosis is usually only too obvious.

PARASITES DETECTABLE IN BLOOD, BONE MARROW OR SPLENIC ASPIRATES

Only brief outlines of the methods used for parasitological diagnoses are given in this chapter. For more detailed accounts, readers are referred to a parasitology textbook. In addition to the *Plasmodia* which give rise to malaria, the other important parasites to be found in the blood are *Leishmaniae*, trypanosomes and microfilaria

MALARIA

Methods for staining and examination of thin and thick blood films for *Plasmodium* are described above; morphological criteria for differentiation of malaria parasites are given in Table 4.3 and illustrated in Figure 4.5. Supplementary screening methods are described in Chapter 22 (p. 537).

LEISHMANIASIS

Leishmania species are transmitted by the bite of an infected female sandfly and are associated with a variety of clinical conditions including visceral, mucous and cutaneous leishmaniasis. Visceral leishmaniasis may present to the haematologist as splenomegaly, hepatomegaly, fever, lymphadeno-

Table 4.3 Morphological differentiation of malaria parasites

	P. falciparum	*P. vivax*	*P. ovale*	*P. malariae*
Infected red cells	Normal size*; Maurer's clefts†	Enlarged; Schüffner's dots‡	Enlarged; oval and fimbriated; Schüffner's dots‡	Normal or microcytic; stippling not usually seen
Ring forms (early trophozoites)	Delicate; frequently 2 or more; accolé forms§; small chromatin dot	Large, thick; usually single (occasionally 2) in cell; large chromatin dot	Thick compact rings	Very small compact rings
Later trophozoites	Compact, vacuolated; sometimes 2 chromatin dots	Amoeboid; central vacuole; light blue cytoplasm	Smaller than *P. vivax*; slightly amoeboid	Band across cell; deep blue cytoplasm
Schizonts	18–24 merozoites filling ⅔ of cell (usually only seen in cerebral malaria)	12–24 merozoites, irregularly arranged	8–12 merozoites filling ¾ of cell	6–12 merozoites in daisy-head around central mass of pigment
Pigment	Dark to black clumped mass	Fine granular; yellow-brown	Coarse light brown	Dark, prominent at all stages
Gametocytes	Crescent or sausage-shaped; diffuse chromatin; single nucleus	Spherical, compact, almost fills cell; single nucleus	Oval; fills ¾ of cell; similar to, but smaller than, *P. vivax*	Round, fills ½ to ⅔ of cell; similar to *P. vivax* but smaller, with no Schüffner's dots

*In *P. falciparum*, it is important to report the percentage of red cells that are infected.

†Large, irregularly shaped, red-staining dots.

‡Fine stippling.

§i.e. marginalized to edge of cell ('appliqué').

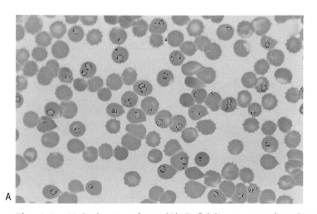
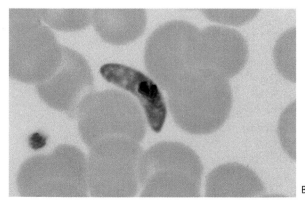

A

B

Fig. 4.5 Malaria parasites. (A) *P. falciparum:* trophozoites; (B) *P. falciparum:* gametocyte; (C) *P. vivax:* trophozoites; (D) *P. ovale:* trophozoites; (E) *P. malariae:* trophozoites; (F) *P. malariae: schizont*; (G) *P. falciparum* and *P. vivax*: mixed infection.

Figures 4.5 (C)–(G), see next page

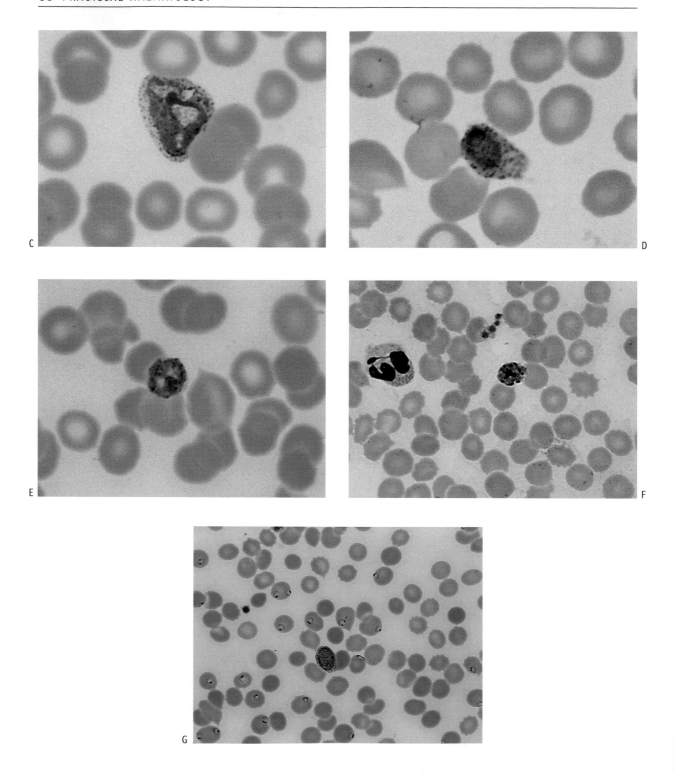

Fig. 4.5 *Continued.*

pathy and pancytopenia and it is being increasingly reported in patients with HIV infection. Serological studies are recommended as the initial diagnostic tests in suspected leishmaniasis. In advanced stages of the disease, parasites can be found in phagocytic cells in spleen, lymph nodes, bone marrow and peripheral blood.

Diagnosis of leishmaniasis in the haematology laboratory

Leishmaniasis is diagnosed in the haematology laboratory by direct visualization of the amastigotes (often referred to as Leishman–Donovan bodies).

Buffy-coat preparations of peripheral blood or aspirates (see p. 57 for preparation of buffy coats) from marrow, spleen, lymph nodes or skin lesions should be spread on a slide to make a thin smear, and stained with Leishman's or Giemsa's stain (pH 7.2) for 20 min (p. 51). Amastigotes are seen within monocytes or, less commonly, in neutrophils in peripheral blood, and in macrophages in aspirates. They are small, round bodies 2–4 μm in diameter with indistinct cytoplasm, a nucleus and a small rod-shaped kinetoplast (Fig. 4.6A). Occasionally amastigotes may be seen lying free between cells.

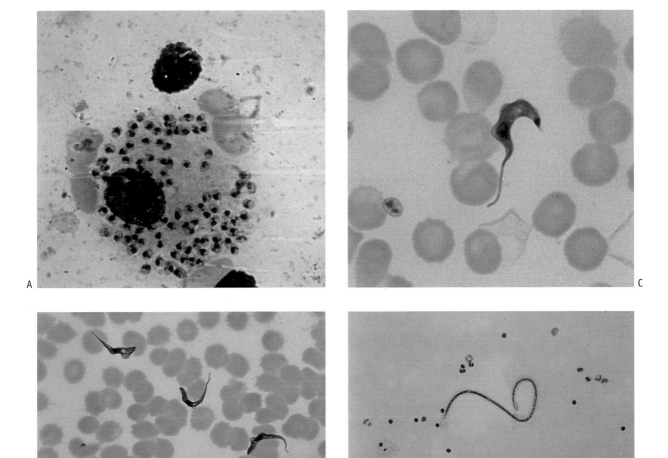

Fig. 4.6 Blood parasites. (A) Leishmaniasis (Leishman–Donovan bodies); (B) Trypanosomiasis (*T. cruzi*); (C) Trypanosomiasis (*T. gambiense*); (D) Microfilaria.

TRYPANOSOMIASIS

African trypanosomiasis (sleeping sickness)

This is caused by *Trypanosoma brucei gambiense* (West Africa and western Central Africa) and *Trypanosoma brucei rhodesiense* (East, Central and Southern Africa); it is transmitted by a few species of tsetse fly. The trypomastigotes can be found in blood, lymph node aspirates and cerebrospinal fluid but repeated examinations and concentration techniques may be needed before they are detected. Serological investigations may also be helpful in diagnosis.

American trypanosomiasis (Chagas' disease)

This is caused by *Trypanosoma cruzi* which is transmitted by the Reduviidae bug, subfamily *Triatominae*. Chagas' disease is only found in tropical and subtropical South and Central American countries. Trypomastigotes can only be found circulating in the blood in the acute form of Chagas' disease. As the trypomastigotes are more fragile than those causing African trypanosomiasis, serology rather than morphology is recommended for initial screening. In the haematology laboratory, tests which detect motile organisms are more sensitive than those which require fixed, stained preparations.

Diagnosis of trypanosomiasis in the haematology laboratory

Care should be taken when handling samples suspected of being infected with trypomastigotes because infection can occur if the organisms penetrate the skin. Several techniques are available for examining specimens for the presence of trypomastigotes.

Wet preparations

If present in high concentrations, trypomastigotes can be seen thrashing amongst the cells on a fresh, unstained wet preparation of blood or lymph node fluid. Preparations should be examined within 4 h of sampling (this time can be extended if a few milligrams of glucose are added to the specimen) using a ×40 objective and a partially closed condenser iris, or dark-field or phase contrast microscopy.

Thick-stained blood films or chancre aspirates

Examination of a thick-stained film allows more of the sample to be examined rapidly, but *T. cruzi* are easily damaged by the spreading of specimens for thick films. Thick films are prepared by spreading a drop of blood on a slide to cover a 15–20 mm diameter area and staining with Giemsa staining technique or Field's rapid technique (p. 53) as for malaria smears. Microscopically, *T. b. gambiense* and *T. b. rhodesiense* cannot be distinguished from each other; they are 13–42 μm long with a single flagellum, a centrally placed nucleus and a small dot-like kinetoplast. *T. cruzi* measures 12–30 μm and has a larger kinetoplast than *T. b. gambiense* and *T. b. rhodesiense* (Fig. 4.6B,C).

Concentration techniques

- Quantitative buffy-coat (QBC) method[36]
  This is described on page 537. After centrifugation, the tube should be left to stand upright for 5 min and the plasma interface area is then examined for motile trypomastigotes. This is considered to be the 'gold standard' for diagnosis.
- Capillary tube method
  Fill one or two micro-haematocrit capillary tubes with EDTA or citrated blood. Seal the ends and centrifuge for about 5 min as for micro-haematocrit. Then lay the capillary tubes adjacent to each other on a microscope slide and secure both ends onto the slide with adhesive tape (Fig. 4.7). Examine the plasma just below the red cell and buffy layer immediately for motile trypomastigotes using a 20× or 10× objective with the condenser iris partially closed or by dark-field microscopy.

FILARIASIS AND LOIASIS

Filariasis involving the lymphatics is the cause of elephantiasis. It is caused by the filarial worms *Brugia malayi*, *Wuchereria bancrofti* and *Brugia timori* whereas filarial infection of the subcutaneous tissues is caused by *Loa loa*. The larvae of these worms, microfilariae, are transmitted by mosquito to humans where they can be found in the blood and where they show periodicity with fluctuating levels at different times of the day (Fig. 4.6D).

Diagnosis of filariasis in the haematology laboratory

Blood concentrations of microfilariae are often higher in capillary blood than venous blood. However, even when blood has been collected at

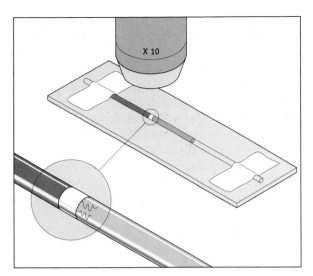

Fig. 4.7 Capillary tube concentration method. Method used for detecting trypomastigotes or microfilariae in blood. See text.

the appropriate time, microfilariae can be scanty, so that serological or rapid immunochromatographic tests, and concentration techniques may be required.

Wet preparation
A thick blood film is prepared from 20 μl blood and stained as for malaria smears (p. 55).

Concentration techniques
- Filtration method
  This is the most sensitive concentration method for microfilariae but samples must be handled gently to preserve the organisms. 10 ml of anti-coagulated blood, followed by 10 ml of methylene blue or azure B saline solution, are passed through a transparent polycarbonate membrane filter of 3 μm porosity attached to a syringe. The filter is placed face upwards on a slide, a drop of saline is added and a cover slip is placed on top. The entire membrane is examined microscopically for motile microfilariae using a ×10 objective and a partially closed condenser iris or dark-field microscopy.
- Quantitative buffy-coat and micro-haematocrit methods
  Microfilariae can be detected using the same methods as for detection of trypomastigotes (see above).

- Lyzed capillary blood
  1 ml of blood is mixed with 9 ml of 2% formalin and centrifuged at 1000 g for 5 min. All the deposit is placed on a slide and 1 drop of Field's stain A or 1% methylene blue is added to facilitate species identification. Motile microfilariae can be seen using a ×10 objective with a partially closed condenser iris or dark-field microscopy.

REFERENCES

1 Wittekind D 1979 On the nature of Romanowsky dyes and the Romanowsky Giemsa effect. Clinical and Laboratory Haematology 1:247.
2 Horobin RW, Walter KJ 1987 Understanding Romanowsky staining:1. the Romanowsky-Giemsa effect in blood smears. Histochemistry 86:331–336.
3 Marshall PN 1977 Methylene blue–azure B–eosin as a substitute for May–Grünwald–Giemsa and Jenner–Giemsa stains. Microscopica Acta 79:153.
4 Wittekind DH, Kretschmer V, Sohmer I 1982 Azure B–eosin Y stain as the standard Romanowsky–Giemsa stain. British Journal of Haematology 5:391.
5 International Committee for Standardization in Haematology 1984 ICSH reference method for staining of blood and bone marrow films by azure B and eosin Y (Romanowsky stain). British Journal of Haematology 57:707.
6 Schenk EA, Willis CT 1989 Note from the Biological Stain Commission: certification of Wright stain solution. Stain Technology 64:152.
7 Wittekind DH 1983 On the nature of Romanowsky–Giemsa staining and its significance for cytochemistry and histochemistry: an overall view. Histochemical Journal 15:1029.
8 Bind M, Huiges W, Halie MR 1985 Stability of azure B–eosin Y staining solutions. British Journal of Haematology 59:73.
9 Hayashi M, Gauthier S, Tatsumi N 1996 Evaluation of an automated slide preparation and staining unit. Sysmex Journal International 6:63–69.
10 Field JW 1940–41 The morphology of malarial parasites in thick blood films. Part IV. The identification of species and phase. Transactions of the Royal Society of Tropical Medicine and Hygiene 34:405.
11 Field JW 1941–42 Further notes on a method of staining malarial parasites in thick films. Transactions of the Royal Society of Tropical Medicine and Hygiene 35:35.

12 British Committee for Standards in Haematology 1997 The laboratory diagnosis of malaria. Clinical and Laboratory Haematology 19:165–170.

13 Warhurst DC, Williams JE 1996 Laboratory diagnosis of malaria (ACP Broadsheet No. 148). Journal of Clinical Pathology 49:533–538.

14 Jahanmehr SAH, Hyde K, Geary CG, et al 1987 Simple technique for fluorescence staining of blood cells with acridine orange. Journal of Clinical Pathology 40:926.

15 Sodeman TM 1970 The use of fluorochromes for the detection of malaria parasites. American Journal of Tropical Medicine 19:40.

16 Melvin DM, Brooke MM 1955 Triton X-100 in Giemsa staining of blood parasites. Stain Technology 30:269.

17 Gleeson RM 1997 An improved method for thick film preparation using saponin as a lysing agent. Clinical and Laboratory Haematology 19:249–251.

18 Zipursky A, Brown E, Palko J, et al 1983 The erythrocyte differential count in newborn infants. American Journal of Pediatric Hematology and Oncology 5:45.

19 Sills RH 1989 Hyposplenism. In: Pochedly C, Sills RH, Schwartz AD (eds) Disorders of the spleen. Marcel Dekker, New York.

20 Bloemendal H (ed) 1977 Cell separation methods. Elsevier-North Holland, Amsterdam.

21 Cutts JH 1970 Cell separation: methods in hematology. Academic Press, New York.

22 Bøyum A 1964 Separation of white blood cells. Nature (London) 204:793.

23 Bøyum A 1984 Separation of lymphocytes, granulocytes and monocytes from human blood using iodinated density gradient media. Methods in Enzymology 108:88.

24 Efrati P, Rozenszajn L 1960 The morphology of buffy coat in normal human adults. Blood 16:1012.

25 Efrati P, Rozenszajn L, Shapira E 1961 The morphology of buffy coat from cord blood of normal human newborns. Blood 17:497.

26 Romsdahl MM, McGrew EA, McGrath RG, et al 1964 Hematopoietic nucleated cells in the peripheral venous blood of patients with carcinoma. Cancer (Philadelphia) 17:1400.

27 Linn YC, Tien SL, Lim LC, et al 1995 Haematophagocytosis in bone marrow aspirate – a review of the clinical course of 10 cases. Acta Haematologica 94:182–191.

28 Ali FMK 1986 Separation of human blood and bone marrow cells. Wright, Bristol.

29 Islam A 1995 A new, fast and convenient method for layering blood or bone marrow over density gradient medium. Journal of Clinical Pathology 48:686–688.

30 Olefsson T, Gartner I, Olsson I 1980 Separation of human bone marrow cells in density gradients of polyvinyl pyrrolidone coated silica gel (Percoll). Scandinavian Journal of Haematology 24:254.

31 Gaudernack G, Leivestand T, Ugelstad J, et al 1993 Isolation of pure functionally active CD8 T cells: positive selection with monoclonal antibodies directly conjugated to monosized magnetic microspheres. Journal of Immunological Methods 90:179–187.

32 Lea T, Vartdal F, Davies C, et al 1985 Magnetic monosized polymer particles for fast and specific fractionation of human mononuclear cells. Scandinavian Journal of Immunology 22:207–216.

33 Bunn A, Gaudernack G, Sandberg S 1990 A new method for isolation of reticulocytes: positive selection of human reticulocytes by immunomagnetic separation. Blood 76:2397–2403.

34 Fleming JA, Stewart JW 1967 A critical and comparative study of methods of isolating tumour cells from the blood. Journal of Clinical Pathology 20:145.

35 Seal SH 1959 Silicone flotation: a simple quantitative method for the isolation of free-floating cancer cells from the blood. Cancer (Philadelphia) 12:590.

36 Bailey W, Smith D 1994 The quantitative buffy coat for the diagnosis of trypanosomes. Tropical Doctor 24:54–56.

5

Blood cell morphology in health and disease

Barbara J. Bain

Examination of a fixed and stained blood film is an essential part of a haematological investigation, and it cannot be emphasized too strongly that, to obtain maximum information from the examination, the films must be well spread, well stained and examined systematically. Details of the recommended technique of examination are given below.

The most important red cell abnormalities, as seen in fixed and stained films, are described and illustrated, and some notes on their significance and diagnostic importance are added. Leucocyte and platelet abnormalities are also described and, where appropriate, are illustrated. The slides were stained with May-Grünwald-Giemsa. Variations in the colours are due to photographic processing and whether a daylight blue filter was used in the microscope.

TECHNIQUE OF EXAMINATION OF BLOOD FILMS

Blood films should be examined systematically, starting with macroscopic observation of the stained film and then progressing from low-power to high-power microscopic examination. It is useless to place a drop of immersion oil randomly on the film and then to examine it using the high-power ×100 objective.

First, the film should be examined macroscopically to assess whether the spreading technique was satisfactory and to judge its staining characteristics and whether there are any abnormal particles present which may represent large platelet aggregates, cryoglobulin deposits or clumps of tumour cells. Either before or after macroscopic assessment, the film should be covered with a cover-glass (cover-slip) using a neutral medium as mountant. Next the film should be inspected under a low magnification (with a ×10 or ×20 objective) in order to: (i) get an idea of the quality of the preparation; (ii) assess whether red cell agglutination, excessive rouleaux formation or platelet aggregation is present; (iii) assess the number, distribution and staining of the leucocytes; and (iv) find an area where the red cells are evenly distributed and are not distorted. A large part of the film should be scanned in order to detect scanty abnormal cells such as occasional granulocyte precursors or nucleated red blood cells.

Having selected a suitable area, a ×40 or ×50 objective or ×60 oil-immersion objective should then be used. A much better appreciation of variation in red cell size, shape and staining can be obtained with one of these objectives than with the ×100 oil-immersion lens. It should be possible to detect features such as toxic granulation or the presence of Howell–Jolly bodies or Pappenheimer bodies. The major part of the assessment of a blood film is usually done at this power. The ×100 objective in combination with ×6 or ×10 eyepieces should be used only for the final examination of unusual cells and for looking at fine details such as punctate basophilia or Auer rods. Whether it is necessary to examine a film with a ×100 objective depends on the clinical features, the blood count and the nature of any morphological abnormality detected at lower power.

As the diagnosis of the type of anaemia or other abnormality present usually depends upon a comprehension of the whole picture which the film presents, the red cells, leucocytes and platelets should all be systematically examined. The film examination also serves to validate the automated blood count, distinguishing for example between true macrocytosis and factitious macrocytosis caused by the presence of a cold agglutinin and, similarly, between true thrombocytopenia and factitious thrombocytopenia caused by platelet aggregation or satellitism.

RED CELL MORPHOLOGY

In health, the red blood cells vary relatively little in size and shape (Fig. 5.1). In well-spread, dried and stained films the great majority of cells have round smooth contours and have diameters within the comparatively narrow range (mean ±2SD) of 6.0 to 8.5 μm. As a rough guide, normal red cell size appears to be about the same as that of the nucleus of a small lymphocyte on the dried film (Fig. 5.1). The red cells stain quite deeply with the eosin component of Romanowsky dyes, particularly at the periphery of the cell in consequence of the cell's normal biconcavity. A small but variable proportion of cells in well-made films (usually less than 10%) are definitely oval rather than round and a very small percentage may be contracted and have an irregular contour or appear to have lost part of their substance as the result of fragmentation (schistocytes). According to Marsh, the percentage of 'pyknocytes'

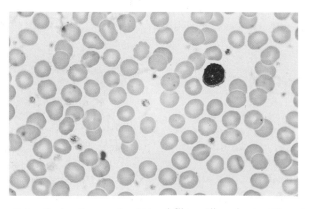

Fig. 5.1 Photomicrograph of blood films. Film of a healthy adult.

(irregularly contracted cells) and schistocytes in normal blood does not exceed 0.1% and the proportion is usually considerably less than this;[1] in normal, full-term infants the proportion is higher, 0.3–1.9%, and in premature infants still higher, up to 5.6%.[1]

Normal and pathological red cells are subject to considerable distortion in the spreading of a film and, as already mentioned, it is imperative to scan films carefully to find an area where the red cells are least distorted before attempting to examine the cells in detail. Such an area can usually be found towards the tail of the film, although not actually at the tail. Rouleaux often form rapidly in blood after withdrawal from the body and may be conspicuous even in films made at a patient's bedside. They are particularly noticeable in the thicker parts of a film that have dried more slowly. Ideally, red cells should be examined in an area in which there are no rouleaux and the red cells are touching but with little overlap. The film in the chosen area must not be so thin as to cause red cell distortion; if the tail of the film is examined, a false impression of spherocytosis may be gained. The varying appearances of different areas of the same blood film are illustrated in Figures 5.2–5.4. The area illustrated in Figure 5.2 would clearly be the best for looking at red cells critically.

The advantages and disadvantages of examining red cells suspended in plasma have been referred to briefly in Chapter 4 (p. 56). By this means, red cells can be seen in the absence of artefacts produced by drying, and abnormalities in size and shape can be better and more reliably appreciated than in films of blood dried on slides. However, the ease and rapidity with which dried films can be made, and their permanence, give them an overwhelming advantage in routine studies.

In disease, abnormality in the red cell picture stems from four main causes:

1. abnormal erythropoiesis which may be effective or ineffective
2. inadequate haemoglobin formation

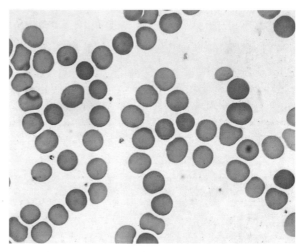

Fig. 5.3 Photomicrograph of a blood film which is too thin. From same slide as Figure 5.2.

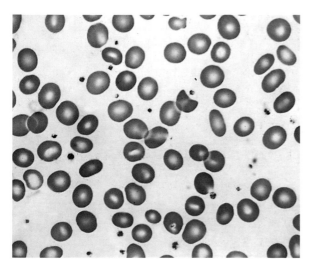

Fig. 5.2 Photomicrograph of a blood film. Ideal thickness for examination.

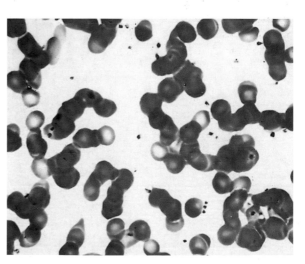

Fig. 5.4 Photomicrograph of a blood film which is too thick. From same slide as Figure 5.2.

3. damage to, or changes affecting, the red cells after leaving the bone marrow, including the effects of reduced or absent splenic function
4. attempts by the bone marrow to compensate for anaemia by increased erythropoiesis.

These processes result, respectively, in the following abnormalities of the red cells:

1. increased variation in size (*anisocytosis*) and shape (*poikilocytosis*) and *punctate basophilia*
2. reduced or unequal haemoglobin content (*hypochromasia* or *anisochromasia* or *dimorphism*)
3. *spherocytosis*, irregular contraction, *elliptocytosis* or fragmentation (*schistocytosis*); the presence of Pappenheimer bodies, Howell–Jolly bodies and

a variable number of certain specific poikilocytes (target cells, acanthocytes and spherocytes)
4. signs of immaturity (*polychromasia* and *erythroblastaemia*).

ABNORMAL ERYTHROPOIESIS

Anisocytosis (ανισοζ, unequal) and poikilocytosis (ποικιλοζ, varied)

These are non-specific features of almost any blood disorder. The terms imply more variation in size or shape than is normally present (Figs 5.5 and 5.6). Anisocytosis may be due to the presence of cells larger than normal (*macrocytosis*) or cells smaller than normal (*microcytosis*) or both; frequently both macrocytes and microcytes are present (Fig. 5.5).

Poikilocytes are produced in many types of abnormal erythropoiesis, e.g. megaloblastic anaemia, iron-deficiency anaemia, thalassaemia, myelofibrosis (both idiopathic and secondary) (Figs 5.7 and 5.8), congenital dyserythropoietic anaemia (Fig. 5.9) and the myelodysplastic syndromes. Elliptocytes and ovalocytes are among the poikilocytes that may be present when there is dyserythropoiesis; they are often present in megaloblastic anaemia (macro-ovalocytes) and in iron-deficiency anaemia ('pencil cells') but they may also be seen in myelodysplastic syndromes and in idiopathic myelofibrosis (see Fig. 5.8). The number of elliptocytes and 'tailed-poikilocytes'

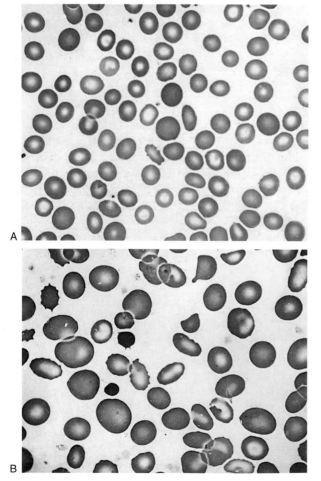

A

B

Fig. 5.5 Photomicrograph of blood films. (A) shows a moderate degree of anisocytosis and anisochromasia; (B) shows a marked degree of anisocytosis caused by the presence of both microcytes and macrocytes.

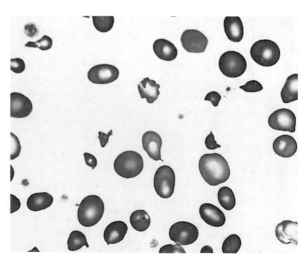

Fig. 5.6 Photomicrograph of a blood film. Shows macrocytes, poikilocytes, red cell fragments (schistocytes) and extreme anisocytosis.

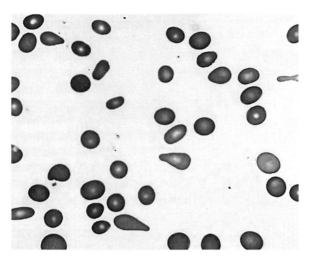

Fig. 5.7 Photomicrograph of a blood film. Idiopathic myelofibrosis. Shows poikilocytosis and moderate anisocytosis.

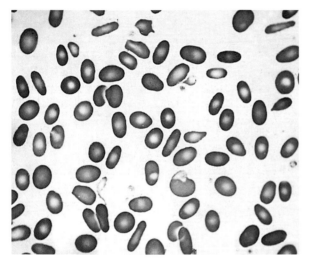

Fig. 5.8 Photomicrograph of a blood film. Idiopathic myelofibrosis. Almost all the cells are elliptical or oval (compare with Fig. 5.7).

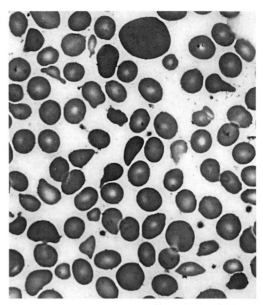

Fig. 5.9 Photomicrograph of a blood film. Congenital dyserythropoietic anaemia type III. Shows moderate anisocytosis, marked poikilocytosis and several unusually large macrocytes.

Macrocytes

Classically found in megaloblastic anaemias (Fig. 5.10), they are also present in some cases of aplastic anaemia, myelodysplastic syndromes and other dyserythropoietic states. In patients being treated with hydroxyurea the red cells are often macrocytic. A common cause of macrocytosis is excess alcohol intake and it occurs in alcoholic and other types of chronic liver disease. In these

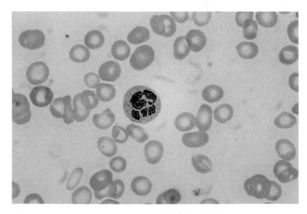

Fig. 5.10 Photomicrograph of a blood film. Megaloblastic anaemia. Shows macrocytes, oval macrocytes and a hypersegmented neutrophil.

(tear-drop poikilocytes) has been observed to correlate with the severity of iron-deficiency anaemia.[2] Poikilocytes are not only characteristic of disordered erythropoiesis but are also seen in various congenital haemolytic anaemias caused by membrane defects and in acquired conditions such as microangiopathic haemolytic anaemia and oxidant damage; in these disorders, the abnormality of shape results from damage to cells after formation and is described below.

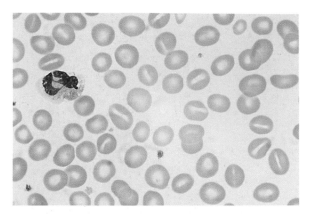

Fig. 5.11 Photomicrograph of a blood film. Liver disease. Shows macrocytosis and stomatocytosis.

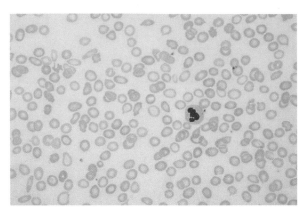

Fig. 5.12 Photomicrograph of a blood film. Iron-deficiency anaemia. Shows hypochromia, microcytosis and poikilocytosis.

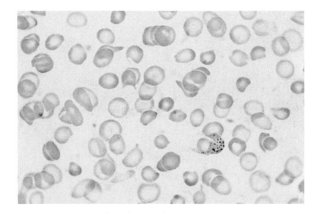

Fig. 5.13 Heterozygous Hb D-Punjab/β° thalassaemia. Shows anisocytosis, poikilocytosis, hypochromia, microcytosis and basophilic stippling.

conditions, the red cells tend to be fairly uniform in size and shape and there may also be stomatocytes (Fig. 5.11). In one rare form of congenital dyserythropoietic anaemia (Type III), some of the macrocytes are exceptionally large (see Fig. 5.9). Another rare cause of macrocytosis is benign familial macrocytosis.[3] Macrocytosis also occurs whenever there is an increased rate of erythropoiesis, because of the presence of reticulocytes. Their presence is suspected in routinely stained films because of the slight basophilia, giving rise to polychromasia (p. 86) and is easily confirmed by special stains (e.g. New methylene blue). These polychromatic macrocytes should be distinguished from other macrocytes since the diagnostic significance is quite different.

Microcytes

The presence of microcytes usually results from a defect in haemoglobin formation. Microcytosis is characteristic of iron-deficiency anaemia (Fig. 5.12), various types of thalassaemia (Fig. 5.13) and severe cases of anaemia of chronic disease. Rarer causes include congenital and acquired sideroblastic anaemias. Microcytosis related to a defect in haemoglobin synthesis should be distinguished from red cell fragmentation or schistocytosis (see p. 78). Both abnormalities can lead to a reduction of the mean cell volume. However, it should be noted that a low mean cell volume is common in association with a defect in haemoglobin synthesis whereas it is uncommon in fragmentation syndromes because the fragments usually comprise only a small percentage of erythrocytes.

Punctate basophilia (basophilic stippling)

Punctate basophilia (or basophilic stippling) means the presence of numerous basophilic granules distributed throughout the cell (Fig. 5.14); in contrast to Pappenheimer bodies (see below), they do not give a positive Perls' reaction for ionized iron. Punctate basophilia has quite a different significance from diffuse cytoplasmic basophilia. It is indicative of disturbed rather than increased erythropoiesis. It occurs in many blood diseases: thalassaemia, megaloblastic anaemias, infections, liver disease, poisoning by lead and other heavy metals, unstable haemoglobins and pyrimidine-5′-nucleotidase deficiency

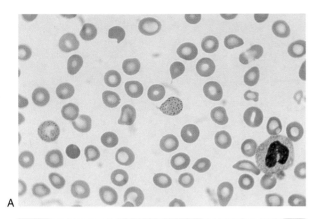

A

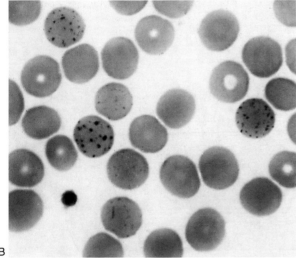

B

Fig. 5.14 Photomicrographs of a blood film. (A) β-Thalassaemia trait shows hypochromia, microcytosis, poikilocytosis and basophilic stippling. (B) Pyrimidine-5′-nucleotidase deficiency. Shows prominent punctate basophilia.

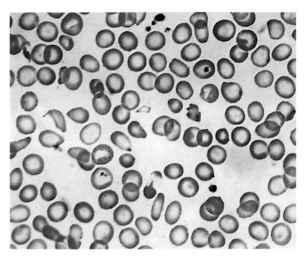

Fig. 5.15 Photomicrograph of a blood film. Iron-deficiency anaemia. Shows a marked degree of hypochromasia, microcytosis and anisocytosis, and a few poikilocytes and red cell fragments.

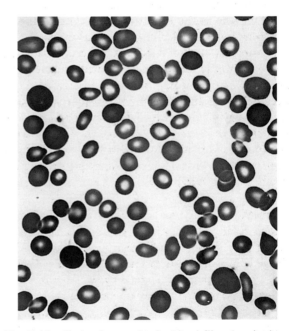

Fig. 5.16 Photomicrograph of a blood film. Acquired sideroblastic anaemia. Shows marked anisocytosis and anisochromasia.

INADEQUATE HAEMOGLOBIN FORMATION

Hypochromasia (hypochromia) (νπορ, under)

The term hypochromasia or now, more often, hypochromia refers to the presence of red cells that stain unusually palely. (In doubtful cases, it is wise to compare the staining of the suspect film with that of a normal film stained at the same time.) There are two possible causes: a lowered haemoglobin concentration and abnormal thinness of the red cells. A lowered haemoglobin concentration results from impaired haemoglobin synthesis. This may stem from failure of haem synthesis – iron deficiency is a very common cause (Fig. 5.15), sideroblastic anaemia (Fig. 5.16) a

rare cause – or failure of globin synthesis as in the thalassaemias (Fig. 5.17). Haemoglobin synthesis may also be impaired in chronic infections and other inflammatory conditions. It cannot be too strongly stressed that a hypochromic blood picture

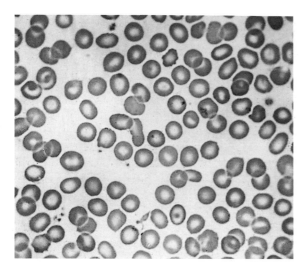

Fig. 5.17 Photomicrograph of a blood film. β Thalassaemia trait. Shows microcytosis, hypochromia and mild poikilocytosis including several target cells.

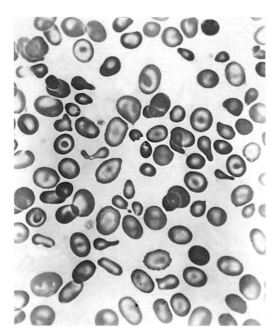

Fig. 5.18 Photomicrograph of a blood film. β Thalassaemia major. Shows hypochromasia and anisocytosis, and numerous poikilocytes (including target cells and red cell fragments).

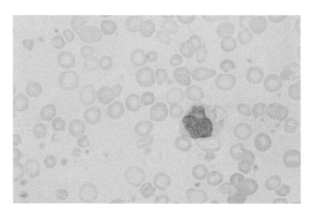

Fig. 5.19 Photomicrograph of a blood film. Iron-deficiency anaemia. Shows a constant gradation of haemoglobinization of cells, i.e. anisochromasia.

does not necessarily mean iron deficiency, although this is the most common cause. In iron deficiency, the red cells are characteristically hypochromic and microcytic, but the extent of these abnormalities depends on the severity; hypochromasia may be minor and be overlooked if the Hb exceeds 100 g/l. In heterozygous α^+ or α^0 thalassaemia, or heterozygous β thalassaemia, hypochromia is often less marked, in relation to the degree of microcytosis, than in iron deficiency. The presence of target cells (see Fig. 5.17) or basophilic stippling also favours a diagnosis of thalassaemia trait rather than iron deficiency. In homozygous β thalassaemia, the abnormalities are greater than in iron deficiency at the same Hb (Fig. 5.18) and nucleated red cells may be present, whereas they are not a feature of iron deficiency.

Anisochromasia (ανισοζ, unequal) and dimorphic red cell population

A distinction should be made between anisochromasia, in which there is abnormal variability in staining of red cells, and a dimorphic picture, in which there are two distinct populations. Anisochromasia, in which some but not all of the red cells stain palely, is characteristic of a changing situation. It can occur during the development or resolution of iron-deficiency anaemia (Fig. 5.19) or the anaemia of chronic disease. In thalassaemia trait, in contrast, anisochromasia is much less common. A dimorphic blood film

can be seen in several circumstances. It can occur when an iron-deficiency anaemia responds to iron therapy, after the transfusion of normal blood to a patient with a hypochromic anaemia (Fig. 5.19) and in sideroblastic anaemia (Fig. 5.20). In acquired sideroblastic anaemia as a feature of myelodysplasia, the two populations of cells are usually hypochromic microcytic and normochromic macrocytic respectively.

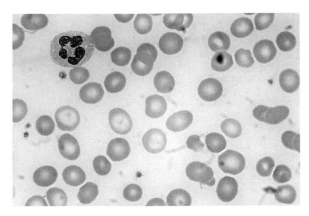

Fig. 5.20 Photomicrograph of a blood film. Acquired sideroblastic anaemia. Shows two distinct populations of cells, hypochromic cells, which also tend to be microcytic, and normocytic normochromic cells.

DAMAGE TO RED CELLS AFTER FORMATION

Poikilocytosis can result not only from abnormal erythropoiesis but also from damage to red cells after their formation. The damage may be consequent on an intrinsic abnormality of the red cell, such as a haemoglobinopathy, a membrane defect or an enzyme defect that renders the cell prone to shape alteration. Poikilocytosis can also result from extrinsic causes, as when a red cell is damaged by drugs, chemicals or toxins, by heat or by abnormal mechanical forces. Poikilocytes of specific shapes suggest different aetiological factors.

Hyperchromasia (hyperchromia) (νπερ, over)

Unusually deep staining of the red cells with a lack of central pallor may be seen in two circumstances; first, in the presence of macrocytes and second, when cells are abnormally rounded. In macrocytosis, as in neonatal blood and megaloblastic anaemias, it is the increased red cell thickness that causes the hyperchromia and the MCHC is normal. When hyperchromia results from cells being of abnormal shape the red cell thickness is greater than normal and the mean cell haemoglobin concentration, when measured by accurate techniques, is increased. Abnormally rounded cells may be either spherocytes or irregularly contracted cells. The distinction between these two cell types is of diagnostic importance.

Spherocytosis (σφαιρα, a sphere)

Spherocytes are cells which are more spheroidal (i.e. less disc-like) than normal red cells but maintain a regular outline. Their diameter is less and their thickness greater than normal. Only in extreme instances are they almost spherical in shape. It is useful to draw a distinction between spherocytes of normal size and microspherocytes; the latter result from red cell fragmentation or from removal of a considerable proportion of the red cell membrane by splenic or other macrophages. Spherocytes may result from genetic defects of the red cell membrane as in hereditary spherocytosis (Fig. 5.21), from the interaction between immunoglobulin- or complement-coated red cells and phagocytic cells, as in ABO haemolytic disease of the newborn (Fig. 5.22) and autoimmune haemolytic anaemia (Fig. 5.23) and from the action of bacterial toxins, e.g. *Clostridium perfringens* lecithinase (Fig. 5.24).

Spherocytes typically appear perfectly round in contour in stained films; they have to be carefully distinguished both from irregularly contracted cells

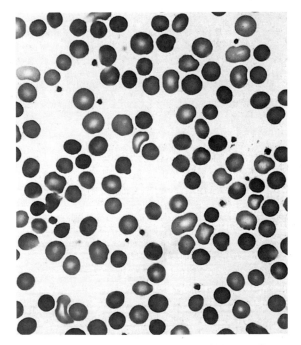

Fig. 5.21 Photomicrograph of a blood film. Hereditary spherocytosis. Shows a moderate degree of spherocytosis and anisocytosis. Note the round contour of the spherocytes.

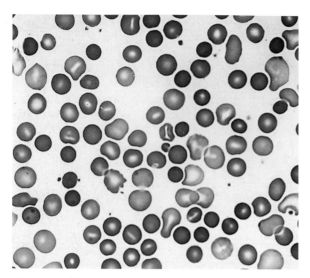

Fig. 5.22 Photomicrograph of a blood film. ABO haemolytic disease of the newborn. Spherocytosis is intense.

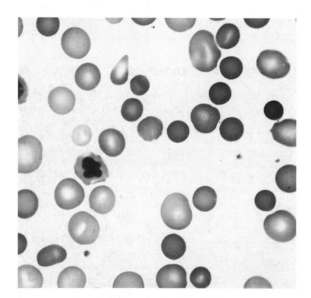

Fig. 5.23 Photomicrograph of a blood film. Auto-immune haemolytic anaemia. Shows a moderate degree of spherocytosis and anisocytosis.

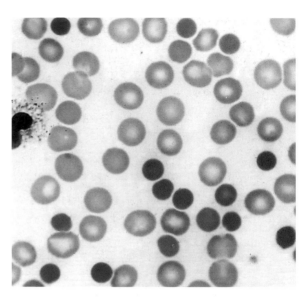

Fig. 5.24 Photomicrograph of a blood film. *Clostridium perfringens* septicaemia. Shows an extreme degree of spherocytosis; note the round contour of the spherocytes. A markedly dimorphic picture.

splenectomized. The blood film of a patient who has been transfused with stored blood may show a proportion of sphero-echinocytes (Fig. 5.27).

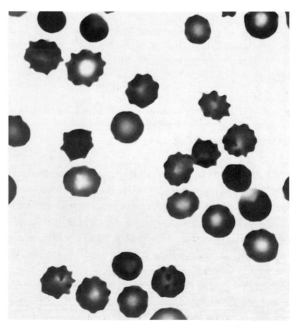

Fig. 5.25 Photomicrograph of a blood film. Acute renal failure following multiple bee stings. Shows crenation leading to finely crenated spheres.

and from 'crenated spheres' or sphero-echinocytes (Fig. 5.25), which are the end-result of crenation (see p. 80). Sphero-echinocytes develop as artefacts especially in blood that has been allowed to stand before films are spread (Fig. 5.26). Sphero-echinocytes are also present in the blood of patients with hereditary spherocytosis who have been

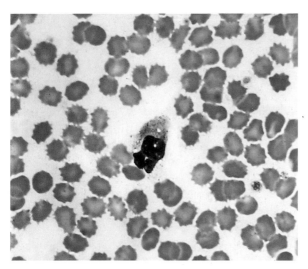

Fig. 5.26 Photomicrograph of a blood film. Normal blood after 18 h at *c* 20°C. Shows a marked degree of crenation.

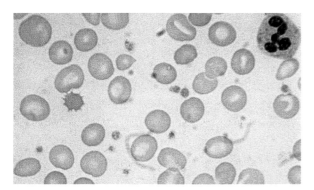

Fig. 5.27 Photomicrograph of a blood film. Post-transfusion, showing one sphero-echinocyte.

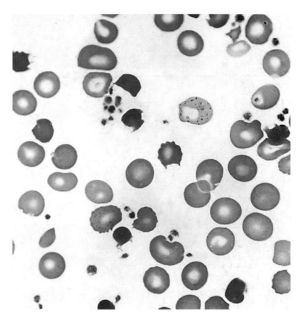

Fig. 5.28 Photomicrograph of a blood film. Haemolytic anaemia caused by an overdose of phenacetin. Shows many markedly and irregularly contracted cells; also punctate basophilia.

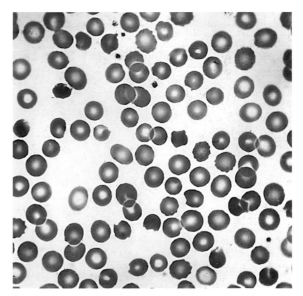

Fig. 5.29 Photomicrograph of a blood film. An unstable haemoglobin haemolytic anaemia (haemoglobin Köln). Shows some moderately contracted cells with somewhat irregular contours.

Irregularly contracted red cells

There are a number of causes of irregularly contracted cells. In drug- or chemical-induced haemolytic anaemias, a proportion of the red cells are smaller than normal and unusually densely stained, i.e. they appear contracted, and their margins are slightly or moderately irregular and may be partly concave (Fig. 5.28). These may be cells from which Heinz bodies have been extracted by the spleen. Similar cells may be seen in films of some unstable haemoglobinopathies before splenectomy, e.g. that caused by the presence of Hb Köln (Fig. 5.29). Heinz bodies are not normally visible in Romanowsky-stained blood films but they may be seen in such films as pale pink-staining bodies in

severe unstable haemoglobin haemolytic anaemias after splenectomy (Fig. 5.30). An extreme degree of irregular contraction is characteristic of severe favism

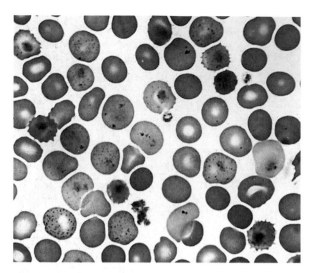

Fig. 5.30 Photomicrograph of a blood film. An unstable haemoglobin haemolytic anaemia (haemoglobin Bristol) after splenectomy. Shows contracted and crenated cells; also punctate basophilia and inclusions (Heinz bodies and Pappenheimer bodies).

or any other very acute haemolytic episode in glucose-6-phosphate dehydrogenase deficient individuals; it is typical to see cells in which the haemoglobin appears to have contracted away from the cell membrane, an appearance sometimes referred to as a hemi-ghost (Fig. 5.31). Irregularly contracted cells

can be seen in small numbers in β thalassaemia trait, in heterozygosity for haemoglobin C and in heterozygosity or homozygosity for haemoglobin E. There may be a considerable number in haemoglobin C homozygosity and in this condition haemoglobin crystal may also be seen (Fig. 5.32).

A type of irregular contraction of unknown origin has been described by the term pyknocytosis.[4] The pyknocytes closely resemble chemically damaged red cells. As already mentioned (p. 67), a small number of pyknocytes may be found in the blood of infants in the first few weeks of life, especially in premature infants. The term 'infantile pyknocytosis' refers to a transient haemolytic anaemia of obscure origin affecting infants in which many pyknocytes are present (Fig. 5.33).[4,5]

Elliptocytosis and ovalocytosis

Elliptocytes are often present in large numbers in hereditary elliptocytosis (Fig. 5.34). In hereditary pyropoikilocytosis, elliptocytes are only one of the many types of poikilocyte present (Fig. 5.35). South-east Asian ovalocytosis is characterized by the presence of a variable number of elliptocytes, macro-ovalocytes and stomatocytes (Fig. 5.36). In all these conditions, the reticulocytes are round in

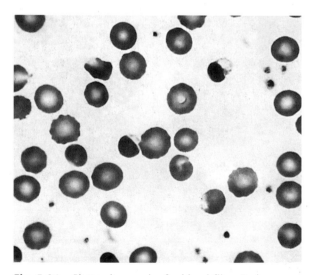

Fig. 5.31 Photomicrograph of a blood film. Favism. Shows numerous markedly contracted cells. Note condensation and contraction of haemoglobin from the cell membrane.

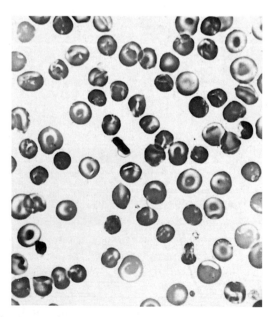

Fig. 5.32 Photomicrograph of a blood film. Haemoglobin C disease (homozygosity for haemoglobin C). Shows many target cells and an intracellular crystal of haemoglobin.

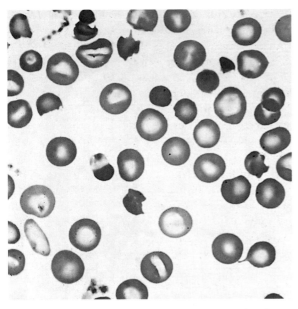

Fig. 5.33 Photomicrograph of a blood film. Infantile pyknocytosis. Shows irregularly contracted cells similar to those seen in chemical- or drug-induced haemolytic anaemias.

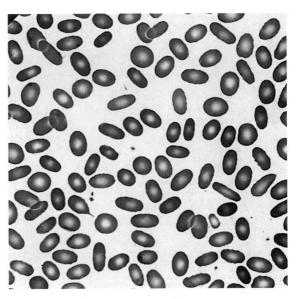

Fig. 5.34 Photomicrograph of a blood film. Hereditary elliptocytosis. Almost all the cells are elliptical.

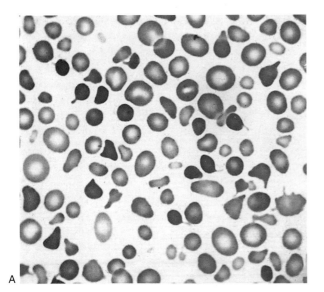

A

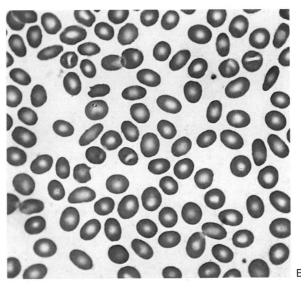

B

Fig. 5.35 Photomicrograph of blood films of a child and the child's mother. (A) Hereditary pyropoikilocytosis in the child. Shows spherocytes and numerous cell fragments, a few ovalocytes and a few elliptocytes. (B) Hereditary elliptocytosis in the mother. Many oval or elliptical cells are present.

contour, i.e. the cell assumes an abnormal shape only in the late stages of maturation. They are therefore acquired defects of red cell shape although the causative condition is inherited.

SPICULATED CELLS AND RED CELL FRAGMENTATION

The terminology applied to spiculated cells is confusing, as the same terms have been used to

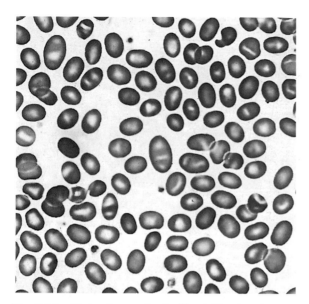

Fig. 5.36 Photomicrograph of a blood film. South-east Asian hereditary ovalocytosis. Some cells show a duplicated central pallor.

designate different types of cell. For this reason it is recommended that the term 'burr cell', originally used by Schwartz & Motto,[6] be abandoned and the terms recommended by Bessis[7] be adopted. On the basis of scanning electron microscopy (see below), he and his colleagues distinguished four types of spiculated cell – schistocyte, keratocyte, acanthocyte and echinocyte. The term echinocyte is used for the crenated cell. It is differentiated from the acanthocyte on the basis of the number, shape and disposition of the spicules.

Schistocytosis (fragmentation) (σχιστοζ, cleft)

Schistocytes or erythrocyte fragments are found in many blood diseases. They are smaller than normal red cells and of varying shape. Sometimes they have sharp angles or spines (spurs), sometimes they are round in contour, usually staining deeply but occasionally palely as the result of loss of haemoglobin at the time of fragmentation. If they are both round and densely staining, they may be referred to as microspherocytes. They occur:

1. in certain genetically determined disorders, e.g. thalassaemias, congenital dyserythropoietic anaemia and hereditary pyropoikilocytosis

2. in acquired disorders of red cell formation when erythropoiesis is megaloblastic or dyserythropoietic
3. as the consequence of mechanical stresses, e.g. in the microangiopathic haemolytic anaemias (Figs 5.37–5.39) and in cardiac haemolytic

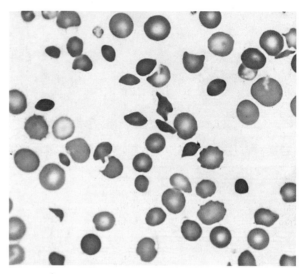

Fig. 5.37 Photomicrograph of a blood film. Microangiopathic haemolytic anaemia; renal cortical necrosis. Shows numerous small poikilocytes and red cell fragments.

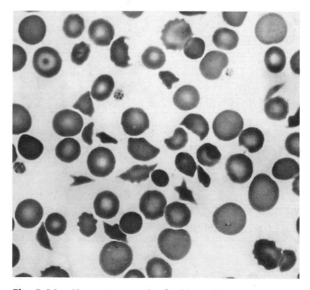

Fig. 5.38 Photomicrograph of a blood film. Microangiopathic haemolytic anaemia; haemolytic-uraemic syndrome. Shows spherocytosis, red cell fragments and marked crenation.

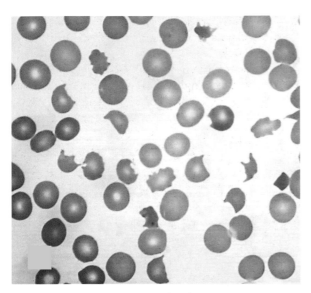

Fig. 5.39 Photomicrograph of a blood film. Microangiopathic haemolytic anaemia; disseminated carcinoma of breast. Shows many bizarre-shaped red cell fragments, one keratocyte and crenation.

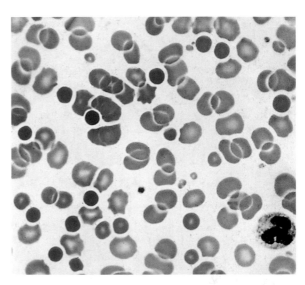

Fig. 5.41 Photomicrograph of a blood film. Severe burns. Shows many very small rounded red cell fragments (microspherocytes) and a little crenation.

In burns, schistocytes are often rounded, being either microspherocytes or very small disc-shaped fragments. In addition, erythrocytes may be seen to be budding off small rounded blebs of cytoplasm.

Not infrequently, as for instance in the haemolytic–uraemic syndrome in children, the blood picture is made more bizarre by the superimposition of varying degrees of echinocytic change (Fig. 5.38).

Keratocytes (κεραζ, horn)

Keratocytes have pairs of spicules, usually either one pair or two pairs. They may be formed either by removal of a Heinz body by the pitting action of the spleen (Fig. 5.42) or by mechanical damage (Fig. 5.43 and 5.44). The terms 'helmet cell' and 'bite cell' have sometimes been used to describe keratocytes.

Acanthocytosis (ακανθα, spine)

The term 'acanthocytosis' was introduced to describe an abnormality of the red cell in which there are a small number of spicules of inconstant length, thickness and shape, irregularly disposed over the surface of the cell (Fig. 5.45). They are often associated with abnormal phospholipid metabolism,[8–10] or with inherited abnormalities of red cell membrane proteins as in the McLeod phenotype, caused by lack of the Kell precursor

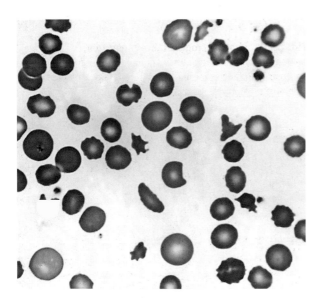

Fig. 5.40 Photomicrograph of a blood film. Post-cardiac surgery haemolytic anaemia. Shows numerous irregularly shaped cell fragments. Note presence of platelets (in contrast to Figs 5.38 and 5.39).

anaemias which are usually caused by a perivalvular leak accompanied by turbulence of left ventricular flow (Fig. 5.40)
4. as the result of direct thermal injury as in severe burns (Fig. 5.41).

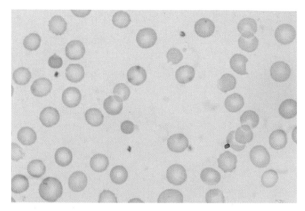

Fig. 5.42 Photomicrograph of a blood film. Keratocytes and irregularly contracted cells in a patient with haemolysis caused by glucose-6-phosphate dehydrogenase deficiency.

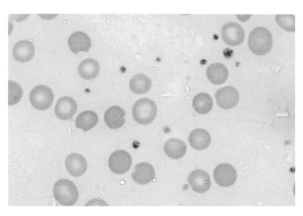

Fig. 5.44 Photomicrograph of a blood film. Two keratocytes in a patient with microangiopathic haemolytic anaemia.

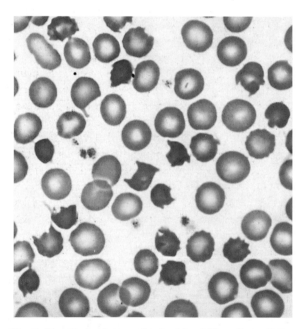

Fig. 5.43 Photomicrograph of a blood film. Haemolytic anaemia caused by an overdose of dapsone. Shows many irregularly contracted cells.

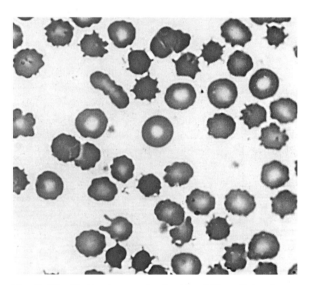

Fig. 5.45 Photomicrograph of a blood film. McLeod phenotype associated with chronic haemolytic anaemia. Acanthocytes are conspicuous.

(Kx).[11] They are present in varying numbers following splenectomy (Fig. 5.46) and in hyposplenism. A similar cell occurs in severe liver disease ('spur cell' anaemia).[12]

Echinocytosis (εχινοζ, sea-urchin (or hedgehog))
Echinocytosis or crenation describes the process by which red cells develop many or numerous short, regular projections from their surface (see Figs 5.25 and 5.26). First described by Ponder[13] as disc–sphere transformation, crenation has many causes. A few crenated cells may be seen in many blood films, even in those from healthy subjects. Crenation regularly develops if blood is allowed to stand overnight at 20°C before films are made (see Fig. 5.26). It may be a marked feature, for obscure and probably diverse reasons, in freshly made blood films made from patients suffering from a variety of illnesses, especially uraemia. It is also

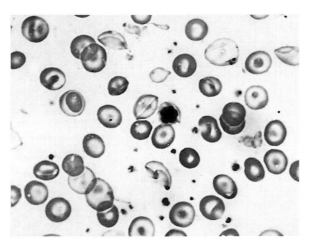

Fig. 5.46 Photomicrograph of a blood film. β-Thalassaemia major, after splenectomy. Shows many target cells and cells grossly deficient in haemoglobin. There are some transfused cells. One normoblast is present.

seen in films from patients undergoing cardio-pulmonary bypass. Marked echinocytosis has been reported in premature infants following exchange transfusion or transfusion of normal red cells.[14] When crenation is superimposed on an underlying abnormality, the red cells may appear bizarre in the extreme.

Crenation also occurs as an artefact if red cells are washed free from plasma and suspended in 9 g/l NaCl between glass surfaces, particularly at a raised pH; in the presence of traces of fatty substances on the slides on which films are made and in the presence of traces of chemicals which at higher concentrations cause lysis.

The end stages of crenation are the 'finely crenated sphere' and the 'spherical form' which closely resemble spherocytes. The disc–sphere transformation may be reversible, e.g. that produced by washing cells free from plasma, and in this respect the contracted 'spherical form' (which has not lost surface) is quite distinct from the 'spherocyte' (which has lost surface), although they may closely resemble one another in stained films.

If echinocytosis is observed in a film it usually represents a storage artefact, caused by delay in making the film. It is a warning that morphological features in the blood film cannot be assessed reliably. If present in films made from fresh blood, it is a clinically significant observation.

MISCELLANEOUS ERYTHROCYTE ABNORMALITIES

Leptocytosis (λεπτοζ, thin)

This term has been used to describe unusually thin red cells, as in severe iron deficiency or thalassaemia in which the cells may stain as rings of haemoglobin with large almost unstained central areas (Fig. 5.46).

Target cells

The term *target cell* refers to a cell in which there is a central round stained area and a peripheral rim of haemoglobinized cytoplasm separated by non-staining or more lightly staining cytoplasm. Target cells result from cells having a surface which is disproportionately large compared with their volume. They may be normal in size, microcytic or macrocytic. They are seen in films in chronic liver diseases in which the cell membrane may be loaded with cholesterol (Fig. 5.47), in hereditary hypobetalipoproteinaemia[15] and in varying numbers in iron-deficiency anaemia and in thalassaemia (see Fig. 5.46). They are often conspicuous in certain haemoglobinopathies, e.g. haemoglobin C disease (see Fig. 5.32), sickle-cell anaemia (Fig. 5.48), sickle-cell/haemoglobin C disease (Fig. 5.49), sickle-cell/β thalassaemia and haemoglobin E disease (Fig. 5.50). Smaller numbers are usual in haemoglobin C trait, haemoglobin E trait and post-splenectomy (Fig. 5.51). Splenectomy in thalassaemia may result in an extreme degree of leptocytosis and target cell formation (see Fig. 5.46).

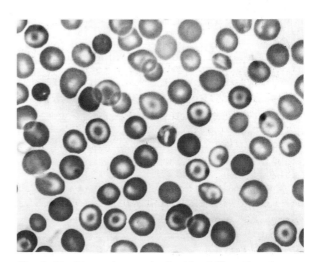

Fig. 5.47 Photomicrograph of a blood film. Chronic obstructive jaundice. Shows many target cells.

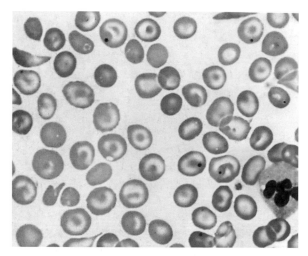

Fig. 5.48 Photomicrograph of a blood film. Sickle-cell anaemia (homozygosity for haemoglobin S). Shows a few sickled cells, target cells and Howell–Jolly bodies.

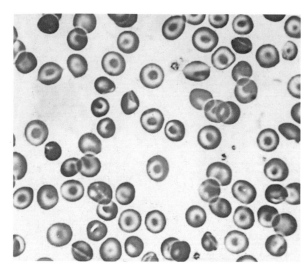

Fig. 5.49 Photomicrograph of a blood film. Sickle-cell/haemoglobin C disease. Shows numerous target cells.

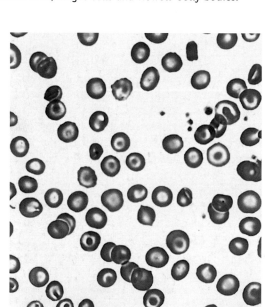

Fig. 5.50 Photomicrograph of a blood film. Haemoglobin E disease (homozygosity for haemoglobin E). Shows large numbers of target cells and small numbers of irregularly contracted cells.

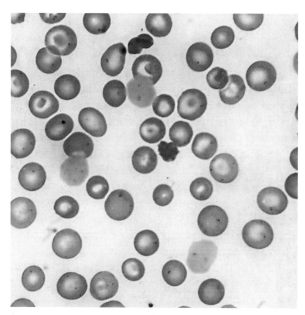

Fig. 5.51 Photomicrograph of a blood film. Pyruvate-kinase deficiency, after splenectomy. Shows macrocytosis, target cells and a markedly crenated cell.

Stomatocytosis (στομα, mouth)

Stomatocytes are red cells in which the central biconcave area appears slit-like in dried films. In 'wet' preparations, the stomatocyte is a cup-shaped red cell. The slit-like appearance of the cell's concavity, as seen in dried films, is thus to some extent an artefact. The term was first used to describe the appearance of some of the cells in a rare type of haemolytic anaemia, hereditary stomatocytosis.[16] They are also a feature of South-east Asian ovalocytosis. They have been described as being particularly frequent in films of Australians

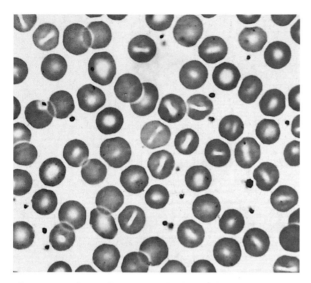

Fig. 5.52 Photomicrograph of a blood film. Stomatocytosis. Many of the cells have a slit-like central unstained area.

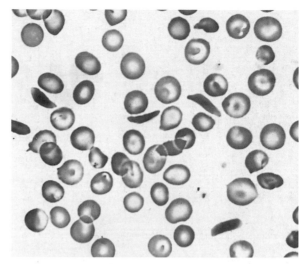

Fig. 5.53 Photomicrograph of a blood film. Sickle-cell anaemia (homozygosity for haemoglobin S). Shows sickled cells and target cells.

of Mediterranean origin.[17,18] Subsequently, stomatocytes were recognized in acquired conditions and occasionally they are prominent (Fig. 5.52). They are observed in liver disease, in alcoholism[19] and occasionally in the myelodysplastic syndromes. There is a suspicion that in some films the occurrence of stomatocytosis is an in vitro artefact since it is known that the change can be produced by decreased pH and as the result of exposure to cationic detergent-like compounds and non-penetrating anions.[20]

Sickle cells

The varied film appearances in sickle-cell anaemia are illustrated in Figures 5.53–5.55. Sickle cells are almost always present in films of freshly withdrawn blood of adults with homozygosity for haemoglobin S. However, sickle cells are usually absent in neonates and are rare in adult patients with a high haemoglobin F percentage. Sometimes many irreversibly sickled cells are present (Fig. 5.53) and in all cases massive sickling takes place when the blood is subjected to anoxia (see p. 251). In films of fresh blood, the sickled cells vary in shape between elliptical forms and sickles. Target cells are also often a feature of blood films from patients with sickle-cell anaemia and Howell–Jolly bodies are found when there is splenic atrophy.

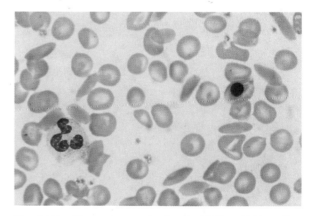

Fig. 5.54 Photomicrograph of a blood film. Sickle-cell anaemia (homozygosity for haemoglobin S). Shows elliptical sickle cells and a nucleated red blood cell.

Haemoglobin C crystals and SC poikilocytes

In patients with homozygosity for haemoglobin, C target cells and irregularly contracted cells are usually both numerous and there may be occasional straight-edged haemoglobin C crystals, either extracellularly (see Fig. 5.32) or within the ghost of a red cell. In patients who are compound heterozygotes for both haemoglobin S and haemoglobin C, the film may resemble that of haemoglobin C disease (see Fig. 5.32). In other patients, there are elliptical cells, rare sickle cells and sometimes distinctive SC poikilocytes (Fig. 5.56).

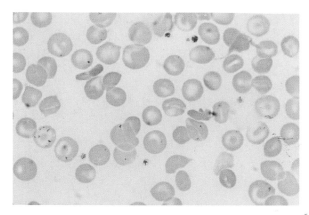

Fig. 5.55 Photomicrograph of a blood film. Sickle-cell anaemia (homozygosity for haemoglobin S). Shows elliptical sickle cells, target cells and Pappenheimer bodies.

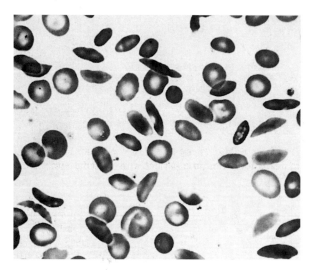

Fig. 5.56 Photomicrograph of a blood film. Sickle-cell/ haemoglobin C disease showing an SC poikilocyte, target cells and severely partially sickled cells.

Erythrocyte inclusions

The possibility of sometimes suspecting the presence of Heinz bodies on a routinely stained film and the detection of haemoglobin crystals within red cells has already been mentioned. Other red cell inclusions include Howell–Jolly bodies and Pappenheimer bodies.

Howell–Jolly bodies

These are nuclear remnants and (usually singly) may be seen in a small percentage of red cells in pernicious anaemia. Cells containing them are regularly

present after splenectomy and where there has been splenic atrophy. Usually only a few such cells are present, but they may be numerous in cases of coeliac disease in which there is splenic atrophy and co-existing folate deficiency (Fig. 5.57).

Pappenheimer bodies

Pappenheimer bodies are small peripherally sited basophilic (almost black) erythrocyte inclusions. Usually only a small number are present in a cell. They are composed of haemosiderin and their presence is related to iron overload and hyposplenism (Figs 5.58 and 5.59). Sometimes they are found in the majority of circulating red cells. Their nature can be confirmed by means of a Perls' stain. They correspond to the siderotic granules of siderocytes and are never distributed in large numbers throughout the cells as in classical punctate basophilia. However, a single cell may show both punctate basophilia and Pappenheimer bodies. On a Perls' stain, the former granules are pink whereas the latter are blue.

Rouleaux and auto-agglutination

The differences between rouleaux and auto-agglutination are described on page 56 and there is usually no difficulty in determining which is which

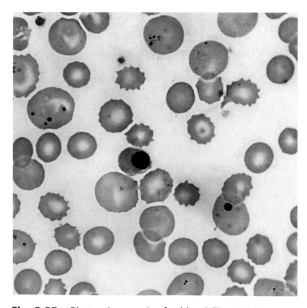

Fig. 5.57 Photomicrograph of a blood film. Coeliac disease. Shows Howell–Jolly bodies, Pappenheimer bodies target cells and crenation, all consequences of splenic atrophy. There is one nucleated red blood cell.

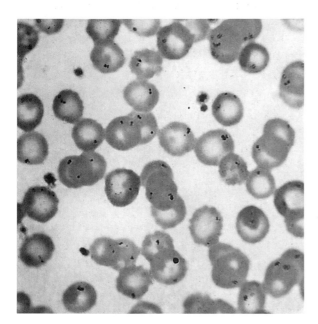

Fig. 5.58 Photomicrograph of a blood film. Pyruvate-kinase deficiency; after splenectomy. Shows many macrocytes, the majority containing Pappenheimer bodies.

in stained films (Figs 5.60 and 5.61). However, in myelomatosis and in other conditions in which there is intense rouleaux formation, the rouleaux may simulate auto-agglutination. Even so, if the film, apparently showing auto-agglutination, is carefully scanned, an area in which rouleaux can be clearly seen will almost certainly be found. Rouleaux occur to some extent in all films, and their presence adds point, as has been mentioned, to the importance of careful selection of the area of film to be examined.

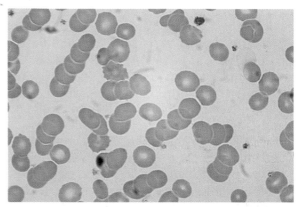

Fig. 5.60 Photomicrograph of a blood film. Increased rouleaux formation in a patient with bacterial infection.

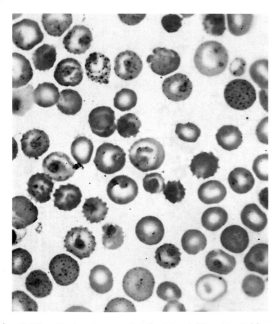

Fig. 5.59 Photomicrograph of a blood film. Unstable haemoglobinopathy (haemoglobin Hammersmith); after splenectomy. There is a remarkable degree of punctate basophilia. Also shows Pappenheimer bodies and circular bodies corresponding to Heinz bodies.

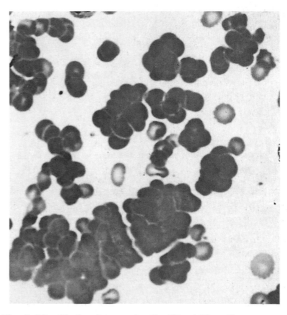

Fig. 5.61 Photomicrograph of a blood film. Shows massive auto-agglutination (compare with Fig. 5.60).

CHANGES ASSOCIATED WITH A COMPENSATORY INCREASE IN ERYTHROPOIESIS

Polychromasia (πολθζ, many)

This term suggests that the red cells are being stained many colours. In practice, it means that some of the red cells stain shades of bluish grey (Fig. 5.62) – these are the reticulocytes. Cells staining shades of blue, 'blue polychromasia', are unusually young reticulocytes. 'Blue polychromasia' is most often seen when there is extramedullary erythropoiesis, as, for instance, in myelofibrosis or carcinomatosis.

Erythroblastaemia

Erythroblasts may be found in the blood films of almost any patient with a severe anaemia; they are, however, very unusual in aplastic anaemia. They are more common in children than in adults and large numbers are a very characteristic finding in haemolytic disease of the newborn. Small numbers can be found in the cord blood of normal infants and quite large numbers in that of premature infants.

When large numbers of erythroblasts are present, many of them are probably derived from extramedullary foci of erythropoiesis, e.g. in the liver and spleen. This seems likely to be true, for instance, in haemolytic disease of the newborn, leukaemia, myelofibrosis and carcinomatosis. In myelofibrosis and carcinomatosis, the number of erythroblasts is often disproportionately high for

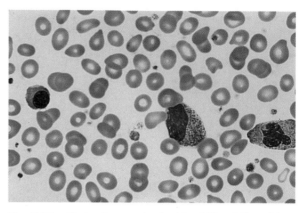

Fig. 5.63 *Photomicrograph of a blood film. Idiopathic myelofibrosis. Shows a leucoerythroblastic blood film, teardrop poikilocytes and ovalocytes.*

the degree of anaemia, and a few immature granulocytes are usually also present (so-called leucoerythroblastic anaemia) (Fig. 5.63).

Erythroblasts can usually be found in the peripheral blood after splenectomy and many may be present in the presence of extramedullary erythropoiesis (Fig. 5.64). Large numbers are frequently seen in the blood films of sickle-cell anaemia patients in painful crises. Small numbers of erythroblasts are not uncommon in blood from patients suffering from cyanotic heart failure or septicaemia.

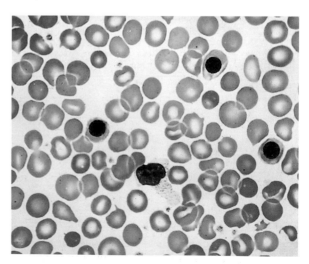

Fig. 5.64 *Photomicrograph of a blood film. Myelofibrosis, after splenectomy. Shows three erythroblasts and moderate anisocytosis and poikilocytosis.*

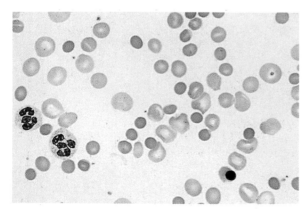

Fig. 5.62 *Photomicrograph of a blood film. Polychromasia. Some red cells stain shades of bluish-grey.*

It should be noted that if the term 'normoblast' is used, it implies that erythroid maturation is normoblastic. 'Erythroblast' is a more general term that also includes megaloblasts.

EFFECTS OF SPLENECTOMY AND HYPOSPLENISM

Some of the changes have already been mentioned, namely, the occurrence of target cells, acanthocytes, Howell–Jolly bodies and Pappenheimer bodies (see Fig. 5.57). In addition, there may be neutrophilia (early after splenectomy), lymphocytosis, thrombocytosis and giant platelets. In haematologically normal people, the blood film features of hyposplenism are very variable, sometimes being striking and sometimes very minor.

SCANNING ELECTRON MICROSCOPY

The morphology of red cells, as illustrated in this chapter, may be distorted by spreading and drying films in the traditional way. A more authentic portrayal of red cell shape in vivo can be seen by scanning electron microscopy. The advent of this technology provided the stimulus and the means for a critical re-examination of red cell morphology. Bessis and his co-workers have published excellent photographs of pathological red cells and proposed a new nomenclature to describe what they have seen.[7,20,21] In this chapter we have generally adopted the terminology that they proposed. They also discussed the difficult question of the in vivo significance of crenation (echinocytic change) observed in vitro. It seems that neither echinocytosis nor acanthocytosis is necessarily associated with increased haemolysis. It cannot be concluded, either, that crenation is occurring in vivo, when the phenomenon is markedly evident in films made on glass slides. To ensure that cells are crenated in any blood sample as it is withdrawn, Brecher & Bessis recommended that the blood be examined immediately between plastic instead of glass cover-slips or slides, to avoid the known 'echinocytogenic' effect of glass surfaces, probably caused by alkalinity.[21]

The specialized procedure of scanning electron microscopy is not practical as a routine but helps in understanding the nature of cells observed in stained blood films. Morphological changes in red cells may be very complex. Echinocytic and stomatocytic change can be superimposed on other pathological forms giving rise to 'sickle-stomatocytes' and 'stomato-acanthocytes'. Acanthocytes can undergo crenation, the product being termed an 'acantho-echinocyte'. Following splenectomy in patients with hereditary spherocytosis, sphero-acanthocytes may be observed.

The appearance of various cells by scanning electron microscopy is illustrated in Figures 5.65–5.72.

MORPHOLOGY OF LEUCOCYTES

This section will include a description of the normal leucocytes, some congenital anomalies and reactive changes that are commonly encountered. To describe adequately the various changes found in malignant conditions would require a lengthy text and many illustrations which arc beyond the scope of this book. They will be referred to briefly here, but for detailed reference readers should consult an atlas on blood cells. For classification of the acute leukaemias, see the original description by the FAB group;[22] and the subsequent revision.[23] There is also a WHO classification.[24]

POLYMORPHONUCLEAR NEUTROPHILS

In normal adults, neutrophils account for more than half the circulating leucocytes. They are the main defence of the body against pyogenic bacterial infections. Normal neutrophils are uniform in size, with an apparent diameter of c 13 μm on a film. They have a segmented nucleus and, when stained, pink/orange cytoplasm with fine granulation (Fig. 5.73). The majority of neutrophils have three nuclear segments (lobes) connected by tapering chromatin strands. The chromatin shows clumping and is usually condensed at the nuclear periphery. A small percentage have four lobes, and

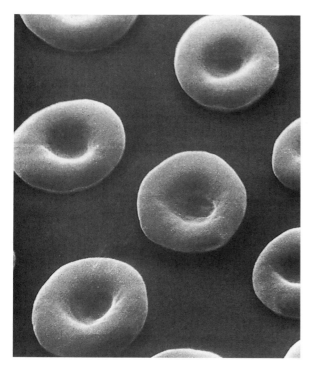

Fig. 5.65 Scanning electron microscope photograph. Normal red cells.

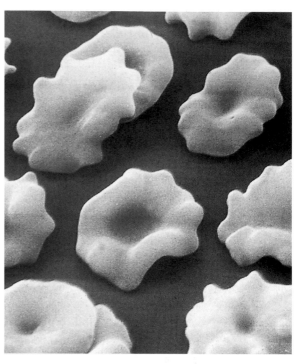

Fig. 5.67 Scanning electron microscope photograph. Normal blood after standing overnight. Note crenation.

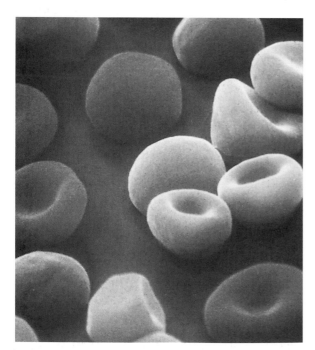

Fig. 5.66 Scanning electron microscope photograph. Hereditary spherocytosis. Note the round shape of spherocytes. (Compare with Fig. 5.65; also see blood film appearances as shown in Fig. 5.21.)

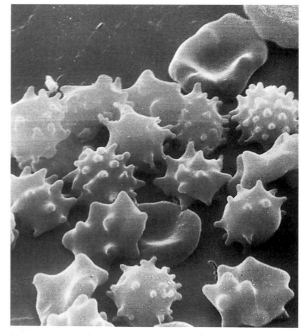

Fig. 5.68 Scanning electron microscope photograph. Acanthocytosis. Some cells also show crenation and contraction. (Compare with Fig. 5.67; see also blood film appearances as shown in Fig. 5.45.)

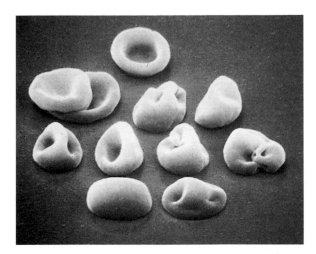

Fig. 5.69 Scanning electron microscope photograph. Drug-induced haemolysis; see blood film appearances shown in Figure 5.43.

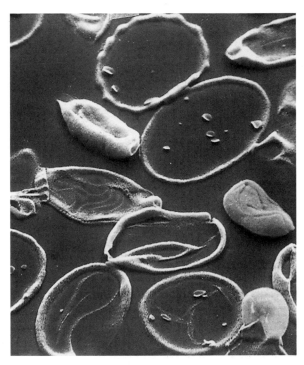

Fig. 5.71 Scanning electron microscope photograph. β-Thalassaemia major, post-splenectomy. Shows cells grossly deficient in haemoglobin; there are also contracted cells and poikilocytes. In the hypochromic cells, inclusions are seen, corresponding to Pappenheimer bodies.

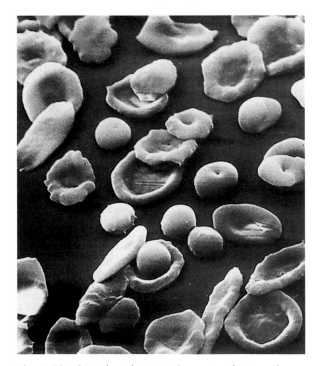

Fig. 5.70 Scanning electron microscope photograph. Iron-deficiency anaemia. (Compare with Fig. 5.71.)

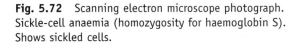

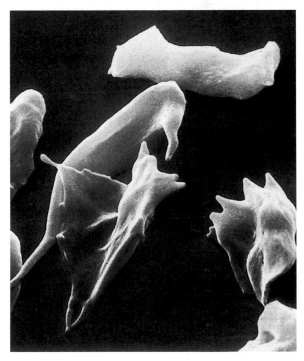

Fig. 5.72 Scanning electron microscope photograph. Sickle-cell anaemia (homozygosity for haemoglobin S). Shows sickled cells.

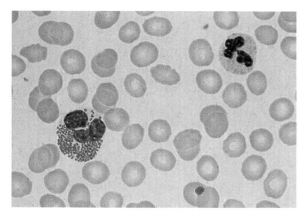

Fig. 5.73 Photomicrograph of a blood film. Normal polymorphonuclear neutrophil and normal eosinophil.

occasionally five lobes may be seen. Up to 8% of circulating neutrophils are unsegmented or partly segmented ('band' forms) (see below).

In women, 2–3% of the neutrophils show an appendage at a terminal nuclear segment. This 'drumstick' is about 1.5 µm in diameter and is connected to the nucleus by a short stalk (see Fig. 00.00). It represents the inactive X chromosome, and corresponds to the Barr body of buccal cells.

Occasionally, red cells will adhere to neutrophils, forming rosettes (Fig. 5.74). The mechanism is unknown but it is likely to be immune; it appears to be of no clinical significance. Leukoagglutination also occurs as an in vitro artefact.[25]

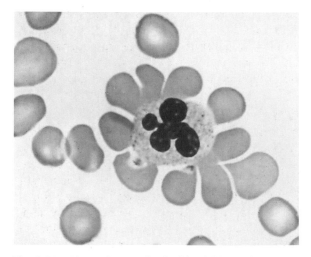

Fig. 5.74 Photomicrograph of a blood film. Adherence of red cells (and two platelets) to a neutrophil. Patient had acquired haemolytic anaemia, with negative direct antiglobulin test.

It is extremely important to ensure the consistency of staining of the blood films using a standardized Romanowsky method (see Ch. 4), as changes in the staining density, colour and appearance of cytoplasmic granulation, if not artefact, may have diagnostic significance. Common neutrophil abnormalities are described below.

Granules

'Toxic' granulation is the term used to describe an increase in staining density and possibly number of granules which occurs regularly with bacterial infection, and often with other causes of inflammation (Fig. 5.75). Fractionally larger, coarser granules may be seen in aplastic anaemia and myelofibrosis. Conversely, poorly staining (hypogranular) and agranular neutrophils occur in the myelodysplastic syndromes (Fig. 5.76) and some forms of myeloid leukaemia.

There are rare inherited disorders which are manifest by abnormal neutrophils. In the *Alder–Reilly anomaly*, the granules are very large, discrete, stain deep red and may obscure the nucleus (Fig. 5.77). Other leucocytes, including some lymphocytes, also show the abnormal granules. In the *Chediak–Higashi syndrome*, there are giant but scanty azurophilic granules (Fig. 5.78), and the other leucocyte types may also be affected. Alder–Reilly neutrophils function normally, but in Chediak–Higashi syndrome, there is a functional defect which is manifested by susceptibility to severe infection.

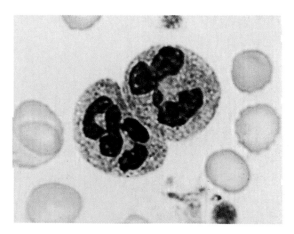

Fig. 5.75 Photomicrograph of a blood film. Severe infection. Neutrophils show toxic granulation.

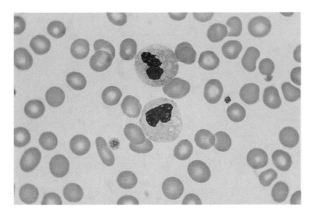

Fig. 5.76 Photomicrograph of a blood film. Myelodysplastic syndrome. Shows a hypogranular neutrophil and a normally granulated neutrophil.

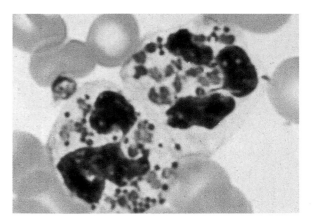

Fig. 5.78 Photomicrograph of a blood film. Chediak–Higashi syndrome. Neutrophils show abnormal granules.

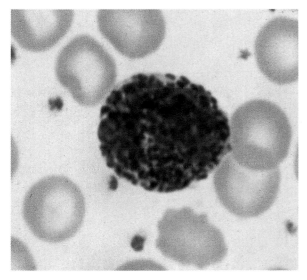

Fig. 5.77 Photomicrograph of a blood film. Alder–Reilly anomaly. The nucleus is obscured by the cytoplasmic granules.

Vacuoles

In blood films spread without delay, the presence of vacuoles in the neutrophils is usually indicative of severe sepsis, when toxic granulation is usually also present. Vacuoles will develop as an artefact with prolonged standing of the blood before films are made (see Fig. 1.3, p. 6).

Bacteria

Very rarely, in the presence of overwhelming septicaemia, bacteria may be seen within vacuoles or lying free in the cytoplasm of neutrophils. When blood is taken from an infected central line, clumps of bacteria may be seen scattered in the film as well as in neutrophils in phagocytic vacuoles (Fig. 5.79). In premature infants with staphylococcal septicaemia, the detection of bacteria in neutrophils helps in early diagnosis.[26]

Döhle bodies

These are small round, or oval pale blue–grey structures, usually found at the periphery of the neutrophil. They consist of ribosomes and endoplasmic reticulum. They are seen in bacterial infections. There is also a benign inherited condition known as *May–Hegglin anomaly* with a similar but not identical morphological structure; in this condition, the May–Hegglin inclusions occur in all types of leucocyte except lymphocytes.

Nuclei

Segmentation of the nucleus of the neutrophil is a normal event as the cell matures from the myelocyte. With the three-lobed neutrophil as a marker, a shift to the left (less mature) or to the right (hypermature) can be recognized (Table 5.1). A left shift with band forms, metamyelocytes and, perhaps, occasional myelocytes, is common in sepsis (Fig. 5.80), when it is usually accompanied by toxic granulation. If promyelocytes and myeloblasts are also present, it is likely to be a feature of a leucoerythroblastic anaemia or leukaemia (Fig. 5.81); occasionally this extreme

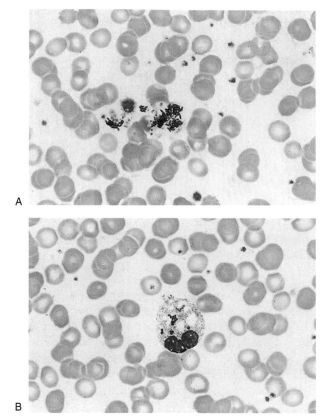

A

B

Fig. 5.79 Photomicrograph of a blood film. Blood collected from infected site, showing bacteria (A) in scattered clumps and (B) in a neutrophil.

Table 5.1 Stages of granulocyte maturation

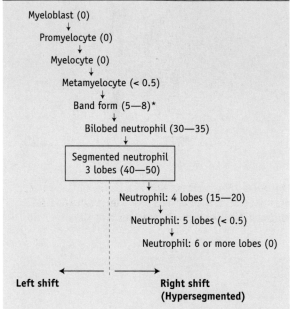

Myeloblast (0)
↓
Promyelocyte (0)
↓
Myelocyte (0)
↓
Metamyelocyte (< 0.5)
↓
Band form (5—8)*
↓
Bilobed neutrophil (30—35)
↓
Segmented neutrophil
3 lobes (40—50)
↓
Neutrophil: 4 lobes (15—20)
↓
Neutrophil: 5 lobes (< 0.5)
↓
Neutrophil: 6 or more lobes (0)

Left shift   **Right shift
(Hypersegmented)**

The figures in brackets give an approximate indication of the number per 100 neutrophils in a normal film. They are intended only as a rough guide.
* However, according to the United States Health and Nutrition Examination surveys, the normal band count is lower, c 0.5% of the neutrophils.[35]

picture may be seen in very severe infections when it is called 'leukaemoid reaction'. A left shift, with a significant number of band forms, occurs normally in pregnancy.

Hypersegmentation

The presence of hypersegmented neutrophils, with five or more nuclear segments, is an important diagnostic feature of megaloblastic anaemias. In florid megaloblastic states, neutrophils are often enlarged and their nuclei may have six or more segments connected by particularly fine chromatin bridges (see Fig. 5.10). A right shift with moderately hypersegmented neutrophils may be seen in uraemia and iron deficiency.[27] Hypersegmentation can be seen after cytotoxic treatment, especially with methotrexate. Patients undergoing hydroxyurea treatment sometimes develop markedly hypersegmented neutrophils.

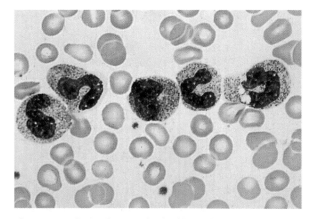

Fig. 5.80 Photomicrograph of a blood film. Infection. Shows left shift of the neutrophils, with toxic granulation.

Pelger cells

The Pelger–Huët anomaly is a benign inherited condition in which neutrophil nuclei fail to segment properly. The majority of circulating neutrophils have only two discrete equal-sized lobes

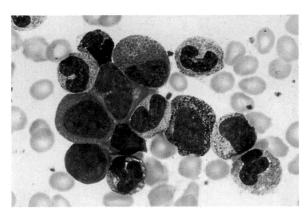

Fig. 5.81 Photomicrograph of a blood film. Chronic granulocytic leukaemia. There is a left shift with band forms, metamyelocytes, myelocytes and one myeloblast.

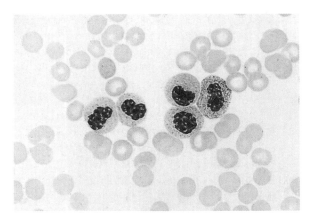

Fig. 5.83 Photomicrograph of a blood film. Chronic granulocytic leukaemia. There are five 'pseudo-Pelger' cells; this abnormality is not seen in the chronic phase of this disease.

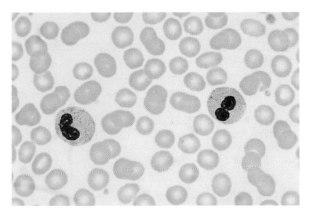

Fig. 5.82 Photomicrograph of a blood film. Pelger–Huët anomaly. Shows hypolobated neutrophils.

connected by a thin chromatin bridge (Fig. 5.82). The chromatin is coarsely clumped and granule content is normal.

A similar acquired morphological anomaly, known as *pseudo-Pelger cells* or the acquired Pelger-Huët anomaly, may be seen in myelodysplastic syndromes, acute myeloid leukaemia with dysplastic maturation and occasionally in chronic granulocytic leukaemia (during the accelerated phase) (Fig. 5.83). In these conditions, the neutrophils are often hypogranular and they tend to have a markedly irregular nuclear pattern.

Pyknotic neutrophils (Apoptosis)
Small numbers of dead or dying cells may normally be found in the blood, especially when there is an infection. They may also develop in normal blood in vitro after standing for 12–18 h, even if kept at 4°C. These cells have round, dense, featureless nuclei and their cytoplasm tends to be dark pink (see p. 6 and Fig. 1.4). It is important not to confuse these cells with normoblasts.

EOSINOPHILS

Eosinophils are a little larger than neutrophils, 12–17 μm in diameter. They usually have two nuclear lobes or segments, and the cytoplasm is packed with distinctive spherical gold/orange (eosinophilic) granules (see Fig. 5.73 and 5.84). The underlying cytoplasm, which is usually

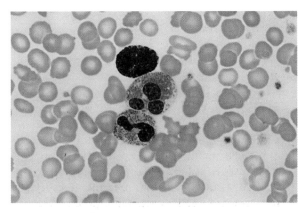

Fig. 5.84 Photomicrograph of a blood film. Normal adult. Shows a basophil, an eosinophil and a neutrophil.

obscured by the granules, is pale blue. Prolonged steroid administration causes eosinopenia. Moderate eosinophilia occurs in allergic conditions; more severe eosinophilia ($20–50 \times 10^9/l$) may be seen in parasitic infections, and even greater numbers in hypereosinophilic syndromes. These are generally of unknown aetiology, although a few cases have been shown to be associated with T-cell lymphoma, B-cell lymphoma or acute lymphoblastic leukaemia. Eosinophilic leukaemia is uncommon, although eosinophils are occasionally a part of the leukaemic population in acute myeloid leukaemia and this is often so in chronic granulocytic leukaemia.

BASOPHILS

Basophils are the rarest (<1%) of the circulating leucocytes. Their nuclear segments tend to fold up on each other, resulting in a compact irregular dense nucleus resembling a closed lotus flower. The distinctive large, variably sized dark blue or purple granules of the cytoplasm (Fig. 5.84) often obscure the nucleus; they are rich in histamine, serotonin and heparin substances. Basophils tend to degranulate, leaving cytoplasmic vacuoles.

Basophils are present in increased numbers in myeloproliferative disorders, and are especially prominent in chronic granulocytic leukaemia; in the latter condition, when basophils are >10% of the differential leucocyte count, this is a sign of impending accelerated phase or blast crisis.

MONOCYTES

Monocytes are the largest of the circulating leucocytes, 15–18 μm in diameter. They have bluish-grey cytoplasm which contains variable numbers of fine reddish granules. The nucleus is large and curved, often in the shape of a horseshoe, but it may be folded or curled (Figs 5.85 and 5.86). It never undergoes segmentation. The chromatin is finer and more evenly distributed in the nucleus than in neutrophil nuclei. An increased number of monocytes occur in some chronic infections and inflammatory conditions such as tuberculosis and Crohn's disease, in chronic myeloid leukaemias (particularly atypical chronic myeloid leukaemia and chronic myelomonocytic leukaemia) and in acute leukaemias with a monocytic component. In

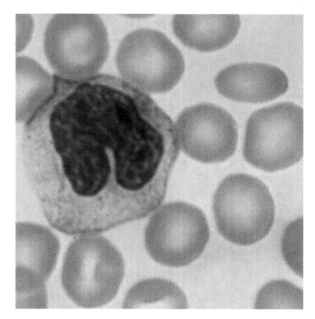

Fig. 5.85 Photomicrograph of a blood film. Healthy adult. Monocyte.

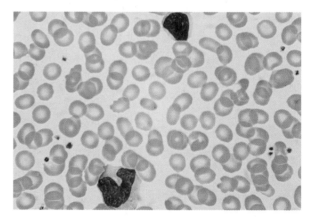

Fig. 5.86 Photomicrograph of a blood film. Healthy adult. Shows a monocyte and a lymphocyte.

chronic myelomonocytic leukaemia, the mature monocyte count may reach as high as $100 \times 10^9/l$. It is occasionally difficult to distinguish monocytes from the large activated T lymphocytes produced in infectious mononucleosis or from circulating high-grade lymphoma cells.

LYMPHOCYTES

The majority of circulating lymphocytes are small cells with a thin rim of cytoplasm, occasionally con-

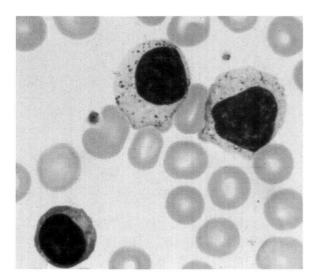

Fig. 5.87 Photomicrograph of a blood film. Shows a small lymphocyte and two large granular lymphocytes with azurophilic granules.

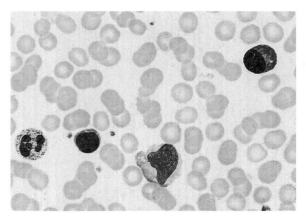

Fig. 5.88 Photomicrograph of a blood film. Viral infection. Shows a Türk cell, a reactive lymphocyte and a small lymphocyte.

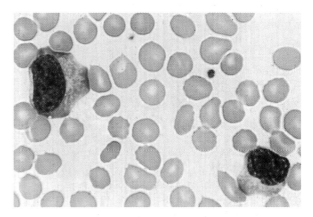

Fig. 5.89 Photomicrograph of a blood film. Infectious mononucleosis. There are two activated lymphocytes ('atypical mononuclear cells').

taining scanty azurophilic granules (see Figs 5.1 and 5.87). Nuclei are remarkably uniform in size (*c* 9 μm in diameter). This provides a useful guide for estimating red cell size (normally *c* 7–8 μm) on the blood film. Some 10% of circulating lymphocytes are larger, with more abundant pale blue cytoplasm containing azurophilic granules (Fig. 5.87). The nuclei of lymphocytes have homogeneous chromatin with some clumping at the nuclear periphery. About 85% of the circulating lymphocytes are T cells or natural killer (NK) cells.

In infections, both bacterial and viral, transforming lymphocytes may be present. These immunoblasts or 'Türk' cells are 10–15 μm in diameter, with a round nucleus and abundant deeply basophilic cytoplasm (Fig. 5.88). They may develop into plasmacytoid lymphocytes and plasma cells and these are occasionally seen in the blood in severe infections. In the absence of infection, multiple myeloma must be excluded. In viral infection, 'reactive lymphocytes' appear in the blood. These have slightly larger nuclei with more open chromatin and abundant cytoplasm which may be irregular. The most extreme examples of these cells are usually found in infectious mononucleosis (Fig. 5.89). These 'glandular fever' cells have irregular nuclei and abundant cytoplasm which is basophilic at the periphery; they have a tendency to adhere to adjacent erythrocytes.

Malignant lymphoid cells vary enormously in their morphology. The commonest malignancy is chronic lymphocytic leukaemia, composed almost exclusively of small lymphocytes (Fig. 5.90), sometimes with a few larger nucleolated cells. In prolymphocytic leukaemia, the majority of cells are a little larger than small lymphocytes with more cytoplasm and usually one distinct nucleolus (Fig. 5.91). Lymphoblasts of acute lymphoblastic leukaemia (Figs 5.92 and 5.93) vary in size from only slightly larger than lymphocytes to cells of 15–17 μm diameter. The nuclei generally have diffuse chromatin but there may be some chromatin condensation in the smaller blasts. The cytoplasm varies from weakly to strongly basophilic.

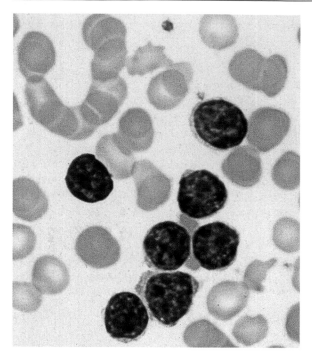

Fig. 5.90 Photomicrograph of a blood film. Chronic lymphocytic leukaemia. The cells are small lymphocytes; note that rouleaux formation is increased.

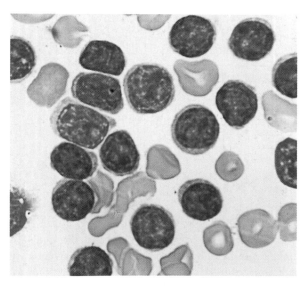

Fig. 5.91 Photomicrograph of a blood film. Prolymphocytic leukaemia. There is a uniform population of prolymphocytes.

Circulating lymphoma cells vary markedly in size, depending on the type of lymphoma. When there is a lymphocytosis, the lymphocytes are

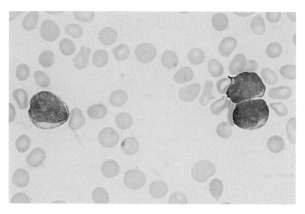

Fig. 5.92 Photomicrograph of a blood film. Philadelphia-positive acute lymphoblastic leukaemia (FAB L1 category). Shows three lymphoblasts.

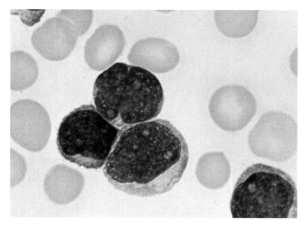

Fig. 5.93 Photomicrograph of a blood film Acute lymphoblastic leukaemia (FAB L1 type). Shows lymphoblasts.

usually far less uniform than in chronic lymphocytic leukaemia, and the lymphoma cells frequently have irregular lobed, indented or cleaved nuclei and relatively scanty agranular cytoplasm that varies in its degree of basophilia. Lobulated lymphocytes are a feature of HTLV-I infection and of adult T-cell leukaemia/lymphoma. However, lymphocytes with definite lobulation are also a common storage artefact in blood kept for 18–24 h at room temperature (see p. 6).

Lymphocytes predominate in the blood films of infants and young children. In this age-range, large lymphocytes and reactive lymphocytes tend to be conspicuous, and a small number of lymphoblasts may also be present.

PLATELET MORPHOLOGY

Normal platelets are 1–3 μm in diameter. They are irregular in outline with fine red granules that may be scattered or centralized. A small number of larger platelets, up to 5 μm in diameter may be seen in normal films. Larger platelets are seen in the blood when platelet production is increased (Fig. 5.94) and in hyposplenism (Fig. 5.95). Thus, for example, in severe immune thrombocytopenia some large platelets will be seen on the film. Very high platelet counts as a feature of a myeloproliferative disorder may be associated with extreme platelet anisocytosis, with some platelets being as large as red cells and often with some agranular or hypogranular platelets

(Fig. 5.96). The platelet count frequently rises with acute inflammatory stress or bleeding, but seldom to more than $1000 \times 10^9/l$. Above this, unless the patient is critically ill, the cause is usually a myeloproliferative disorder.

Characteristic morphological features are seen in two inherited platelet disorders associated with bleeding. These are the *Bernard–Soulier syndrome* in which there are giant platelets with defective ristocetin response, and *grey platelet syndrome* in which the platelets lack granules and have a ghost-like appearance on the stained blood film (Fig. 5.97). Thrombocytopenia may also be present in the May–Hegglin anomaly (see p. 91).

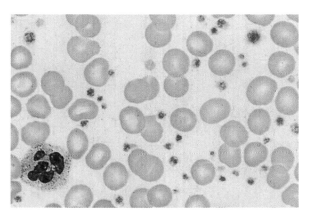

Fig. 5.94 Photomicrograph of a blood film. Essential thrombocythaemia. Shows platelet anisocytosis and increased numbers of platelets.

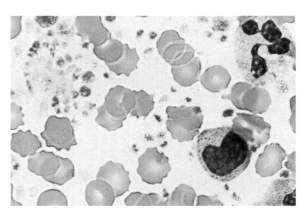

Fig. 5.96 Photomicrograph of a blood film. Myeloproliferative disorder. Shows platelet anisocytosis with some giant platelets.

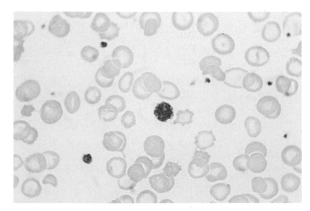

Fig. 5.95 Photomicrograph of a blood film. Hyposplenism in coeliac disease. Shows giant platelet.

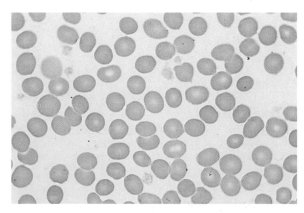

Fig. 5.97 Photomicrograph of a blood film. Grey platelet syndrome. Shows agranular platelets.

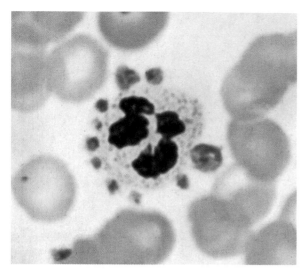

Fig. 5.98 Photomicrograph of a blood film. Shows adhesion of platelets to neutrophil (platelet satellitism).

In about 1% of individuals EDTA anti-coagulant causes platelet clumping, resulting in pseudo-thrombocytopenia.[28] This phenomenon may be detected when it gives rise to a 'flag' on an automated blood cell counter; it is identifiable on the blood film. It is not associated with any coagulation disturbance and platelet function is normal. Occasionally, EDTA may also inhibit the staining of platelets.[29]

Occasionally, platelets may be seen adhering to neutrophils (Fig. 5.98).[30–33] This has been reported in patients who have demonstrable anti-platelet auto-antibodies,[34] but it is more commonly seen in apparently healthy individuals. It is not seen in films made directly from blood which has not been anticoagulated.

REFERENCES

1 Marsh GW 1966 Abnormal contraction, distortion and fragmentation in human red cells. London University MD thesis.
2 Rodgers MS, Chang C-C, Kass L 1999 Elliptocytosis and tailed poikilocytes correlate with severity of iron-deficiency anemia. American Journal of Clinical Pathology 111:672–675.
3 Sechi LA, De Carll S, Catena C, et al 1996 Benign familial macrocytosis. Clinical and Laboratory Haematology 18:41–43.
4 Tuffy P, Brown AK, Zuelzer WW 1959 Infantile pyknocytosis: a common erythrocyte abnormality of the first trimester. American Journal of Diseases of Children 98:227.
5 Keimowitz R, Desforges JF 1965 Infantile pyknocytosis. New England Journal of Medicine 273:1152.
6 Schwartz SO, Motto SA 1949 The diagnostic significance of 'Burr' red blood cells. American Journal of Medical Sciences 218:563.
7 Bessis M 1972 Red cell shapes. An illustrated classification and its rationale. Nouvelle Revue Française d'Hématologie 12:721.
8 Estes JW, Morley TJ, Levine IM et al 1967 A new hereditary acanthocytosis syndrome. American Journal of Medicine 42:868.
9 Mier M, Schwartz SO, Boshes B 1960 Acanthrocytosis [sic], pigmented degeneration of the retina and ataxic neuropathy: a genetically determined syndrome with associated metabolic disorder. Blood 16:1586.
10 Salt HB, Wolfe OH, Lloyd JK, et al 1960 On having no beta-lipoprotein. A syndrome comprising a-beta-lipoprotinaemia, acanthocytosis, and steatorrhoea. Lancet ii:325.
11 Winner BM, Marsh WL, Taswel HF, et al 1977 Haematological changes associated with the McLeod phenotype of the Kell blood group system. British Journal of Haematology, 36:219.
12 Silber R, Amorosi EL, Howe J, et al 1966 Spur-shaped erythrocytes in Laennec's cirrhosis. New England Journal of Medicine 275:639.
13 Ponder E 1948 Hemolysis and related phenomena. Grune & Stratton, New York.
14 Feo CJ, Tchernia G, Subtu E, et al 1978 Observation of echinocytosis in eight patients: a phase contrast and SEM study. British Journal of Haematology 40:519.
15 Crook M, Williams W, Schey S 1998 Target cells and stomatocytes in heterozygous familial hypobetalipoproteinaemia. European Journal of Haematology, 60: 68–69.
16 Lock SP, Sephton Smith R, Hardisty RM 1961 Stomatocytosis: a hereditary red cell anomaly associated with haemolytic anaemia. British Journal of Haematology 7:303.
17 Ducrou W, Kimber RJ, 1969 Stomatocytes, haemolytic anaemia and abdominal pain in Mediterranean migrants: some examples of a new syndrome? Medical Journal of Australia ii:1087.
18 Norman JG 1969 Stomatocytosis in migrants of Mediterranean origin. Medical Journal of Australia i:315.
19 Douglass C, Twomey J 1970 Transient stomatocytosis with hemolysis: a previously unrecognized complication of alcoholism. Annals of Internal Medicine 72:159.

20 Weed RI, Bessis M 1973 The discocyte-stomatocyte equilibrium of normal and pathologic red cells. Blood 41:471.

21 Brecher G, Bessis M 1972 Present status of spiculated red cells and their relationship to the discocyte–echinocyte transformation: a critical review. Blood 40:333.

22 Bennett JM, Catovsky D, Daniel MT, et al 1976 Proposals for the classification of the acute leukaemias (FAB cooperative group). British Journal of Haematology 33:451.

23 Bennett JM, Catovsky D, Daniel MT, et al 1985 Proposed revised criteria for the classification of acute myeloid leukemia. Annals of Internal Medicine 103:626.

24 Harris NL, Jaffe ES, Diebold J, et al 1999 World Health Organization classification of neoplastic diseases of the hematopoietic and lymphoid tissues: report of the Clinical Advisory Committee Meeting – Airlie House, Virginia, November 1997. Journal of Clinical Oncology 17:3835.

25 Deal J, Hernandez AM, Pierre RV 1995 Ethylenediamine tetraacetic acid-associated leukoagglutination. American Journal of Clinical Pathology 103: 338–340.

26 Howard MR, Smith RA 1999 Early diagnosis of septicaemia in preterm infants from examination of the peripheral blood films. Clinical and Laboratory Haematology 21:365–368.

27 Westerman DA, Evans D, Metz J 1999 Neutrophil hypersegmentation in iron deficiency anaemia: a case control study. British Journal of Haematology 107:512–515.

28 Gowland E, Kay HEM, Spillman JC, et al 1969 Agglutination of platelets by a serum factor in the presence of EDTA. Journal of Clinical Pathology 22:460.

29 Stavem P, Berg K 1973 A macromolecular serum component acting on platelets in the presence of EDTA – 'Platelet stain preventing factor'. Scandinavian Journal of Haematology 10:202.

30 Crome PE, Barkhan P 1963 Platelet adherence to polymorphs. British Medical Journal ii:871.

31 Field EJ, Macleod I 1963 Platelet adherence to polymorphs. British Medical Journal ii:388.

32 Greipp PR, Gralnick HR 1976 Platelet to leucocyte adherence phenomena associated with thrombocytopenia. Blood 47:513.

33 Skinnider LF, Musclow CE, Kahn W 1978 Platelet satellitism – an ultrastructural study. American Journal of Hematology 4:179.

34 White LA, Brubaker LH, Aster RH, et al 1978 Platelet satellitism and phagocytosis by neutrophils: association with antiplatelet antibodies and lymphoma. American Journal of Hematology 4:313.

35 Van Assendelft OW, McGrath C, Murphy RS, et al 1977 The differential distribution of leukocytes. In: Koepke JA (ed) CAP Aspen conference: Differential leukocyte counting. College of American Pathologists, Northfield, IL.

Bone marrow biopsy
Imelda Bates

Biopsy of the bone marrow is an indispensable adjunct to the study of diseases of the blood and may be the only way in which a correct diagnosis can be made. Marrow can be obtained by needle aspiration, percutaneous trephine biopsy or surgical biopsy. If performed correctly, *bone marrow aspiration* is simple and safe; it can be repeated many times and performed on outpatients. It seems to be safe in almost all circumstances, even when thrombocytopenic purpura is present. However, it should never be attempted when there is a major disorder of coagulation such as in haemophilia, without appropriate cover and checking by coagulation factor assay prior to the procedure. *Trephine biopsy* is a little less simple, but it too can be performed on outpatients.

The disadvantage of bone marrow aspiration in comparison with trephine biopsy is that the arrangement of the cells in the marrow and the relationship between one cell and another is disrupted by the process of aspiration, and, in fibrotic marrows, little but blood may be aspirated. On the other hand, when marrow is aspirated, individual cells are well preserved. After staining, subtle differences between cells can be recognized usually to a far greater degree than is possible with sectioned material. The great value of trephine biopsy is that it can provide information about the structure of relatively large pieces of marrow. At the same time,

morphological features of individual cells may be identified by making an imprint from the material obtained.

Studies on large numbers of cases have demonstrated that trephine biopsy specimens are superior to films of aspirated material in some circumstances (e.g. for diagnosing marrow involvement by lymphoma or non-haematological neoplastic diseases). However, the simple procedure of marrow aspiration seldom fails to provide important information in patients who have a blood disease.[1,2] The two techniques have an important and complementary role in clinical investigation.

ASPIRATION OF THE BONE MARROW

Satisfactory samples of bone marrow can usually be aspirated from the sternum, iliac crest or anterior or posterior iliac spines. The iliac spines have the advantage that if no material is aspirated, a trephine biopsy can be performed immediately. These sites may, however, be technically difficult in obese or immobile subjects, and puncture of the sternum may occasionally be necessary. The sternum should, in general, not be used in children. In adults, unless the needle is correctly inserted is the sternum, there is a danger of perforating the inner cortical layer and damaging the underlying large blood vessels and right atrium, with serious consequences.

Performing a bone marrow aspiration

Only needles designed for the purpose should be used for marrow aspiration (see below). The operator should always wear surgical gloves to biopsy bone marrow, and take great care to avoid needle-stick injuries. To perform a marrow aspiration, clean the skin in the area with 70% alcohol (e.g. ethanol) or 0.5% chlorhexidine (5% diluted 1 in 10 in ethanol). Infiltrate the skin, subcutaneous tissue and periosteum overlying the selected site with a local anaesthetic such as 2–5 ml 2% lignocaine. With a boring movement, pass the needle perpendicularly into the cavity of the ilium at the centre of the oval posterior superior iliac spine or 2 cm posterior and 2 cm inferior to the anterior superior iliac spine. When the bone has been penetrated, remove the stilette, attach a 2 or 5 ml syringe and suck up marrow contents. As a rule, material can be sucked into the syringe without difficulty; occasionally it may be necessary to re-insert the stilette and to push the needle in a little further and to suck again. Failure to aspirate marrow – a 'dry tap' – suggests bone marrow fibrosis or infiltration.

Bone marrow clots faster than peripheral blood so films should be made from the aspirated material without delay at the bedside (see p. 105). The remainder of the material may then be delivered into a bottle containing an appropriate amount of EDTA anticoagulant and used later to make more films. Preservative-free heparin should be used rather than EDTA if phenotyping or cytogenetic studies are needed. Some material can be preserved in fixative rather than anticoagulant for preparation of histological sections (p. 109). Fix some of the films in absolute methanol as soon as they are dry for subsequent staining by a Romanowsky method or Perls' stain for iron. These films are also suitable for cytochemical staining (Ch. 13). If there has been a 'dry tap', insert the stilette into the needle and push any material in the lumen of the needle on to a slide; in lymphomas and carcinomas, especially, sufficient material can thus be obtained to make a diagnosis.[3]

Puncture of the ilium

The usual sites for puncture in adults are the posterior, and less commonly, the anterior iliac spine. If serial punctures are being performed, a different site should be selected for each, in order to avoid aspirating marrow which has been diluted by haemorrhage resulting from previous punctures. The posterior iliac spine overlies a large marrow-containing area and relatively large volumes of marrow can be aspirated from this site.[4] Posterior iliac puncture can be carried out with the patient lying sideways, as for a lumbar puncture, or prone. The anterior superior iliac spine may be easier to locate in very obese individuals and the bone overlying it is said to be thinner than that of the iliac crest.[5]

Puncture of the sternum

As stated above, this must be performed with care to avoid pushing the aspiration needle through the bone. The usual site for puncture is the manubrium or the first or second parts of the body of the sternum. The manubrium is formed of rather denser bone than the body of the sternum, and, in elderly subjects at least, it tends to contain more fatty marrow than is found elsewhere in the sternum. The thickness of the cortex here varies from 0.2 mm to 5.0 mm so it may be difficult to be certain that the needle point has reached the cavity of the bone.

The site for puncture of the manubrium should be about 1 cm above the sternomanubrial angle and slightly to one side of the mid-line; if the body of the bone is to be punctured, this should be done opposite the second intercostal space slightly to one side of the mid-line. It is essential to use a needle with a guard which cannot slip such as a Klima type. After piercing the skin and subcutaneous tissues, when the needle-point reaches the periosteum, adjust the guard on the needle to allow it to penetrate for about 5 mm further. Then push the needle with a boring motion into the cavity of the bone. It is usually easy to appreciate when the cavity of the bone has been entered. Aspiration is then carried out as described above.

Puncture of spinous processes

Good samples of marrow may be obtained from adults by puncturing the spines of lumbar vertebrae.[6] Puncture is not difficult since the bones lie superficially, but rather more pressure is required than for ilial or sternal puncture. Pass the needle into the spine of a lumbar vertebra slightly lateral to the mid-line in a direction at right angles to the skin surface, with the patient either sitting up or lying on his or her side as for a lumbar puncture.

Comparison of different sites for marrow puncture

There is considerable variation in the composition of cellular marrow withdrawn from adjacent or different sites. Aspiration from only one site may give misleading information;[7] this is particularly true in aplastic anaemia as the marrow may be affected patchily.[8,9] In general, however, the overall cellularity, the haemopoietic maturation pathways and the balance between erythropoiesis and leucopoiesis are similar at all sites.[10,11] In practice, it is an advantage to have a choice of several sites for puncture, particularly when puncture at one site results in a 'dry tap' or when only peripheral blood is withdrawn. Aspiration at a different site may yield cellular marrow or strengthen suspicion of a widespread change affecting the bone marrow, such as fibrosis or hypoplasia. In aplastic anaemia, several punctures may be necessary in order to arrive at the diagnosis.

ASPIRATION OF THE BONE MARROW IN CHILDREN

Iliac puncture, particularly in the region of the posterior spine, is usually the method of choice in children. Occasionally, in an older child who is obese the posterior iliac spine cannot be felt. In this case, a satisfactory sample can usually be obtained from the anterior ilium. In small babies, marrow can be withdrawn from the medial aspect of the upper end of the tibia just below the level of the tibial tubercle. This site should be used with caution, as it is vulnerable to fractures and laceration of the adjacent major blood vessels. In older children, the tibial cortical bone is usually too dense and the marrow within is normally less active. It must be remembered that sternal puncture in children should be avoided because the bone is thin and the marrow cavities are small.

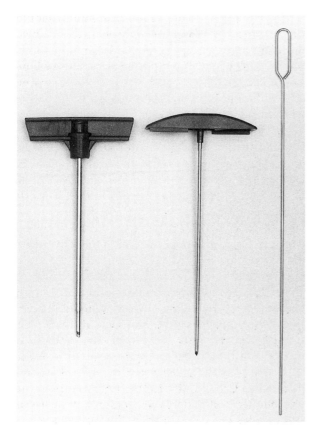

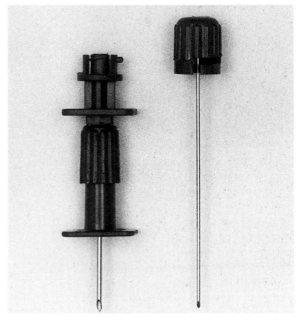

Fig 6.1 Disposable bone marrow needles. For aspiration (left) and trephine biopsy (right) (reduced ×0.75).

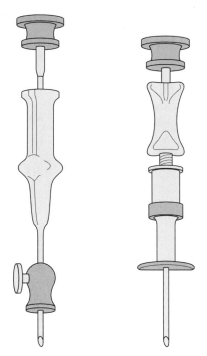

Fig 6.2 Marrow puncture needles. Salah (left) and Klima (right) (reduced ×0.75).

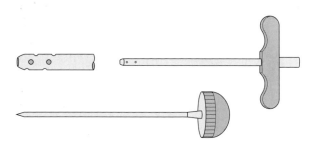

Fig 6.3 Islam's bone marrow aspiration needle. The dome-shaped handle and T-bar are intended to provide stability and control during operation.

MARROW PUNCTURE NEEDLES

Several types of disposable bone marrow aspiration and trephine biopsy needles are available; their design is similar to the traditional re-usable needles (Fig. 6.1). Needles should be stout and made of hard stainless steel, about 7–8 cm in length, with a well-fitting stilette, and must be provided with an adjustable guard. For re-usable needles, the point of the needle and the edge of the bevel must be kept well sharpened. The most common re-usable needles are the Salah and Klima needles (Fig. 6.2).

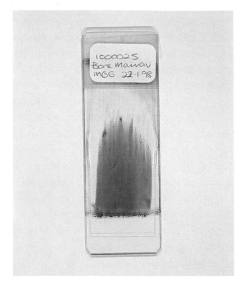

Fig 6.4 Film of aspirated bone marrow. The marrow particles are easily visible, mostly at the tail of the film (×1.5).

A slightly larger needle with a T-bar handle at the proximal end has been developed by Islam (Fig. 6.3). It is said to provide a better grip, to be more manoeuvrable and to be more successful for biopsies of excessively hard (e.g. osteosclerosis) or soft (e.g. profound of bone osteoporosis).[12,13] A modified version of the Islam needle has multiple holes in the distal portion of the shaft in addition to the opening at the tip, in order to overcome sampling error when the marrow is not uniformly involved in a pathological lesion.[14]

PROCESSING OF ASPIRATED BONE MARROW

There is little advantage in aspirating more than 0.3 ml of marrow fluid from a single site for morphological examination as this increases peripheral blood dilution. If large amounts of marrow are needed for several tests, such as immunophenotyping, cytogenetics and molecular studies, the syringe can be detached from the aspiration needle, and the stilette replaced, leaving the aspiration needle in the bone. After the marrow smears have been prepared, the syringe can be re-attached to the needle and another 5–10 ml of marrow aspirated.

It is good practice to obtain a sample of peripheral blood from the patient at the same time as the bone marrow so that both specimens can be examined and stored together. This can be done simply by preparing some films from blood obtained from a finger prick after completing the bone marrow sampling or by venepuncture so that a full blood count can be obtained.

Preparing films from bone marrow aspirates

Make films, 3–5 cm in length, of the aspirated marrow using a smooth-edged glass spreader of not more than 2 cm in width (Fig. 6.4). The marrow fragments are dragged behind the spreader and leave a trail of cells behind them. If there are insufficient fragments, they can be concentrated. This is not usually necessary for marrows which are very cellular such as in acute and chronic myeloid leukaemia and megaloblastic anaemia. Concentration of marrow can be achieved by delivering single drops of aspirate on to slides about 1 cm from one end. Most of the blood is quickly sucked off from the edge of the drop with the marrow syringe or a fine plastic pipette. The irregularly shaped marrow fragments tend to be left behind on the slide and smears can then be prepared as above.

After drying, fix the films of bone marrow and stain them with Romanowsky dyes, as for peripheral blood films (p. 51). However, a longer fixation time (at least 20 min in methanol) is essential for high quality staining. Films can also be stained by Perls' method to demonstrate the presence or absence of iron (see p. 270).

The preparation can be considered satisfactory only when marrow particles and free marrow cells can be seen in stained films. It is in the cellular trails that differential counts should be made, commencing from the marrow fragment and working back towards the head of the film; in this way, smaller numbers of cells from the peripheral blood are included in a differential count.

When the aspirated marrow is taken into an anticoagulant in a tube (e.g. dried EDTA) care should be taken that appropriate amounts are used for the volume of marrow to be anticoagulated. When films of marrow containing a gross excess of anticoagulant are spread (as when a few drops of marrow are added to a tube containing sufficient EDTA to prevent the clotting of 5 ml of blood),

masses of pink-staining amorphous material may be seen and some of the erythroblasts and reticulocytes may clump together.

Concentration of bone marrow by centrifugation

Centrifugation can be used to concentrate the marrow cells and to assess the relative proportions of marrow cells, peripheral blood and fat in aspirated material. While concentration of poorly cellular samples is useful, especially when an abnormal cell is present in small numbers,[15] it is unnecessary when the aspirated material is of average or increased cellularity. Volumetric data, too, are of little value in individual patients because of the wide range of values encountered even in health. Methods for separation of marrow cells are described on page 111.

Preparation of films of post-mortem bone marrow

Films made of bone marrow obtained postmortem are seldom satisfactory. When the marrow is spread in the ordinary way, the majority of the cells tend to break up and appear as smears. The rate and pattern of cellular autolysis during the first 15 h after death has been studied and the differences between the changes of post-mortem autolysis and those which occur in life as a result of blood diseases have been defined.[16] Blood cells are much better preserved if a small piece of marrow is suspended in 1–2 ml of 5% bovine albumin (1 volume 30% albumin, 5 volumes 9 g/l NaCl).[17] The suspension is then centrifuged and the deposited marrow cells are resuspended in a volume of supernatant approximately equal to, or slightly less than, that of the deposit. Films are made of this suspension in the usual way.

EXAMINATION OF ASPIRATED BONE MARROW

Quantitative cell counts on aspirated bone marrow

A number of values for the cell content of aspirated normal bone marrow have been given in the literature.[18–21] The percentage of marrow in the sternum of healthy adults that is cellular rather than fatty was given by Berman & Axelrod as

48–79%.[22] But quantitation of the cell content of aspirated marrow is not reliable in view of the tendency of the marrow to be aspirated in the form of particles of varying size as well as free cells, and the uncontrollable factor of dilution with peripheral blood, which according to some authors may amount to 40–100% in 0.25–0.5 ml bone marrow samples.[23]

Quantitative cell counts on aspirated marrow are therefore difficult to interpret. For practical purposes, the degree of marrow cellularity can be assessed within broad limits as increased, normal or reduced by inspection of a stained film containing marrow particles. As a rough guide, if less than 25% of the particle is occupied by haemopoietic cells, it is hypocellular, and if more than 75–80%, it is hypercellular. Less subjective quantitative measurement can be obtained by 'point counting' of sections;[24,25] a normal range of 30–80% has been reported in the anterior iliac spine.[24]

Physiological variation in the cell content has to be taken into account. The cellularity of the marrow is affected by age. In adults, a smaller proportion of the marrow cavity is occupied by haemopoietic marrow than in children and the proportion of fat cells to cellular marrow is increased. In one study, by means of point counting of sections from the iliac crest, the range of cellularity in children under 10 years was reported as 59–95% with a mean of 79%; at 30 years, the mean was 50%, and at 70 years, it was 30% with a range of 11–47%.[24] The decrease in cellularity in elderly subjects is even more marked in the manubrium sterni. The marrow undergoes slight to moderate hyperplasia in pregnancy.[26]

Differential cell counts on aspirated bone marrow

For general purposes, it is not usually necessary to document the proportion of every stage of each cell type on the marrow slide. A 200–500 cell differential using the categories erythroid, myeloid, lymphoid and plasma cells is generally adequate providing that a systematic scheme for examining the morphology of these, and all other, cells is also used (p. 108). In some conditions, such as chronic myeloid leukaemia and myelodysplastic syndrome, detailed differential counts are important since the results may indicate prognosis

and affect treatment. Occasionally, it may be important to specifically count one cell type (e.g. blasts in acute leukaemia for assessing response to chemotherapy). Follow-up bone marrows should always be compared with previous bone marrow films in order to assess the course of a disease or the effect of treatment.

Sources of error and physiological variations

Because of the naturally variegated pattern of the bone marrow, the irregular distribution of the marrow cells when spread in films and the variable amount of dilution with blood, differential cell counts on marrow aspirated from normal subjects vary widely. Counting cells in the trails left behind marrow particles as they are spread on the slide minimizes the dilutional effect of blood. When there is an increase in associated reticulin, some cell types may resist aspiration or remain embedded in marrow fragments, and will therefore be under-represented in the differential count. The chance aspiration of a lymphoid follicle would result in an abnormally high percentage of lymphocytes.[27] Megakaryocytes in particular are irregularly distributed and tend to be carried to the tail of the film.

Ideally, differential counts should be performed on sectioned material but difficulties in identification make this impractical. Methacrylate embedding offers a better opportunity for correctly identifying cells. The incidence of the various cell types is usually expressed as percentages. The normal values for cell differentials in bone marrow (Table 6.1) can only be taken as an approximate guide.[20,21] Glaser et al gave figures for the cellular composition of the bone marrow in normal infants, children and young adults, based on 151 samples.[28] Variation is marked in the first year, particularly so in the first month. The percentage of erythroblasts falls from birth, and at 2 to 3 weeks they constitute only c 10% of the nucleated cells. Myeloid cells (granulocyte precursors) increase during the first 2 weeks of life, following which a sharp fall occurs at about the 3rd week, but by the end of the 1st month c 60% of the cells are myeloid. Lymphocytes constitute up to 40% of the nucleated cells in the marrow of small infants; the mean value at 2 years is c 20%, falling to c 15% during the rest of childhood. The percentage of

Table 6.1 Normal ranges for differential counts on aspirated bone marrow

	95% Range	Mean[21]	Mean[20]
Myeloblasts	0–3	1.4	0.4
Promyelocytes	3–12	7.8	13.7*
Myelocytes (neutrophil)	2–13	7.6	–
Metamyelocytes	2–6	4.1	–
Neutrophils	22–46	32.1[M]; 37.4[W]	35.5
Myelocytes (eosinophil)	0–3	1.3	1.6
Eosinophils	0.3–4	2.2	1.7
Basophils	0–0.5	0.1	0.2
Lymphocytes	5–20	13.1	16.1
Monocytes	0–3	1.3	2.5
Plasma cells	0–3.5	0.6	1.9
Erythroblasts**	5–35	28.1[M]; 22.5[W]	23.5
Megakaryocytes	0–2		0.5
Macrophages	0–2	0.4	2.0

*Includes all 'immature neutrophils'.
[M] = Men; [W] = Women.
** Hammersmith Hospital data:
    Proerythroblasts   0.5–5
    Early erythroblasts   2–20
    Late erythroblasts   2–10.

plasma cells is especially low from infancy up to the age of 5 years.[29]

The hyperplasia which occurs in pregnancy affects both erythropoiesis and granulopoiesis, the latter proportionately less, though with some increase in the relative proportion of immature cells.[26] The hyperplasia is maximal in the third trimester; a return to normal begins in the puerperium but is not completed until at least 6 weeks postpartum.

Cellular ratios

Ratios based on a count of 200–500 cells can provide useful qualitative information. The myeloid:erythroid ratio has been widely used and is the ratio of neutrophil and neutrophil precursor cells to erythroid precursors. The inclusion of eosinophils and basophils is controversial but in practice makes little difference to the overall ratio which varies from 2:1 to 4:1.[30] As an alternative, the leuco-erythrogenetic ratio can be calculated: for this, mature cells are excluded; the normal ratio has been reported as 0.56–2.67:1.[31] The myeloid:lymphoid ratio varies widely, 1–17:1, and the lymphoid:erythroid ratio has a similarly wide variation, 0.2–4.0:1.[32]

REPORTING BONE MARROW ASPIRATE FILMS

A systematic examination of the marrow aspirate, combined with a knowledge of the clinical context, provides the best chance of arriving at a diagnosis. Choose several of the best spread stained films which contain easily visible marrow particles. Several particles should then be examined with a low-power (×10) objective to estimate whether the marrow is hypocellular, normocellular or hypercellular (Fig. 6.5). Megakaryocytes and clumps of non-haemopoietic cells (as in metastatic carcinoma cells) should be looked for at this stage of the examination; they are most often found towards the tail of the film.

Select for detailed examination – still using the ×10 objective – a highly cellular area of the film where the nucleated cells are well stained and well spread. Areas such as these can usually be found towards the tails of films behind marrow particles. The cells in these cellular areas should then be examined with a higher power (e.g. ×40) objective and subsequently, if necessary, with the ×100 oil-immersion objective. It is important always to examine marrows in a systematic fashion as it is

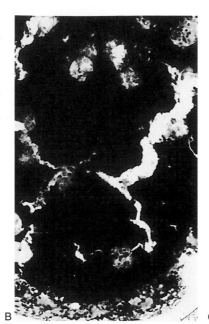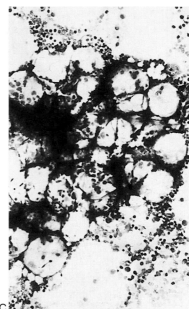

Fig 6.5 Film of aspirated bone marrow. Photomicrographs of particles illustrating cellularity: (A) normal; (B) hypercellular; (C) hypocellular.

easy to overlook subtle abnormalities. A suggested scheme for this is outlined below.

Systematic scheme for examining bone marrow aspirate films

Low power (×10)

- **Determine cellularity** by examining several particles.
- **Identify megakaryocytes** and note morphology and maturation sequence (higher power may be needed for smaller immature megakaryocytes and micromegakaryocytes).
- Look for clumps of **abnormal cells** that could indicate infiltration by metastatic tumour (higher power needed to examine content and morphology of clumps).
- Identify **macrophages** and examine at higher power for evidence of haemophagocytosis, malaria pigment and bacterial or fungal infections which may be present in the cytoplasm.

Higher power (×40, ×100 oil immersion)

- Identify all stages of **maturation of myeloid and erythroid cells**. This is usually easiest to achieve by starting with mature red cells and

working backwards to the most immature cells. Repeat the process for the myeloid series starting with mature neutrophils. Maturation abnormalities, such as giant pronormoblasts or evidence of dysfunctional maturation, including nuclear-cytoplasmic asynchrony, will suggest specific diagnoses such as *Parvovirus* infection, myelodysplastic syndrome or megaloblastic anaemia, respectively. Changes in the proportion of primitive to mature myeloid cells may reflect response to treatment in leukaemia or recovery from agranulocytosis, and the actual percentage of blast cells may be of significance in the differentiation of refractory anaemias and in assessing leukaemia prognosis.

- Determine the **myeloid:erythroid ratio** (p. 107). While a lack of myeloid cells may be obvious without performing a formal differential count, it is easy to overlook an increase in erythroid cells which might suggest blood loss or peripheral destruction.

- Perform a **differential count** (p. 106) using the categories erythroid, myeloid, lymphoid, plasma cell and 'others' simultaneously noting any morphological abnormalities. The normal lymphocyte percent in the marrow is 5–20%;

moderate increases to 30–40%, which may indicate a significant disorder such as lymphoma, are not likely to be identified simply by rapidly surveying the slide. The proportion of lymphoid cells is an important indicator of prognosis in chronic lymphocytic leukaemia.[33] Plasma cells should be less than 5%; in plasma cell dyscrasias, they may be increased, occur in clumps or have an abnormal morphological appearance.

- Look for areas of bone marrow **necrosis**. In necrotic areas, the cells stain irregularly, with blurred outlines, cytoplasmic shrinkage and nuclear pyknosis. Bone marrow necrosis may occur in sickle cell disease; it also occurs occasionally in lymphomas, acute lymphoblastic and chronic lymphocytic leukaemia, myeloproliferative diseases and metastatic carcinoma as well as in septicaemia, tuberculosis and anorexia nervosa.[34–38] In anorexia, there may be gelatinous transformation of the ground substance of the marrow.[37]

- Assess the **iron content** of macrophages and look for iron granules in erythroid cells on a slide stained with Perls' stain. In sideroblastic anaemia, the granules incompletely encircle the nucleus. Abnormal patterns of iron staining may also be seen in dyserythropoietic anaemias such as the thalassaemias.

Reporting results

It is helpful to report bone marrow films on a printed form on which the report and conclusion can be set out in an ordered fashion (Fig. 6.6). Where a computerized reporting system is in use, it is useful to have a template with headings to ensure that the marrow reports are systematic and consistent. A list of the various descriptive comments which may be used should be provided in coded form to facilitate data entry. Report summaries should be intelligible to clinicians who are not haematology specialists.

PREPARATION OF SECTIONS OF ASPIRATED BONE MARROW FRAGMENTS

In situations where it is not possible to obtain a trephine biopsy (see below), the small fragments obtained by marrow aspiration can be fixed, stained and examined.[39] Such samples are useful for assessing cellularity and for detecting granulomas and tumour cells.

PERCUTANEOUS TREPHINE BIOPSY OF THE BONE MARROW

Trephine biopsies of the bone marrow are invaluable in the diagnosis of conditions which yield a 'dry tap' on bone marrow aspiration (e.g. myelofibrosis, infiltrations) or when disrupted architecture of the marrow is an important diagnostic feature (e.g. Hodgkin's disease, lymphoma). Like marrow aspirations, they can be carried out at the bedside or in outpatients. The posterior iliac spine is the usual site though the anterior iliac spine can also be used. The posterior iliac spine is said to provide samples that are longer and larger, while the aspiration is less uncomfortable for the patient.[40]

The trephine specimen is obtained by inserting the biopsy needle into the bone and using a to-and-fro rotation to obtain a core of tissue. The main problems with this method are that the specimen may be crushed thereby distorting the architecture, and it is difficult to detach the core of bone from inside the marrow space. Trephine biopsy needles, both re-usable and disposable, have been specifically designed to overcome these problems. The Jamshidi needle[41] has a tapering end to reduce crush artefact (Fig. 6.7) and the Islam trephine[42] has a core-securing device (Fig. 6.8). If larger specimens are needed, trephine needles which have bores of 4–5 mm may be used.[43,44] Other needles which are occasionally used for trephine biopsy specimens are a 2 mm bore 'microtrephine' needle[45] and a Vim–Silverman needle.[46] However, compared to other needles, these yield smaller specimens of marrow which are prone to fracturing.

For the investigation of thrombocytopenia and neutropenia in small preterm neonates, sections of aspirated bone marrow can be obtained which allow assessment of marrow cellularity and architecture.[47] A 19 G, half-inch Osgood needle*

---

*Popper and Sons, New Hyde Park; New York.

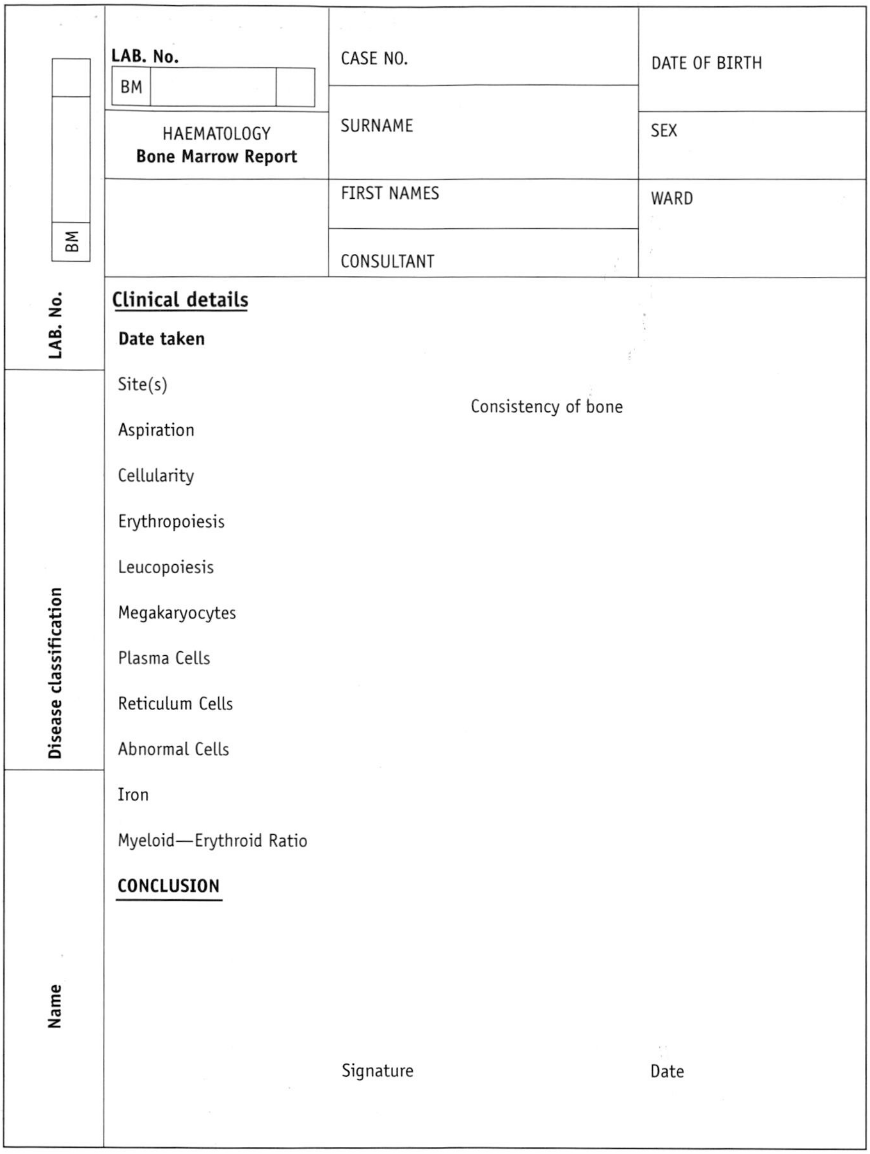

	LAB. No. BM	CASE NO.	DATE OF BIRTH
	HAEMATOLOGY **Bone Marrow Report**	SURNAME	SEX
		FIRST NAMES	WARD
		CONSULTANT	

Clinical details

Date taken

Site(s)

Aspiration

Cellularity

Erythropoiesis

Leucopoiesis

Megakaryocytes

Plasma Cells

Reticulum Cells

Abnormal Cells

Iron

Myeloid—Erythroid Ratio

CONCLUSION

Consistency of bone

Signature   Date

(left margin labels: LAB. No. / BM / LAB. No. / Disease classification / Name)

Fig 6.6 Example of report form for bone marrow films.

is introduced 2 cm below the tibial tuberosity. The trocar is removed and the hollow needle advanced by twisting 2–3 mm into the marrow space. A syringe is used to apply suction to the needle until marrow appears and then the needle and syringe are withdrawn. The marrow clot is gently dislodged with the tip of a needle and placed into fixative. The specimen is processed as if it was an adult biopsy except that decalcification is not required.

Imprints from bone marrow trephine biopsy specimens

Whenever a trephine biopsy is obtained, imprints can be taken before the specimen is transferred into fixative. This is particularly useful if the bone marrow aspirate is inadequate. The bony core is gently dabbed or rolled across the slide which is then fixed and stained as for bone marrow smears (p. 51). This allows immediate examination of cells which fall out of the specimen onto the

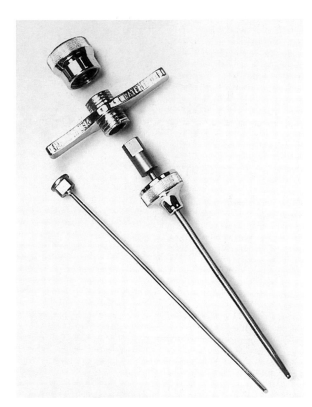

Fig 6.7 Jamshidi trephine for bone marrow biopsy.

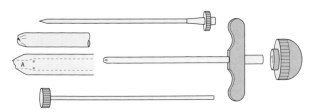

Fig 6.8 Islam trephine for bone marrow biopsy. The distal cutting edge is shaped to hold the core secure during extraction of the material.

slide, and may provide a diagnosis several days before the trephine biopsy specimen has been processed.

Processing of bone marrow trephine biopsy specimens

The specimen should be fixed in 10% formal saline, buffered to pH 7.0, or preferably in Helly's fluid (potassium dichromate 2.5 g, mercuric chloride 5 g, formalin (40% formaldehyde) 5 ml, water 100 ml) for 12–48 h prior to decalcifying, dehydrating and embedding in paraffin wax by the usual histological procedures. Cell shrinkage and distortion from the decalcification process may distort cellular detail. These disadvantages can be overcome by methyl methacrylate ('plastic') embedding.[48] Details of the preparation of sections of bone marrow biopsies can be found in the eighth edition of *Practical Haematology* (p. 185) and in Bain et al.[49]

Staining of sections of bone marrow trephine biopsy specimens

Bone marrow sections should be routinely stained with haematoxylin and eosin (H&E), and a silver impregnation method for reticulin. Sections can also be stained with Romanowsky dyes such as May–Grünwald–Giemsa and for iron by Perls' reaction. H&E staining is excellent for demonstrating the cellularity and pattern of the marrow and for revealing pathological changes such as fibrosis or the presence of granulomata or carcinoma cells. Figure 6.9 shows the extent to which the cellularity of the marrow varies in health. Haemopoietic cells may be more easily identified in a Romanowsky-stained preparation (Figs 6.10 and 6.11). Both paraffin- and plastic-embedded specimens are suitable for immunohistochemistry.

Silver impregnation stains the glycoprotein matrix which is associated with connective tissue. The bone marrow always contains a small amount of this material which is referred to as 'reticulin' and is an early form of collagen.[50] The reticulin content of iliac bone marrow is shown in Figure 6.12. An increase in marrow reticulin appears as an increase in the number and thickness of fibres. Increased reticulin deposition can occur in myeloproliferative disorders, particularly those associated with proliferation of megakaryocytes, and in lymphoproliferative disorders, secondary carcinoma with marrow infiltration, osseous disorders such as hyperparathyroidism and Paget's disease, and in inflammatory reactions.[51-53] In myelofibrosis or myelosclerosis, a more 'mature' form of collagen is present which, unlike reticulin, is visible on H&E staining (Fig. 6.13).

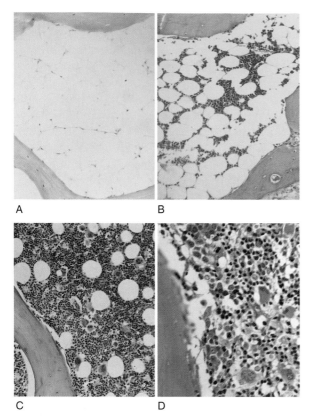

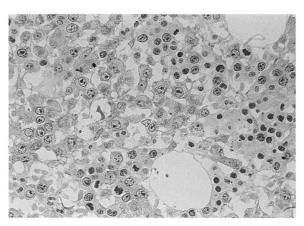

Fig 6.11 Photomicrograph of section of bone marrow. Iliac crest biopsy. Methacrylate embedding. Myeloblastic leukaemia. Stained by May–Grünwald–Giemsa.

Fig 6.9 Photomicrographs of sections of bone marrow. Iliac crest bone marrow illustrating range of cellularity: (A) hypocellular; (B) and (C) normal cellularity; (D) hypercellular.

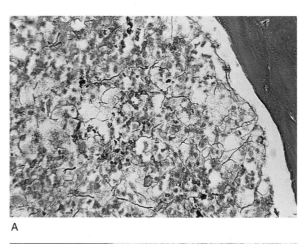

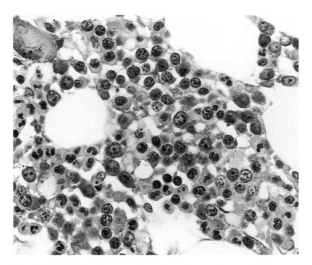

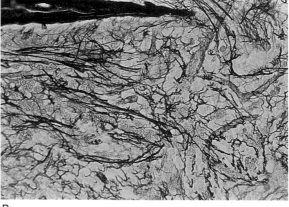

Fig 6.10 Photomicrograph of section of normal bone marrow. Iliac crest biopsy. Methacrylate embedding. Stained by May–Grünwald– Giemsa.

Fig 6.12 Photomicrographs of sections of bone marrow. Iliac crest biopsy. Stained for reticulin by silver impregnation method: (A) normal; (B) chronic myelofibrosis.

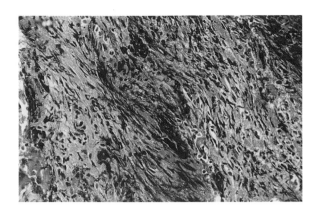

Fig 6.13 Photomicrographs of sections of bone marrow. Iliac crest biopsy; fibroblast proliferation and collagen in myelofibrosis. Haematoxylin-Eosin stain.

REFERENCES

1 Dee JW, Valdivieso M, Drewinko B 1976 Comparison of the efficacies of closed trephine needle biopsy, aspirated paraffin-embedded clot section and smear preparation in the diagnosis of bone marrow involvement by lymphoma. American Journal of Clinical Pathology 65:183.

2 Pasquale D, Chikkappa G 1981 Comparative evaluation of bone marrow aspirate particle smears, biopsy imprints, and biopsy sections. American Journal of Hematology 22:381.

3 Engeset A, Nesheim A, Sokolowski J 1979 Incidence of 'dry tap' on bone marrow aspirations in lymphomas and carcinomas. Diagnostic value of the small material in the needle. Scandinavian Journal of Haematology 22:417.

4 Berman HR, Kelly KH 1956 Multiple marrow aspiration in man from the posterior ilium. Blood 11:370.

5 Leffler RJ 1957 Aspiration of bone marrow from the anterior superior iliac spine. Journal of Laboratory and Clinical Medicine 50:482.

6 Loge JP 1948 Spinous process puncture. A simple clinical approach for obtaining bone marrow. Blood 3:198.

7 Hashimoto M 1960 The distribution of active marrow in the bones of normal adults. Kyushu Journal of Medical Science 11:103.

8 Ferrant A 1980 Selective hypoplasia of pelvic bone marrow. Scandinavian Journal of Haematology 25:12.

9 Lewis SM 1965 Course and prognosis in aplastic anaemia. British Medical Journal i:1027.

10 Bennike T, Gormsen H, Møller B 1956 Comparative studies of bone marrow punctures of the sternum, the iliac crest and the spinous process. Acta Medica Scandinavica 155:377.

11 Fadem RS, Yalow R 1951 Uniformity of cell counts in smears of bone marrow particles. American Journal of Clinical Pathology 27:541.

12 Islam A 1991 New sternal puncture needle. Journal of Clinical Pathology 44:690.

13 Jacobs P 1995 Choice of needle for bone marrow trephine biopsies. Hematology Reviews 9:163–168.

14 Islam A 1983 A new bone marrow aspiration needle to overcome the sampling errors inherent in the technique of bone marrow aspiration. Journal of Clinical Pathology 36:954.

15 Fillola GM, Laharrague PF, Corberand JX 1992 Bone marrow enrichment technique for detection and characterization of scarce abnormal cells. Nouvelle Revue Française d'Hématologie 34:337.

16 Hoffman SB, Morrow GW Jnr, Pease GL, et al 1964 Rate of cellular autolysis in postmortem bone marrow. American Journal of Clinical Pathology 41:281.

17 Berenbaum MC 1956 The use of bovine albumin in the preparation of marrow and blood films. Journal of Clinical Pathology 9:381.

18 Osgood EE, Seaman AJ 1944 The cellular composition of normal bone marrow as obtained by sternal puncture. Physiological Reviews 24:46.

19 Vaughan SL, Brockmyre F 1947 Normal bone marrow as obtained by sternal puncture. Blood, Special Issue No 1:54.

20 Den Ottolander GJ 1996 The bone marrow aspirate of healthy subjects. British Journal of Haematology. 95:574–575.

21 Bain B 1996 The bone marrow aspirate of healthy subjects. British Journal of Haematology 94:206–209.

22 Berman L, Axelrod AR 1950 Fat, total cell and megakaryocyte content of sections of aspirated marrow of normal persons. American Journal of Clinical Pathology 20:686.

23 Berlin NI, Hennessy TG, Gartland J 1950 Sternal marrow puncture: the dilution with peripheral blood as determined by P[32] labelled red cells. Journal of Laboratory and Clinical Medicine 36:23.

24 Hartsock RJ, Smith EB, Petty CS 1965 Normal variations with aging of the amount of hematopoietic tissue in bone marrow from the anterior iliac crest. American Journal of Clinical Pathology 43:326.

25 Kerndrup G, Pallesen G, Melsen F et al 1980 Histological determination of bone marrow cellularity in iliac crest biopsies. Scandinavian Journal of Haematology 24:110.

26 Lowenstein L, Bramlage CA 1957 The bone marrow in pregnancy and the puerperium. Blood 12:261.

27 Maeda K, Hyun BH, Rebuck JW 1977 Lymphoid follicles in bone marrow aspirates. American Journal of Clinical Pathology 67:41.

28 Glaser K, Limarzi LR, Poncher HG 1950 Cellular composition of the bone marrow in normal infants and children. Pediatrics 6:789.

29 Steiner ML, Pearson HA 1966 Bone marrow plasmacyte values in childhood. Journal of Pediatrics, 68:562.

30 Buckley PJ 1991 Examination and interpretation of bone marrow biopsies and aspirate smears. In: Hoffman R, Benze E, Shattil S, et al (eds) Hematology. Basic principles and practice. Churchill Livingstone, New York, ch 58, p 1804.

31 Pontoni L 1936 Su alcuni rapporti citologici ricavati dal mielogramma; metodica e valutazione fisopatognostica generale. Haematologica 17:833.

32 Frisch B, Lewis SM 1974 The bone marrow in aplastic anaemia: diagnostic and prognostic features. Journal of Clinical Pathology 27:231.

33 Rozman C, Montserrat E, Rodriguez-Fernandez JM et al 1984 Bone marrow histologic pattern – the best single prognostic parameter in chronic lymphocytic leukemia: a multivariate survival analysis of 329 cases. Blood 64:642.

34 Conrad ME, Carpenter JT 1979 Bone marrow necrosis. American Journal of Hematology 7:181.

35 Kiraly JF, Wheby MS 1976 Bone marrow necrosis. American Journal of Medicine 60:361.

36 MacFarlane SD, Tauro GP 1986 Acute lymphocytic leukaemia in children presenting with bone marrow necrosis. American Journal of Hematology 22:341.

37 Smith RRL, Spivak JL 1985 Marrow cell necrosis in anorexia nervosa and involuntary starvation. British Journal of Haematology 60:525.

38 Vesterby A, Jensen OM 1985 Aseptic bone/bone marrow necrosis in leukaemia. Scandinavian Journal of Haematology 35:354.

39 Raman K 1955 A method of sectioning aspirated bone-marrow. Journal of Clinical Pathology 8:265.

40 Hernándes-Garciá MT, Hernández-Nieto L, Pérez-González E et al 1993 Bone marrow trephine biopsy: anterior superior iliac spine versus posterior superior iliac spine. Clinical and Laboratory Haematology 15:15.

41 Jamshidi K, Swaim WR 1971 Bone marrow biopsy with unaltered architecture: a new biopsy device. Journal of Laboratory and Clinical Medicine 77:335.

42 Islam A 1981 A new bone marrow biopsy needle with core securing device. Journal of Clinical Pathology 35:359.

43 Landys K 1980 A new trephine for closed bone marrow biopsy. Acta Haematologica 64:216.

44 Williams JA, Nicholson GI 1963 A modified bone-biopsy drill for outpatient use. Lancet i:1408.

45 Türkel H, Bethell FH 1943 Biopsy of bone marrow performed by a new and simple instrument. Journal of Laboratory and Clinical Medicine 28:1246.

46 Conrad ME, Crosby WH 1961 Bone marrow biopsy: modification of the Vim–Silverman needle. Journal of Laboratory and Clinical Medicine 57:642.

47 Sola M, Rimsza L, Christensen R 1999 A bone marrow biopsy technique suitable for use in neonates. British Journal of Haematology 107:458–460.

48 Frish B, Lewis SM, Burkhardt R, et al 1985 Biopsy pathology of bone and bone marrow. Chapman and Hall, London.

49 Bain B, Clark DC, Lampert IO, Wilkins BS 2000 Bone marrow pathology, 3rd edn. Blackwell Science, Oxford.

50 Bentley SA, Alabaster O, Foidart JM 1981 Collagen heterogeneity in normal human bone marrow. British Journal of Haematology 48:287.

51 Frisch B, Bartl R 1985 Histology of myelofibrosis and osteomyelosclerosis. In: Lewis SM (ed) Myelofibrosis: pathophysiology and clinical management. Marcel Dekker, New York, p 51–86.

52 Lennert K, Nagai K, Schwarze EW 1975 Patho-anatomic features of the bone marrow. Clinics in Haematology 4:331.

53 McCarthy DM 1985 Fibrosis of the bone marrow; content and causes. British Journal of Haematology 59:1.

7

Iron-deficiency anaemia and iron overload

Mark Worwood

INTRODUCTION

The adult body contains 3–4 g of iron, mostly in haemoglobin, and the major pathways of iron metabolism also involve haemoglobin. Every day about 30 mg Fe is required to make haemoglobin in new red cells and most of this iron is obtained from iron released during the breakdown of life-expired red cells. Adult males lose only about 1 mg Fe/day and absorb a similar amount from food. Losses in young women are greater because of menstruation and childbirth and iron deficiency is more common in women because iron absorption from food does not always compensate for the increased losses. After the menopause, female iron stores approach male levels.

Normal iron status implies erythropoiesis which is not limited by iron supply and this means that there is a small reserve of 'storage iron' in the tissues (ferritin) to cope with normal physiological variation. Sufficient storage iron to survive an acute loss of blood is also an advantage.

Apart from too little or too much iron in the body there is also the possibility of maldistribution. An example is anaemia associated with inflammation or infection, where there is a partial failure of erythropoiesis and of iron release from the phagocytic cells in liver, spleen and bone marrow which results in accumulation of iron as ferritin and haemosiderin in these cells. Thus determination of iron status requires an estimate of the amount of haemoglobin iron (usually by measuring the haemoglobin concentration in the blood, see Ch. 3) and the level of storage iron (measuring serum ferritin concentration). Iron deficiency should be suspected in hypochromic, microcytic anaemia but in the early stages of iron deficiency red cells may be normocytic and normochromic. Another feature of iron deficiency is an increased concentration of protoporphyrin in the red cells; normally, there is a small amount, but defective haem synthesis results in an accumulation of a significant amount in the red cells (see p. 161).

Additional assays are sometimes required. In genetic haemochromatosis, early iron accumulation is indicated by an increased transferrin saturation. The serum ferritin concentration increases later as the level of stored iron increases. In the anaemia of chronic disease, patients often have normal serum ferritin concentrations even in the absence of storage iron in the bone marrow (Ch. 4). In this situation, the assay of serum transferrin receptor concentration can detect tissue iron deficiency.

SERUM FERRITIN

With the recognition that the small quantity of ferritin in human serum (15–300 µg/l in men) reflects body iron stores, measurement of serum ferritin has been widely adopted as a test for iron deficiency and iron overload.

The first reliable method to be introduced was an immunoradiometric assay[1] in which excess radio-labelled antibody is reacted with ferritin, and antibody not bound to ferritin is removed with an immunoadsorbent. This assay was supplanted by the two-site immunoradiometric assay[2] which is sensitive and convenient. Since then the principle of this assay has been extended to non-radioactive labelling, including enzymes (enzyme-linked immunoassay, ELISA). The method described below is of this type.

ENZYME IMMUNOASSAY FOR FERRITIN

Reagents and materials

Ferritin. This may be prepared from iron-loaded human liver or spleen obtained at operation (spleen) or post-mortem. The permission of the patient or the patient's relatives should be obtained for removal of tissue and its use in preparation of ferritin. Tissue should be obtained as soon as possible after death and may be stored at –20°C for 1 year. Remember the risk of infection when handling tissues and extracts. Ferritin is purified by methods which exploit its stability at 75°C. Further purification is obtained by chromatography and either by ultracentrifugation[3] or by precipitation from cadmium sulphate solution.[4] Purity should be assessed by polyacrylamide gel electrophoresis[3] and the protein content determined by the method of Lowry et al as described by Worwood.[3] Human ferritin may be stored at 4°C, at concentrations of

1–4 mg protein/ml, in the presence of sodium azide as a preservative, for up to 3 years. Such solutions should not be frozen. Ferritin, from human liver or spleen, may be obtained from several suppliers of laboratory reagents. This may be used as a standard after calibration against the international standard[4] (see later).

Antibodies to human ferritin. High affinity antibodies to human liver or spleen ferritin are suitable. Polyclonal antibodies may be raised in rabbits or sheep by conventional methods[5] and the titre checked by precipitation with human ferritin.[3] An IgG-enriched fraction of antiserum is required for labelling with enzyme in the assay. The simplest method is to precipitate IgG with ammonium sulphate.[6] Monoclonal antibodies which are specific for 'L' subunit rich ferritin (liver or spleen ferritin) are also suitable. Suitable antibodies (including a preparation labelled with horseradish peroxidase) may also be obtained from Dako Ltd, High Wycombe, Bucks, UK.

Conjugation of antiferritin IgG preparation to horseradish peroxidase[7]

1. Dissolve 4 mg of horseradish peroxidase (Sigma Type VI P-8375) in 1 ml of water and add 200 µl of freshly prepared 0.1 mol/l sodium periodate solution. The solution should turn greenish-brown. Mix gently by inverting and leave for 20 min at room temperature, mixing gently every 5 min. Dialyse overnight against 1 mmol/l sodium acetate buffer, pH 4.4.

2. Add 20 µl of 0.2 mol/l sodium carbonate buffer, pH 9.5 to a solution of antiferritin IgG fraction (8 mg in 1 ml). Add 20 µl of 0.2 mol/l

sodium carbonate buffer, pH 9.5 to the horse-radish peroxidase solution to raise the pH to 9.0–9.5 and immediately mix the two solutions. Leave at room temperature for 2 h and mix by inversion every 30 min.

3. Add 100 μl of freshly prepared sodium boro-hydride solution (4 mg/ml in water) and stand at 4°C for 2 h. Dialyse overnight against 0.1 mol/l borate buffer, pH 7.4.

4. Add an equal volume of 60% glycerol in borate buffer to the conjugate solution and store at 4°C.

Assay reagents

Buffer A. Phosphate buffered saline, pH 7.2, containing 0.05% Tween 20. Prepare a 10 times concentrated (1.5 mol/l) stock solution by dissolving sodium chloride, 80 g; potassium chloride, 2 g; anhydrous disodium phosphate, 11.5 g and anhydrous potassium phosphate (KH_2PO_4), 2 g in 1 litre of water. Store at room temperature. Prepare Buffer A by diluting 100 ml of stock solution to 1 litre with water and adding 0.5 ml of Tween 20. Store at 4°C for up to 2 weeks.

Buffer B. Prepare by dissolving 5 g of bovine serum albumin (BSA; Sigma A-7030) in 1 litre of buffer A. Store at 4°C for up to 2 weeks.

Buffer C. Carbonate buffer, 0.05 mol/l, pH 9.6. Dissolve sodium carbonate, 1.59 g and sodium bicarbonate, 2.93 g in 1 litre of water and store at room temperature.

Buffer D. Citrate phosphate buffer, 0.15 mol/l, pH 5.0. Dissolve 21 g of citric acid monohydrate in 1 litre of water and store at 4°C. Dissolve 28.4 g of anhydrous disodium phosphate in 1 litre of water and store at room temperature. Prepare fresh buffer on the day of assay by mixing 49 ml of citric acid solution with 51 ml of phosphate solution.

Substrate solution. Prepare immediately before use by adding 33 μl of hydrogen peroxide, 30%, to 100 ml of buffer D and mixing well. Add 1 tablet containing 30 mg of *o*-phenylenediamine dihydro-chloride (Sigma P 8412) and mix.

Sulphuric acid. Purchase as a 4 M solution.

Preparation and storage of a standard ferritin solution. Dilute a solution of human ferritin to approximately 200 μg/ml in water. Measure the protein concentration by the method of Lowry after diluting further to 20–50 μg/ml. Then dilute the ferritin solution (approx. 200 μg/ml) to a concentration of 10 μg/ml in 0.05 mol/l sodium barbitone solution containing 0.1 mol/l NaCl, 0.02% NaN_3, BSA (5 g/l) and adjusted to pH 8.0 with 5 mol/l HCl. Deliver 200 μl into small plastic tubes, cap tightly and store at 4°C for up to 1 year. For use, dilute in Buffer B to 1000 μg/l, then prepare a range of standard solutions between 0.2 and 25 μg/l. Calibrate this working standard against the WHO standard for the assay of serum ferritin (reagent 94/572, recombinant human L type ferritin).

Coating of plates. 96-well microtitre plates for immunoassay are required. Do not use the outer wells until you have established the assay procedure and can check that all wells give consistent results. Coat the plates by adding to each well 200 μl of antiferritin IgG preparation diluted to 2 μg/ml in Buffer C. Cover the plate with a lid and leave overnight at 4°C. On the day of the assay, empty the wells by sharply inverting the plate and dry by tapping briefly on paper towels. Block unreacted sites by adding 200 μl of 0.5% (w/v) BSA in Buffer C. After 30 min at room temperature, wash each plate three times by filling each well with Buffer A (using a syringe and needle) and emptying and draining as described above. Plates may be stored, dry, at 4°C for up to 1 week.

Preparation of test sera. Collect venous blood and separate the serum. Samples may be stored for 1 week at 4°C or for 2 years at –20°C. Plasma obtained from EDTA or heparinized blood is also suitable. For assay, dilute 50 μl of serum to 1 ml with Buffer B. Further dilutions may be made in the same buffer if required.

Assay procedure

The use of a multi-channel pipette for rapid addition of solutions is recommended. Standards and sera, in duplicate, should be added to each plate within 20 min.

Add 200 μl of standard solution or diluted serum to each well. Cover the plate and leave at room temperature on a draught-free bench away from direct sunlight for 2 h. Empty the wells by sharply inverting the plate and drain by standing on paper towels with occasional tapping for 1 min. Wash three times by filling each well with Buffer A, leaving for 2 min at room temperature and draining as described above. Dilute the conjugate in 1% BSA in Buffer A. The optimal dilution (of the order of 10^3–10^4 times) must be ascertained by experiment.

Add 200 µl of diluted horseradish peroxidase conjugate to each well and leave the covered plate for a further 2 h at room temperature. Wash three times with Buffer A. Add 200 µl of substrate solution to each well. Incubate the plate for 30 min in the dark. Stop the reaction by adding 50 µl of 4 M sulphuric acid to each well. Read the absorbance at 492 nm within 30 min, using an automatic plate reader. Alternatively, transfer 200 µl from each well to a tube containing 800 µl of water and read the absorbance in a spectrophotometer.

Calculation of results

Calculate the mean absorbance for each point on the standard curve and plot against ferritin concentration using semilogarithmic paper. Read concentrations for the serum from this curve. If results are captured on a file and calculated with a computer program, the log-logit plot provides a linear dose response. For serum ferritin concentrations >200 µg/l, re-assay at a dilution of 100 times or greater. Control sera should be included in each assay.

Selecting an assay method

The following notes may be of use for those considering introducing the ferritin assay into a clinical laboratory by purchasing a commercially available kit.

1. Limit of detection. For some early radio-immunoassays, the limits of detection approached 10 µg/l and this caused difficulties in using the assay for detection of iron deficiency. Most current assays have a lower limit of about 1 µg/l.

2. The 'high-dose hook'. This is a problem peculiar to labelled antibody assays, particularly two-site immunoradiometric assays.[8,9] This causes sera with very high ferritin concentrations to give anomalous readings in the lower part of the standard curve. Most current commercial assays are not affected. Because of the wide range of serum ferritin concentrations which may be encountered in hospital patients (0–40 000 µg/l), it is good practice to dilute and re-assay any samples giving readings above the working range of the assay.

3. Interference by non-ferritin proteins in serum. This may occur with any method but particularly with labelled antibody assays. Serum proteins may inhibit the binding of ferritin to the solid phase when compared with the binding in buffer solution alone. Such an effect may be avoided by diluting the standards in a buffer containing a suitable serum or by diluting serum samples as much as possible. For example, in the assay described above, the sample is diluted 20 times with buffer. Another cause of error, which is difficult to detect, is interference by anti-immunoglobulin antibodies.[10] These antibodies bind to the animal immunoglobulins used to detect the antigen and form artefactual 'sandwiches'. Such antibodies are found in about 10% of patients and normal subjects. Interference may be reduced by adding the appropriate species of animal immunoglobulins to block the cross-reaction but this is not always successful.[11] One solution is to use antibodies from different species as solid-phase and then the labelled antibodies. Thus one may use a polyclonal, rabbit antiferritin to coat plates in the ELISA with a polyclonal sheep antiferritin labelled with horseradish peroxidase as the second antibody. Rabbit serum (0.5%) replaces BSA in buffer B.

4. Reproducibility. Most assays are satisfactory, but this must always be established for any method introduced into the laboratory. With microtitre plate assays there may be 'edge' effects (differences between readings for inner and outer wells).

5. Dilution of serum samples. It should be established that both standard and serum samples dilute in parallel over a 100-fold range.

6. Accuracy. The use of the WHO standard ferritin preparation is recommended (see above).

Evaluation reports of various immuno-assay systems are available from the Medical Devices Agency (Hannibal House, London SE1 6TQ) for the following systems: Abbott Imx, Abbott AxSYM and Chiron ACS:180 (MDA/97/41), Roche Elecsys 2010 (MDA/98/56) and Wallac Auto DELFIA (MDA/00/32) Beckman Coulter

Access (MDA/00/18). All provide excellent assays for serum ferritin.

Interpretation of results

The use of serum ferritin for the assessment of iron stores has become well established.[12] In most normal adults, serum ferritin concentrations lie within the range 15–300 µg/l. During the first months of life, mean serum ferritin concentrations change considerably, reflecting changes in storage iron concentration. Concentrations are lower in children than in adults and from puberty to middle life are higher in men than in women. In adults, concentrations of <15 µg/l indicate an absence of storage iron. Reference ranges quoted by kit manufacturers vary and this is partly due to the selection of 'normal' subjects. Sometimes subjects with iron-deficiency anaemia are included and sometimes they are excluded. The interpretation of serum concentration in many pathological conditions is less straightforward, but concentrations of less than 15 µg/l indicate depletion of storage iron. In children, mean levels of storage iron are lower and a threshold of 12 µg/l has been found to be appropriate for detecting iron deficiency.[13]

Iron overload causes high concentrations of serum ferritin but these may also be found in patients with liver disease, infection, inflammation or malignant disease. Careful consideration of the clinical evidence is required before it is concluded that a high serum ferritin concentration is primarily the result of iron overload and not due to tissue damage or enhanced synthesis of ferritin. A normal ferritin concentration provides good evidence against iron overload but does not exclude genetic haemochromatosis. This is because haemochromatosis is a late-onset condition and iron stores may remain within the normal range for many years.

Serum ferritin concentrations are high in patients with advanced haemochromatosis but the serum ferritin estimation should not be used alone to screen the relatives of patients or to assess re-accumulation of storage iron after phlebotomy. This is because the early stages of iron accumulation are detectable by a decreased unsaturated iron-binding capacity and increased transferrin saturation although the serum ferritin concentration may be within the normal range. In this situation the measurement of serum iron and total iron-binding capacity provides useful clinical information not given by the ferritin assay.

In patients with acute or chronic disease, interpretation of serum ferritin concentrations is less straightforward[14] and patients may have serum ferritin concentrations of up to 100 µg/l despite an absence of stainable iron in the bone marrow. There is evidence that ferritin synthesis[15] is enhanced by interleukin-1 – the primary mediator of the acute phase response. In patients with chronic disease, the following approach should be adopted: low serum ferritin concentrations indicate absent iron stores, values within the normal range either low or normal levels, and high values indicate either normal or high levels. In terms of adequacy of iron stores for replenishing haemoglobin in anaemic patients, the degree of anaemia must also be considered. Thus a patient with a haemoglobin concentration of 100 g/l may benefit from iron therapy if the serum ferritin concentration is <100 µg/l, as below this level there is unlikely to be sufficient iron available for full regeneration. Here measurement of serum transferrin receptor concentration may be of value (see p. 124).

Immunologically, plasma ferritin resembles the 'L-rich' ferritins of liver and spleen and only low concentrations are detected with antibodies to heart or HeLa cell ferritin, ferritins rich in 'H' subunits. The heterogeneity of serum ferritin on isoelectric focusing is largely due to glycosylation and the presence of variable numbers of sialic acid residues and not variation in the ratio of H to L subunits.[16] Attempts to assay for 'acidic' (or 'H'-rich) isoferritins in serum as tumour markers have not been successful.[17,18] The iron content of serum ferritin is low[12] and its measurement is not diagnostically useful.[19]

SERUM IRON

ESTIMATION OF SERUM IRON

Introduction

Iron is carried in the plasma bound to the protein transferrin (mol mass 80 000). This molecule binds two atoms of Fe^{3+} and delivers iron to cells by interaction with the membrane transferrin receptor.

The method below is a modification of that recommended by the International Committee for

Standardization in Haematology (ICSH) and is based on the development of a coloured complex when ferrous iron is treated with a chromagen solution.[20]

Reagents and materials

All reagents must be of analytical grade with the lowest obtainable iron content.

Preparation of glassware. It is essential to avoid contamination by iron. If possible, use disposable plastic tubes and bottles. If glassware is to be used, wash in a detergent solution; soak in 2 mol/l HCl for 12 h and finally rinse in iron-free water.

Protein precipitant. 100 g/l trichloracetic acid (0.61 M) and 30 ml/l thioglycollic acid in 1 mol/l HCl. This solution may be stored in the dark for 2 months. Ascorbic acid is an alternative reducing agent although there may be more interference from copper.[19] However, any benefit from reduced copper interference is outweighed by the associated health and safety problems of working with thioglycollic acid. To 45 ml 1 mol/l HCl in a 50 ml screw-cap tube add 5 ml 6.1 mol/l trichloracetic acid solution (Sigma 490–10). Add 200 mg ascorbic acid and mix. Make a fresh solution when required and discard after 4 h.

Chromogen solution. In 100 ml 1.5 mol/l sodium acetate dissolve 25 mg of ferrozine (monosodium 3-(2-pyridyl)-5, 6-bis(4-phenylsulphonic acid)-1, 2, 4-triazine). Store in the dark for up to 4 weeks.

Iron Standard 80 μmol/l. Add 22.10 ml of deionized water in a universal container (the easiest way is by weight). Add 200 μl 2 mol/l HCl and mix. Add 100 μl of Iron Standard Solution (1000 μg Fe/ml in 1% HCl, Aldrich No. 30, 595–2) and mix. Store for up to 2 months at room temperature.

Iron-free water. Use deionized water for the preparation of all solutions.

Method

Place 0.5 ml of serum (free of haemolysis), 0.5 ml of working iron standard and 0.5 ml of iron-free water (as a blank), respectively, in each of three 1.5 ml plastic Eppendorf tubes with lids. Add 0.5 ml of protein precipitant to each and replace the lid. Mix the contents vigorously, e.g. with a vortex mixer, and allow to stand for 5 min. Centrifuge the tube containing the serum at 13 000 g for 4 min (in a microfuge) to obtain an optically clear supernatant. To 0.5 ml of this supernatant, and to 0.5 ml of each of the other mixtures add 0.5 ml of the chromogen solution with thorough mixing. After standing for 10 min, measure the absorbance in a spectrophotometer against water at 562 nm. If a microfuge is not available, use double the volume of serum and reagents in a 3 ml plastic tube with lid and centrifuge at 1500 g for 15 min in a bench centrifuge.

If EDTA-plasma is used, the colour develops more slowly and the preparation should be allowed to stand for at least 15 min before measuring the absorbance. The use of EDTA-plasma is not recommended. Iron chelators such as desferrioxamine also delay colour development.[21]

Calculation

$$\text{Serum iron } (\mu mol/l) = \frac{(A_{562} \text{ test} - A_{562} \text{ blank})}{(A_{562} \text{ standard} - A_{562} \text{ blank})} \times 80$$

The method described by the ICSH (Expert Panel on Iron) specifies thioglycollic acid as a reducing agent. This reduces possible interference by copper.

ALTERNATIVE PROCEDURE: SERUM IRON WITHOUT PROTEIN PRECIPITATION

This is a microtitre plate method developed from the assay of Persijn et al.[22]

Reagents and materials

Iron Standard. 80 μmol/l (see above). Dilute with an equal volume of water to make the 40 μmol/l standard

Phosphate–ascorbate buffer (stock). Add approx. 200 ml of deionized water to an acid-washed plastic beaker. Add 17.5 g sodium dihydrogen orthophosphate ($NaH_2PO_2 2H_2O$) to the water and dissolve fully by stirring (plastic stirrer). Adjust the pH to 5.0 using 2M NaOH solution (2 g NaOH in 25 ml water). Make the volume up to 250 ml and add 25 ml of the buffer to ten universal containers. Store for up to 1 month at room temperature. Prior to use, add 50 mg of ascorbic acid to each universal container required and shake to dissolve. Discard after 4 h.

Chromogen solution. Dissolve 50 mg of ferrozine (see p. 120) in 25 ml deionized water and shake to dissolve. Store for up to 1 month in the dark.

Microtitre trays. Optical grade, with flat-bottomed wells.

Control serum. Suitable control sera are Lyphochek (Biorad).

Method

Add 80 µl of deionized water ('0') standard solution (40, 80), controls (C1, C2) and samples (S1, S2 etc.) to the microtitre plate.

Plate map

Add 80 µl of phospate-ascorbate buffer to each well, using a multi-channel pipette. Tap the tray to mix. Leave for 20 min. During this time take an initial absorbance reading of the tray at 560–570 nm on a microtitre plate reader. Add 40 µl of chromagen solution to each well, then tap the tray to mix. Cover with a film or lid. Incubate for 40 min at 37°C. Take a second absorbance reading. Calculate the net absorbance values.

Calculations

Calculate the difference in Absorbance (A) between the final and initial readings for each standard (A_{40} A_{80}) and serum (A_{sample}).

The approximate values are 0.015–0.03 for the water blank (zero standard) and 0.25–0.28 for the 40 µmol Fe/l standard. Subtract the mean net value of the zero standard (A_0) (final − initial reading) from each standard or sample (A_{sample}). The net value of the 80 µmol/l standard should be 2 × that of the 40 µmol/l standard.

Serum iron concentrations are:

$$\frac{A_{sample} - A_0}{A_{40} - A_0} \times 40 \ \mu mol/l$$

The data may be downloaded from the plate reader and imported into a suitable statistical program, e.g. Minitab or Excel, for these calculations.

Automated methods

Procedures for measuring serum iron are available for most clinical chemistry analysers. Their performance was reviewed by Tietz et al[23] who found differences between the various methods particularly at low values of serum iron concentration. Serum iron concentrations may also be measured by atomic absorption spectroscopy but this has the disadvantage of measuring any haem iron present as a result of haemolysis.

SERUM IRON CONCENTRATIONS IN HEALTH AND DISEASE[21]

Jacobs et al[24] measured serum iron concentrations in a random sample of 517 women and 499 men in the general population. Serum iron concentrations approximate to a normal distribution. The mean (± SD) of 16.1 ± 7.4 µmol/l in women is slightly lower than in men (18.0 ± 6.3 µmol/l). These figures do not refer to 'iron replete'

	1	2	3	4	5	6	7	8	9	10	11	12
A	0	80	C1	S1	S5	S9	S13	S17	S21	S25	S29	S33
B	0	80	C1	S1	S5	S9	S13	S17	S21	S25	S29	S33
C	0	80	C1	S2	S6	S10	S14	S18	S22	S26	S30	S34
D	0	80	C1	S2	S6	S10	S14	S18	S22	S26	S30	S34
E	40	0	C2	S3	S7	S11	S15	S19	S23	S27	S31	S35
F	40	0	C2	S3	S7	S11	S15	S19	S23	S27	S31	S35
G	40	0	C2	S4	S8	S12	S16	S20	S24	S28	S32	S36
H	40	0	C2	S4	S8	S12	S16	S20	S24	S28	S32	S36

Plate map

subjects, as subjects with absent iron stores or with frank anaemia are included. In the first month of life mean concentration of serum iron is higher (22 µmol/l) than in adults, falls to about 12 µmol/l by the age of 1 year, and remains at that level throughout childhood.[25,26]

Measurement of the serum iron concentration alone provides little useful clinical information because, although methodological variation is low, there is considerable variation from hour to hour

and day to day in normal individuals.[13] Low concentrations are found in patients with iron-deficiency anaemia, in chronic disease (including inflammation, infection and cancer) and during acute phase response, including after surgery. Low serum iron concentrations do not, therefore, necessarily indicate an absence of storage iron. High concentrations are found in liver disease, hypoplastic anaemias, ineffective erythropoiesis and iron overload.

IRON-BINDING CAPACITY, SERUM TRANSFERRIN AND TRANSFERRIN SATURATION

TOTAL IRON-BINDING CAPACITY

In the plasma, iron is bound to transferrin and the total iron-binding capacity (TIBC) is a measure of this protein. The additional iron-binding capacity of transferrin is known as the 'unsaturated iron-binding capacity' (UIBC). The serum iron concentration plus the UIBC together give TIBC.

Iron-binding capacity is usually measured by adding an excess of iron and measuring the iron retained in solution after the addition of a suitable reagent such as light magnesium carbonate, or an ion-exchange resin which removes excess iron. All methods are empirical, and none is completely satisfactory. The method described below was developed by the ICSH.[26]

ESTIMATION OF TOTAL IRON-BINDING CAPACITY

Principle. Excess iron as ferric chloride is added to serum. Any iron which does not bind to transferrin is removed with excess magnesium carbonate. The iron concentration of the iron-saturated serum is then measured.

Reagents

Basic magnesium carbonate, $MgCO_3$, 'light grade'.

Saturating solution (100 µmol Fe/l). Add 17.7 ml deionized water to a universal container (by weight is most convenient). Add 100 µl 1 mol/l HCl. Add 100 µl of iron Standard Solution (1000 µg Fe/ml in 1% HCl, (see p. 120)). Mix and store for up to 2 months at room temperature.

The 'saturating iron solution' contains 5.6 µg Fe/ml (100 µmol Fe/l).

Method

Place 0.5 ml of serum (EDTA-plasma should not be used) in a 1.5 ml Eppendorf tube and add 0.5 ml of saturating iron solution. Mix carefully by hand and leave at room temperature for 15 min. Use a plastic scoop or tube to add 100 mg (± 15 mg) of light magnesium carbonate and cap the tube. Shake vigorously and allow to stand for 30 min with occasional mixing. Centrifuge at 13 000 *g* for 4 min (microfuge). If the supernatant contains traces of magnesium carbonate, remove the supernatant and recentrifuge. Carefully remove 0.5 ml of the supernatant and treat as serum for the iron estimation described above. Multiply the final result by 2.

DETERMINATION OF UNSATURATED IRON-BINDING CAPACITY

The UIBC may be determined by methods which detect iron remaining, and able to bind to chromogen, after adding a standard and excess amount of iron to the serum.[22] The UIBC is the difference between the amount added and the amount binding to the chromogen.

Reagents and materials

Saturating solution 2000 µmol/l Add 7.95 ml of deionized water to a universal container (by weight is most convenient). Add 1.0 ml of Iron Standard Solution (1000 µg Fe/ml in 1% HCl (see p. 120)). Mix. Store for up to 2 months at room temperature.

Tris–ascorbate–iron buffer (stock) Add approx. 200 ml of deionized water to a weighed acid-washed plastic beaker. Add 6.8 g tris to the water and fully dissolve by stirring with a plastic stirrer. Adjust the pH to 7.8 using 2M HCl. Adjust the volume to 250 ml using water (by weight), mix, and add 24.5 ml (24.5 g) into universal containers. Store for up to 1 month at room temperature. Prior to use, add 50 mg of ascorbic acid to each universal container required and dissolve by mixing, then add 0.5 ml of the saturating solution. Discard after 4 h.

Chromogen solution. See page 121.

Microtitre trays. See page 121.

Control serum. See page 121.

Method

Add 80 µl of deionized water ('0'), control (C1, C2) and sample (S1, S2 etc.) to the microtitre plate.

Add 160 µl of tris–ascorbate–iron buffer to each well, using a multi-channel pipette. Tap the tray to mix. Leave the tray for 20 min. During this time, take an initial reading $A_{initial}$ of the $A^{560–570\,nm}$. Add 40 µl of chromogen solution to each sample and tap the tray to mix; and cover with a film or lid. Incubate for 40 min at 37°C. Take a final absorbance reading (A_{final}).

Calculations

The saturating solution added to each well (160 µl) contains 6.4 nmol Fe. Calculate the absorbance reading corresponding to 6.4 nmol Fe from the mean value of the readings in column 1 as $A_{final} - A_{initial}$ (A_s). This absorbance value may be compared with the serum iron 40 µmol/l standard value (from the iron determination). Divide A_s by the net 40 µmol/l standard reading and then multiply by 40 (see p. 121). The figure obtained should be 75–80 µmol/l.

Once A_s has been calculated, it is used in the following equation:

For controls 1 & 2 and samples, UIBC =

$$\frac{[1 - (A_{final} - A_{initial})]}{A_s} \times 80\ \mu mol/l$$

As with the serum iron determination, data may be imported into a statistical program for calculation. As with the serum iron determination, protocols for clinical chemistry analysers sometimes include a method for UIBC.

Determination of total iron-binding capacity

TIBC = serum iron + UIBC (µmol/l)

SERUM TRANSFERRIN

An alternative approach is to measure transferrin directly by an immunological assay. This avoids some of the spuriously high values of TIBC found when the transferrin is saturated and non-

	1	2	3	4	5	6	7	8	9	10	11	12
A	0	C1	S1	S5	S9	S13	S17	S21	S25	S29	S33	S37
B	0	C1	S1	S5	S9	S13	S17	S21	S25	S29	S33	S37
C	0	C1	S2	S6	S10	S14	S18	S22	S26	S30	S34	S38
D	0	C1	S2	S6	S10	S14	S18	S22	S26	S30	S34	S38
E	0	C2	S3	S7	S11	S15	S19	S23	S27	S31	S35	S39
F	0	C2	S3	S7	S11	S15	S19	S23	S27	S31	S35	S39
G	0	C2	S4	S8	S12	S16	S20	S24	S28	S32	S36	S40
H	0	C2	S4	S8	S12	S16	S20	S24	S28	S32	S36	S40

Plate map

therefore be directly compared. Changes in normal range with age have been described by Choi et al.[37] Concentrations decline from birth to adulthood but do not differ significantly between male and female subjects.

Performance

Åkesson et al[38] evaluated the Orion, Ramco and R&D kits. They found acceptable intra-assay variation but regression analysis of serum samples showed a lower comparability for Orion compared to the other two kits.

Worwood et al[39] found similar imprecision but noted some assay drift particularly for the R&D assay. Kuiperkramer et al,[40] Åkesson et al[41] and Worwood et al[39] all comment on the differences in both units and absolute amounts for serum transferrin receptor concentrations. For the four kits evaluated, there are four different units (nmol/l, µg/ml, mg/l, kU/l) and four different normal ranges (despite the equivalence of µg/ml and mg/l).

Samples. The information provided by the manufacturers shows good recovery of standard and linearity, but some problems with interference. Although serum is the preferred matrix, the R&D and Ramco assays give the same results with EDTA, heparin and citrate plasma. Orion state that EDTA-plasma is not acceptable. It is recommended that sera are stored for no more than 2 days at room temperature, 7 days at 2–8°C, 6 months at –20°C and 1 year at –70°C. Repeated freezing and thawing are not advisable. Moderate haemolysis is not a problem. There is no interference at serum bilirubin concentrations of <1700 µmol/l (R&D) or 280 µmol/l (Orion). However, Ramco noted that addition of bilirubin at a concentration of 17 µmol/l (10 µg/ml) caused a 16% increase in apparent serum transferrin receptor concentration. This represents a bilirubin concentration of only about twice the upper limit of normal.

Transferrin receptors in diagnosis
Erythropoiesis. The function of the transferrin receptor in delivering iron to the immature red cell immediately suggested an application in the clinical laboratory for the assay of circulating transferrin receptors. The use of the assay to monitor changes in the rate of erythropoiesis has been explored.[33]

Iron deficiency. The major application of the serum transferrin receptor assay has been to detect patients with an absence of stored iron (ferritin and haemosiderin in cells). Not only are circulating transferrin receptor levels raised in patients with simple iron deficiency but also in patients with the anaemia of chronic disease who lack stainable iron in the bone marrow and may not have sufficient iron to regenerate a normal haemoglobin level even when the process of chronic inflammation, infection or cancer has ended.[32] Detection of a lack of storage iron has been difficult in patients with the anaemia of chronic disease because serum iron concentrations are low regardless of iron stores and serum ferritin concentrations, although reflecting the level of iron stores, are higher than in patients not suffering from chronic disease.[42] However, there is less correlation between bone marrow iron stores and serum transferrin receptor levels for more heterogeneous groups of patients.[43,44]

Serum transferrin receptor measurements have also been shown to provide a sensitive indicator of iron deficiency in pregnancy although questions remain about the decreased erythropoiesis in early pregnancy as this may mask iron deficiency at this time.[38] Van den Broek et al[45] found that measurement of serum transferrin receptors did not enhance the sensitivity and specificity for the detection of iron-deficiency anaemia in pregnant women from Malawi where anaemia and chronic disease are very prevalent.

Iron overload. Huebers et al[46] and Baynes et al[47] reported normal concentrations of serum transferrin receptors in patients with genetic haemochromatosis (although some had been venesected) and also in African iron overload.[47] In contrast, Khumalo et al[48] and Looker et al[49] found lower mean values of serum transferrin receptors in subjects with a raised transferrin saturation. However, there was considerable overlap with the normal range of serum transferrin receptor concentration and measurement of serum transferrin receptors in iron overload is unlikely to be of diagnostic value.

Acknowledgment. I am grateful to Kymberley Carter and Richard Ellis for their work in developing the microtitre plate assays for serum iron and UIBC.

REFERENCES

1 Addison GM, Beamish MR, Hales CN, et al 1972 An immunoradiometric assay for ferritin in the serum of normal subjects and patients with iron deficiency and iron overload. Journal of Clinical Pathology 25:326–329.

2 Miles LEM, Lipschitz DA, Bieber CP, et al 1974 Measurement of serum ferritin by a 2-site immunoradiometric assay. Analytical Biochemistry 61:209–224.

3 Worwood M 1980 Serum ferritin. In: JD Cook JD (ed) Methods in Haematology. Churchill Livingstone, New York, vol 1:59.

4 International Committee for Standardization in Haematology (Expert Panel on Iron) 1985 Proposed international standard human ferritin for the serum ferritin assay. British Journal of Haematology 61:61–63.

5 Dresser DW 1986 Immunization of experimental animals. In: Weir DM (ed) Handbook of Experimental Immunology Vol 1: Immunocytochemistry. Blackwell Science, Oxford, p. 8.1–8.21.

6 Johnson GD, Holborow EJ 1986 Preparation and use of fluorochrome conjugates. In: Weir DM (ed) Handbook of Experimental Immunology Vol 1: Immunocytochemistry. Blackwell Science, Oxford, p. 28.1–28.21.

7 Wilson MB, Nakane PK 1978 Recent developments in the periodate method of conjugating horseradish peroxidase (HRPO) to antibodies. In: Knapp W, Houlbar K, Wick G (eds) Immunoflurescence and related staining techniques. Elsevier/North-Holland, Amsterdam, p 215–224.

8 Perera P, Worwood M 1984 Antigen binding in the two-site immunoradiometric assay for serum ferritin: the nature of the hook effect. Annals of Clinical Biochemistry 21:393–397.

9 Robard D, Feldman Y, Jaffe ML, et al 1978 Kinetics of two-site immunoradiometric ('sandwich') assays – II. Studies on the nature of the 'high-dose hook' effects. Immunochemistry 15:77–82.

10 Boscato LM, Stuart MC 1988 Heterophillic antibodies: a problem for all immunoassays. Clinical Chemistry 34:27–33.

11 Zweig MH, Csako G, Benson CC, et al 1987 Interference by anti-immunoglobulin G antibodies in immunoradiometric assays of thyrotropin involving mouse monoclonal antibodies. Clinical Chemistry 33:840–844.

12 Worwood M 1982 Ferritin in human tissues and serum. Clinics in Haematology 11:275.

13 British Nutrition Foundation 1995 Iron: nutritional and physiological significance. Chapman and Hall, London, p 23–32.

14 Witte DL 1991 Can serum ferritin be effectively interpreted in the presence of the acute-phase response? Clinical Chemistry 37:484–485.

15 Rogers JT, Bridges KR, Durmowiez GP, et al 1990 Translational control during the acute phase response. Journal of Biological Chemistry 265:14572–14578.

16 Worwood M 1986 Serum ferritin (Editorial review). Clinical Science 70:215–220.

17 Cavanna F, Ruggeri G, Iacobello C, et al 1983 Development of a monoclonal antibody against human heart ferritin and its application in an immunoradiometric assay. Clinica Chimica Acta 134:347–356.

18 Jones BM, Worwood M, Jacobs A 1980 Serum ferritin in patients with cancer: determination with antibodies to HeLa cell and spleen ferritin. Clinica Chimica Acta 106:203–214.

19 Neilsen P, Günther U, Dürken M, Fischer R, Düllmann J 2000 Serum ferritin iron in iron oveload and liver damage: correlation to body iron stores and diagnostic relevance. Journal of Laboratory and Clinical medicine 135: 413–418.

20 International Committee for Standardization in Haematology (Expert Panel on Iron) 1990 Revised recommendations for the measurement of serum iron in human blood. British Journal of Haematology 75:615–616.

21 Bothwell TH, Charlton RW, Cook JD, et al 1979 Iron metabolism in man. Blackwell Scientific, Oxford.

22 Persijn J-P, van der Slik W, Riethorst A 1971 Determination of serum iron and latent iron-binding capacity (LIBC). Clinical Chimica Acta 35:91–98.

23 Tietz NW, Rinker AD, Morrison SR 1996 When is a serum iron really a serum iron? A follow-up study on the status of iron measurements in serum. Clinical Chemistry 42:109–111.

24 Jacobs A, Waters WE, Campbell H, et al 1969 A random sample from Wales. III. Serum iron, iron binding capacity and transferrin saturation. British Journal of Haematology 17:581–587.

25 Koerper MA, Dallman PR 1977 Serum iron concentration and transferrin saturation in the diagnosis of iron deficiency in children: normal development changes. Journal of Pediatrics 91:870–874.

26 Saarinen UM, Siimes MA 1977 Development changes in serum iron, total iron-binding capacity, and transferrin saturation in infancy. Journal of Pediatrics 91:875–877.

27 International Committee for Standardization in Haematology 1978 The measurement of total and unsaturated iron-binding capacity in serum. British Journal of Haematology 38:281–290.

28 Beilby J, Olynyk J, Ching S, et al. 1992 Transferrin index: an alternative method for calculating the iron saturation of transferrin. Clinical Chemistry 38:2078–2081.

29 Huebers HA, Eng MJ, Josephson BM, et al 1987 Plasma iron and transferrin iron-binding capacity evaluated by colorimetric and immunoprecipitation methods. Clinical Chemistry 33:273–277.

30 Bandi ZL, Schoen I, Bee DE 1985 Immunochemical methods for measurement of transferrin in serum: effects of analytical errors and inappropriate reference intervals on diagnostic utility. Clinical Chemistry 31:1601–1605.

31 Bainton DF, Finch CA 1964 The diagnosis of iron deficiency anemia. American Journal of Medicine 37:62–70.

32 Edwards CQ, Kushner JP 1993 Current concepts – screening for hemochromatosis. New England Journal of Medicine 328:1616.

33 Feelders RA, Kuiperkramer EPA, Van Eijk HG 1999 Structure, function and clinical significance of transferrin receptors. Clinical Chemistry and Laboratory Medicine 37:1–10.

34 Klausner R, Rouault TA, Hartford JB 1993 Regulating the fate of mRNA: the control of cellular iron metabolism. Cell 72:19–28.

35 Kohgo Y, Niitsu Y, Kondo H, et al 1987 Serum transferrin receptor as a new index of erythropoiesis. Blood 70: 1955–1958.

36 Cook JD, Skikne BS, Baynes RD 1993 Serum transferrin receptor. Annual Review of Medicine 44:63–74.

37 Choi JW, Pai SH, Im MW, et al 1999 Change in transferrin receptor concentrations with age. Clinical Chemistry 45:1562–1563.

38 Åkesson A, Bjellerup P, Berglund M, et al 1998 Serum transferrin receptor: a specific marker of iron deficiency in pregnancy. American Journal of Clinical Nutrition 68:1241–1246.

39 Worwood M, Ellis RD, Bain BJ 2000 Evaluation report: serum transferrin receptor assays. MDA/00/09. Medical Devices Agency, London.

40 Kuiperkramer EPA, Huisman CMS, VanRaan J, et al 1996 Analytical and clinical implications of soluble transferrin receptors in serum. European Journal of Clinical Chemistry and Clinical Biochemistry 34:645–649.

41 Åkesson A, Bjellerup P, Vahter M 1999 Evaluation of kits for measurement of the soluble transferrin receptor. Scandinavian Journal of Clinical and Laboratory Investigation 59:77–81.

42 Worwood M 1997 Influence of disease on iron status. Proceedings of the Nutrition Society 56:409–419.

43 Means RT, Allen J, Sears DA, et al 1999 Serum soluble transferrin receptor and the prediction of marrow iron results in a heterogeneous group of patients. Clinical and Laboratory Haematology 21:161–167.

44 Worwood M, Darke C 1993 Serum ferritin, blood donation, iron stores and haemochromatosis. Transfusion Medicine 3:21.

45 Van den Broek NR, Letsky EA, White SA, et al 1998 Iron status in pregnant women: which measurements are valid? British Journal of Haematology 103:817–824.

46 Huebers HA, Beguin Y, Pootrakul P, et al 1990 Intact transferrin receptors in human plasma and their relation to erythropoiesis. Blood 75:102–107.

47 Baynes RD, Cook JD, Bothwell TH et al 1994 Serum transferrin receptor in hereditary hemochromatosis and African siderosis. American Journal of Hematology 45:288–292.

48 Khumalo H, Gomo ZAR, Moyo VM, et al 1998 Serum transferrin receptors are decreased in the presence of iron overload. Clinical Chemistry 44:40–44.

49 Looker AC, Loyevsky M, Gordeuk VR 1999 Increased serum transferrin saturation is associated with lower serum transferrin receptor concentration. Clinical Chemistry 45:2191–2199.

8

Investigation of megaloblastic anaemia

Roger J. Amos

INTRODUCTION

Megaloblastic anaemia can be suspected from the presence in a blood film of oval, macrocytic red cells, pear-shaped poikilocytes or hypersegmented neutrophils with >5 nuclear lobes. The latter may be difficult to recognize in neutropenic patients or in those with severe infection. However, the first indication of the diagnosis in many cases is the finding of a raised mean cell volume, often without anaemia. There are many other conditions which may produce a macrocytosis apart from megaloblastic anaemia, including myelodysplasia, aplastic anaemia and other primary bone marrow disorders, excess alcohol intake, hypothyroidism and a young red cell population secondary to haemolysis or acute blood loss; it is important to remember also that a peripheral blood macrocytosis may be masked by concomitant iron deficiency or thalassaemia trait. A bone marrow aspirate is always useful but, is particularly important in mild or doubtful cases, confirming the diagnosis of megaloblastic anaemia by the presence of megaloblasts and giant metamyelocytes. It is noteworthy that megaloblastosis may be partially or completely concealed by iron deficiency and megaloblasts may also be seen in some rare, inherited disorders, such as orotic aciduria or the Lesch–Nyhan syndrome and may follow treatment with cytotoxic drugs including cytosine arabinoside, hydroxyurea and methotrexate.

The assay of serum cobalamin (vitamin B_{12}) together with serum and red cell folate provides the additional evidence for a firm diagnosis to be made and allows identification of the specific vitamin deficiency. The serum B_{12} assay is particularly important in the diagnosis of vitamin B_{12} neuropathy, as this is often associated with little haematological abnormality. As will be discussed, other factors may affect the measured levels of vitamin B_{12} and folate apart from their tissue concentration; it is important therefore that vitamin assays are not interpreted in isolation but in the light of other clinical and haematological data. Depletion of vitamin B_{12} bound to transcobalamin II (TC II) occurs early in B_{12} deficiency[1] and an assay of TC II bound B_{12} may help clarify the significance of equivocal serum B_{12} levels; however, a sensitive assay is required to reliably measure the small amounts of vitamin B_{12} involved.

The deoxyuridine (dU) suppression test is a specific and sensitive indicator of both vitamin B_{12} and folate deficiency[2] and may be abnormal before obvious morphological changes develop.[3] When performed at the same time as a bone marrow aspirate, it provides rapid confirmation of 'biochemical megaloblastosis' and also indicates which vitamin deficiency is present.

Serum methylmalonic acid and homocysteine are both increased in vitamin B_{12} deficiency when their measurement is a sensitive marker of B_{12} depletion,[4] and serum homocysteine is increased in folate deficiency. Previously, measurement of the accumulation of these substrates involved their assay in urine by colorimetric, chromatographic or enzymatic techniques, with or without oral preloading. However, there was considerable overlap between deficient and normal patients and the methods were of limited diagnostic use. The development of sensitive techniques to measure the small quantities of these metabolites in serum using gas chromatography–mass spectrometry or high-pressure liquid chromatography has renewed interest in their clinical use. When measured by a sensitive technique, metabolite concentrations can be used for the primary diagnosis of a deficiency state, to distinguish between vitamin B_{12} and folate deficiency and to monitor the response to treatment.[5] Current methodologies are not suitable for general laboratory use and will not be discussed further here; however, it is likely that automated, more generally applicable methods, will be available in the near future when these assays will become important diagnostic tools in the investigation of megaloblastic anaemia.

Having made the diagnosis of vitamin B_{12} or folate deficiency, the elucidation of the cause of the deficiency state depends both on the clinical picture and on the results of laboratory tests. For B_{12} deficiency, these include measurement of the absorption of vitamin B_{12}, other tests of intestinal absorption, the demonstration of antibodies to intrinsic factor or gastric parietal cells, and measurement of gastric secretion of intrinsic factor. The estimation of serum B_{12} binding capacity and transcobalamins are occasionally helpful. For folate deficiency, if malabsorption is suspected, the presence of IgA endomyseal antibodies is a sensitive and specific marker for gluten-induced enteropathy, provided that IgA deficiency has been excluded; a jejunal biopsy may still be required in some cases. Features of splenic atrophy in the blood film, in the absence of a previous splenectomy, suggest gluten-induced enteropathy. If inborn errors involving the metabolic utilization of vitamin B_{12} or folate are suspected, assay of vitamin B_{12} or folate co-enzymes together with somatic cell complementation studies using cultured skin fibroblasts may be required to make a specific diagnosis.

A review by the British Committee for Standards in Haematology provides guidelines for the investigation of cobalamin and folate deficiencies.[6] In this chapter, the assay of serum vitamin

B_{12}, serum and red cell folate is considered first, followed by the dU suppression test and finally some of the tests to determine the cause of a particular deficiency state.

ASSAY OF SERUM VITAMIN B_{12}, SERUM AND RED CELL FOLATE

These vitamin assays remain the routine procedures for determining vitamin status. The original assays were based on the specific growth requirements of certain microorganisms, but these have been largely superseded by radiodilution assays and more recently by non-isotopic immunoassays. These different techniques will be discussed in turn.

MICROBIOLOGICAL ASSAYS

Principle of microbiological assay

Certain microorganisms (e.g. *Euglena gracilis* and *Lactobacillus casei*) require specific factors for growth which they cannot synthesize. The assay medium for *E. gracilis* contains all the essential growth factors, with the exception of B_{12} which is provided by the standards and test sera. The growth of the organism is directly proportional to the concentration of B_{12}. Likewise, *L. casei* requires folate, which is provided by the standards and test sera in the microbiological assay for folic acid. The microbiological assays are generally considered to be technically demanding and labour intensive, their turn-round times are comparatively long and the growth of the test organism may be inhibited by antibiotics or antimetabolites in the test sera. Nevertheless, they are suitable for the economic processing of large numbers of samples particularly utilizing semi-automated and microplate technology.[7]

Microbiological assay of serum vitamin B_{12}

Several methods are available, using *E. gracilis*, *Lactobacillus leichmannii*, *Escherichia coli* and *Ochromonas malhamensis*. The *E. gracilis* method is sensitive, accurate and especially suitable for the assay of a large number of specimens although it has been largely confined to use in centres with a particular interest in B_{12} metabolism.[8] It was the assay method chosen to assign a potency value to the British Standard for human serum B_{12}[9] and is described in the sixth edition of this book.

Microbiological assay of serum and red cell folate

The folate activity of serum is due mainly to the presence of 5-methyltetrahydrofolate (methyl-THF). Because this compound is a growth requirement for *L. casei*, this organism is used for the assay of naturally occurring folates in serum and in red cells.

Methyl-THF is labile, but can be protected during assay with ascorbic acid.[10] Serum to which 5 mg/ml of ascorbic acid has been added can be stored at –20°C for up to 2 months without loss of folate activity. Haemolysis must be avoided when serum is separated because red cells contain 30 times more folic acid than serum; as a result, even minimal haemolysis will increase the serum folate concentration significantly. The presence of lysis in a plasma sample can be readily determined and quantified with the low haemoglobin Hemocue (se p. 152).

The assay of red cell folate is critically dependent on pre-analytic variables, particularly the preparation and storage of the haemolysate. Consistency and attention to detail are essential for accurate results.[11] Whole blood anticoagulated with EDTA, can be stored for up to 1 week at 4°C before the haemolysate is made. The lysate is prepared by adding 0.1 ml of whole blood, of known packed cell volume, to 1.9 ml of 10 g/l freshly prepared, aqueous ascorbic acid, with incubation for 60 min at 20°C or room temperature, in the dark. The ascorbate not only preserves folate but the low pH (approximately 4.6) allows the polyglutamate forms of folate to be deconjugated by plasma folate polyglutamate hydrolase. Folate activity can either be assayed straight away or the haemolysate can be stored at 4°C and assayed within 24 h without loss of activity. The lysate may be stored for up to 5 months at –20°C although a single freeze–thaw cycle does result in some loss of activity.

One of the major disadvantages of microbiological assay is that antibiotics or antimetabolites may inhibit the growth of the assay microorganism. The growth of *L. casei*[12d] is inhibited by penicillins, tetracycline, erythromycin, streptomycin, lincomycin, rifampicin, trimethoprim and sulphonamides. Methotrexate and pyrimethamine also inhibit the assay. However, alkylating agents do not usually inhibit the assay at conventional doses whereas some antimetabolites, e.g. cytosine arabinoside and hydroxyurea, do. Drug inhibition will depend on the dose as well as on the nature of the drug. Serious inhibition is evident if the growth of the organism is less in the test serum than in the blank (zero folic acid) standard tube; inhibition can also be detected by assay of a mixture of the patient's serum and a normal serum, or of a higher dilution of the patient's serum. Inhibition is rarely observed with haemolysate assays because of their higher dilution.

RADIOISOTOPE DILUTION ASSAYS

Principle of radioisotope dilution assays

A known amount of radioactive 'hot' analyte is diluted by the non-radioactive 'cold' analyte in the test serum, which has been released from any serum binders by heat or chemical means. A measured volume of the mixture of 'hot' and 'cold' analyte is bound to a binding protein, which is added in an amount insufficient to bind all the 'hot' analyte. The bound analyte is then separated from the free and its radioactivity counted. This count will be inversely proportional to the analyte concentration in the test serum, as the higher the analyte concentration in the test serum, the greater will be the dilution of the radioactively labelled analyte and thus less radioactivity will be attached to the binding protein. By comparison with standards of known analyte content, the analyte content of the serum can be calculated. Radionuclide methods have the advantage over microbiological assays in that they are simpler and more rapid and the results are unaffected by antibiotics and other drugs which may affect a microbiological assay organism. However, the strict regulations involving storage, use and disposal of radioactivity are a disadvantage.

Measurement of serum B_{12} by radioisotope dilution assay

Assay of serum B_{12} by radionuclide dilution (competitive binding) was first described over 40 years ago.[13] Many variations have since been reported and commercial kits have extended the use of the test. Radioimmunoassay which is sensitive and spe-

cific has been developed[14,15] using antibodies raised in rabbits against the monocarboxylic acid derivative of cyanocobalamin conjugated to human serum albumin. Donkey anti-rabbit gammaglobulin coated magnetic particles used to separate the bound from free B_{12} are an improvement.[16] The presence of intrinsic factor antibodies does not appear to affect the assays.[17] In many assays, only 200 µl of test material is required and it is possible to use serum or plasma from heparinized or EDTA-anticoagulated blood. Variations at each assay step can affect the results.

Extraction of B_{12} from serum transcobalamins

Boiling or autoclaving at an acid pH with removal of the protein precipitate by filtration or centrifugation was first used and is the most satisfactory method of extraction.[17,18] The pH of the extract does not require adjustment for a subsequent binding stage by intrinsic factor (IF). Denaturation of the transcobalamin serum binders by boiling at pH 9.2–11.7 or by treatment at room temperature with pH 12.9–13.0, without removal of the protein products, is used in many commercial methods, but with both techniques the residue gives a varying amount of non-specific binding (NSB) which may be excessive with certain test sera, e.g. those with high transcobalamin levels as in chronic myeloid leukaemia. Dithiothreitol (DTT) reduces NSB. The effect of NSB on the measured serum vitamin B_{12} concentration depends on the separation stage (see below). Alkaline extraction, by whatever method, will require subsequent adjustment of the pH to that optimal for the binding stage.

Binding agent

Vitamin B_{12} contains a nucleotide, 5,6-dimethylbenzimidazole, which is attached to the corrin ring through a ribose group and directly to the central cobalt atom. Corrinoids are compounds containing the corrin ring with either altered side chains and/or lacking the specific B_{12} nucleotide. They are commonly called B_{12} analogues and are microbiologically inactive. It is essential that the binding agents used in the assay system distinguish between vitamin B_{12} and vitamin B_{12} analogues.

IF of human or porcine origin is commonly used as the B_{12} binder. The IF may be purified (e.g. by affinity chromatography), or contaminating R binder may be rendered inactive by blocking with the addition of excess cobalamin analogue, e.g. cobinamide,[19] or the IF may be coupled to a solid phase carrier, prior to the assay, at a pH which prevents R binder uptake of vitamin B_{12}.[20] Carriers used include polyacrylamide beads, glass particles, microcrystalline cellulose and magnetic particles. All these methods improve the binding specificity of the IF. The specificity of pure and blocked IF can be demonstrated by the addition of $10\,\mu g/l$ cobinamide dicyanide (Sigma) to sera; cross-reactivity should be minimal with no significant increase in the assay value. Other binders which have been used instead of IF include normal human serum,[21] unsaturated TC I[22] and the R binders of saliva[23] and of chicken serum.[24] These, however, give higher results than when IF is used, estimating both B_{12} and the microbiologically inert cobalamin analogues, i.e. total corrinoids, whereas pure IF binds only cobalamins.[25,26] The first commercial kits used crude IF preparations, sometimes giving falsely normal results, attributed to such analogues.

B_{12} standards

For non-commercial methods, the pharmaceutical preparation of cyanocobalamin (Duncan Flockhart) $250\,\mu g/ml$ is satisfactory. The cobalamins in the test sera are converted to the cyano form during the extraction process. The standards usually range from 50 or 100 to $2000\,\mu g/l$. With heat extraction, aqueous standards are usually satisfactory, but a protein matrix, to 'balance' that of the test serum, is required for alkaline extracts. The *Biorad* standards containing B_{12} and folic acid in human serum albumin are suitable (see p. 136).

Radioisotope tracer

[57]Co-labelled cyanocobalamin is used in all methods. CN([57]Co) cobalamin, $0.05\,\mu g$ in 1 ml with activity 370–740 kBq, is available from Kodak Clinical Diagnostic Ltd (product number CT2). Good precision is required to diagnose B_{12} deficiency at the lower end of the normal reference range, and the amount of tracer added should be such that 40–50% is bound at this level.[27]

Separation of free from bound B_{12}

Charcoal coated with albumin or haemoglobin is used to separate free and bound B_{12} although it is messy and invariably takes up some bound B_{12}.[28] Alternative agents are Sephadex gel and DEAE-cellulose.[29,30] Following centrifugation, the supernatant containing the bound B_{12} is decanted into counting tubes without disturbing the deposit. Centrifugation in solid phase methods leaves the free B_{12} in the supernatant and the deposit in the assay tube is counted, sometimes after washing.[31] The removal of the supernatant calls for care and a standard technique. Tween 20 may enhance the pelleting of the deposit.[31] Bound [57]Co-B_{12} is counted because the bound B_{12} gives the highest counts at lower B_{12} concentrations. B_{12} bound non-specifically remains in the supernatant in the liquid systems, adds to the counts of that specifically bound and gives apparently lower serum B_{12} levels, whereas in solid phase systems the non-specifically bound B_{12} is discarded, giving apparently higher serum B_{12} levels. The zero standard will allow correction for NSB only when the protein content of the standards is the same as that in the test material.

Calculation of results

The bound B_{12} in the standards and test sera are counted in a γ-counter, a curve relating counts to B_{12} concentration in the standards is drawn and the unknowns are read from this. However, with the usual workload this needs to be done automatically or semi-automatically. Computerized programs are available with modern counters. The choice of methods for expressing results has been reviewed by Ekins.[32] The most popular is the percentage binding, $(B/B_0) \times 100$, where B is the count of the test serum and B_0 the count of the zero standard on the ordinate axis of logarithmic graph paper. The B_{12} concentration is then read on the log abscissa axis.

Measurement of serum folate by radioisotope dilution assay

The development of commercial radioisotope dilution (RID) kits followed upon the discovery of suitable folate binders and the production of γ-emitting iodinated folate compounds. The principle of the assay is the same as for serum B_{12} and the procedures are similar.

Extraction of folate from the serum binder

In contrast to microbiological assay, the folate has to be released by heat or alkaline denaturation of the endogenous binder. Ascorbic acid must not be added to sera for preservation of folate during extraction (and storage) if the sample is also to be used for B_{12} assay because it destroys B_{12}. Dithioreital (DTT) is used in most combined B_{12} and folate assays to keep the folate in the reduced, stable form. Without it, stored sera may give low results.[33]

Binding agent

β-lactoglobulin isolated from cow's milk is commonly used as a binding agent.[34] Methyl-THF has been used as the standard in the binding reaction for assay of endogenous folates. However, it is unstable and folic acid is more stable with a greater affinity for the milk binder. At pH 9.3 ± 0.1, the binding affinities are similar, and it is essential that this pH is strictly maintained at the binding stage of the procedure.[35] Porcine serum is a less satisfactory binder.

Folate standards

As described above, methyl-THF is unstable and the majority of assay methods use folic acid standards, which may cause underestimation of serum folate.[36]

Radioactive tracer

^{125}I-labelled folic acid is generally used.

Separation of free from bound folate

The liquid and solid phase methods used for B_{12} are satisfactory for folate assays. Many of the assay kits measure both serum B_{12} and serum folate.

Measurement of red cell folate by radioisotope dilution assay

Whereas *L. casei* responds equally to both tri- and mono-glutamates, the affinity of the binder for folates varies with the number of glutamate residues. Reproducible assays can only be obtained by release and conversion of the protein-bound folate polyglutamates, mainly methyl-THF with four or five additional glutamate moieties, to a monoglutamate form. Adequate dilution of the red cells,[37] a pH between 3 and 6,[38] plasma folate polyglutamate hydrolase, and ascorbic acid to preserve the reduced form[39] are required. Sodium ascorbate does not lyse the red cells completely. Inadequate lysis and deconjugation give falsely low results.[40,41] The preparation of the haemolysate is described above; some commercial kits use different concentrations of ascorbic acid, require the

addition of protein diluent before assaying and use a different dilution.

AUTOMATED NON-ISOTOPIC ASSAYS

Baxter Stratus automated fluorometric enzyme-linked immunoassay for vitamin B_{12} and folate

The vitamin B_{12} assay uses the principle of sequential binding between natural B_{12} in the sample, or an enzyme-linked B_{12} to porcine intrinsic factor (pIF). Cyanocobalamin is used for calibration and enzyme labelling and potassium cyanide to convert sample B_{12} to the more stable cyanocobalamin. Endogeneous B_{12} binders are denatured at alkaline pH and the treated sample is neutralized in the presence of pIF:mouse anti-pIF complex, and reacts on glass fibre paper with immobilized goat anti-mouse immunoglobulin. Conjugase consisting of alkaline phosphatase-labelled B_{12} is added and it reacts with unoccupied sites on the immobilized pIF. Enzyme substrate 4-methylumbelliferyl phosphate is added and the reaction rate, which is inversely proportional to the concentration of B_{12} in the sample, is measured by an optical system that monitors the reaction rate by fluorimetry. The first result is obtained in 6–8 min and thereafter at 1-min intervals. Statistical evaluation and graphics of control values are easily obtained using the software on the microprocessor.

The folate assay employs the principle of sequential binding of natural sample folate and an enzyme-linked folate conjugate to bovine milk-derived folate binding protein (FBP). A stable form of folate, folic acid, is used for calibrators and enzyme labelling. The serum folate is reduced and extracted from endogenous serum binders at alkaline pH eliminating the necessity of boiling. The extracted sample is neutralized and then adjusted to a pH which facilitates equal folate affinity for immobilized mouse monoclonal anti-FBP/FBP complexed with goat anti-mouse IgG, Fc fragment specific, on glass fibre paper. Free folate combines with folate binding proteins. Alkaline phosphatase conjugase covalently linked to folate is added and combines with unoccupied binding sites on the FBP. The substrate 4-methylumbelliferyl phosphate initiates enzyme activity and the reaction rate is measured by fluorimetry. The rate is inversely proportional to the concentration of folate present in the sample; the first result is obtained in 6–8 min and thereafter at 1-min intervals.

Ciba–Corning ACS: 180 assay

This is a fully automated random access system allowing the use of primary bar-coded collection tubes with a 15-min assay time using the same Ciba–Corning Magic Lite chemiluminescent reaction as is used in the manual Magic Lite assays which have been available since 1986. The B_{12} and folate assays are competitive assays in which B_{12} or folate from the sample competes with the Lite reagent, namely B_{12} or folate bound to acridinium ester, for a limited amount of purified intrinsic factor/purified bovine milk-binding protein covalently coupled to paramagnetic particles (Solid Phase). Sodium hydroxide and DTT release the B_{12}/folate from endogenous binding proteins in the sample. The chemiluminescent reaction is measured and the photon output (relative light units) quantitated. An indirect relationship exists between the amount of B_{12} and folate and the relative light units detected. Quality control statistics and charts are produced automatically.

Abbott fluorescent microparticle enzyme assay using IMX analyser

In the vitamin B_{12} assay,[42] the sample is treated at pH >12.5 to release B_{12} bound to serum transcobalamins and to convert all forms to cyanocobalamin. The analyte is bound at a lower pH by purified pIF immobilized on polymeric microspheres. The microspheres and bound analyte are separated from the reaction mixture by irreversible binding to a glass fibre matrix. Alkaline phosphatase conjugate is added and binds to the B_{12}/IF complex. A substrate 4-methylumbelliferyl phosphate is converted by alkaline phosphatase to form a fluorescent product, 4-methylumbelliferone, which is generated in inverse proportion to the amount of B_{12} in the original sample. The fluorescence is read by the IMX. Twenty four samples can be assayed in 60 min.

The folate assay utilizes ion capture technology. A high molecular weight quaternary ammonium compound imparts a positive charge to the glass fibre matrix, which can then capture by electrostatic interaction negatively charged polyanion-analyte complexes. Folate is bound by a soluble affinity reagent composed of FBP affinity coupled to mouse monoclonal antibodies, which are in turn covalently bound to carboxymethylamylose (polyanion), imparting a positive charge. Unoccupied FBP sites bound to the matrix are then measured using a conjugate of pteroic acid and alkaline phosphatase, which generates a fluorescent signal on the addition of the substrate 4-methylumbelliferyl. The strength of the fluorescence is then inversely proportional to the concentration of folate.

WHICH ASSAY METHOD?

The choice of assay method should be based upon technical performance, clinical value and compatibility with current laboratory procedures. Consideration may need to be given to the turnround time required by requesting clinicians and the need to be cost efficient. Whatever methodology is chosen, the accuracy, precision and sensitivity of the assays should be known.

A laboratory setting up a B_{12} assay would not now normally introduce a microbiological method since radioassays are generally satisfactory and more convenient. The automated non-isotopic methods, although expensive, produce results quickly, often provide random access and require less highly trained personnel for routine operation. They also avoid the strict regulations governing the storage, use and disposal of radioactive isotopes. The accuracy of a B_{12} assay can be judged by assay of reference sera and by its performance in external quality assessment schemes, in which the mean from a large number of participants appears to be the true value.[33] The accuracy of most radioassay kits is acceptable. A satisfactory assay gives a CV of 5% or less with within-batch duplicates and 10% or less with between-batch duplicates. All manufacturers claim that these levels can be reached. A laboratory carrying out other in-house B_{12} investigations may wish to establish its own method for serum B_{12} assay. The solid phase, boil technique of Muir & Chanarin[31] is recommended although the bead preparation is both time-consuming and not inexpensive and the boil technique with charcoal separation of Gutcho & Mansbach[43] is also recommended.

Both the serum and red cell folate assays show considerable variation in accuracy, though the correlation between them is reasonable and a whole blood folate standard reference preparation is now available (p 603). Some laboratories may wish to measure only serum or red cell folate, but because of the limitations of both (see p. 137), it is advisable to assay both, or to measure the red cell folate if the serum folate is low.

Table 8.1 lists the kits in use in the UK. Kits using solid phase binders for B_{12} and folate assays are preferable since they reduce the number of assay steps and are as satisfactory as charcoal separation. A boil technique with a solid phase binder was generally considered the best for detecting B_{12} deficiency.[17] However, good correlation is obtained using both an established radioassay and the new non-isotopic methods, all the latter being no-boil. Table 8.2 lists the automated non-isotopic methods. The features mentioned previously which affect radioassays and the references to their performance should help in the choice of an appropriate kit. The protocol should be studied before a trial kit is obtained. A new kit requires full evaluation including the assay of sera of low B_{12} and folate content. Whichever method is chosen, each laboratory should establish its own normal reference range.

QUALITY CONTROL AND REFERENCE MATERIALS FOR VITAMIN B_{12} AND FOLATE ASSAYS

Sera and haemolysates of known B_{12} and folate content must be included in each assay. For quality control it is usual to collect pools of low, intermediate and normal values, to store these in 1 ml volumes at $-20°C$ and to thaw one for each assay. Their vitamin content is determined by assay alongside samples of known concentration from another laboratory or samples from previous external quality assessment surveys. Alternatively, commercial controls are now widely available, several

Table 8.1 Commercial kits for B_{12} and folate radioassays

Manufacturer	Kit		Extraction pH	Binding pH	Separator	Relative accuracy(%)***			Selected references
						B_{12}	Serum folate	Red cell folate	
1 Kodak Clinical Diagnostics	B_{12}/folate*	A	12.9	9.5	Charcoal	90		155	18,33,76
2 Becton Dickinson	B_{12}	B	9.3	9.3	Charcoal				19,77,78
3 Becton Dickinson	Simultrac B_{12}/folate	B	9.3	9.3	Charcoal	93	80	115	17,18,25,33
4 Becton Dickinson	Simultrac-S B_{12}/folate	B	9.3	9.3	Solid phase	99	82	85	33
5 Becton Dickinson	Simultrac-SNB B_{12}/folate	A	12–13	9.3	Solid phase	94	96	104	33
6 Becton Dickinson	Folic acid	B	9.3	9.3					33,76,77,78
7 Biorad	Quantaphase B_{12}/folate+	B	11.7	9.2	Polymer beads	100	98	73	33,77,78
8 Diagnostic Products Inc.	Dualcount SP	A	13.0	9.3	Cellulose particles	92	96	135	25,77,78
9 Diagnostic Products Inc.	Dualcount SP	B	9.4		Cellulose particles				25,77,78
10 Ciba–Corning	Magic B_{12}/folate	B	9.2		Paramagnetic particles				76
11 Ciba–Corning	Magic B_{12}/folate	A	12–13	9.3	Paramagnetic particles				
12 Ciba–Corning	MagicLite B_{12}**	A	12–13	9.3	Paramagnetic particles				
13 Ciba–Corning	MagicLite folate**	A	12–13	9.3	Paramagnetic particles				

A, alkaline denaturation; B, boil. The binder in all kits is IF, purified except in Simultrac kits when R is blocked by analogue in tracer.
*Reagents for a single B_{12} or folate assay are available.
**Non-isotopic.
***Microbiological assay = 100%.

Table 8.2 Automated non-isotopic no-boil B_{12} and folate assays

Manufacturer	Assay system	Principle
Ciba–Corning	ACS: 180	Chemiluminescence using intrinsic factor/milk binder coupled to paramagnetic particles
Baxter immunoassay	STRATUS	Fluorometric enzyme linked
Abbott Laboratories assay	B_{12} IMX Folate IMX	Micro-particle enzyme intrinsic factor Ion capture FBP assay
Biorad	RADIAS	ELISA-based immunoassay

companies offering free statistical analysis on an individual basis as well as a comparison with laboratories worldwide. International reference reagents for human serum B_{12} and whole blood folate have been developed by ICSH and established by WHO[44,45] (see p. 607); they can be used for checking the accuracy of an assay; an equivalent serum B_{12} British Standard is also available.[9] Recovery experiments with the addition of B_{12} and folic acid to normal samples are of some value, although they do not assess the extraction stage in B_{12} assays or the haemolysate preparation in folate assays. The repeat assay of three to five sera from the previous batch and plotting the mean or median of each batch (providing the samples come from an unchanging population) help to assure reproducibility of the assay. Participation in an external quality assessment scheme is essential to monitor technical performance.[46]

INTERPRETATION OF ASSAY RESULTS

Serum vitamin B_{12} assay

Vitamin B_{12} in serum is found predominantly as methylcobalamin bound to carrier proteins called transcobalamins (TCs). A normal serum B_{12} level excludes significant tissue B_{12} deficiency except in the rare inherited syndrome of TC II deficiency, or when TC I levels are increased as in chronic myeloid leukaemia and following nitrous oxide anaesthesia when intracellular B_{12} is inactivated. A fall in the concentration of serum B_{12} is an early sign of defi-

ciency and may be found before cellular changes appear in the marrow and blood. A low serum B_{12} level is not, however, specific for B_{12} deficiency and may also be found in approximately one-third of patients with severe folate deficiency, as well as during normal pregnancy, in myelomatosis or TC I deficiency and sometimes for no apparent reason.

An increase in the vitamin B_{12} level may be found with acute liver cell damage and in the myeloproliferative conditions, particularly chronic myeloid leukaemia, primary proliferative polycythaemia (polycythaemia vera) and myelofibrosis.

Serum and red cell folate assay

Folic acid in serum is found as methyl-THF and falls rapidly with a reduction in folate intake or with negative folate balance. Serum folate may therefore be low without significant tissue deficiency.[12e] The concentration of folate within red cells (largely folate polyglutamates) shows better correlation with megaloblastic change,[39] although it is not a specific sign of folate deficiency, since it is also low in about two-thirds of patients with severe vitamin B_{12} deficiency.[12f] This is because of the requirement for vitamin B_{12} in the conversion of methyl-THF to tetrahydrofolate which is the preferred substrate for folate polyglutamate synthesis.[47–49] Red cell folate may also be normal, despite folate deficiency, when there is a reticulocytosis, since reticulocytes have a higher folate content than mature red cells, or following a recent blood transfusion or when the deficiency state develops rapidly.[39]

DEOXYURIDINE SUPPRESSION TEST[2]

Principle

Pre-incubation of normal bone marrow with an appropriate concentration of dU suppresses the subsequent incorporation of tritiated thymidine (^3H-TdR) into DNA. This suppression is less in patients with B_{12} or folate deficiency. This is due to failure of the thymidylate synthesis reaction in which deoxyuridine monophosphate (dUMP) is methylated to thymidine monophosphate (dTMP), the methyl donor being the folate co-enzyme 5,10-methylene tetrahydrofolate (in the polyglutamate form). dU suppression is normal when the cause of the megaloblastic anaemia is neither B_{12} nor folate deficiency, nor any other defect in thymidylate synthesis.[50,51]

Materials

Bone marrow. $10-50 \times 10^6$ nucleated cells or 0.5–2.0 ml of aspirated marrow, in EDTA. It is preferable to test the marrow freshly but it can be left overnight at 18–25°C without affecting the results significantly.

Blood. 10 ml of heparinized blood.

Reagents

Hanks balanced salt solution (GIBCO Cat. No. 041–4020) ready for use.

KCl 0.6 mol/l. 4.473 g in 100 ml of water.

Phosphate buffered saline, pH 7.4. Add 90 ml of 0.15 mol/l, $NaH_2PO_4.H_2O$ (23.4 g/l) and 410 ml of 0.15 mol/l Na_2HPO_4 (21.3 g/l) to 500 ml of 9.0 g/l NaCl (saline).

Perchloric acid, 0.5 mol/l. Make up 20.8 ml of concentrated perchloric acid to 500 ml with water.

Hydroxocobalamin, 1000 µg/ml.

Folinic acid (calcium leucovorin) (Lederle), 3 mg/ml.

5-Methyltetrahydrofolic acid (Sigma), 1 mg. Reconstitute with 33 µl of saline immediately before use.

Tritiated thymidine-TRA 120 (Amersham), 185 GBq/mmol. Dilute 100 µl to 10 ml with saline (1 µCi/0.2 µmol/100 µl).

Deoxyuridine (Sigma), 100 mmol/l. Prepare a working solution of 11.4 mg in 0.5 ml of saline. This is stable at 4°C.

Scintillation fluid, e.g. Packard emulsifier scintillator 299™ Cat. No. 6013079.

Method

Whenever possible, except when stated, carry out all procedures at 4°C.

Wash marrow once in buffered Hanks solution, centrifuging at 4°C at $1000\,g$ for 5 min.

Lyse the red cells by adding 3 ml of cold water; mix for 30 s; add 1.0 ml of 0.6 mol/l KCl; add 1–2 ml of buffered Hanks solution to maintain the pH, and then centrifuge at $1000\,g$ for 5 min.

Wash the deposit with buffered Hanks solution, centrifuging at $1000\,g$ for 5 min.

Discard the supernatant. Repeat the lysing process if a visible button of red cells remains.

Suspend the pellets in 1 ml of Hanks solution, checking that there are no clumps in the final suspension. If necessary, pass the suspension through a 19-G needle attached to a 1 ml syringe.

Count the number of cells present and express the number as $\times 10^6$/ml.

Add 1 volume of autologous plasma to 4 volumes of Hanks solution and dilute the cells with this solution to obtain $1-3 \times 10^6$ cells/ml.

Set up the plastic centrifuge tubes as shown in Table 8.3.

Transfer the tubes into an ice-bath.

Centrifuge at $1000\,g$ for 5 min and discard the supernatant.

Vortex-mix and wash the pellets once with 2.0 ml of cold phosphate buffered saline and discard the supernatant.

Mix and add 2 ml of the perchloric acid to each pellet.

Mix and stand in the ice-bath for 10 min. Centrifuge and discard the supernatant. If necessary, the pellets can be left overnight at this stage.

Mix, add 0.5 ml of the perchloric acid, mix and place the tubes in a water-bath at 80°C for 20 min.

Centrifuge at 18–25°C and $1000\,g$ for 5 min.

Transfer 100 µl of the supernatant into counting vials. Add 5 ml of scintillation fluid; allow to equilibrate for 30 min and count for 200 s.

Calculate % counts per min using the counts of ^{3}H-TdR alone as 100%.

Interpretation of results

1. dU suppression in normal marrow <8%.
2. dU suppression in megaloblastic marrow >8%.
3. Correction, partial or complete, with added B_{12} but not with methyl-THF, in B_{12} deficiency.

Table 8.3 Preparation of assay tubes for the deoxyuridine suppression test

Tubes	Saline (μl)	Vitamin B$_{12}$ (μl)	Folinic acid (μl)	5-Methyl-THF (μl)	Cells* (ml)	dU* (μl)	^{3}H-TdR** (μl)
1 & 2	20	–	–	–	1	–	100
3 & 4	10	–	–	–	1	10	100
5 & 6	–	10	–	–	1	10	100
7 & 8	–	–	10	–	1	10	100
9 & 10	–	–	–	10	1	10	100

*Mix and incubate all tubes at 37°C for 15 min with shaking.
**Mix and incubate all tubes at 37°C for 1 h with shaking.

4. Correction with added folinic acid (5-formyl THF) to <5% in both B$_{12}$ and folate deficiencies.
5. Correction, partial, with added methyl-THF in folate deficiency.
6. There may be partial correction with both B$_{12}$ and methyl-THF in mixed B$_{12}$ and folate deficiency.

A microtitre plate method is reported to be less cumbersome and more economic in sample requirement, thus allowing more replicate tests.[52] The use of peripheral blood lymphocytes has been criticized since normal cultured cells develop folate deficiency.[2]

INVESTIGATION OF THE ABSORPTION OF VITAMIN B$_{12}$

An important step in the study of patients suffering from B$_{12}$ deficiency is to establish whether or not they have the capacity to absorb the vitamin normally. This is best accomplished with the aid of vitamin B$_{12}$ labelled by a radionuclide of cobalt. Originally, ^{60}Co was employed, but the shorter-lived radionuclides, ^{58}Co (half-life 71 days) and ^{57}Co (half-life 270 days) are more suitable. ^{57}Co emits γ-rays of several energies, the most important being of 122 keV, and no particulate energies are emitted. It can be used in larger tracer doses than ^{58}Co and is the isotope of choice when a well-type scintillation counter is used. ^{58}Co can be used with all counting methods, but its counting efficiency is low and relatively large amounts must be given to obtain adequate count rates, especially for measuring blood radioactivity. Radionuclide labelled cyanocobalamin is used routinely.

Either the urinary excretion (Schilling) test[53] or whole-body counting test is utilized to assess the absorption of the test dose of radionuclide labelled vitamin B$_{12}$.[19,54] The hepatic uptake and faecal excretion methods are obsolete and the estimation of plasma radioactivity is unreliable; these methods are not described here. If absorption of vitamin B$_{12}$ is found to be subnormal by either method, the test can be repeated with the simultaneous administration of intrinsic factor* mixed with the dose of radioactively labelled B$_{12}$.[55] The urinary excretion test has been recommended by the International Committee for Standardization in Haematology as being the most convenient and reliable in practice.[56]

URINARY EXCRETION (SCHILLING) TEST[53,56]

Give an oral dose of 1.0 μg (37 kBq) of radioactive B$_{12}$ either ^{57}Co or ^{58}Co** in about 200 ml of water to a patient who has fasted overnight and, at the same time, give 1 mg of non-radioactive hydroxocobalamin or cyanocobalamin intramuscularly (a flushing dose). The patient should fast for a further 2 h. Collect all the urine for 24 h and measure the radioactivity of this urine and of a standard, where the standard consists of a similar dose of radioactive B$_{12}$ suitably diluted in water. Calculate the percentage dose excreted in the urine as follows:

---

* Human recombinant intrinsic factor is available from Biofac A/S, 350 Endlandsweg, DK 2770 Kastrup, Copenhagen Fax: 45 7010 3020 E-mail: biofac @ biofac.dk
** E.g. Amersham International:

   Co^{57}-B$_{12}$, Code CR51P; Co^{58}-B$_{12}$, Code CR3P.

$$\frac{\text{Total cpm in 24 h urine}}{\text{cpm in standard (= test dose)}} \times 100.$$

It is more convenient and cheaper to prepare 10 test doses at one time. Vial CR3P (Amersham) contains c 10 µg of vitamin B_{12} with activity c 0.37 MBq (10 µCi). Using sterile containers:

1. Dilute the contents to 100 ml in water.
2. Take 100 µl for the standard and dilute to 100 ml in water; this standard is a 1 in 10 000 dilution of the test dose.
3. Dispense the remainder in 10 ml volumes.
4. Store doses and standard at 4°C.
5. Mix the 24 h urine collection well and estimate the radioactivity in equal volumes of urine and standard.
6. Calculate the percentage of the test dose excreted as follows:

$$\frac{\text{Urine cpm} \times \text{Urine volume (ml)}}{\text{Standard cpm} \times \text{Dilution of standard}} \times 100$$

The dual isotope (Dicopac) kit of free ^{58}Co-B_{12} and ^{57}Co-B_{12} bound to intrinsic factor is no longer available.

Interpretation of results

With hydroxycobalamin, the normal urinary excretion is >10% of the test dose in the first 24 h; in patients with pernicious anaemia or with B_{12} deficiency associated with intestinal malabsorption, the excretion is usually <5%, whereas in patients with dietary deficiency of vitamin B_{12}, absorption will be normal. Results with cyanocobalamin are generally lower than with hydroxycobalamin.[57,59] Absorption can be increased in pernicious anaemia by the simultaneous administration of IF, whereas absorption remains subnormal if malabsorption is due to an intestinal defect. The second test dose, with IF, can be given 48 h after the first, provided that an additional flushing injection is given 24 h after the first oral dose.

The method is generally reliable, the results are clear-cut and the technique is simple; however, reliable results depend on a complete collection of urine. Low results may be found in patients with renal disease, when excretion may be delayed. In such cases, urine should be collected for 48 h. The need for large flushing doses of B_{12} is a disadvantage in that they may interfere with other metabolic studies. Deficiency of vitamin B_{12} or folate may themselves cause temporary malabsorption of B_{12}.[58] It is advisable therefore either to carry out all tests of absorption when patients are vitamin replete or to repeat tests with discrepant results after replacement therapy for 2 months.

Achlorhydria secondary to atrophic gastritis or following partial gastrectomy may be associated with normal absorption of aqueous vitamin B_{12} but malabsorption of protein-bound B_{12}.[60] Tests of vitamin B_{12} absorption with the B_{12} attached to binders in egg yolk[61] and in chicken serum[62] have been described. These so-called 'food Schilling tests' may help to diagnose food B_{12} malabsorption when the results of conventional Schilling tests are normal.

WHOLE BODY COUNTING

The advantage of this method is that a 'flushing' dose of B_{12} does not have to be given.[63] However, it does require specialized equipment and, normally, a low-background room, although a system has been described which can be used in the absence of a low-background room and accurate measurements of ^{58}Co absorption have been reported.[63] ^{57}Co-B_{12} can also be used[64] and a double isotope test has been described.[65] Whole body counts are performed on a scanning bed moving at a fixed rate past four static sodium iodide crystal detectors vertically opposed in pairs. Counting times of 4.5 min are suitable. Counts are performed immediately before and after the test dose has been given, taking care that there is no external contamination with radioactive B_{12}. The counts are then repeated 14 days later. The % retention of the dose is calculated correcting for any variation in natural background and radionuclide decay.

Interpretation of results

Normal subjects absorb >30% and usually >50% of a 1 µg dose of vitamin B_{12}. Patients with pernicious anaemia usually absorb <20%; repeating the test with additional IF should result in an increase in the retention of the dose by >15%.

ESTIMATION OF INTRINSIC FACTOR IN GASTRIC JUICE[66]

Direct estimation of the intrinsic factor (IF) content of gastric juice is useful in the diagnosis of pernicious anaemia, particularly when there is associated small intestinal disease which complicates the interpretation of B_{12} absorption studies.

Principle

B_{12} binding by gastric juice is due to its content of IF and R proteins (salivary and gastric). Normally more than 90% is due to IF. This can be estimated by determining the difference in the binding capacity of gastric juice with and without neutralization of the IF by serum IF antibody (IFA).[67] An alternative assay in which the non-IF binding is neutralized by the addition of B_{12} analogue (e.g. cobinamide) gives comparable results, does not depend upon the availability of IFA of a certain potency and is simpler. This latter technique is described here.

Reagents

Buffer. 0.01 mol/l Tris-HCl, pH 8.0 containing 0.15 mol/l NaCl and 50 μg/ml 22% bovine albumin.

Activated albumin-coated charcoal (25 g/l). Heat 2.5 g of activated charcoal (Norit A: Merck; Sigma) at 110°C overnight. Suspend in 50 ml of water. Add 6.8 ml of 22% bovine albumin in 50 ml of water and mix well for 10 s. The coating is done immediately before use.

Vitamin B_{12}. Dilute ^{57}Co-B_{12} (Code CT2) 45–85 ng B_{12}, 370–740 kBq (10–20 μCi),* with water to 1 ng/l. Store in the dark at 4°C. This is stable for 3 months. For the assay, add non-radioactive cyanocobalamin to give a solution containing 200 ng/l.

Cobinamide. Make up a stock solution of 10 mg/l. Store at 4°C. For use, dilute to give 50 ng in 100 μl.

Collection of gastric juice. Collect into an ice-cooled container the basal secretion for 1 h followed by a further hour collection after subcutaneous administration of pentagastrin as a stimulus (8 μg/kg body weight). Centrifuge at 1000 *g* for 15 min to separate the mucus. Record the pH. Take clear juice, add sufficient 5 mol/l NaOH to obtain a pH of 11.0, stand for 20 min at room temperature to inactivate peptidases and then neutralize to pH 7.0 with 1 mol/l HCl. Measure the volume. It may be stored for some months at –20°C without loss of activity.

Method

Set up controls and samples, in duplicate, as shown in Table 8.4. Mix and incubate at *c* 20°C for 30 min. Add 100 μl of ^{57}Co-B_{12} to each tube. After mixing, again leave at *c* 20°C for 10 min. Add 1.5 ml of coated charcoal suspension to all tubes except A. Mix and incubate for 10 min. Centrifuge the tubes and deliver 2 ml into counting vials. Measure the radioactivity and average the counts.

Calculation

By definition 1 unit (u) of IF binds 1 ng of B_{12}.

$$\text{Units IF/ml gastric juice} = \frac{D - B}{C - A} \times 10 \times 20$$

The total binding capacity of a gastric juice may be determined by omitting the cobinamide in the assay.

Interpretation of results

The normal range varies widely from 15 to 115 u/ml with a total secretion per hour of 500 to several thousand units.[12b] In females, the concentration is the same as in males, but because of a smaller

Table 8.4 Preparation of control and sample tubes for the estimation of intrinsic factor in gastric juice

Tube	Buffer (ml)	Gastric juice (μl)	Cobinamide (μl)
A Untreated	3.7	0	0
B Charcoal control	2.2	0	100
C Standard	2.0	100	100
D Test	2.0	100	100

* Lifescreen, Watford, UK.

volume of gastric juice, there is only half the total secretion. The concentration in pernicious anaemia is usually zero and never more than 10 u/ml, with a total secretion of less than 250 u in 1 h.

INTRINSIC FACTOR ANTIBODIES[12g]

Two types of antibody to IF have been detected in the sera of patients with pernicious anaemia. Type I (blocking antibody) prevents the attachment of B_{12} to IF, while Type II (precipitating antibody) prevents the attachment of IF or the IF-B_{12} complex to the ileal receptors. Type I antibody is present in over two-thirds of cases of pernicious anaemia; Type II antibody probably occurs with equal frequency[68] and has been reported to be even more frequent.[69] The presence of IF antibodies in a patient under investigation for pernicious anaemia confirms the diagnosis and renders a B_{12} absorption test unnecessary. IF antibodies occur only rarely in conditions other than pernicious anaemia, e.g. they have been described in a few patients with thyroid disorders, diabetes mellitus and the Eaton–Lambert myasthenic syndrome. The gastric juice in pernicious anaemia almost always contains IF antibodies, but tests for these are not carried out routinely and will not be described here.

ESTIMATION OF TYPE I INTRINSIC FACTOR ANTIBODY

Reagents

Normal gastric juice. Determine the IF content. Dilute in 0.154 mol/l NaCl to give a solution containing 25 μ/ml. Store at −20°C in volumes suitable for a batch of tests.

Normal serum. Pool the sera from six or more normal subjects.

^{57}Co-B_{12}. 50 μg/l. Code CT2.*

Albumin-coated charcoal. 25 g/l (see p. 141).

Method
Set out a series of tubes, in duplicate, as shown in Table 8.5. Mix and incubate at room temperature for 30 min with periodic mixing. Add 5 ng of ^{57}Co-B_{12} in 100 μl volumes to all tubes. Incubate at room temperature for 10 min. Add 1.5 ml of charcoal suspension to tube B onwards. Mix and incubate at room temperature for 5 min. Centrifuge at 1500 g for 15 min and transfer 2 ml of the supernatant to counting vials. Measure the radioactivity and calculate the ratio of normal to test serum counts.

Interpretation of results
Negative sera, ratio <1.02; Positive sera, ratio >1.10.

Ratios between these figures are termed indeterminate and the test should be repeated using 500 μl volumes of the test and normal sera. These ratios are given as guidelines, and each laboratory should determine its own normal range.

In this method, the proportion of IF in ng to serum in ml is 4:1.[70] The sensitivity of the test can be enhanced by reducing this proportion but preliminary treatment of the sera with a microfine

Table 8.5 Estimation of Type I intrinsic factor antibody. Preparation of control and sample tubes

Tube	0.154 mol/l NaCl (ml)	Gastric juice (μl)	Normal serum (μl)	Test serum (μl)
A Radioactive control	3.7	0	0	0
B Charcoal control	2.2	0	0	0
C Normal serum pool	1.85	50	300	0
D Positive serum	1.85	50	0	300
E Test serum	1.85	50	0	300

* Lifescreen, Watford, UK.

silica QUSO is required to neutralize the effect of the contained transcobalamins.[71]

ESTIMATION OF TYPE II INTRINSIC FACTOR ANTIBODY

Reagents

Barbitone buffer, pH 8.3. 0.04 mol/l sodium diethyl barbitone, 100 ml; 0.2 mol/l HCl 6.21 ml. Make up the solution freshly every 4 weeks, and keep at 4°C.

Anhydrous sodium sulphate.   300 g/l and 150 g/l.

Albumin-coated charcoal.   See page 141.

Gastric intrinsic factor-^{57}Co-B$_{12}$ complex.   For every 1 ml of normal gastric juice, add an excess of ^{57}Co-B$_{12}$, e.g. 200 ng. Leave at *c* 20°C for 30 min, and then remove excess (free) B$_{12}$ by adding 1 ml of charcoal suspension. After a further 10 min at *c* 20°C, centrifuge the suspension for 15 min at 1500 *g*; dispense the supernatant in 2 ml volumes and store at –20°C.

Method

Place 0.3 ml of serum, including negative and positive control sera, in 10 ml centrifuge tubes. Add 0.5 ml of barbitone buffer and 1.0 ml of IF-^{57}Co-B$_{12}$ complex, diluted 1 to 5 with saline. Incubate at 37°C for 30 min. Add 2 ml of 300 g/l sodium sulphate, warmed to 37°C. After mixing, incubate for a further 10 min, and then centrifuge the suspensions at 1500 *g* for 15–20 min. Discard the supernatant and add 1 ml of 150 g/l sodium sulphate and centrifuge twice. After discarding the supernatant, add 3.5 ml of saline to each tube to dissolve the precipitate. Place 3 ml volumes from each tube in counting vials and count the radio-activity. A radioactive control containing 1.0 ml of the diluted IF-^{57}Co-B$_{12}$ complex and 2.0 ml of water is also set up and counted.

Interpretation of results

Precipitating antibodies are indicated by a high count in the precipitate, usually ten times higher than that of the negative controls. A sensitive radioimmune assay using ^{125}I-labelled IF[68] and an ELISA technique[72] for the simultaneous detection of Type I and II antibodies have been reported recently. Using this technique,[69] Type II antibodies were detected in 39 of the 40 sera containing Type II antibodies only, suggesting that the occurrence of Type-II antibodies both alone and in combination with Type I is a more common feature than has been previously recognized.

INTRINSIC FACTOR ANTIBODY KITS

A radioisotope competitive binding assay kit, which detects binding antibodies only, is available from Diagnostic Products Corporation Ltd. An ELISA kit, which detects both Type-I and Type-II antibodies, is available from Cambridge Life Sciences.

PARIETAL CELL ANTIBODIES

These are present in the sera of about 90% of patients with pernicious anaemia but also occur in other conditions and increase in frequency with age so that about 15% of elderly individuals may exhibit them. They are usually detected by an immunofluorescence technique, using human or rat stomach.

PLASMA (OR SERUM) B$_{12}$ BINDING CAPACITY[12a,67]

The total B$_{12}$ binding capacity (TBBC) of plasma comprises the sum of the serum B$_{12}$ concentration and the plasma unsaturated binding capacity (UBBC). 80% or more of the serum B$_{12}$ is bound to transcobalamin I (TC I), a small fraction is bound to TC II and TC III is virtually unsaturated. TC I and TC III (R binders) are both glycosolated proteins and differ only in their sugar moiety. Chronic myeloid leukaemia, myelofibrosis and other myeloproliferative conditions are characterized by increased levels of TC I and therefore an increased concentration of serum B$_{12}$; primary liver cancer may be associated with the synthesis of large quantities of an abnormal form of TC I. Congenital absence of R binders results in a very low serum B_{12} but no evidence of B_{12} deficiency and no adverse effects. It is suggested that some low B_{12} levels, without any evidence of B_{12} deficiency, may be due to a decrease in R binder concentration.[73]

TC II delivers B_{12} to the tissues. Rare congenital absence or functional abnormality results in fulminating pancytopenia and megaloblastosis usually within 2 months of birth. The serum B_{12} is normal, the UBBC is reduced, B_{12} absorption is reduced and the dU suppression test is abnormal and corrected by B_{12}.

Estimation of the UBBC of an individual TC requires a separation technique; the adsorption of TC II to silica powder[74] is a suitable procedure. Estimation of the UBBC and of its components needs care in the collection of the sample. To minimize release of TC I and TC III from granulocytes, blood should be added to an anticoagulant mixture of 1 mg EDTA and 2 mg sodium fluoride per ml blood.[75] If serum is used, this should be separated within 2 h of blood collection.

ESTIMATION OF UNSATURATED B_{12} BINDING CAPACITY

Principle
The UBBC is measured by noting the quantity of ^{57}Co-B_{12} taken up by a unit of plasma or serum. The total B_{12} binding capacity is the sum of the serum B_{12} concentration and ^{57}Co-B_{12} uptake.

Requirements
^{57}Co-B_{12} Code CT2 (Lifescreen, Watford, UK). Dilute ^{57}Co-B_{12} specific activity c 6.6–8.1 MBq/µg in non-radioactive cyanocobalamin (Duncan Flockhart) to give a concentration of 2 µg/l as follows:

Dilute cyanocobalamin 1000 µg/ml 1 in 100 in water and add 50 µl to 1 ml ^{57}Co-B_{12}. Make this up to 5 ml, mix and aliquot into 0.3 ml amounts and store at −20°C. On day of assay thaw, add 14.7 ml of water and mix.

Table 8.6 Preparation of tubes for the estimation of plasma B_{12} binding capacity

Tube	Saline (ml)	Plasma (ml)
A Standard	2.5	0
B Supernatant control	0.5	0
C Test	0	0.5

Albumin-coated charcoal
Suspend 1 g of activated charcoal (DARCO G60; Merck Ltd) in 20 ml water and dispense 0.67 ml of 30% BSA in a further 20 ml of water. Add the albumin to the charcoal suspension with constant mixing for 10 s. Prepare fresh for each assay.

Method
Set up a series of conical centrifuge tubes containing plasma or 9 g/l NaCl as shown in Table 8.6. Add 1 ml of ^{57}Co-B_{12} to each tube. After mixing and incubating at c 20°C for 30 min, add 2 ml of charcoal suspension to each tube except A. After standing for 10 min, centrifuge the tubes at 1500 g for 10 min. Pipette 3 ml volumes of the supernatant into counting vials. Measure the radioactivity and correct for background counts.

Calculation
$$UBBC\ (ng/l) = \frac{C - B}{A} \times ng/l\ ^{57}Co\text{-}B_{12} \times plasma\ dilution$$

If the UBBC is equal to or greater than the amount of ^{57}Co-B_{12} added, the test should be repeated after appropriately diluting the plasma with saline.

Normal range
The normal range for serum UBBC is 670–1200 ng/l; that of plasma collected into EDTA-sodium fluoride is 505–1208 ng/l.[75]

TRANSCOBALAMIN SEPARATION

A variety of techniques are available for the separation and measurement of TCs I, II and III, each being based on some physicochemical difference between the proteins. The method described here[74] is simple to perform and reliable. It should be noted, however, that as cobalamin is added to a volume of serum to saturate available binders, a functionally ineffective TC II would not be detected.

SEPARATION OF TRANSCOBALAMIN II FROM TRANSCOBALAMINS I AND III

Requirements

Microfine precipitated silica (non-crystalline) QUSO (Croxton and Garry, Surrey).

Method

After counting the UBBC add 90 mg of QUSO to each sample and blank, mix, centrifuge at $1500\,g$ for 10 min and remove the supernatant into 10 ml flat-bottomed polystyrene tubes. Count both sets of tubes on a γ-counter. Calculations for separated TC II and TCs I and III are the same as for the UBBC.

SEPARATION OF TRANSCOBALAMINS I AND III

Requirements

1. Diethylaminoethyl cellulose fibrous anion exchanger (Whatman DE23).
2. 0.06 mol/l Phosphate buffer pH 6.3.
3. Stock solution (A) KH_2PO_4 8.165 g in 1 litre water.
4. Stock solution (B) Na_2HPO_4 8.517 g in 1 litre water.

5. To prepare buffer for assay, mix 162 ml (A) with 38 ml (B).
6. 0.02 mol/l Phosphate buffer pH 6.3.
7. Add 10 ml of 0.06 mol/l buffer as prepared above to 20 ml of water mix and discard 2 ml.
8. Add 2.4 g of DE23 to 28 ml of 0.02 mol/l buffer and allow to equilibrate for at least 10 min.

Method

TCs I and III are taken up by DE23. TC III is eluted off by the 0.06 mol/l buffer leaving TC I on the DE23.

To each tube containing supernatant after removal from TC II, add 2 ml of pre-wetted DE23 and leave the tubes to mix on a rotary mixer for 10 min. Add 5 ml of 0.06 mol/l buffer and continue mixing for a further 10 min. Centrifuge at $1500\,g$ for 10 min; discard supernatant. Add 5 ml of fresh 0.06 mol/l buffer, mix for 10 min, centrifuge, discard supernatant and repeat once more. Count the tubes containing TC I on a γ-counter and calculate as before. The TC III values are obtained by subtracting TC I from the TC-I and III result.

Normal range

UBBC 520–1132 ng/l.
TC I 49–132 ng/l.
TC II 402–930 ng/l.
TC III 80–280 ng/l.

RESPONSE TO TREATMENT AS AN AID TO DIAGNOSIS

Assessment of the response to specific treatment should be an integral part of the diagnosis of megaloblastic anaemia. By convention, day 0 is the day on which the haematinic is given. An optimal response is shown by the red cell count rising, depending upon the severity of the anaemia, to at least 3.0×10^{12}/l by the 15th day after the start of therapy. The reticulocyte count starts to rise on days 2 to 3 and the maximum count occurs between days 5 and 7. The size of the reticulocyte peak is related to the initial red cell count; the more anaemic the patient, the higher the reticulocyte peak. Neutropenia and thrombocytopenia normally correct within the first few days of treatment and hypersegmented neutrophils decline in

number after day 10 and are absent by day 14. In patients with little or no anaemia, therapeutic doses of the deficient vitamin should correct the MCV within 3 to 4 months. Erythropoiesis in the marrow rapidly becomes normoblastic; there is an obvious improvement by 12 h with a normal appearance by 36–48 h. Giant metamyelocytes may still be present up to 12 days after treatment.

Failure of an optimal haematological response should prompt reevaluation of the data and reconsideration of the diagnosis. However, the response to the correct specific therapy will be impaired by other factors, including co-existing infection, hypothyroidism or iron deficiency as well as by unrelated bone marrow disorders such as myelodysplasia.

A haematological response to pharmacological doses of folic acid (5 mg daily) occurs in B_{12} deficient megaloblastic anaemia. However, B_{12} neuropathy is aggravated or may even be precipitated, by such treatment. Vitamin B_{12} deficiency should always be excluded before folic acid is given alone.

REFERENCES

1 Herzlich B, Herbert V 1988 Depletion of serum holotranscobalamin II. An early sign of negative vitamin B_{12} balance. Laboratory Investigations 58:332.

2 Wickramasinghe SN, Matthews JH 1988 Deoxyuridine suppression: biochemical basis and diagnostic applications. Blood Reviews 2:168.

3 Carmel R, Karnaze DS 1985 The deoxyuridine suppression test identifies subtle cobalamin deficiency in patients without typical megaloblastic anemia. Journal of the American Medical Association 253:1284.

4 Lindenbaum J, Healton EB, Savage DG, et al 1988 Neuropsychiatric disorders caused by cobalamin deficiency in the absence of anaemia or macrocytosis. New England Journal of Medicine 318:1720.

5 Green R 1995 Metabolic assays in cobalamin and folate deficiencies. In: Wickramasinghe SN (ed) Baillière's Clinical Haematology: Megaloblastic anaemia. 8:533.

6 Amos RJ, Dawson DW, Fish DI, et al 1994 Guidelines on the investigation and diagnosis of cobalamin and folate deficiencies. Clinical and Laboratory Haematology 16:101.

7 O'Broin SD, Kelleher BP 1992 Microbiological assay on microtitre plates of folate in serum and red cells. Journal of Clinical Pathology 45:344.

8 Anderson BB 1964 Investigation into the *Euglena* method for the assay of vitamin B_{12} in serum. Journal of Clinical Pathology 17:14.

9 Curtis AD, Mussett MV, Kennedy DA 1986 British Standard for human serum vitamin B_{12}. Clinical and Laboratory Haematology 8:135.

10 Waters AH, Mollin DL 1961 Studies on the folic acid activity of human serum. Journal of Clinical Pathology 14:335.

11 Gilois CR, Stone J, Lai AP, et al 1990 Effect of haemolysate preparation on measurement of red cell folate by radioisotope assay. Journal of Clinical Pathology 43:160.

12 Chanarin I 1979 The megaloblastic anaemias, 2nd edn. (a) p 59, (b) p 87, (c) p 121, (d) p 190, (e) p 193, (f) p 194, (g) p 362. Blackwell Scientific, Oxford.

13 Barakat RM, Ekins RP 1961 Assay of vitamin B_{12} in blood. Lancet ii:25.

14 Rothenberg SP, Marcoulis GP, Schwarz S et al 1984 Measurement of cyanocobalamin in serum by a specific radioimmunoassay. Journal of Laboratory and Clinical Medicine 103:959.

15 O'Sullivan JJ, Leeming RJ, Lynch SS, et al 1992 Radioimmunoassay that measures serum vitamin B_{12} Journal of Clinical Pathology 45:328.

16 Fish DI, Dawson DW 1983 Comparison of methods used in commercial kits for the assay of serum vitamin B_{12}. Clinical and Laboratory Haematology 5:271.

17 Cooper BA, Fehedy V, Blanshay P 1986 Recognition of deficiency of vitamin B_{12} using measurement of serum concentration. Journal of Laboratory and Clinical Medicine 107:447.

18 Lee-Owen V, Bolton AE, Carr PJ 1979 Formation of a vitamin B_{12}-serum complex on heating at alkaline pH. Clinica Chimica Acta 93:239.

19 Bain B, Broom GW, Woodside J, et al 1982 An assessment of a radioisotope assay for vitamin B_{12}, using an intrinsic factor preparation with R protein blocked by cobinamide. Journal of Clinical Pathology 35:1110.

20 Shum RY, O'Neill BJ, Streeter AM 1971 Effect of pH changes on the binding of vitamin B_{12} by intrinsic factor. Journal of Clinical Pathology 24:239.

21 Raven JL, Robson MB, Morgan JO, et al 1972 Comparison of three methods for measuring vitamin B_{12} in serum: radioisotopic, *Euglena gracilis* and *Leichmannii*. British Journal of Haematology 22:21.

22 Rothenberg SP 1968 A radioassay for serum B_{12} using unsaturated transcobalamin I as the binding protein. Blood 31:44.

23 Carmel R, Coltman CA 1969 Radioassay for serum vitamin B_{12} with the use of saliva as the vitamin B_{12} binder. Journal of Laboratory and Clinical Medicine 74:967.

24 Green R, Newark PA, Musso AM, et al 1974 The use of chicken serum for the measurement of serum vitamin B_{12} by radioisotope dilution. Description of method and comparison with microbiological assay results. British Journal of Haematology 27:507.

25 Chen IW, Silberstein ES, Maxon HR et al 1981 Clinical significance of serum vitamin B_{12} measured by radioassay using pure intrinsic factor. Journal of Nuclear Medicine 22:447.

26 Herbert V, Colman N, Palat D, et al 1984 Is there a 'gold standard' for human serum vitamin B_{12} assay? Journal of Laboratory and Clinical Medicine 104:829.

27 Robard D 1978 Data processing for radioimmunoassays: an overview. In: Natelson S, Pesce A, Dietz A (eds) Clinical Immunochemistry.

American Association for Clinical Chemistry, Washington, p. 477.

28 Adams JF, McEwain FC 1974 The separation of free and bound vitamin B_{12}. British Journal of Haematology 26:581.

29 Frenkel EP, White JD, Reisch JS, et al 1973 Comparison of two methods of the radioassay of vitamin B_{12} in serum. Clinical Chemistry 19:1327.

30 Tibbling G 1969 A method for determination of vitamin B_{12} in serum by radioassay. Clinica Chimica Acta 23:209.

31 Muir M, Chanarin I 1983 The assay of serum cobalamin by solid phase saturation analysis. In: Hall CA (ed) Methods in Hematology, Vol. 10: The Cobalamins. Churchill Livingstone, Edinburgh, p. 85

32 Ekins RP 1974 Radioimmunoassay and saturation analysis. Basic principles. British Medical Bulletin 30:3.

33 Dawson DW, Fish DI, Frew IDO et al 1987 Laboratory diagnosis of megaloblastic anaemia: current methods assessed by external quality assurance trials. Journal of Clinical Pathology 40:393.

34 Ghitis J 1966 The labile folate of milk. American Journal of Clinical Nutrition 18:452.

35 Givas J, Gutcho S 1975 pH dependence of the binding of folate to milk binder in radioassay of folates. Clinical Chemistry 21:427.

36 Mitchell GA, Pochron SP, Smutny PV et al 1976 Decreased radioassay values for folate after serum extraction when pteroylglutamic acid standards are used. Clinical Chemistry 22:647.

37 Bain BJ, Wickramasinghe SN, Broom GW, et al 1984 Assessment of the value of a competitive protein binding radioassay of folic acid in the detection of folic acid deficiency. Journal of Clinical Pathology 37:888.

38 Omer A 1969 Factors influencing the release of assayable folate from erythrocytes. Journal of Clinical Pathology 22:217.

39 Hoffbrand AV, Newcombe BFA, Mollin DL 1966 Method of assay of red cell folate activity and the value of the assay as a test for folate deficiency. Journal of Clinical Pathology 19:17.

40 Netteland B, Bakke OM 1977 Inadequate sample-preparation technique as a source of error in determination of erythrocyte folate by competitive binding of radioassay. Clinical Chemistry 23:1505.

41 Shane B, Tamura T, Stokstad ELR 1980 Folate assay: a comparison of radioassay and microbiological methods. Clinica Chimica Acta 100:13.

42 Kuemmerie GL, Boltinghouse GL, Delby SM et al. 1992 Automated assay of vitamin B_{12} by the Abbott IMX analyser. Clinical Chemistry 38:2073.

43 Gutcho S, Mansbach L 1977 Simultaneous radioassay of serum vitamin B_{12} and folic acid. Clinical Chemistry 23:1609.

44 International Committee for Standardization in Haematology 1981 Proposed serum standard for human serum vitamin B_{12} assay. British Journal of Haematology 64:809.

45 WHO Expert Committee on Biological Standards 1998 Fourth-sixth report, p. 25. WHO Technical Report Series No. 872.

46 Mollin DL, Hoffbrand AV, Ward PG et al 1980 Interlaboratory comparison of serum vitamin B_{12} assay. Journal of Clinical Pathology 33:243.

47 Cook TD, Cichowicz DJ, George S, et al 1987 Mammalian folipolyglutamate synthetase. 4. In vitro and in vivo metabolism of folates and analogues and regulation of folate homeostasis. Biochemistry 26:530.

48 Hoffbrand AV, Jackson BFA 1993 Correction of the DNA synthesis depletion in vitamin B_{12} deficiency by tetrahydrofolate: evidence in favour of the methyl-folate trap hypothesis as the cause of megaloblastic anaemia in vitamin B_{12} deficiency. British Journal of Haematology 83:643.

49 Lavoie A, Tripp E, Hoffbrand AV 1974 The effect of vitamin B_{12} deficiency on methylfolate metabolism and pteryolpolyglutamate synthesis in human cells. Clinical Science and Molecular Medicine 47:617.

50 Ganeshaguru K, Hoffbrand AV 1978 The effect of deoxyuridine, vitamin B_{12}, folate and alcohol on the uptake of thymidine and on the deoxyuridine triphosphate concentration in normal and megaloblastic cells. British Journal of Haematology 40:29.

51 Metz J, Kelly A, Swett VC, et al 1968 Deranged DNA synthesis by bone marrow from vitamin B_{12}-deficient humans. British Journal of Haematology 14:575.

52 Matthews J, Wickramasinghe SN 1986 A method for performing deoxyuridine suppression on microtitre plates. Clinical and Laboratory Haematology 8:61.

53 Schilling RF 1953 Intrinsic factor studies. II. The effect of gastric juice on the urinary excretion of radioactivity after the oral administration of radioactive vitamin B_{12}. Journal of Laboratory and Clinical Medicine 42:860.

54 Cottrall MF, Wells DG, Trott NG et al 1971 Radioactive vitamin B_{12} absorption studies: comparison of the whole-body retention, urinary excretion and eight-hour plasma levels of radioactive vitamin B_{12}. Blood 38:604.

55 McDonald JWD, Barton WB 1975 Spurious Schilling test results obtained with intrinsic factor

enclosed in capsules. Annals of Internal Medicine 83:827.

56 International Committee for Standardization in Haematology 1981 Recommended method for the measurement of vitamin B_{12} absorption. Journal of Nuclear Medicine 22:1091.

57 Wallis J, Clark DM, Bain BJ 1986 The use of hydroxocobalamin in the Schilling test. Scandinavian Journal of Haematology 37:337–340.

58 Herbert V 1969 Transient (reversible) malabsorption of vitamin B_{12}. British Journal of Haematology 17:213.

59 England JM, Snashall EA, De Silva PM 1981 Comparison of the DICOPAC with the conventional Schilling test. Journal of Clinical Pathology 34:1191.

60 Doscherholmen A, McMahon J, Ripley D 1978 Inhibitory effect of eggs in vitamin B_{12} absorption: description of a simple ovalbumin ^{57}Co-vitamin B_{12} absorption test. British Journal of Haematology 33:261.

61 Doscherholmen A, Silvis S, McMahon J 1983 Dual Schilling test for measuring absorption of food-bound and free vitamin B_{12} simultaneously. American Journal of Clinical Pathology 80:490.

62 Dawson DW, Sawers AH, Sharma RK 1984 Malabsorption of protein bound vitamin B_{12}. British Medical Journal 288:675.

63 Callender ST, Witts LJ, Warner GT et al 1966 The use of a simple wholebody counter for haematological investigations. British Journal of Haematology 12:276.

64 Tait CE, Hesp R 1976 Measurement of ^{57}Co-vitamin B_{12} uptake using a static whole-body counter. British Journal of Radiology 49:948.

65 Briedis D, Mcintyre PA, Judisch J et al 1973 An evaluation of a dual isotope method for the measurement of vitamin B_{12} absorption. Journal of Nuclear Medicine 14:135.

66 Begley JA, Trachtenberg A 1979 An assay for intrinsic factor based on blocking of the R binder of gastric juice by cobinamide. Blood 53:788.

67 Gottlieb C, Lau KS, Wasserman LR, et al 1965 Rapid charcoal assays for intrinsic factor (IF), gastric juice unsaturated B_{12} binding capacity, antibody to IF and serum unsaturated B_{12} binding capacity. Blood 25:6.

68 Conn DA 1986 Detection of Type I and Type II antibodies to intrinsic factor. Medical Laboratory Sciences 43:148.

69 Waters HM, Dawson DW, Howarth JE et al 1993 High incidence of Type II auto-antibodies in pernicious anaemia. Journal of Clinical Pathology 46:45.

70 Shackleton PJ, Fish DI, Dawson DW 1989 Intrinsic factor antibody tests. Journal of Clinical Pathology 42:210.

71 Nimo RE, Carmel R 1987 Increased sensitivity of detection of the blocking (type I) anti-intrinsic factor antibody. American Journal of Clinical Pathology 88:729.

72 Waters HM, Smith C, Howarth JE et al 1989 A new enzyme immunoassay for the detection of total Type I and Type II intrinsic factor antibody. Journal of Clinical Pathology 42:307.

73 Carmel R 1988 R-binder deficiency. A clinically benign cause of cobalamin deficiency. Journal of the American Medical Association 250:1886.

74 Jacob E, Herbert V 1975 Measurement of unsaturated 'granulocyte-related' (TCI and TCIII) and 'liver-related' (TCII) B_{12} binders by instant batch separation using a microfine precipitate of silica (QUSO G32). Journal of Laboratory and Clinical Medicine 88:505.

75 Scott JM, Bloomfield FJ, Stebbins R et al 1974 Studies on derivation of transcobalamin III from granulocytes. Enhancement by lithium and elimination by fluoride of in vitro increments in vitamin B_{12}-binding capacity. Journal of Clinical Investigation 53:228.

76 Gilois CR, Dunbar DR 1987 Measurement of low serum and red cell folate levels; a comparison of analytical methods. Medical Laboratory Sciences 44:33.

77 Oxley DK 1984 Serum vitamin B_{12} assays. Archives of Pathology Laboratory Medicine 108:277.

78 Reynoso G, MacKenzie JR 1982 Are ligand assay methods specific for cobalamin? American Journal of Clinical Pathology 78:621.

9

Laboratory methods used in the investigation of the haemolytic anaemias

S. Mitchell Lewis & David Roper

Normally, effete red cells undergo lysis at the end of their life-span of *c* 120 days. In haemolytic anaemia, the red cell life-span is shortened. The causes can be divided into three groups:

1. defects within red cells from dysfunction of enzyme-controlled metabolism, abnormal haemoglobins and thalassaemias
2. loss of structural integrity of red cell membrane and cytoskeleton in hereditary spherocytosis, elliptocytosis, paroxysmal nocturnal haemoglobinuria (PNH), immune and drug-associated antibody damage
3. damage by outside factors such as mechanical trauma, microangiopathic conditions, thrombotic thrombocytopenic purpura and chemical toxins.

At the end of a normal life-span, red cells are destroyed within the reticulo-endothelial (RE) system in the spleen, liver and bone marrow. In some haemolytic anaemias, the haemolysis may occur predominantly in the RE system (extravascular) and the plasma haemoglobin concentration is barely raised; in other disorders, a major degree of haemolysis takes place within the bloodstream (intravascular haemolysis): the plasma haemoglobin rises substantially, and in some cases the amount of haemoglobin so liberated may be sufficient to lead to haemoglobin being excreted in the urine (haemoglobinuria). However, there is often a combination of both mechanisms. The two pathways by which haemoglobin derived from effete red cells is metabolized are illustrated in Figure 9.1.

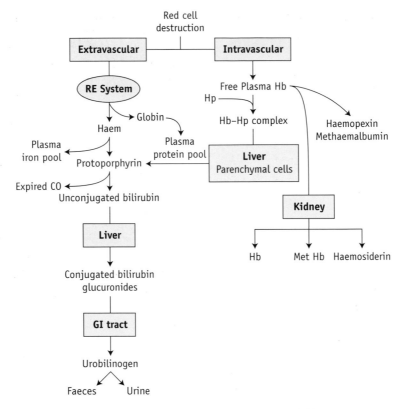

Fig. 9.1   Catabolic pathway of haemoglobin.

INVESTIGATION OF HAEMOLYTIC ANAEMIA

The clinical and laboratory phenomena of increased haemolysis reflect the nature of the haemolytic mechanism, where the haemolysis is taking place and the response of the bone marrow to the anaemia resulting from the haemolysis, namely, erythroid hyperplasia and reticulocytosis.

The investigation of patients suspected of suffering from a haemolytic anaemia comprises several distinct stages: recognizing the existence of increased haemolysis; determining the type of haemolytic mechanism; and making the precise diagnosis. In practice, the procedures are often telescoped, for the diagnosis in some instances may be obvious to the experienced observer from a glance down the microscope at the patient's blood film.

The following practical scheme of investigation is recommended. The tests are arranged in order of importance and practicability.

Is there evidence of increased haemolysis?

1. Hb estimation; reticulocyte count; inspection of a stained blood film for the presence of spherocytes, elliptocytes, irregularly-contracted cells, schistocytes or auto-agglutination (see Ch. 5).
2. Test for increased unconjugated serum bilirubin and urinary urobilinogen excretion; measurement of haptoglobin or haemopexin.
3. Detection of urinary haemoglobin or haemosiderin.
4. Measurement of life-span of patient's red cells (see Ch. 15).
5. Determination of sites of haemolysis by radionuclide scan or surface counting if splenectomy is contemplated (see Ch. 15).

What is the type of haemolytic mechanism?

1. Direct antiglobulin test (DAT) with broad-spectrum serum.
2. Osmotic fragility and glycerol lysis test.
3. Test for haemosiderin and Hb in urine; estimation of plasma Hb; Schumm's test.

What is the precise diagnosis?

Which further test should be done depends upon the results of the tests which have already been carried out. Not all are appropriate in every case.

1. If a hereditary haemolytic anaemia is suspected:

Osmotic-fragility determination after 24 h incubation at 37°C; autohaemolysis test ± the addition of glucose; red cell instability at 45°C; screening test for red cell G6PD deficiency; red cell pyruvate kinase assay; assay of other red cell enzymes involved in glycolysis; estimation of red cell glutathione (see Ch. 10).

Electrophoresis for abnormal haemoglobins; estimation of % Hb A_2; estimation of % Hb F; tests for sickling; tests for unstable haemoglobin; MCV and MCH (see Ch. 12).

Demonstration of the proteins of the red cell membrane and cytoskeleton (spectrin, etc.) by gel electrophoresis and by specific radioimmunoassay.

2. If an auto-immune acquired haemolytic anaemia is suspected:

Direct antiglobulin test using anti-immunoglobulin and anti-complement sera; tests for auto-antibodies in the patient's serum; titration of cold agglutinins; Donath–Landsteiner test; electrophoresis of serum proteins; demonstration of thermal range of auto-antibodies; tests for agglutination and/or lysis of enzyme-treated cells by auto-antibodies; tests for lysis of normal cells by auto-antibodies (see Ch. 11).

3. If the haemolytic anaemia is suspected of being drug-induced:

Screening test for red cell G6PD; glutathione stability test; staining for Heinz bodies; identification of methaemoglobin (Hi) and sulphaemoglobin (SHb); tests for drug-dependent antibodies.

4. If mechanical stress is suspected:

Red cell morphology; platelet count; renal function tests; coagulation screen; fibrinogen assay; test for fibrinogen/fibrin degradation products (see Ch. 16).

5. In all instances of haemolytic anaemia of obscure type and in aplastic anaemia:

Investigations for PNH, e.g. acidified serum test (Ham's test), sucrose lysis test (see Ch. 11).

ESTIMATION OF PLASMA HAEMOGLOBIN

Methods are based on (a) peroxidase reaction and (b) direct measurement of haemoglobin by spectrophotometry*. In the peroxidase method, the catalytic action of haem-containing proteins brings about the oxidation of benzidine compounds by hydrogen peroxide to give a green colour which changes to blue and finally to reddish violet. The intensity of reaction may be compared in a spectrophotometer with that produced by solutions of known Hb. Methaemalbumin and Hb are measured together. Formerly, the test used benzidene,[1] but this is a carcinogenic substance and in many countries its use is prohibited without a special licence. Tetramethylbenzidine is an analogue which is more readily available, but it is also hazardous to some degree, and it must be handled with great care.

When the plasma Hb is >50 mg/l, it can be measured by a modification of the haemiglobincyanide method for whole blood[2] or as HbO_2 by any spectrometer at 540 nm. Lower concentrations can also be measured reliably, as described below, provided that the spectrometer plots of concentration/absorbance give a linear slope passing through the origin. A pink tinge to the plasma is detectable by eye when the Hb is above 200 mg/l.

Sample collection

Every effort must be made to prevent haemolysis during the collection and manipulation of the

---

*Also termed "spectrometry"

blood. A clean venepuncture is essential; a relatively wide-bore needle should be used and a plastic syringe should be allowed to fill spontaneously with blood without negative pressure. When the required amount of blood has been withdrawn, the needle should be detached with care and 9 volumes of blood added to 1 volume of 32 g/l sodium citrate. Haemolysis may be reduced to a minimum if the blood is collected through a wide-bore needle direct into a siliconized centrifuge tube containing heparin and the plasma separated without delay.

PEROXIDASE METHOD[3]

Reagents

Benzidine compound. Dissolve 1 g of 3,3′,5,5′-tetramethylbenzidine in 90 ml of glacial acetic acid and make up to 100 ml with water. The solution will keep for several weeks in a dark bottle at 4°C.

Hydrogen peroxide. Dilute 1 volume of 3% ('10 vols') H_2O_2 with 2 volumes of water before use.

Acetic acid. 100 g/l glacial acetic acid.

Standard. A blood sample of known Hb content is diluted with water to a final concentration of 200 mg/l. It is convenient to use a HiCN standard solution (p. 21) as the source of Hb.

Method

Add 20 μl of plasma to 1 ml of the benzidine reagent in a large glass tube. At the same time, set up a control tube, in which 20 μl of water are substituted for the plasma, and a standard tube, containing 20 μl of the Hb standard. Add 1 ml of the H_2O_2 solution to each tube and mix the contents well.

Allow the mixture to stand at *c* 20°C for 20 min and then add 10 ml of the acetic acid solution to each tube and, after mixing, allow the tubes to stand for a further 10 min. Compare the coloured solutions at 600 nm, using the colour developed by the control tube as a blank. If the Hb of the plasma to be tested is abnormally high, it can be measured by the method used with whole blood (see below).

SPECTROPHOTOMETRIC METHOD

1. From a normal blood sample, prepare an 80 g/l haemolysate (see p. 21).
2. Dilute 1:100 with phosphate buffer, pH 8, to obtain a haemoglobin concentration of 800 mg/l. By six consecutive double dilutions with phosphate buffer, make a set of seven lysate standards with values from 800 to 12.5 mg/l.
3. Read the absorbance of each solution at 540 nm, with water as a blank. Prepare a calibration graph by plotting the readings of absorbance (on y axis) against haemoglobin concentration (on x axis) on arithmetic graph paper, and draw the slope. Check that the slope passes through the xy origin.
4. Read the absorbance of the plasma directly at 540 nm with a water blank, and read the haemoglobin concentration from the calibration graph. If absorbance is greater than the maximum value plotted on the graph, repeat the reading with a sample diluted with buffer.

Low haemoglobin HemoCue

This is a modification of the HemoCue (p. 23) which can reliably measure plasma haemoglobin at or above 100 mg/l.[34]

Range

10–40 mg/l; lower levels may be obtained when blood is collected into a siliconized centrifuge tube with heparin (see above).

Significance of raised plasma haemoglobin

Haemoglobin liberated from the intravascular or extravascular breakdown of red cells interacts with the plasma haptoglobins to form a haemoglobin–haptoglobin complex[4] which, because of its size, does not undergo glomerular filtration, but it is removed from the circulation by, and degraded in, RE cells. Hb in excess of the capacity of the haptoglobins to bind it passes into the glomerular filtrate; it is then partly excreted in the urine in an uncomplexed form, resulting in haemoglobinuria, and partly reabsorbed by the proximal glomerular tubules where it is broken down into haem, iron and globin. The iron is retained in the cells and eventually excreted in the urine (haemosiderin). The haem and globin are reabsorbed into the plasma.

The haem complexes with albumin forming methaemalbumin (see p. 156) and with haemopexin (see p. 157); the globin competes with Hb to form a complex with haptoglobin. In effect, the plasma haemoglobin level is significantly raised in haemolytic anaemias when haemolysis is sufficiently severe for the available haptoglobin to be fully bound. The highest levels are found when haemolysis takes place predominantly in the bloodstream (intravascular haemolysis). Thus, marked haemoglobinaemia, with or without haemoglobinuria, may be found in paroxysmal nocturnal haemoglobinuria, paroxysmal cold haemoglobinuria, the cold-haemagglutinin syndrome, blackwater fever, and in march haemoglobinuria and in other mechanical haemolytic anaemias, e.g. that after cardiac surgery. In warm-type auto-immune haemolytic anaemias, sickle-cell anaemia and severe β thalassaemia, the plasma haemoglobin level may be slightly or moderately raised, but in hereditary spherocytosis, in which haemolysis occurs predominantly in the spleen, the levels are normal or only very slightly raised.

Haem within the proximal tubular epithelium undergoes further degradation to bilirubin with liberation of iron, some of which is retained intracellularly bound to proteins as ferritin and haemosiderin. When haemolysis is severe, the excess of haemoglobin which occurs in the glomerular filtrate will lead to an accumulation of intracellular haemosiderin in the glomerular tubular cells; when these cells slough, haemosiderin will appear in the urine (see p. 157).

It cannot be over-emphasized that the presence of excess Hb in the plasma is a reliable sign of intravascular haemolysis only if the observer can be sure that the lysis has not been caused during or after the withdrawal of the blood. It is also necessary to exclude colouring of the plasma from certain foods and food additives.

Increased levels may occur as a result of violent exercise.[5,6] They also occur in runners and joggers from mechanical trauma caused by continuous impact of the soles of the feet with hard ground.[7]

ESTIMATION OF SERUM HAPTOGLOBIN

Haptoglobin is a glycoprotein which is synthesized in the liver. It consists of two pairs of α chains and two pairs of β chains. Free haemoglobin, as a result of haemolysis, readily dissociates into dimers of α and β chains; the α chains bind avidly with the β chains of haptoglobin in plasma or serum to form a complex which can be differentiated from free haemoglobin by column chromatographic separation[8] or by its altered rate of migration on electrophoresis.[9]

Direct measurement of haptoglobin is also possible by turbidimetry[10] or nephelometry,[11] and by radial immunodiffusion.[12] The methods described below are cellulose-acetate electrophoresis and radial immunodiffusion.

ELECTROPHORESIS METHOD [9,13]

Principle
Known amounts of haemoglobin are added to serum. The Hb-haptoglobin complex is separated by electrophoresis on cellulose acetate; the presence of bound and free Hb is identified in each sample and the amount of haptoglobin is estimated by noting where free haemoglobin appears.

Reagents
Buffer (pH 7.0, ionic strength 0.05). $Na_2HPO_4.H_2O$ 7.1 g/l, 2 volumes; $NaH_2PO_4.H_2O$ 6.9 g/l, 1 volume. Store at 4°C.

Haemolysates. Prepare as described on page 240. Adjust the Hb to 30 g/l with water and dilute this preparation further with water to obtain a batch of solutions with haemoglobin concentrations of 2.5, 5, 10, 20 and 30 g/l. These solutions are stable at 4°C for several weeks.

Stain. Dissolve 0.5 g of *o*-dianisidine (3,3′-dimethoxybenzidine) in 70 ml of 95% ethanol; prior to use, add together 10 ml of acetate buffer, pH 4.7 (sodium acetate 2.92 g, glacial acetic acid 1 ml, water to 1 litre), 2.5 ml of 3% (10 volumes) H_2O_2 and water to 100 ml.

Clearing solution. Glacial acetic acid 25 ml, 95% ethanol 75 ml.

Acetic acid rinse. Glacial acetic acid, 50 ml/l.

Method

Serum is obtained from blood allowed to clot undisturbed at 37°C. As soon as the clot starts to retract, remove the serum by pipette and centrifuge it to rid it of suspended red cells. The serum may be stored at −20°C until used.

Mix well 1 volume of each of the diluted haemolysates with 9 volumes of serum. Allow to stand for 10 min at room temperature.

Impregnate cellulose acetate membrane filterstrips (12 × 2.5 cm) in buffer solution and blot to remove all obvious surface fluid. Apply 0.75 µl samples of the serum-haemolysate mixtures across the strips as thin transverse lines. As controls, include strips with serum alone and haemoglobin lysate alone. Electrophorese at 0.5 mA/cm width. Good separation patterns about 5–7 cm in length should be obtained in 30 min (Fig. 9.2).

After electrophoresis is completed, immerse the membranes in freshly prepared *o*-dianisidine stain for 10 min. Then rinse with water and immerse in 50 ml/l acetic acid for 5 min. Remove the membranes and place in 95% ethanol for exactly 1 min. Transfer the membranes to a tray containing freshly prepared clearing solution and immerse for exactly 30 s. While still in the solution, position the membranes over a glass plate placed in the tray. Remove the glass plate with the membranes on it, drain the excess solution from the membranes, transfer the glass plate to a ventilated oven preheated to 100°C, and allow the membranes to dry for 10 min.

Interpretation. The patterns of free Hb and Hb-haptoglobin complex migration are shown in Figure 9.2. Hb-haptoglobin complex appears in the α_2 globulin position. When there is more haemoglobin than can be bound to the haptoglobin the free Hb migrates in the β globulin position. The amount of haptoglobin present in the serum is determined semi-quantitatively as between the lowest concentration of haemoglobin which shows only a free Hb band and the adjacent strip which shows a band of Hb-haptoglobin complex. In the total absence of haptoglobin, a Hb band alone will be seen even at 2.5 g/l. In severe intravascular haemolysis with depleted haptoglobin, a stained band may also appear in the albumin position due to metahaemalbumin.

The concentration of haptoglobin can be determined quantitatively with a densitometer. The test is carried out as described above, but only one haemolysate is required with a Hb of 30–40 g/l. After the plate has cooled, the membranes are scanned by a densitometer at 450 nm with a 0.3 mm slit width. The density of the haptoglobin band is calculated as a fraction of the total Hb in the electrophoretic strip:

$$\text{Haptoglobin (g/l)} = \text{Haptoglobin fraction} \times \text{Hb (g/l)}$$

RADIAL IMMUNODIFFUSION (RID) METHOD

Principle

The test serum samples and reference samples of known haptoglobin concentration are dispensed into wells in a plate of agarose gel containing a monospecific antiserum to human haptoglobin. Precipitation rings form by the reaction of haptoglobin with the antibody; the diameter of each ring is proportional to the concentration of haptoglobin in the sample.

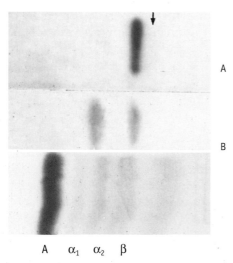

A

B

A α_1 α_2 β

Fig. 9.2 Demonstration of serum haptoglobin.
(A) Serum from case of haemolytic anaemia with no haptoglobin: the added haemoglobin is demonstrated as a band in the β-globulin position. (B) Normal serum with added haemoglobin: there are bands in the β-globulin (Hb) and α_2-globulin (Hb-haptoglobin complex) positions, respectively. The line of origin is indicated by the arrow. The pattern of serum electrophoresis is shown below (A, albumin; α_1, α_2 and β, components of globulin).

---

*Gel plates containing the antiserum are available commercially.

Reagents

Single diffusion plates. Dissolve agarose (20 g/l) in boiling phosphate buffered water pH 7.4 (p. 605). Allow to cool to 50°C. Add 5% sheep or goat anti-human haptoglobin antiserum diluted in buffered water, pH 7.4. Mix well but without creating bubbles. Pour the gel onto thin plastic trays (plates) to a thickness of less than 1 mm. After the gel has set, cut out a series of wells *c* 2 mm in diameter, about 2 cm apart. Extract the core by a pipette tip with a negative pressure pump. Cover the plates with fitted lids and store in sealed packets at 4°C until used.

Reference sera. Preparations of human serum with stated haptoglobin concentration are available commercially. They should be stored at 4°C.

Test serum. This can be kept at 4°C for 2 to 3 days, but if not used within this time, store at –20°C. Thaw completely and mix well immediately before use.

Method

Allow the plate (in its sealed packet) and the sera to equilibrate at room temperature for 15 min. Remove the lid from the plate. Check for moisture; if present, allow to evaporate. Add 5 µl of each serum into one of the wells in the plate. Stand for about 10 min to ensure that the serum is completely absorbed into the gel. Then cover the plate, return it to its container and reseal the packet. Leave on a level surface at room temperature for 18 h. From measurements of the reference sera, construct a reference curve on log-linear graph paper by plotting haptoglobin concentration on the vertical axis (logarithmic scale) and the diameter of the rings on the horizontal scale (linear scale). Measure the diameter of the precipitation ring formed by the test serum and express concentration in g/l (Fig. 9.3).

Normal ranges

By direct measurement, results are expressed as haptoglobin concentration; slightly different normal reference values have been reported for the different methods:[10,11,14,15]

RID 0.8–2.7 g/l
Nephelometry 0.3–2.2 g/l
Turbidimetry 0.5–1.6 g/l.

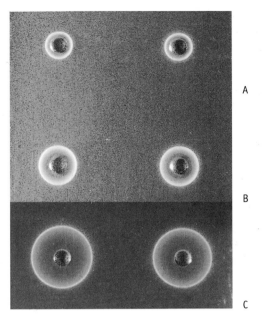

Fig. 9.3 Demonstration of serum haptoglobin. Radial immunodiffusion: (A) low; (B) normal; (C) increased concentrations.

When measured as Hb binding capacity, in normal sera haptoglobins will bind 0.3–2.0 g of Hb/l; levels are higher in men than in women.[14]

Significance

Haptoglobins begin to be depleted when the daily Hb turnover exceeds about twice the normal.[9] This occurs irrespective of whether the haemolysis is predominantly extravascular or intravascular; but rapid depletion, often with the formation of methaemalbumin, occurs as a result of small degrees of intravascular haemolysis, even when the daily total Hb turnover is not increased appreciably above normal. Low concentrations of haptoglobins, in the absence of increased haemolysis, may be found in hepatocellular disease, and are characteristic of congenital ahaptoglobinaemia which occurs in about 2% of Caucasians and a larger number of Blacks.[16] Low concentrations may also be found in megaloblastic anaemias probably because of increased haemolysis, and following haemorrhage into tissues.

The haptoglobin–haemoglobin complex is cleared by the RE system, mainly in the liver. The rate of removal is influenced by the concentration of free haemoglobin in the plasma: at levels below 10 g/l, the clearance $T_{1/2}$ is 20 min; at higher concentrations, clearance is considerably slower.

Increased haptoglobin concentrations may be found in pregnancy, chronic infections, malignancy, tissue damage, Hodgkin's disease, rheumatoid arthritis, systemic lupus erythematosus, biliary obstruction and as a consequence of steroid therapy or the use of oral contraceptives. Under these circumstances, a normal haptoglobin concentration does not exclude increased haemolysis.

EXAMINATION OF PLASMA (OR SERUM) FOR METHAEMALBUMIN

A simple but not very sensitive method is to examine the plasma using a hand spectroscope.

Free the plasma from suspended cells and platelets by centrifuging at 1200–1500 *g* for 15–30 min. Then view it in bright daylight with a hand spectroscope using the greatest possible depth of plasma consistent with visibility. Methaemalbumin gives a rather weak band in the red (at 624 nm) (Fig. 9.4). As HbO_2 is usually present as well, its characteristic bands in the yellow–green may also be visible. The position of the methaemalbumin absorption band in the red can be readily differentiated from that of methaemoglobin (Hi) by means of a reversion spectroscope.

Presumptive evidence of the presence of small quantities of methaemalbumin, giving an absorption band too weak to recognize, can be obtained by extracting the pigment by ether and then converting it to an ammonium haemochromogen which gives a more intense band in the green (Schumm's test).

SCHUMM'S TEST

Method

Cover the plasma (or serum) with a layer of ether. Add a one-tenth volume of saturated yellow ammonium sulphide and mix it with the plasma. Then view it with a hand spectroscope. If methaemalbumin is present, a relatively intense narrow absorption band will be seen in the green (at 558 nm) (Fig. 9.4).

Significance of methaemalbuminaemia

Methaemalbumin is found in the plasma when haptoglobins are absent in haemolytic anaemias in which lysis is predominantly intravascular. It was first observed by Fairley & Bromfield in blackwater fever.[17] It is a haem–albumin compound formed subsequent to the degradation of Hb liberated into plasma. In contrast to haptoglobin-bound Hb and haemopexin-bound haem, the haem–albumin complex is thought to remain in

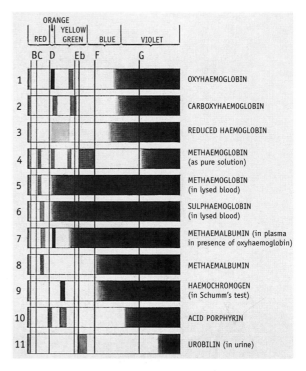

Fig. 9.4 Absorption spectra of derivatives of human haemoglobin. The absorption bands are shown in relation to the Fraunhofer lines, the positions of which are as follows: B at 686.7 nm, C at 656.3 nm, D at 589 nm, E at 527 nm, b at 518.4 nm, F at 486.1 nm and G at 430.8 nm.

circulation until the haem is transferred from albumin to the more highly avid haemopexin.[18]

QUANTITATIVE ESTIMATION OF METHAEMALBUMIN BY A SPECTROPHOTOMETRIC METHOD

To 2 ml of plasma (or serum) add 1 ml of iso-osmotic phosphate buffer, pH 7.4. Centrifuge the mixture for 30 min at 1200–1500 *g* and measure its absorbance in a spectrophotometer at 569 nm. Add *c* 5 mg of solid sodium dithionite to the supernatant diluted plasma. Shake the tube gently to dissolve the dithionite and leave for 5 min to allow complete reduction of the methaemalbumin. Remeasure the absorbance. The difference between the two readings represents the absorbance owing to methaemalbumin; its concentration can be read off from a calibration graph.

The calibration graph is constructed as follows: solutions containing 10–100 mg/l methaemal-bumin are obtained by dissolving appropriate amounts of haemin (bovine or equine) in a minimum volume of 40 g/l human serum albumin. The absorbance of each solution is measured in a spectrophotometer at 569 nm, and a graph drawn from the figures obtained.

DEMONSTRATION OF HAEMOSIDERIN IN URINE

Method

Centrifuge 10 ml of urine at 1200 g for 10–15 min. Transfer the deposit to a slide, spread out to occupy an area of 1–2 cm and allow to dry in the air. Fix by placing the slide in methanol for 10–20 min and then stain by the method used to stain blood films for siderocytes (p. 270). Haemosiderin, if present, appears in the form of isolated or grouped blue-staining granules, usually from 1–3 µm in size (Fig. 9.5); they may be both intracellular and extra-cellular. If haemosiderin is present in small amounts, and especially if distributed irregularly on the slide, or if the findings are difficult to interpret, the test should be repeated on a fresh sample of urine collected into an iron-free container and centrifuged in an iron-free tube. (For the preparation of iron-free glassware, see p. 609.)

Significance of haemosiderinuria
Haemosiderinuria is a sequel to the presence of Hb in the glomerular filtrate. It is a valuable sign of chronic intravascular haemolysis, for the urine will be found to contain iron-containing granules even if there is no haemoglobinuria at the time. However, haemosiderinuria is not found in the urine at the onset of a haemolytic attack even if this is accompanied by haemoglobinaemia and haemoglobinuria, as the haemoglobin has first to be absorbed by the cells of the renal tubules. The intracellular breakdown of Hb liberates iron which is then re-excreted. Haemosiderinuria may persist for several weeks after a haemolytic episode.

DEMONSTRATION OF SERUM HAEMOPEXIN

Haemopexin is a transport glycoprotein of molecular weight 70 000, synthesized in the liver. Haem derived from Hb, which fails to bind to haptoglobin, complexes with either albumin or haemopexin. The latter has a much higher affinity, and only when all the haemopexin has been used up will the haem combine with albumin to form methaemalbumin. When complexed, the haem-haemopexin complex is eliminated from the circulation, e.g. by the liver Kupffer cells.

In normal adults of both sexes, its concentration is 0.5–1 g/l;[18] in newborn infants, there is much less, *c* 0.3 g/l, but adult levels are reached by the end of the first year of life. In severe intravascular haemolysis, haemopexin levels are low or zero when haptoglobin is depleted. With less severe haemolysis, although haptoglobin is likely to be reduced or absent, haemopexin may be normal or only slightly lowered, and it has been suggested that the haemopexin level gives a more reliable measure of haemolysis than does the haptoglobin level. Haem binds in a 1:1 molar ratio to haemopexin; 6 µg/ml of free haem is required to deplete the normal binding levels of haemopexin. Haemopexin seems to be disproportionately low in thalassaemia major, and low levels may be found in certain pathological conditions other

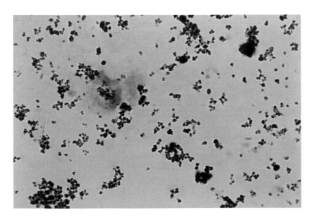

Fig. 9.5 Photomicrograph of urine deposit stained by Perls' reaction.

than haemolytic disease, namely, renal and liver diseases. The concentration is raised in diabetes mellitus, infections and carcinoma.[18]

Haemopexin can be measured by starch-gel electrophoresis[19] or immunochemically by radial immunodiffusion.[20]

CHEMICAL TESTS OF HAEMOGLOBIN CATABOLISM

Measurement of serum or plasma bilirubin, urinary urobilin and faecal urobilinogen can provide important information in the investigation of haemolytic anaemias. In this section, their interpretation and significance in haemolytic anaemias will be described, but as the tests are, nowadays, seldom performed in a haematology laboratory, for details of the techniques readers are referred to textbooks of clinical chemistry, e.g. that by N.W. Tietz.[15]

SERUM BILIRUBIN

Bilirubin is present in serum in two forms: as unconjugated prehepatic bilirubin and bilirubin conjugated to glucuronic acid. Normally, the serum bilirubin concentration is <17 µmol/l (10 mg/l) and mostly unconjugated. As illustrated in Figure 9.1, when there is increased red cell destruction, the protoporphyrin gives rise to an increased amount of unconjugated bilirubin and carbon monoxide. The bilirubin is then conjugated in the liver and this bilirubin glucuronide is excreted into the intestinal tract. Bacterial action converts bilirubin glucuronide to urobilin and urobilinogen. In haemolytic anaemias, the serum bilirubin usually lies between 17 and 50 µmol/l (10–30 mg/l) and most is unconjugated. Sometimes the level may be normal, despite a considerable increase in haemolysis. Levels >85 µmol/l (50 mg/l) and/or a large proportion of conjugated bilirubin suggest liver disease. In haemolytic disease of the newborn (HDN), the bilirubin level is an important factor in determining whether an exchange transfusion should be carried out, as high values of unconjugated bilirubin are toxic to the brain and can lead to kernicterus. In normal newborn infants, the level often reaches 85 µmol/l, whilst in HDN infants levels of 350 µmol/l are not uncommon and need to be urgently lowered by exchange transfusion.

Moderately raised serum bilirubin levels are frequently found in dyshaemopoietic anaemias, e.g.

pernicious anaemia, where there is ineffective erythropoiesis. Although part of the bilirubin comes from red cells which have circulated, a major proportion is derived from red cell precursors in the bone marrow which have failed to complete maturation.

Total bilirubin can be measured by direct reading spectrophotometry at 454 (or 461) and 540 nm; the former are the selected wavelengths for bilirubin whilst the latter automatically corrects for any interference by free haemoglobin. The instrument can be standardized with bilirubin solutions of known concentration or with a coloured glass standard. Another direct reading method is by reflectance photometry on a drop of serum which is added to a reagent film.

An alternative 'wet chemistry' method is by the reaction with aqueous diazotized sulphanilic acid. A red colour is produced which is compared in a photoelectric colorimeter with that of a freshly prepared standard or read in a spectrophotometer at 600 nm. Only conjugated bilirubin reacts directly with this aqueous reagent; unconjugated bilirubin, which is bound to albumin, requires either the addition of ethanol to free it from albumin or an accelerator such as methanol or caffeine to enable it to react. The method of Michaelsson et al[21] in which caffeine benzoate is used as the accelerator possibly has advantages. A positive urine spot test indicates a condition in which there is an elevated serum conjugated bilirubin.

Bilirubin is destroyed by exposure to direct sunlight or any other source of ultraviolet (UV) light, including fluorescent lighting. Solutions are stable for 1 to 2 days if kept at 4°C in the dark.

UROBILIN AND UROBILINOGEN

Urobilin and its reduced form urobilinogen are formed by bacterial action on bile pigments in the intestine. The excretion of faecal urobilinogen in health is 50–500 µmol (30–300 mg) per day. It is increased in patients with a haemolytic anaemia.

Quantitative measurement of faecal urobilinogen should, in theory, provide an estimate of the total rate of bilirubin production. This is, however, a crude method of assessing rates of haemolysis, and minor degrees are more reliably demonstrated by red cell life-span studies. Urobilinogen excretion is also increased in dyshaemopoietic anaemias such as pernicious anaemia because of ineffective erythropoiesis.

The amount of urobilinogen in the urine in health is up to 6.7 μmol (4 mg) per day. But this is not a reliable index of haemolysis, for excessive urobilinuria can be a consequence of liver dysfunction as well as of increased red cell destruction.

For estimation in the faeces, the bile-derived pigments (stercobilin) are reduced to urobilinogen which is extracted with water. The solution is then treated with Ehrlich's dimethylaminobenzaldehyde reagent to produce a pink colour which can be compared with either a natural or an artificial standard in a quantitative assay.

QUALITATIVE TEST FOR UROBILINOGEN AND UROBILIN IN URINE

Schlesinger's zinc test

To 5 ml of urine, add 2 drops of 0.5 mol/l iodine to convert urobilinogen to urobilin. After mixing and standing for 1–2 min, add 5 ml of a 100 g/l suspension of zinc acetate in ethanol and centrifuge the mixture. A green fluorescence becomes apparent in the clear supernatant if urobilin or urobilinogen is present. If a spectroscope is available, the fluid may be examined for the broad absorption band (caused by urobilin) at the green-blue junction (see Fig. 9.4). Urobilinogen can also be detected in freshly voided urine by commercially available reagent strip methods.

PORPHYRINS

Haem synthesis is initiated by succinyl co-enzyme A and glycine, activated by the rate-limiting enzyme ALA-synthase. This produces δ-aminolaevulinic acid (ALA), which is the precursor of the porphyrins (Fig. 9.6). The three porphyrins of clinical importance in man are: protoporphyrin, uroporphyrin and coproporphyrin together with their precursor ALA. Protoporphyrin is widely distributed in the body and, in addition to its main role as a precursor of haem in Hb and myoglobin, it is a precursor of cytochromes and catalase. Uroporphyrin and coproporphyrin, which are precursors of protoporphyrin, are normally excreted in small amounts in urine and faeces. Red cells normally contain a small amount of coproporphyrin (5–35 nmol/l) and protoporphyrin (0.2–0.9 μmol/l). Deranged haem synthesis (e.g. sideroblastic anaemias, lead toxicity) and iron-deficiency anaemia result in an increased concentration of protoporphyrin in the red cells.

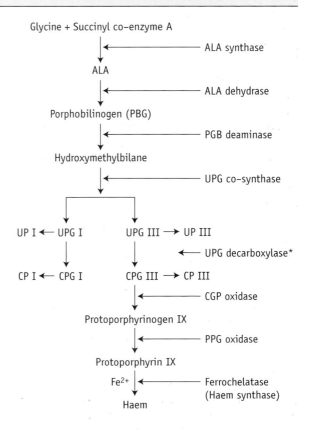

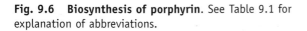

Fig. 9.6 Biosynthesis of porphyrin. See Table 9.1 for explanation of abbreviations.

acts on both isomer I and isomer III

ESTIMATION OF RED CELL PORPHYRINS

Principle

Porphyrins are extracted from washed red cells by a mixture of ethyl acetate and acetic acid. The preparation is treated with ether. Coproporphyrin is extracted from the ethereal solution by 0.1 mol/l HCl and protoporphyrin by 1.5 mol/l HCl. The porphyrin concentration in each extract is determined by a spectrophotometric method. Details of the procedure are given by Moore.[22]

DEMONSTRATION OF PORPHOBILINOGEN IN URINE

Principle

Ehrlich's dimethylaminobenzaldehyde reagent reacts with porphobilinogen to produce a pink aldehyde compound which can be differentiated from that produced by urobilinogen by the fact that the porphobilinogen compound is insoluble in chloroform.

Ehrlich's reagent. Dissolve 0.7 g of *p*-dimethyl-aminobenzaldehyde in a mixture of 150 ml of 10 mol/l HCl and 100 ml of water.

Method

The test is best carried out on a freshly passed specimen of urine. Mix a few ml of urine and an equal volume of Ehrlich's reagent in a large test-tube. Add 2 volumes of a saturated solution of sodium acetate. The urine should then have a pH of about 5.0, giving a red reaction with Congo red indicator paper.

If a pink colour develops in the solution, add a few ml of chloroform and shake the mixture thoroughly to extract the pigment. The colour owing to urobilinogen or indole will be extracted by the chloroform, whereas that owing to porphobilinogen will not, and remains in the supernatant aqueous fraction. When present, the concentration of porphobilinogen in the urine may be estimated quantitatively by a spectrophotometric method at 555 nm.[22]

Aminolaevulinic acid

When ALA is present in the urine, it can be concentrated with acetyl acetone. It then reacts with Ehrlich's reagent in the same way as porphobilin-ogen to give a red solution with an absorbance maximum at 553 nm. It can be separated from porphobilinogen by ion exchange resins and estimated quantitatively by a spectrophotometric method.[22]

DEMONSTRATION OF PORPHYRINS IN URINE

Principle

Porphyrins exhibit pink-red fluorescence when viewed by UV light (at 405 nm). Uroporphyrin can be distinguished from coproporphyrin by the different solubilities of the two substances in acid solution.

Method

Mix 25 ml of urine with 10 ml of glacial acetic acid in a separating funnel and extract twice with 50 ml volumes of ether. Set the aqueous fraction (Fraction 1) aside. Wash the ether extracts in a separating funnel with 10 ml of 1.6 mol/l HCl and collect the HCl fraction (Fraction 2). View both fractions in UV light (at 405 nm) for pink-red fluorescence. Its presence in Fraction 1 indicates uroporphyrin; in Fraction 2, coproporphyrin. The presence of the porphyrins should be confirmed spectroscopically (see below).

If uroporphyrin has been demonstrated, the reaction can be intensified by the following procedure. Adjust the pH of Fraction 1 to 3.0–3.2 with 0.1 mol/l HCl and extract the fraction twice with 50 ml volumes of ethyl acetate. Combine the extracts and extract three times with 2 ml volumes of 3 mol/l HCl. View the acid extracts for pink-red fluorescence in UV light and spectroscopically for acid porphyrin bands.

SPECTROSCOPIC EXAMINATION OF URINE FOR PORPHYRINS

This is carried out on extracts, made as described above, or on urine which is acidified with a few drops of 10 mol/l HCl. If porphyrins are present, a narrow band will appear in the orange at 596 nm and a broader band in the green at 552 nm (see Fig. 9.4). Qualitative tests are adequate for screening purposes. Accurate determinations require spectrophotometry or fluorimetry. Porphyrins are stable in EDTA blood for up to 8 days at room temperature if protected from light. Urine should be collected in a brown bottle, or if in a clear container, kept in a light-proof bag. If the urine is rendered alkaline to pH 7 to 7.5 with sodium bicarbonate, porphyrins will not be lost for several days at room temperature.

Significance of porphyrins in blood and urine

Normal red cells contain <650 nmol/l of protoporphyrin and <64 nmol/l of coproporphyrin.[22] Increased amounts are present during the first few months of life. At all ages, there is an increase in red cell protoporphyrin in iron-deficiency anaemia or latent iron deficiency, in lead poisoning, thalassaemia, some cases of sideroblastic anaemia and the anaemia of chronic infection.

Normally, a small amount of coproporphyrin is excreted in the urine (<430 nmol/day). This is demonstrable by the qualitative test described above, the intensity of pink-red fluorescence being proportional to the concentration of coproporphyrin. The excretion of coproporphyrin is increased when erythropoiesis is hyperactive, e.g. in haemolytic anaemias, polycythaemia and in pernicious anaemia, sideroblastic anaemias, etc. It is high in liver disease; renal impairment results in diminished excretion. In lead poisoning, there is an increase in red cell protoporphyrin and coproporphyrin, with excretion of exceptionally high levels of urinary ALA, coproporphyrin III and uroporphyrin I.

Normally, porphobilinogen cannot be demonstrated in urine, and only traces of uroporphyrin (<50 nmol/day), not detectable by the qualitative test described above, are present.[22] ALA excretion is <40 μmol/day; it is increased in lead poisoning.

The increase in urinary coproporphyrin excretion occurring in the above conditions is known as 'porphyrinuria'. There is no increase in uroporphyrin excretion. The porphyrias, on the other hand, are a group of disorders associated with abnormal porphyrin metabolism.

There are several forms of porphyria, caused by specific enzyme defects, each with a different clinical and biochemical manifestation.[23] The commonest type is acute intermittent porphyria in which the defect in the enzyme porphobilinogen deaminase presents in one of three ways: in type 1, there is decreased enzyme activity together with reduced amount of the enzyme in the red cells; type 3 also exhibits reduced red cell enzyme activity but normal amount of enzyme in the red cells; type 2 demonstrates decreased enzyme activity in lymphocytes and liver cells, but normal red cell activity. The different mutations of the porphobilinogen deaminase in the three types can be identified by DNA hybridization using specific oligonucleotides.[24]

The commonest hepatic type is *porphyria cutanea tarda*, which results in photosensitivity, dermatitis and, often, hepatic siderosis; it is due to a defect in uroporphyrinogen decarboxylase. There are two erythropoietic types: *congenital erythropoietic porphyria*, caused by defective uroporphyrinogen cosynthase and *erythropoietic protoporphyria*, caused by defective ferrochelatase (Table 9.1). In the former, uroporphyrin and coproporphyrin are present in red cells and urine in increased amounts; in the latter, increased protoporphyrin is found in the red cells, but the urine is normal. In erythropoietic porphyria, haemolytic anaemia may occur. The patterns of excretion of porphyrin and precursors and the clinical effects in the different types of porphyria are shown in Table 9.1.

RECOGNITION AND MEASUREMENT OF ABNORMAL HAEMOGLOBIN PIGMENTS

Methaemoglobin (Hi), sulphaemoglobin (SHb) and carboxyhaemoglobin (HbCO) are of clinical importance, and each has a characteristic absorption spectrum demonstrable by simple spectroscopy or, more definitely, by spectrophotometry. If the absorbance of a dilute solution of blood (e.g. 1 in 200) is measured at wavelengths between 400 and 700 nm, characteristic absorption spectra are obtained (Fig. 9.7). In practice, the abnormal substance represents usually only a fraction of the total Hb (except in coal-gas poisoning), and its identification and accurate measurement may be difficult. Hi can be measured more accurately than SHb.

Table 9.1 Distribution of porphyrins in red cells, urine and faeces in different forms of porphyria

Disease	Clinical effect	Enzyme defect[+]	Red cells	Urine	Faeces
Acute intermittent porphyria	(a)	PBG deaminase		PBG ALA	
Congenital erythropoietic porphyria	(b)	UPG III cosynthase	UP I CP I	UP I CP I	UP I CP I
Acquired cutaneous hepatic porphyria (symptomatic)	(b)	UPG decarboxylase		UP I CP III	
Hereditary coproporphyria	(a), (b)	CPG oxidase		CP III	CP III
Variegate porphyria (South African genetic)	(a), (b)	PPG oxidase		PBG* ALA*	CP III PP
Erythropoietic protoporphyria	(b)	Ferrochelatase	PP		PP

[+]See Figure 9.6.
* Mainly during acute attacks.
(a) Gastrointestinal and/or nervous system disorders.
(b) Photosensitive dermatitis.
ALA, δ-aminolaevulinic acid; PBG, porphobilinogen; UP, uroporphyrin; CP, coproporphyrin; PP, protoporphyrin; UPG, uroporphyrinogen; CPG, coproporphyrinogen; PPG, protoporphyrinogen.

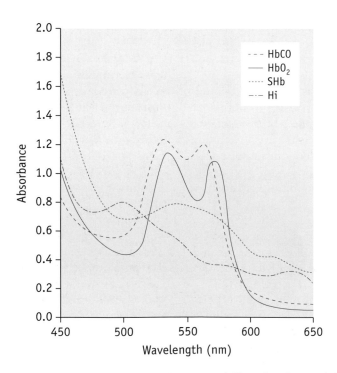

Fig. 9.7 Absorption spectra of various haemoglobin pigments. HbCO, carboxyhaemoglobin; HbO_2, oxyhaemoglobin; SHb, sulphaemoglobin; Hi, methaemoglobin.

SPECTROSCOPIC EXAMINATION OF BLOOD FOR METHAEMOGLOBIN AND SULPHAEMOGLOBIN

Method

Dilute blood 1 in 5 or 1 in 10 with water and then centrifuge. Examine the clear solution, if possible in daylight, using a hand spectroscope. It is important that the greatest possible depth or concentration of solution consistent with visibility should be examined and that a careful search should be made (with varying depths or concentrations of solution) for absorption bands in the red part of the spectrum at 620–630 nm. If bands are seen in the red, add a drop of yellow ammonium sulphide to the solution. A band caused by Hi, but not that caused by SHb, will disappear. For comparison, lysed blood may be treated with a few drops of potassium ferricyanide (50 g/l) solution which will cause the formation of Hi; SHb may be prepared by adding to 10 ml of a 1 in 100 dilution of blood 0.1 ml of a 1 g/l solution of phenylhydrazine hydrochloride and a drop of water which has been previously saturated with hydrogen sulphide. The spectra of the unknown and the known pigments may then be compared in a reversion spectroscope. The absorption band in the red caused by Hi is at 630 nm (compare with methaemalbumin at 624 nm) (see Fig. 9.4).

Hi and SHb are formed intracellularly; they are not found in plasma except under very exceptional circumstances, e.g. when their formation is associated with intravascular haemolysis.

MEASUREMENT OF METHAEMOGLOBIN IN BLOOD

Principle

Hi has a maximum absorption at 630 nm. When cyanide is added, this absorption band disappears and the resulting change in absorbance is directly proportional to the concentration of Hi. Total Hb in the sample is then measured after complete conversion to HiCN by the addition of ferricyanide-cyanide reagent. The conversion will measure HbO_2 and Hi but not SHb. Thus, the presence of a large amount of SHb will result in an erroneously low measurement of total Hb.

The method described below is based on that of Evelyn & Malloy.[25] Turbidity of the haemolysate

can be overcome by the addition of a non-ionic detergent such as Nonidet P40[26] (see p. 20).

Reagents

Phosphate buffer: 0.1 mol/l, pH 6.8.
Potassium cyanide: 50 g/l.
Potassium ferricyanide: 50 g/l.
Non-ionic detergent (see p. 20): 10 ml/l.

Method

Lyse 0.2 ml of blood in a solution containing 4 ml of buffer and 6 ml of detergent solution. Divide the lysate into two equal volumes (A and B). Measure the absorbance of A in a spectrophotometer at 630 nm (D_1). Add 1 drop of potassium cyanide solution and measure the absorbance again, after mixing (D_2). Add 1 drop of potassium ferricyanide solution to B, and after 5 min, measure the absorbance at the same wavelength (D_3). Then add 1 drop of potassium cyanide solution to B and after mixing make a final reading (D_4). All the measurements are made against a blank containing buffer and detergent in the same proportion as present in the sample.

Calculation

$$\text{Methaemoglobin (\%)} = \frac{D_1 - D_2}{D_3 - D_4} \times 100$$

The test should be carried out within 1 h of collecting the blood. After dilution, the buffered lysate can be stored for up to 24 h at 2–4°C without significant auto-oxidation of Hb to methaemoglobin.

SCREENING METHOD FOR DETERMINATION OF SULPHAEMOGLOBIN IN BLOOD

Principle

An absorbance reading at 620 nm measures the sum of the absorbance of HbO_2 and SHb in any blood sample. In contrast to HbO_2, the absorption band caused by SHb is unchanged by the addition of cyanide. The residual absorbance, as read at 620 nm, is therefore proportional to the concentration of SHb.

The absorbance of the HbO_2 alone at 620 nm can only be inferred from a reading at 578 nm, and a conversion factor, A^{578}/A^{620}, has to be determined experimentally for each instrument on a series of normal blood samples.[26] The absorbance of SHb is obtained by subtracting the absorbance of the HbO_2 from that of the total Hb. This provides an approximation only, but it may be regarded as adequate for clinical purposes in the absence of a more reliable method.

Method

Mix 0.1 ml of blood with 10 ml of a 20 ml/l solution of a non-ionic detergent (Sterox SE or Nonidet P40). Record the absorbance (A) at 620 nm (total Hb). Add 1 drop of 50 g/l potassium cyanide and after standing for 5 min, record A at 620 nm and at 578 nm.

Calculation

Sulphaemoglobin (SHb) (%) $= 2 \times \dfrac{A^{620}SHb}{A^{620}HbO_2}$

where $A^{620}HbO_2 = \dfrac{\text{Absorbance read at 578 nm}}{\text{Conversion factor,}}$

and $A^{620}SHb = A^{620}$ total Hb $- A^{620}HbO_2$

Significance of methaemoglobin and sulphaemoglobin in blood

Hi is present in small amounts in normal blood, and constitutes 1–2% of the total Hb. Its concentration is very slightly higher in infants, especially in premature infants, than in older children and adults.[27] Excessive formation of Hi occurs as the result of oxidation of Hb by drugs and chemicals such as phenacetin, sulphonamides, aniline dyes, nitrates and nitrites.

The Hi produced by drugs is chemically normal and the pigment can be reconverted to HbO_2 by reducing agents such as methylene blue.

Other (rare) types of methaemoglobinaemia are caused by inherited deficiency of the enzyme NADH-methaemoglobin reductase and by inherited haemoglobin abnormalities (types of Hb M). The absorption spectra of the Hb Ms differ from that of normal Hi and they react slowly and incompletely with cyanide; their concentration cannot be estimated by the method of Evelyn & Malloy.[25]

Methaemoglobinaemia leads to cyanosis which becomes obvious with as little as 15 g Hi per litre, i.e. c 10%.

SHb is usually formed at the same time as Hi; it represents a further and irreversible stage in Hb degradation. It is present as a rule at a much lower concentration than is Hi.

DEMONSTRATION OF CARBOXYHAEMOGLOBIN

Principle

HbO_2, but not HbCO, is reduced by sodium dithionite and the percentage of HbCO in a mixture can be determined by reference to a calibration graph.

Calibration graph

Dilute 0.1 ml of normal blood in 20 ml of 0.4 ml/l ammonia and divide into two parts. To each add 20 mg of sodium dithionite. Then bubble pure CO into one for 2 min, so as to provide a 100% solution of HbCO.

Add various volumes of the HbCO solution to the reduced Hb solution to provide a range of concentrations of HbCO. Within 10 min of adding the dithionite, measure the absorbance of each solution at 538 nm and 578 nm. Plot the quotient A^{538}/A^{578} on arithmetical graph paper against the % HbCO in each solution.

Method[26,28]

Dilute 0.1 ml of blood in 20 ml of 0.4 ml/l ammonia and add 20 mg of sodium dithionite. Measure the absorbance in a spectrophotometer at 538 nm and 578 nm within 10 min. Calculate the quotient A^{538}/A^{578} and read the % HbCO in the blood from the calibration curve[26] or calculate it from the equation.[28]

$$\% \text{ HbCO} = \left\{ \frac{2.44 \times A^{538}}{A^{578}} \right\} - 2.68$$

Significance of carboxyhaemoglobin in circulating blood

Carbon monoxide has an affinity for Hb c 200 times that of oxygen. This means that even low concentrations of CO rapidly lead to the formation of HbCO. Less than 1% of HbCO is present in normal blood and up to 10% in smokers.[29,30] There is also an increased production, and excretion in the lungs, in haemolytic anaemias. A high concentration in blood from inhalation of the gas causes tissue anoxia and may lead to death. Recovery can take place, as HbCO dissociates in time in the presence of high concentrations of oxygen.

IDENTIFICATION OF MYOGLOBIN IN URINE

Myoglobin is the principal protein in muscle, and may be released into the circulation when there is cardiac or skeletal muscle damage. Some may be excreted in the urine where its concentration can be measured by a specific and relatively sensitive radioimmunoassay.[31] As the absorption spectra of myoglobin and Hb are similar, although not identical, it is not possible to distinguish them readily by spectroscopy or even by spectrophotometry; but they can be separated by column chromatography.[32] The following is a simple screening test for identifying the presence of myoglobin in urine; it is based on the fact that Hb and myoglobin are precipitated in urine at different degrees of ammonium sulphate saturation. First, it is necessary to demonstrate by precipitation with sulphosalicylic acid that the pigment in the urine is a protein.

Method[33]

Add 3 ml of a 30 g/l solution of sulphosalicylic acid to 1 ml of urine. Mix well and filter. If the pigment is a protein, it will be precipitated. (If the filtrate retains the abnormal colour, this must be due to a non-protein pigment, perhaps a porphyrin.) If the pigment has been shown to be protein, add 2.8 g of ammonium sulphate to 5 ml of urine (= 80% saturation). Shake the mixture to dissolve the ammonium sulphate, then filter or centrifuge. In myoglobinuria, the filtrate will be abnormally coloured; in haemoglobinuria, the filtrate will be of normal colour and the precipitate coloured.

Normal range[15]

Men, <80 μg/l; women, <60 μg/l; increasing slightly in older age. Children have very low values.

REFERENCES

1 Crosby WH, Furth FW 1956 A modification of the benzidine method for measurement of hemoglobin in plasma and urine. Blood 11:380–383.
2 Moore GL, Ledford ME, Merydith A 1981 A micromodification of the Drabkin hemoglobin assay for measuring plasma hemoglobin in the range of 5 to 2000 mg/dl. Biochemical Medicine 26:167–173.
3 Standefer JC, Vanderjogt D 1977 Use of tetramethyl benzidine in plasma hemoglobin assay. Clinical Chemistry 23:749–751.
4 Laurell CB, Nyman N 1957 Studies on the serum haptoglobin level in hemoglobinemia and its influence on renal excretion of hemoglobin. Blood 12:493–506.
5 Chaplin H, Cassell M, Hanks GE 1961 The stability of the plasma hemoglobin level in the normal human subject. Journal of Laboratory and Clinical Medicine 57:612–619.
6 Vanzetti G, Valente D 1965 A sensitive method for the determination of hemoglobin in plasma. Clinica Chimica Acta 11:442–446.
7 Davidson RJL 1969 March or exertional haemoglobinuria. Seminars in Haematology 6:150–161.
8 Ratcliff AP, Hardwicke J 1964 Estimation of serum haemoglobin-binding capacity (haptoglobin) on Sephadex G 100. Journal of Clinical Pathology 17:676–679.
9 Brus I, Lewis SM 1959 The haptoglobin content of serum in haemolytic anaemia. British Journal of Haematology 5:348–355.
10 Viedma JA 1987 Immunoturbidimetry of haptoglobin and transferrin in the EPOS 5060 analyzer. Clinical Chemistry 33:1257.
11 Van Lente F, Marchand A, Galen RS 1979 Evaluation of a nephelometric assay for haptoglobin and its clinical usefulness. Clinical Chemistry 25:2007–2010.
12 Vaerman J-P 1981 Single radial immunodiffusion. Methods in Enzymology 73:291–305.
13 Valeri CR, Bond JC, Flower K, et al. 1965 Quantitation of serum hemoglobin-binding capacity using cellulose acetate membrane electrophoresis. Clinical Chemistry 11:581–588.
14 Nyman M 1959 Serum haptoglobin: methodological and clinical studies. Scandinavian Journal of Clinical and Laboratory Investigation 11 (Suppl. 39):1–169.
15 Tietz NW 1986 Textbook of clinical chemistry. WB Saunders, Philadelphia.
16 Nagel RL, Gibson QH 1971 The binding of hemoglobin to haptoglobin and its relation to subunit dissociation of hemoglobin. Journal of Biological Chemistry 246:69–73.
17 Fairley NH, Bromfield RJ 1934 Laboratory studies in malaria and blackwater fever. Part III. A new blood pigment in blackwater fever and other biochemical observations. Transactions of the Royal Society of Tropical Medicine and Hygiene 28:307–334.
18 Muller-Eberhard U 1970 Hemopexin. New England Journal of Medicine 283:1090–1094.
19 Heide K, Haupt H, Störiko K, et al. 1964 On the heme-binding capacity of hemopexin. Clinica Chimica Acta 10:460–469.
20 Hanstein A, Muller-Eberhard U 1968 Concentration of serum hemopexin in healthy children and adults and in those with a variety of hematological disorders. Journal of Laboratory and Clinical Medicine 71:232–239.

21 Michaelsson M, Nosslin B, Sjölin S 1965 Plasma bilirubin determination in the newborn infant. A methodological study with special reference to the influence of haemolysis. Paediatrica 35:925–931.

22 Moore MR 1983 Laboratory investigation of disturbances of porphyrin metabolism. Association of Clinical Pathologists Broadsheet No. 109. British Medical Association, London.

23 Bottomley SS, Muller-Eberhard U 1988 Pathophysiology of heme synthesis. Seminars in Haematology 25:282–302.

24 Sassa S 1996 Diagnosis and therapy of acute intermittent porphyria. Blood Reviews 10:53–58.

25 Evelyn KA, Malloy HT 1938 Microdetermination of oxyhemoglobin, methemoglobin and sulfhemoglobin in a single sample of blood. Journal of Biological Chemistry 126:655–662.

26 Van Kampen EJ, Zijlstra WG 1965 Determination of hemoglobin and its derivates. Advances in Clinical Chemistry 8:141–187.

27 Kravitz H, Elegant LD, Kaiser E, et al. 1956 Methemoglobin values in premature and mature infants and children. American Journal of Diseases of Children 91:1–5.

28 Van Assendelft OW 1970 Spectrophotometry of haemoglobin derivatives. Royal VanGorcum Ltd, Assen, The Netherlands.

29 Shields CE 1971 Elevated carbon monoxide level from smoking in blood donors. Transfusion (Philadelphia) 11:89–93.

30 Russell MAH, Wilson C, Cole PV, et al. 1973 Comparison of increases in carboxyhaemoglobin after smoking 'extra mild' and 'non mild' cigarettes. Lancet ii:687–690.

31 Stone MJ, Willerson JT, Waterman MR 1982 Radioimmunoassay of myoglobin. Methods in Enzymology 84:172–177.

32 Cameron BF, Azzam SA, Kotite L, et al. 1965 Determination of myoglobin and hemoglobin. Journal of Laboratory and Clinical Medicine 65:883–890.

33 Blondheim SH, Margoliash E, Shafrir E 1958 A simple test for myohemoglobinuria (myoglobinuria). Journal of the American Medical Association 167:453–454.

34 Morris LD, Pont A, Lewis SM 2001 Use of a new HemoCue system for measuring haemoglobin at low concentrations. Clinical and Laboratory Haematology 23:91–96.

10

Investigation of the hereditary haemolytic anaemias: membrane and enzyme abnormalities

David Roper,   Mark Layton   &   S. Mitchell Lewis

The various initial steps to be taken in the investigation of a patient suspected of having a haemolytic anaemia are outlined in Chapter 9 and the changes in red cell morphology which may be found in haemolytic anaemias are illustrated in Chapter 5. In this chapter are described procedures useful in investigating haemolytic anaemias suspected of being due to defects within the red cell membrane or deficiency of enzymes important in red cell metabolism.

The precise identification of an enzyme defect is beyond the scope of most haematological laboratories; it may require the isolation and purification of the enzyme and the determination and delineation of its kinetic and structural properties. In a service laboratory, it is sufficient to identify the general nature of the defect, whether it be in the membrane or the metabolic pathways of the red cell. In the case of putative metabolic defects, an attempt should be made, where possible, to pinpoint the enzyme involved. In the first part of this chapter are described screening tests for spherocytosis, including hereditary spherocytosis (HS), and for glucose 6-phosphate dehydrogenase (G6PD) deficiency. In the later sections are described specific enzyme assays, and the measurement of 2,3-diphosphoglycerate (DPG) and reduced glutathione (GSH).

Most of the enzyme assays have been standardized by the International Council for Standardization in Haematology (ICSH). Commercial kits are also available for some quantitative assays and screening tests. These are noted in the relevant sections.

INVESTIGATION OF MEMBRANE DEFECTS

The osmotic fragility test gives an indication of the surface area/volume ratio of erythrocytes. Its greatest usefulness is in the diagnosis of hereditary spherocytosis. The test may also be used in screening for thalassaemia. Red cells that are spherocytic, for whatever cause, take up less water in a hypotonic solution before rupturing than normal red cells.

Other tests which demonstrate red cell membrane defects include glycerol lysis time, cryohaemolysis, autohaemolysis and, more specifically, membrane protein analysis.

colleagues modified the original test further by decreasing the pH.[10] There is some loss of specificity for HS with the acidified glycerol lysis-time test (AGLT) compared with the original method but in practice this loss is unimportant.

ACIDIFIED GLYCEROL LYSIS-TIME TEST[10]

Principle
Glycerol present in a hypotonic buffered saline solution slows the rate of entry of water molecules into the red cells so that the time taken for lysis may be more conveniently measured. Like the osmotic-fragility test, differentiation can be made between spherocytes and normal red cells.

Reagents

Phosphate buffered saline (PBS).   Add 9 volumes of 9.0 g/l (154 mmol/l) NaCl to 1 volume of 100 mmol/l phosphate buffer (2 volumes of Na_2HPO_4, 14.9 g/l added to 1 volume of KH_2PO_4, 13.61 g/l). Adjust the pH to 6.85 ± 0.05 at room temperature (15–25°C). This adjustment must be accurate.

Glycerol reagent (300 mmol/l).   Add 23 ml of glycerol (27.65 g AR grade) to 300 ml of PBS and bring the final volume to 1 litre with water.

Method
Add 20 μl of whole blood, anticoagulated with EDTA, to 5.0 ml of PBS, pH 6.85. Mix the suspension carefully.

Transfer 1.0 ml to a standard 4-ml cuvette of a spectrometer equipped with a linear-logarithmic recorder. Fix the wavelength at 625 nm and start the recorder. Add 2.0 ml of the glycerol reagent rapidly to the cuvette with a 2.0-ml syringe or automatic pipette and mix well.

The rate of haemolysis is measured by the rate of fall of turbidity of the reaction mixture. The results are expressed as the time required for the optical density to fall to half the initial value ($AGLT_{50}$). The test can also be carried out using a colorimeter and stopwatch.

Results
Normal blood takes more than 1800 s (30 min) to reach the $AGLT_{50}$. The time taken is similar for blood from normal adults, newborn infants and cord samples. In patients with HS, the range of the $AGLT_{50}$ is 25–150 s. A short $AGLT_{50}$ may also be found in chronic renal failure, chronic leukaemias, auto-immune haemolytic anaemia and in some pregnant women.

Significance of the AGLT
The same principles apply as with the osmotic-fragility test. Cells with a high volume to surface area ratio resist swelling for a shorter time than normal cells. This applies to all spherocytes, whether the spherocytosis is caused by HS or other mechanisms. The test is particularly useful in screening family members of patients with HS where morphological changes are too small to indicate clearly whether the disorder is present or not.

CRYOHAEMOLYSIS

Principle
Whereas osmotic fragility is abnormal in any condition where spherocytes occur, it has been suggested that cryohaemolysis is specific for HS.[11] This appears to be due to the fact that the latter is dependent on factors that are related to molecular defects of the red cell membrane rather than to changes in the surface area to volume ratio. The test can be carried out on EDTA blood up to 1 day old.

Reagent

Buffered 0.7 mol/l sucrose.   23.96 g sucrose in 100ml of 50 mmol/l phosphate buffer, pH 7.4 (p. 605). This can be stored frozen in 2-ml aliquots in tubes ready for use.

Method[11]

1. Centrifuge the blood and wash the red cells three times with cold (4°C) 9 g/l NaCl. Make a suspension of 50–70% cells in the saline and keep on ice until tested.
2. Prepare 2-ml volumes of reagent, thawing if frozen, and stand for 10 min in a 37°C waterbath to equilibrate.
3. Pipette 50 μl of the cell suspension into each of two tubes of the warmed-reagent, vortex

immediately for a few seconds and then incubate for exactly 10 min at 37°C.

4. Without delay, transfer the tubes to an ice-bath for another 10 min, vortex for a few seconds and then centrifuge to sediment the remaining cells. Transfer some of the supernatant to a clean tube.

5. Prepare a 100% haemolysate solution by pipetting 50 μl of the original sample into 2 ml of water. Centrifuge and dilute 200 μl of the supernatant in 4 ml of water.

6. Read absorbance at 540 nm of the test and the 100% lysis samples.

Calculation

% cryohaemolysis = [A^{540} test/A^{540} haemolysate] × 21.

Interpretation

The normal range is 3–15%; in hereditary spherocytosis, there is >20% lysis.

AUTOHAEMOLYSIS (SPONTANEOUS HAEMOLYSIS DEVELOPING IN BLOOD INCUBATED AT 37°C FOR 48 HOURS)

The autohaemolysis test is useful as an initial screen in suspected cases of haemolytic anaemia. It provides information about the metabolic competence of the red cells and helps to distinguish membrane and enzyme defects if the results of the tests are taken together with other observations such as morphology, inheritance and the presence or absence of associated clinical disorders.[12]

Principle

Aliquots of blood are incubated both with and without sterile glucose solution at 37°C for 48 h. After this period, the amount of spontaneous haemolysis is measured colorimetrically.

Method

It is essential to use aseptic techniques in setting up the autohaemolysis test in order to maintain sterility throughout the incubation period.

Use sterile defibrinated blood and deliver four 1-ml or 2-ml samples into sterile 5-ml capped bottles. Retain a portion of the original sample; separate and store this as the pre-incubation serum.

Add to two of the bottles 50 or 100 μl of sterile 100 g/l glucose solution so as to provide a concentration of glucose in the blood of at least 30 mmol/l. Make sure that the caps of the bottles are tightly closed and place the series of bottles in the incubator at 37°C. A sample from a known normal individual should be run in parallel as a control.

After 24 h, thoroughly mix the content by gentle swirling. After incubating for 48 h, inspect the samples for signs of infection, thoroughly mix again, then from each bottle remove a sample for the estimation of the PCV and Hb and centrifuge the remainder to obtain the supernatant serum.

Estimate the spontaneous lysis by means of a colorimeter or in a spectrometer at 540 nm.

As a rule, it is convenient to make a 1 in 10 dilution of the incubated serum in cyanideferricyanide (Drabkin's) solution (see p. 20) unless there is marked haemolysis, when a 1 in 25 or 1 in 50 dilution is more suitable. A corresponding dilution of the pre-incubation serum is used as a blank and a 1 in 100 or 1 in 200 dilution of the whole blood in Drabkin's solution indicates the total amount of Hb present and serves as a standard.

Calculate the percentage lysis, allowing for the change in PCV resulting from the incubation as follows:[12]

$$\text{Lysis (\%)} = \frac{R_t - B}{R_0} \times \frac{D_o}{D_t} \times (1 - PCV_t) \times 100,$$

where R_o = reading of diluted whole blood; R_t = reading of diluted serum at 48 h; B = reading of blank; PCV_t = packed cell volume at time T; D_o = dilution of whole blood (e.g. 1 in 200 = 0.005), and D_t = dilution of serum (e.g. 1 in 10 = 0.1).

The reading at time t is multiplied by $(1 - PCV_t)$ so as to give the concentration which would be found if the liberated haemoglobin was dissolved in whole blood, i.e. in both plasma and red cell compartments, not in the plasma compartment alone.

Normal range of autohaemolysis

Lysis at 48 h. Without added glucose, 0.2–2.0%; with added glucose, 0–0.9%.

The results obtained are sensitive to slight differences in technique and each laboratory should use a carefully standardized procedure and establish its own normal range. If the amount of liberated haemoglobin is small, it is more accurate (although more time consuming) to measure lysis by a chemical method rather than by a direct spectrometric method (see p. 151). It can also be measured directly by a simple and rapid procedure with a *HemoCue Plasma/Low Hb system*.[13]

Significance of increased autohaemolysis

Little or no lysis takes place when normal blood is incubated for 24 h under sterile conditions and the amount present after 48 h is small.[12] If glucose is added so that it is present throughout the incubation, the development of lysis is markedly slowed. The amount of autohaemolysis which occurs after 48 h with and without glucose is determined by the properties of the membrane and the metabolic competence of the red cell. In membrane disorders such as HS, the rate of glucose consumption is increased to compensate for an increased cation leak through the membrane.[6b] During the 48 h incubation, glucose is therefore used up relatively rapidly so that energy production fails more quickly than normal unless glucose is added. This is one factor which contributes to the increased rate of autohaemolysis in HS. Usually, but not always, the addition of glucose to the blood decreases the rate of autohaemolysis in HS. This was referred to as Type-1 autohaemolysis.[12] When the utilization of glucose via the glycolytic pathway is impaired, as in PK deficiency, the rate of autohaemolysis at 48 h is usually increased and glucose fails to correct or may even aggravate lysis (Type-2 autohaemolysis).[6c] Although a similar result may be seen in severe HS (Type B), in the absence of spherocytosis failure of glucose to diminish autohaemolysis is a strong indication of a glycolytic block. Blood from patients with G6PD deficiency or other disorders of the pentose phosphate pathway may undergo a slight increase in autohaemolysis, (without additional glucose) which is corrected by the addition of glucose. Commonly, the result is normal but examination of the incubated blood may show an increase in methaemoglobin (Hi) (see below). Not all glycolytic enzyme deficiencies give a Type 2 reaction so that a Type 1 result does not exclude the possibility of such a defect.

In the acquired haemolytic anaemias, the results of the autohaemolysis test are variable and generally not very helpful in diagnosis. In the auto-immune haemolytic anaemias, lysis may be increased in the absence of additional glucose but the effect of added glucose is unpredictable. In paroxysmal nocturnal haemoglobinuria (PNH), the autohaemolysis of aerated defibrinated blood is usually normal.

Autohaemolysis may be increased in haemolytic anaemias caused by oxidant drugs or when there are defects in the reducing power of the red cell. Heinz bodies and/or Hi will be detectable at the end of incubation. Normally, red cells produce less than 4% Hi after 48 h incubation and Heinz bodies are not seen. Red cells containing an unstable haemoglobin also contain Heinz bodies at the end of the incubation period and increased amounts of Hi.

The nucleosides adenosine, guanosine and inosine, like glucose, diminish the rate of autohaemolysis when added to blood. Remarkably, adenosine triphosphate (ATP) strikingly retards haemolysis in PK deficiency, although glucose itself is ineffective.[14] ATP does not pass the red cell membrane.

The autohaemolysis test lacks specificity. This has drawn much criticism upon the test, including the suggestion that it has no place in the screening of blood for inherited defects.[15] The best way to detect metabolic defects in red cells is undoubtedly to measure glucose consumption, lactate production and the contribution to metabolism of the pentose phosphate pathway. These measurements are, unfortunately, difficult and are likely to be undertaken only by specialized laboratories. The autohaemolysis test does provide some information about the metabolic competence of the red cells and helps to distinguish membrane defects from enzyme defects.

In summary, we feel that the autohaemolysis test is still useful in the investigation of patients who have or who may have *chronic haemolytic anaemia* for the following reasons:

1. If the result is entirely normal, an intrinsic red cell abnormality is unlikely.
2. If abnormal haemolysis is fully corrected by glucose, a metabolic abnormality is unlikely and a membrane abnormality is likely.

3. If abnormal haemolysis shows little or no correction by glucose, a metabolic abnormality is very likely, *provided* obvious features of spherocytosis are not present on the blood film.

Thus, in our experience a combination of red cell morphology with the results of the autohaemolysis tests makes it possible to differentiate membrane abnormalities from enzyme deficiencies in the vast majority of cases.

MEMBRANE PROTEIN ANALYSIS

Defects of red cell membrane proteins which constitute the cytoskeleton are associated with congenital haemolytic anaemias accompanied by characteristic morphological features. Their analysis is generally only possible in the setting of a reference laboratory. SDS-polyacrylamide gel electrophoresis of the membranes will identify qualitative and quantitative alterations in the specific proteins. Densitometry of protein bands on the gel gives an overall profile, showing spectrin, ankyrin, band 3 (the anion transport protein) and protein 4.2. Spectrin variants may be detected after limited trypsin digestion of spectrin extracted from the red cell membranes; an increase in spectrin dimer is indicative of an unstable tetramer, leading to susceptibility to red cell fragmentation in hereditary elliptocytosis and hereditary pyropoikilocytosis.[16]

A flow cytometric method based on binding of a fluorescent dye (eosin-5-maleimide) to intact red cells has recently been described.[17] The dye binds to Lys-430 on the extracellular domain of band 3 on intact red cells, and there is a reduction in fluorescence intensity from red cells with deficiency of band 3, spectrin or protein 4.2. This provides useful information in cases of HS, congenital

dyserythropoietic anaemia Type II and South-east Asian ovalocytosis.

Membrane protein defects implicated in hereditary haemolytic anaemias are listed in Table 10.3.

Table 10.3 Haemolytic anaemias associated with defects of red cell membrane proteins[16]

Band	Protein	Haemolytic anaemia
1	α Spectrin	HE HS HPP
2	β Spectrin	HE HS
2.1	Ankyrin	HS
3	Anion exchanger	HS SAO, CDAII
4.1	Protein 4.1	HE
4.2	Pallidin	HS
7	Stomatin	HStom
PAS-1	Glycophorin A	CDAII
PAS-2	Glycophorin C	HE

HS, hereditary spherocytosis; HE, hereditary elliptocytosis; HPP, hereditary pyropoikilocytosis; SAO, south-east Asia ovalocytosis; HStom, hereditary stomatocytosis; CDAII, congenital dyserythropoietic anaemia Type II.

DETECTION OF ENZYME DEFICIENCIES IN HEREDITARY HAEMOLYTIC ANAEMIAS

It is feasible for most haematological laboratories to identify the enzyme deficiencies of G6PD and PK, and to indicate where the probable defect lies in less common disorders. Detailed investigation of the aberrant enzymes and of the metabolism of the abnormal cells is probably best undertaken by specialized laboratories. Comprehensive accounts of methods available for studying red cell metabolism are to be found in *Red Cell Metabolism, a Manual of Bio-chemical Methods*, by Beutler[18] and the ICSH recommendations.[19]

There are two stages in the diagnosis of red cell enzyme defects: first, screening procedures and, second, specific enzyme assays. The simple nonspecific screening procedures such as the osmoticfragility and autohaemolysis tests, which have already been described, may indicate the presence of a metabolic disorder and simple biochemical tests are available to show whether the disorder is in the pentose phosphate or the Embden–Meyerhof pathways; these intermediate stages of glycolysis are illustrated in Figure 10.4.

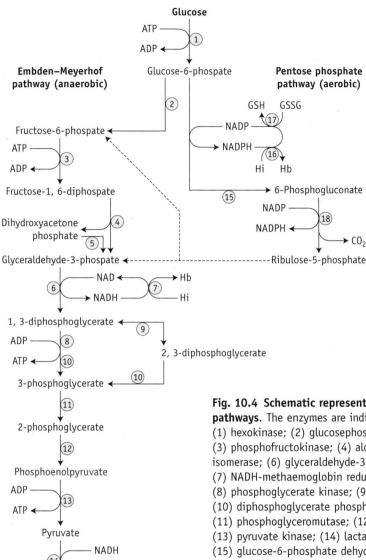

Fig. 10.4 Schematic representation of red cell glycolytic pathways. The enzymes are indicated as follows: (1) hexokinase; (2) glucosephosphate isomerase; (3) phosphofructokinase; (4) aldolase; (5) triose phosphate isomerase; (6) glyceraldehyde-3-phosphate dehydrogenase; (7) NADH-methaemoglobin reductase; (8) phosphoglycerate kinase; (9) diphosphoglyceromutase; (10) diphosphoglycerate phosphatase; (11) phosphoglyceromutase; (12) enolase; (13) pyruvate kinase; (14) lactate dehydrogenase; (15) glucose-6-phosphate dehydrogenase; (16) NADPH-methaemoglobin reductase; (17) glutathione reductase; (18) 6-phosphogluconate dehydrogenase. For explanation of abbreviations, see page 195).

These investigations may be augmented by quantitation of the major red cell metabolites 2,3-DPG, ATP and GSH which are present at millimolar concentrations and which can be assayed conveniently by spectrometric techniques. Metabolic block in the Embden–Meyerhof pathway is most accurately pinpointed by measurement of the concentration of glycolytic intermediates with demonstration of accumulation of metabolites proximal and depletion of metabolites distal to the defective step (Fig. 10.4). These assays, which are generally con-fined to specialized laboratories, must be performed on deproteinized red cell extracts immediately after preparation.

SCREENING TESTS FOR G6PD DEFICIENCY AND OTHER DEFECTS OF THE PENTOSE PHOSPHATE PATHWAY

Many variants of the red cell enzyme, G6PD, have been detected and the methods used to identify variants have been standardized.[20] Inheritance is sex-linked as the enzyme is controlled by one gene locus in the X chromosome. Variants which have deficient activity produce one of several types of clinical disorder. The two most common variants are the Mediterranean type which has very low activity and which may lead to favism, i.e. acute intravascular haemolysis following the ingestion of broad beans, and the A-type found in black populations in West Africa and the USA which leads to primaquine sensitivity. Both groups are susceptible to haemolysis produced by oxidant drugs and infections.

Much less frequently a chronic, non-spherocytic haemolytic anaemia is produced by rare variants of the enzyme. Severe neonatal jaundice with anaemia occurs in about 5% of patients who have major deficiencies of enzyme activity.

G6PD deficiency in hemizygous (male) or homozygous (female) individuals may be readily detected by screening tests but it is more difficult to detect heterozygous (female) carriers. Other defects of the pentose phosphate pathway (see p. 178) also lead to deficiency in the reducing power of the red cell. The clinical syndromes associated with these defects include intravascular haemolysis, with or without methaemoglobinaemia, in response to oxidative drugs.

G6PD catalyses the oxidation of glucose-6-phosphate (G6P) to 6-phosphogluconate (6PG) with the simultaneous reduction of nicotine adenine dinucleotide phosphate (NADP) to reduced NADP (NADPH):

$$G6P + NADP \xrightarrow{\text{G6PD}} 6PG + NADPH$$

In a second, consecutive, oxidative reaction 6PG is converted to 6-phosphogluconolactone, with reduction of a further molecule of NADP to NADPH. The lactone then undergoes decarboxylation to ribulose 5-phosphate through a reaction catalysed by a specific lactonase, but which can also take place spontaneously. Thus the overall reaction catalysed by 6PG dehydrogenase (6PGD), can be written as:

$$6PG + NADP \xrightarrow{\text{6PGD}} 6PGD\ Ru5P + CO_2 + NADPH$$

The release of CO_2 drives the reaction to the right so that in practice the pathway is not reversible.

NADPH is an important reducing compound for the conversion of oxidized glutathione (GSSG) to glutathione (GSH) (see Fig. 10.4) and, under conditions of stress, the reconversion of Hi to Hb. Screening tests for G6PD deficiency depend upon the inability of cells from deficient subjects to convert an oxidized substrate to a reduced state. The substrates used may be the natural one of the enzyme, NADP, or other naturally occurring substrates linked by secondary reactions to the enzyme, for example GSSG or Hi or artificial dyes such as methylene blue. The reaction is demonstrated by fluorescence,[21] colour change when a dye is used[22] or deposit of a dye, e.g. a blue ring of formazan from diphenyltetrazolium bromide in the presence of phenazine methosulphate.[23]

Which screening test is used in any particular laboratory will depend upon a number of factors such as cost, time required, temperature and humidity and availability of reagents. Two tests that are commonly used and which are generally reliable are described here.

FLUORESCENT SCREENING TEST FOR G6PD DEFICIENCY

The method is that of Beutler & Mitchell[21] modified on the recommendation of the ICSH.[19]

Principle
NADPH, generated by G6PD present in a lysate of blood cells, fluoresces under long-wave UV light. In G6PD deficiency, there is an inability to produce sufficient NADPH; this results in a lack of fluorescence.

Reagents

D-Glucose-6-Phosphate, 10 mmol/l. Dissolve 305 mg of the disodium salt, or an equivalent amount of the potassium salt, in 100 ml of water.

NADP+, 7.5 mmol/l. Dissolve 60 mg of NADP+, disodium salt, in 10 ml of water.

Saponin. 750 mmol/l (10 g/l).

Tris-HCl buffer, pH 7.8. See page 606.

Oxidized glutathione (GSSG), 8 mmol/l. Dissolve 49 mg of GSSG in 10 ml of water.

Mix the reagents in the following proportion: 2 volumes of G6P; 1 volume of NADP+, 2 volumes of saponin; 3 volumes of buffer; 1 volume of GSSG; 1 volume of water.

The combined reagent is stable at –20°C for 2 or more years and for 2 months at least if kept at 4°C. Azide may be added to prevent growth of contaminants without loss of activity. 100-µl volumes of the reagent may be placed in appropriate small tubes and kept at –20°C ready to use.

Method

Thaw out sufficient tubes to set up test and controls. Allow reagent to reach room temperature before use.

Add 10 µl of whole blood, either anticoagulated (EDTA, heparin, ACD or CPD) or added before clotting, to 100 µl of the reagent mixture and keep at room temperature (15–25°C).

Apply 10 µl of the reaction mixture on to a Whatman No. 1 filter paper at the beginning of the reaction and again after 5–10 min. A shorter interval may be appropriate at a high ambient temperature (c 25–30°C). Allow to air dry thoroughly before examining the spots under UV light. Record whether fluoresence is present (+) or absent (–). Always set up samples of normal blood and known G6PD-deficiency blood in parallel.

If the samples are to be collected away from the laboratory, place about 10 µl of blood on Whatman No. 1 filter paper and allow it to dry. Cut out the disc of dried blood in the laboratory and add it to the reaction mixture. A sample of normal blood should always be tested as a positive fluorescence (i.e. normal) control.

The test can be carried out on blood stored in ACD (provided it is sterile) for up to 21 days at 4°C and for about 5 days at room temperature.

Interpretation

Fluorescence is produced by NADPH formed from NADP⁺ in the presence of G6PD. Some of the NADPH produced is oxidized by GSSG, but this reaction, catalyzed by glutathione reductase, is normally slower than the rate of NADPH production. Red cells with less than 20% of normal G6PD activity do not cause fluorescence.

Like all screening tests, this method is useful when large numbers of samples are to be tested but the result must be interpreted with caution in an individual patient. The main causes of erroneous interpretations are as follows:

1. *False-normal.* If there is reticulocytosis, a vivid fluorescence may be seen with a genetically G6PD-deficient blood sample, because young red cells have more G6PD activity. If the test is carried out during an acute haemolytic episode the patient's blood should be retested when the reticulocyte count has returned to normal.
2. *False-deficient.* If the patient is anaemic, very little fluorescence may be seen despite the G6PD being genetically normal, simply because there are relatively few red cells in the 10 µl of blood used.

Although it is possible to correct for either or both of these contingencies, it is best, if in doubt, to proceed directly to a quantitative enzyme assay (see below).

The test is meant to give only a + or – (normal or deficient) result, by comparison with the controls, and it does not make sense to grade by eye the intensity of fluorescence. If a control G6PD-deficient sample is not available, the appearance of the 'zero time' spot can be used for reference. The threshold for a 'deficient' result can be worked out by making dilutions of a normal blood sample in saline, and is best set by regarding as deficient the fluorescence obtained when G6PD activity is 20% of normal or less (corresponding to a 1 in 5 dilution of normal blood). This means that very mildly deficient variants, and a substantial proportion of heterozygotes (see p. 181), will be missed. However, clinically important haemolysis is unlikely to occur in subjects who have more than 20% G6PD activity, and therefore this seems an appropriate (though arbitrary) threshold for a diagnostic laboratory. Because the test depends on visual inspection, it is best to select the time of incubation in relation to ambient temperature in preliminary trials. NADPH production is a cumulative process. Therefore, given enough time, a G6PD-deficient sample will fluoresce! The time allowed for the reaction should be one at which the contrast in fluorescence between a G6PD-normal and a G6PD-deficient sample is maximal.

METHAEMOGLOBIN REDUCTION TEST

The method was developed by Brewer et al in 1962.[22]

Principle

Sodium nitrite converts Hb to Hi. When no methylene blue is added, methaemoglobin persists, but incubation of the samples with methylene blue allows stimulation of the pentose phosphate pathway in subjects with normal G6PD levels. The Hi is reduced during the incubation period. In G6PD-deficient subjects, the block in the pentose phosphate pathway prevents this reduction.

Reagents

Sodium nitrite. 180 mmol/l.

Dextrose. 280 mmol/l. Dissolve 5 g of AR dextrose and 1.25 g of $NaNO_2$ in 100 ml of water.

Methylene blue. 0.4 mmol/l. Dissolve 150 mg of methylthionine chloride (methylene blue chloride, Sigma) in 1 litre of water.

Nile blue sulphate. 22 mg in 100 ml of water. This may be used as an alternative to methylene blue. It is the better reagent if the test is to be combined with the Hi elution test (see p. 182).

The reagents may be used in a variety of ways to suit the convenience of the laboratory. A batch of tubes may be prepared in advance of use by mixing equal volumes of the reagents (sodium nitrite with methylene blue or Nile blue sulphate) and pipetting 0.2 ml of the combined reagent into individual glass tubes. Glass tubes must be used because plastic may adsorb some reagents. The contents of the tubes are allowed to evaporate to dryness at room temperature (15–25°C) or in an oven at a temperature not exceeding 37°C. The tubes must then be tightly stoppered. The reagent will keep for 6 months at room temperature. The reagents may, however, be used fresh, without drying.

Method

Use anticoagulated blood (EDTA or ACD) and test the samples preferably within 1 h of collection if left on the bench or within 6 h if kept at 4°C. Blood in ACD, however, can be stored for up to 1 week, but will be unsatisfactory if there is any haemolysis. With blood from severely anaemic patients, adjust the PCV to 0.40 ± 0.05.

Add 2 ml of blood to the tube containing 0.2 ml of the combined reagent either freshly prepared or dried. Close the tube with a stopper and gently mix the contents by inverting it 15 times.

Prepare control tubes by adding 2 ml of blood to a similar tube without reagents (normal reference tube) and to a tube containing 0.1 ml of sodium nitrite–dextrose mixture without methylene blue ('deficient' reference tube).

Incubate the samples at 37°C for 90 min. If the blood has been heparinized, incubation should be continued for 3 h.

After the incubation, pipette 0.1-ml volumes from the test sample, the normal reference tube and the deficient reference tube into 10 ml of water in separate, clear glass test-tubes of identical diameter. Mix the contents gently. Compare the colours in the different tubes (see below).

Interpretation

Normal blood yields a colour similar to that in the normal reference tube – a clear red. Blood from deficient subjects gives a brown colour similar to that in the deficient reference tube. Heterozygotes give intermediate reactions.

Although this method is longer than the fluorescent test, its advantages include the fact that it is extremely cheap, and that the only equipment required is a water-bath. In addition, the test can be complemented by cytochemical analysis which lends itself to detecting G6PD deficiency in patients with reticulocytosis and in heterozygotes.

DETECTION OF HETEROZYGOTES FOR G6PD DEFICIENCY

Females heterozygous for G6PD deficiency have two populations of cells, one with normal G6PD activity and the other deficient. This is the result of inactivation of one of the two X chromosomes in individual cells early in the development of the embryo. All progeny cells (i.e. somatic cells) in females will have the characteristics of only the active X chromosome.[24] The total G6PD activity of blood in the female will depend on the proportion of normal to deficient cells. In most cases, the activity will be between 20 and 80% of the normal. However, a few heterozygotes (about 1%) may have almost only normal or almost only G6PD-deficient cells.

Screening tests for G6PD deficiency fail to demonstrate most heterozygotes. The deficient red cells may, however, be identified in blood films by a cytochemical elution procedure based on the methaemoglobin reduction test.[25]

Test kits

Several commercial kits are available for detection of G6PD deficiency. Sigma 203* is a fluorescent spot test and Sigma 400* is based on reduction of the dye dichloroindophenol to a colourless state in the presence of phenazine methosulphate.

The Quantase kit** is a photometric method in which NADPH produced by oxidation of G6P to 6PG is measured by an increase in absorption at 340 nm.

Quality control. Each test or batch of tests should include a normal and a G6PD-deficient sample. Sheep blood is a useful source of naturally deficient blood. Where possible, participation in an external quality assessment (or proficiency testing) scheme is also recommended.

METHAEMOGLOBIN ELUTION TEST

Principle

HbO_2 cannot be eluted from red cells in the presence of H_2O_2 presumably because of its peroxidase activity. HiCN has no peroxidase activity and is eluted. This property has been adapted for use in a differential staining technique so that individual cells retaining HbO_2 in the methaemoglobin elution test are stained and Hi-containing cells appear as ghosts.[25]

An alternative cytochemical method is described in Chapter 13 (p. 276).

Reagents

Potassium cyanide. 400 mmol/l. Dissolve 260 mg of KCN in 10 ml of water. Under no circumstances should this solution be pipetted by mouth.

Elution fluid. Mix 80 ml of ethanol (96%), 16 ml of 200 mmol/l citric acid (3.84 g in 100 ml of water) and 5 ml of H_2O_2 (30% v/v). The solution is only active for 1 day.

Staining fluid. Haematoxylin, 7.5 g/l in 96% (v/v) ethanol.

Counterstain. Aqueous erythrosin, 1 g/l or aqueous eosin, 20 g/l.

---

*Sigma–Aldrich; **England & Quantase, Cumbernauld, Scotland.

Method

Use the incubated samples from the reduction test (see p. 181). For preference, use samples incubated with Nile blue sulphate rather than methylene blue. Ideally, the samples should be oxygenated during incubation by bubbling 95% O_2–5% CO_2 mixtures through them continuously. However, it is equally adequate to blow air gently through the samples with a pipette from time to time.

After 2–3 h, add 20 µl of KCN solution to 1 ml of the incubated mixture and mix gently. Make blood films on clean, dry glass slides.

Dry the films quickly in air. Immerse the slides in the elution fluid and agitate them up and down for 1 min.

Wash the slides first in methanol and then in water for 3 s each.

Stain the films for 2 min with haematoxylin, rinse in tap water, then counterstain with the erythrosin for 2 min.

Rinse the slides in tap water and allow to dry in the air.

Examine the films under the microscope and count the proportion of stained (HbO_2) cells to ghosts (Hi cells).

Interpretation and comments

In females heterozygous for G6PD deficiency, the proportion of G6PD-deficient (ghost) cells varies from case to case: while usually 40–60% of the cells are deficient, the proportion may be much less and in extreme cases even only as few as 2–3% are deficient. Apparently normal subjects may, in a few instances, have a small residue of Hi-containing cells after the Hi reduction test, but this rarely exceeds 5% of the cells. Nearly all heterozygotes can be reliably detected if Nile blue sulphate is used and there is good oxygenation of the samples in the initial incubation. Nile blue sulphate increases the sensitivity of the test because the reduced form of the dye, which is produced in any normal cells that are present, diffuses less readily out of these cells than reduced methylene blue. An artefactual reduction of Hi in G6PD-deficient cells from inward diffusion of an extrinsic reducing compound is thus less likely.

PYRIMIDINE-5′-NUCLEOTIDASE SCREENING TEST

Pyrimidine-5′-nucleotidase (P5N) was first described by Valentine et al[26] as a cytosolic enzyme in human red cells. Deficiency of P5N-1 (uridine monophosphate hydrolase-1), which shows autosomal recessive inheritance, is associated with congenital haemolytic anaemia. Heterozygotes are clinically and haematologically normal and typically have about half the normal red cell P5N activity. Homozygous P5N deficiency, in which enzyme activity is generally 5–15% of normal, results in a chronic non-spherocytic haemolytic anaemia. This is characterized by mild to moderate haemolysis, pronounced basophilic stippling visible in up to 5% of red cells, and marked increase in both red cell glutathione and pyrimidine nucleotides. Osmotic fragility is normal. The rate of autohaemolysis is increased with little or no reduction in lysis by added glucose.[6c]

P5N deficiency appears to be one of the more common causes of hereditory non-spherocytic haemolytic anaemia. As lead is an inhibitor of P5N, an acquired deficiency occurs in lead toxicity and this may be important in the pathogenesis of the associated anaemia. The ultimate diagnostic test is a quantitative assay of P5N activity; but the finding of supranormal levels of red cell nucleotides (mostly pyrimidines) is strongly suggestive, and can be used for screening.

Activity of P5N may be quantitatively measured by a colorimetric method[26] or by a radiometric method.[27] For the screening of P5N deficiency, the method recommended by ICSH is the determination of the UV spectra of a blood extract.[28]

Principle

The nucleotide pool of normal red cells consists largely (>96%) of purine (adenine and small amounts of guanine) derivatives. The levels of cytidine and uridine are normally extremely low. However, in P5N-deficient cells, more than 50% of this pool consists of pyrimidine nucleotides.

In acidic solutions, cytidine nucleotides have an absorbance maximum at approximately 280 nm, while adenine, guanine and uridine nucleotides absorb maximally at 260 nm. The ratio of absorbance at 260 nm to absorbance at 280 nm reflects the relative abundance of cytidine nucleotides; the absorbance ratio is lower when pyrimidine derivatives are higher.

Reagents

Sodium chloride solution, NaCl, 9 g/l.

Perchloric acid, 4%. 28.6 ml of a 70% perchloric acid solution are diluted to a final volume of 500 ml with water.

Glycine buffer. 1 mol/l pH 3.0. 7.51 g of glycine are dissolved in about 80 ml of water, the pH is adjusted to 3.0 with concentrated HCl and the solution made up to a final volume of 100 ml with water.

Method [28]

Sample preparation. Centrifuge blood freshly collected in EDTA at 1200 g for 5 min, remove the plasma, and wash the cells three times with ice-cold 9 g/l NaCl solution. Add 1 ml of a 50% suspension of the washed red cells to 4 ml of ice-cold 4% perchloric acid (PCA) solution and then shake vigorously for 30 s. Transfer the clear supernatant obtained after centrifugation at 1200 g for 15 min to a small test tube. Prepare a sham extract by adding 1 ml of 9 g/l NaCl to 4 ml of 4% PCA solution.

Add 500 μl of water and 300 μl of 1 mol/l glycine buffer to each of two cuvettes. In order to correct for optical differences between the cuvettes, read the sample cuvette against the blank at 260 and at 280 nm, giving readings B^{260} and B^{280}. Add 200 μl of the red cell extract to the sample cuvette and 200 μl of the sham extract to the blank cuvette. With the spectrometer zeroed at 260 nm on the blank cuvette, read the sample cuvette to obtain the value S^{260}. Repeat the process at 280 nm to obtain the reading S^{280}.

The A^{260}/A^{280} absorbance ratio (R) is calculated by subtracting the cuvette blank readings (positive or negative) at 260 and 280 nm from the readings obtained on the red cell extract when blanked against the sham extract:

$$R = \frac{S^{260} - B^{260}}{S^{280} - B^{280}}$$

Interpretation

The A^{260}/A^{280} absorbance ratio of freshly collected washed red cells has been reported to be 3.11 ± 0.41 (mean ± SD). Absorbance ratios of less than 2.29 imply that the concentration of cytidine nucleotide is increased and suggest a reduced level of P5N. Selective accumulation of pyrimidines owing to putative defect in CDP-choline phosphotransferase has been reported in rare patients with a disorder that resembles P5N deficiency characterized by haemolytic anaemia and basophilic stippling.

RED CELL ENZYME ASSAYS

As is illustrated in Figure 10.4, a large number of enzymes play a part in the metabolism of glucose in the red cell, and genetically-determined variants of almost all the enzymes are known to occur. This means that in investigating a patient suspected of suffering from a hereditary enzyme-deficiency haemolytic anaemia, multiple enzyme assays may be needed to identify the defect. In practice, however, G6PD deficiency and PK deficiency should be excluded first, because of the relative frequency (common in the case of G6PD, not rare in the case of PK) with which variants of these enzymes are associated with deficiency and increased haemolysis.

Many methods are available for assaying each enzyme, and for this reason the International Council for Standardization in Haematology has produced simplified methods suitable for diagnostic purposes.[29] These methods are not necessarily the most appropriate for detailed study of the kinetic properties of the variant enzymes but they are relatively simple to set up and allow comparison of results between different laboratories.

GENERAL POINTS OF TECHNIQUE

Collection of blood samples

Blood samples may be anticoagulated with heparin (10 iu/ml blood), EDTA (1.5 mg/ml blood) or ACD (for formulae and volumes see p. 603). In any of these anticoagulants, all normal enzymes are stable for 6 days (and most for 20 days) at 4°C and for 24 h at 25°C. However, enzyme variants in samples from patients may be less stable. Therefore, we recommend that ACD is used as anticoagulant and that the samples are tested promptly. Ideally, samples of blood should be transferred to central laboratories in tubes surrounded by wet ice (4°C). Frozen samples are unsuitable because the cells are lysed by freezing. Further details of enzyme stability were given by Beutler.[18] Approximately 1 ml of blood is required for each enzyme assay.

Separation of red cells from blood samples

Leucocytes and platelets generally have higher enzyme activities than red cells. Moreover, with many enzyme deficiency, notably PK deficiency, the decrease in enzyme activity may be much less pronounced in leucocytes and platelets than in red cells or even absent. It is, therefore, necessary to prepare red cells as free from contamination as possible. Various methods are suitable (see ICSH[29]); two are described below.

Washing the red cells

Centrifuge the anticoagulated blood at 1200–1500 g for 5 min and remove the plasma together with the buffy coat layer.

Re-suspend the cells in 9 g/l NaCl (saline) and repeat the procedure three times. This will remove about 80–90% of the leucocytes.

This simple method is adequate in most instances when more complicated manoeuvres are impracticable, but it has the disadvantage that some of the reticulocytes and young red cells are lost together with the buffy coat. In addition, the remaining leucocytes may still be sufficient to cause misleading results, for instance in PK deficiency. Therefore, ideally the method below should be adopted.

Filtration through microcrystalline cellulose mixtures

Pure red cell suspensions can be made from whole blood by filtering the blood through a mixed bed of microcrystalline cellulose (mean size 50 μm) and α-cellulose. Mix approximately 0.5 g of each type of cellulose with 20 ml of ice-cold saline; this gives sufficient slurry for 3 to 5 columns. The barrel of a 5-ml syringe is used as a column. The outlet of the syringe is blocked with absorbent cotton wool, equal in volume to the 1-ml mark on the barrel. Pour the well-shaken slurry into the column to give a bed volume of 1–2 ml after the saline has run through. Wash the bed with 5 ml of saline to remove any 'fines'. When the saline has run through, pipette 1–2 ml of whole blood onto the column, taking care not to disturb the bed. Collect the filtrate, and once the blood has completely run into the bed, wash the column through with 5–7 ml of saline. The column should be made freshly for each batch of enzyme assays and used promptly.

By this method, about 99% of the leucocytes and about 90% of the platelets are removed. About 97% of the red cells are recovered and reticulocytes are not removed selectively. The procedure should not alter the age or size of distribution of the recovered red cells compared to native blood. This should be checked with each new batch of cellulose by counting reticulocytes.

Wash the cells collected from the column twice in 10 volumes of ice-cold saline and finally re-suspend them in the saline to give a 50% suspension.

Determine the haemoglobin and/or red cell count in a sample of the suspension.

Preparation of haemolysate

Mix 1 volume of the washed or filtered suspension with 9 volumes of lysing solution consisting of 2.7 mmol/l EDTA, pH 7.0 and 0.7 mmol/l 2-mercaptoethanol (100 mg of EDTA disodium salt and 5 μl of 2-mercaptoethanol in 100 ml of water); adjust the pH to 7.0 with HCl or NaOH.

Ensure complete lysis by freeze-thawing. Rapid freezing is achieved using a dry-ice acetone bath or methanol which has been cooled to −20°C. Thawing is achieved in a water-bath at 25°C or simply in water at room temperature. Usually the haemolysate is ready for use without further centrifugation, but a 1-min spin in a microfuge is preferable in order to remove any turbidity (this may be unsuitable for some red cell enzymes which are stroma-bound). Dilutions, when necessary, are carried out in the lysing solution. The haemolysate should be prepared freshly for each batch of enzyme assays. Most enzymes in haemolysates are stable for 8 h at 0°C, but it is best to carry out assays immediately. G6PD is one of the least stable enzymes in this haemolysate and its assay should be conducted within 1 or 2 h of the lysate being prepared. The storing of frozen cells or haemolysates is not recommended; it is preferable to store whole blood in ACD.

Control samples

Control samples should always be assayed at the same time as the test samples even when a normal range for the various enzymes has been established.

Take the control samples of blood at the same time as the test samples and treat them in the same way. When receiving samples from outside sources, always ask for a normal 'shipment control' to be included.

Reaction buffer

The ICSH recommendation is for a Tris-HCl/EDTA buffer which is appropriate for all the common enzyme assays. The buffer consists of 1 mol/l Tris-HCl and 5 mmol/l Na_2EDTA, the pH being adjusted to 8.0 with HCl.

Dissolve 12.11 g of Tris (hydroxymethyl) methylamine and 168 mg of Na_2 EDTA in water; adjust the pH to 8.0 with 1 mol/l HCl and bring the volume to 100 ml at 25°C.

Only two assays will be described in detail – those for G6PD and PK. However, the principles of these assays apply to all other enzyme assays. The assays are carried out in a spectrometer at a wavelength of 340 nm unless otherwise indicated. A final reaction mixture of 1.0 ml (or 3.0 ml) is suitable, the quantities given in the text being for 1.0-ml reaction mixtures unless otherwise stated. All dilutions of auxiliary enzymes are made in the lysing solution and all working materials should be kept in an ice-bath until ready for use. The assays are carried out at a controlled temperature, 30°C being the most appropriate. Cuvettes loaded with the assay reagents should be pre-incubated at this temperature for 10 min before starting the reaction. In most cases, the reaction is started by the addition of substrate. Many spectrometers have a built-in or attached recorder, by which the absorbance changes can be conveniently measured. If no recorder is available, visual readings should be made every 60 s. In any case, the reaction should be followed for 5–10 min, and it is essential to ensure that during this time the change in absorbance is linear with time.

G6PD ASSAY

The reactions involving G6PD have already been described (p. 178). The activity of the enzyme is assayed by following the rate of production of NADPH which, unlike NADP, has a peak of UV light absorption at 340 nm.

Method
Assay conditions. The assays are carried out at 30°C, the cuvettes containing the first four reagents and water being incubated for 10 min before starting the reaction by adding the substrate, as shown in Table 10.4. A commercial kit (Sigma–Aldrich) is also available.

The change in absorbance following the addition of the substrate is measured over the first 5 min of the reaction. The value of the blank is subtracted from the test reaction, either automatically or by calculation.

Calculation of enzyme activity
The activities of the enzymes in the haemolysate are calculated from the initial rate of change of NADPH accumulation:

G6PD activity in the lysate (in mol/ml)

$$= \Delta A/min \times \frac{10^3}{6.22}$$

where 6.22 is the mmol extinction coefficient of NADPH at 340 nm and 10^3 is the factor appropriate for the dilutions in the reaction mixture. Results are expressed per 10^{10} red cells, per ml red cells or per g haemoglobin by reference to the respective values obtained with the washed red cell suspension. However, the ICSH recommendation is to express values per g haemoglobin, and it is ideal to determine the haemoglobin concentration of the haemolysate directly. When doing this, use a haemolysate to Drabkin solution ratio of 1:25.

G6PD is very stable and, with most variants, venous blood may be stored in ACD for up to 3 weeks at 4°C without loss of activity.

Table 10.4 Glucose 6-phosphate dehydrogenase assay

Reagents	Assay (μl)	Blank (μl)
Tris-HCl EDTA buffer, pH 8.0	100	100
MgCl$_2$, 100 mmol/l	100	100
NADP, 2 mmol/l	100	100
1:20 Haemolysate	20	20
Water	580	680
Start reaction by adding: G6P, 6 mmol/l	100	–

Some enzyme-deficient variants lose activity more rapidly, and this will cause deficiency to appear more severe than it is. Therefore, for diagnostic purposes, a delay in assaying well-conserved samples should not be a deterrent.

Normal values
The normal range for G6PD activity should be determined in each laboratory. If the ICSH method is used, values should not differ widely from the given valves. Results are expressed in enzyme units (eu) which are the μmoles of substrate converted per min.

For adults, these values are 8.83 ± 1.59 eu/g haemoglobin at 30°C. However, newborns and infants may have enzyme activity which deviates appreciably from the adult value.[29,30] In one study, the newborn mean activity was about 150% of the adult mean.[31]

Interpretation of results
In assessing the clinical relevance of a G6PD assay, three important facts must be borne in mind:

1. As already stated (p. 181), the gene for G6PD is on the X-chromosome, and therefore males, having only one G6PD gene, can be only either normal or deficient hemizygotes. By contrast, females, who have two allelic genes, can be either normal homozygotes or heterozygotes with 'intermediate' enzyme activity or deficient homozygotes.
2. Red cells are likely to haemolyse on account of G6PD deficiency only if they have less than about 20% of the normal enzyme activity.
3. G6PD activity falls off markedly as red cells age. Therefore, whenever a blood sample has a young red cell population, G6PD activity will be higher than normal, sometimes to the extent that a genetically deficient sample may yield a value within the normal range. This will be usually, but not always, associated with a high reticulocytosis.

In practice, the following notes may be useful:
1. In males, diagnosis does not present difficulties in most cases, because the demarcation between normal and deficient subjects is sharp. There are very few acquired situations in which G6PD activity is decreased (one is pure red cell aplasia where there is reticulocytopenia); whereas

an increased G6PD activity is found in all acute and chronic haemolytic states with reticulocytosis. Therefore a G6PD value below a well-established normal range always indicates G6PD deficiency. A value in the low–normal range in the face of reticulocytosis should also raise the suspicion of G6PD deficiency, because with reticulocytosis G6PD activity should be *higher* than normal. In such suspicious cases, G6PD deficiency can be confirmed by repeating the assay when the reticulocytosis has subsided, or by assaying older red cells after density fractionation, or by family studies.

2. In females, all the same criteria apply, with the added consideration that heterozygosity can *never* be rigorously ruled out by a G6PD assay: for this purpose, the cytochemical test described on page 182 is more useful than a spectrometric assay, and a counsel of perfection is to use the two in conjunction with each other and with family studies. However, in most cases, a normal value in a female means that she is a normal homozygote, and a value below 10% of normal means that she is a deficient homozygote (see Table 10.5): but a few heterozygotes may fall in either of these ranges, because of the 'extreme phenotypes' that can be associated with an unbalanced ratio of the mosaicism consequent on X-chromosome inactiv-ation. Any value between 10 and 90% of normal usually means a heterozygote, except for the complicating effect of reticulocytosis. As far as the clinical significance of heterozygosity for G6PD deficiency is concerned, it is important to remember that, because of mosaicism, a fraction of red cells in heterozygotes (on the average, 50%) is as enzyme-deficient as in a hemizygous male, and therefore susceptible to haemolysis. The severity of potential clinical complications is roughly proportional to the fraction of deficient red cells. Therefore, within the heterozygote range, the actual value of the assay (or the proportion of deficient red cells estimated by the cytochemical test) correlates with the risk of haemolysis.

IDENTIFICATION OF G6PD VARIANTS

There are many variants of G6PD in different populations with enzyme activities ranging from nearly zero to 400–500% of normal activity (see full details in ref. 32). Classification and provisional identification of variants are based on their physicochemical and enzymic characteristics.[33] Criteria were laid down by a WHO scientific group in 1967[20] for the minimum requirements for identification of such variants and these recommendations have been revised recently.[34] The tests are carried out on male hemizygotes and are:

- red cell G6PD activity
- electrophoretic migration
- Michaelis constant (K_m) for G6PD
- relative rate of utilization of 2-deoxyG6P (2dG6P)
- thermal stability.

The full amino-acid sequence of G6PD has been established and definitive identification can be made by sequence analysis at the DNA level.[35,36] Diagnosis of G6PD deficiency by molecular analysis may be clinically useful when a patient has received a large volume of transfused blood or when a reticulocytosis results in a normal enzyme assay level; also, heterozygous deficient females can readily be identified (see Ch. 21).

Table 10.5 Glucose 6-phosphate dehydrogenase in various clinical situations (activity in enzyme units (eu) per g haemoglobin)

Male genotypes Female genotypes	Gd+ Gd+/Gd+	Gd− Gd−/Gd−	Gd+/Gd−
In health	7–10	<2	2–7
In increased haemolysis unrelated to G6PD deficiency	15	4	4–9
During recovery from G6PD-related anaemia	–	6.5	6–10

The values quoted are examples.
Gd+ designates a gene encoding normal G6PD; *Gd−* designates a gene encoding a variant associated with G6PD deficiency.

PYRUVATE KINASE ASSAY

Many variants of PK have deficient enzyme activity in vivo.[37,38] In most cases, deficient activity can be identified by simple enzyme assay. However, PK activity in red cells is subject to regulation by a number of effector molecules. With some PK variants, the maximum velocity (V_{max}) of the enzyme is normal or nearly so, but at the low-substrate concentrations found in vivo PK activity may be sufficiently low to cause haemolysis, either because affinity for the substrates, phosphoenolpyruvate (PEP) and ADP, is low or because binding of the important allosteric ligand, fructose-1,6-diphosphate, is altered. Some of these unusual variants can be identified by carrying out the enzyme assay not only under standard conditions but also at low substrate concentrations. Functional PK deficiency can also be identified by finding high concentrations of the substrates immediately above the block in the glycolytic pathway, particularly DPG.[39] (For measurement of DPG, see p. 191.)

PK deficiency is inherited as an autosomal recessive condition.

Method
The preparation of haemolysate, buffer and lysing solution is exactly the same as for the G6PD assay. In the PK assay, it is particularly important to remove as many contaminating leucocytes and platelets as possible because these cells may be unaffected by a deficiency affecting the red cells and contain high activities of PK. The principle of the assay is as follows:

$$PEP + ADP \xrightarrow{PK} pyruvate + ATP$$

The pyruvate so formed is reduced to lactate in a reaction catalysed by lactate dehydrogenase with the conversion of NADH to NAD:

$$pyruvate + NADH \xrightarrow{LDH} lactate + NAD$$

In order to ensure that this secondary reaction is not rate-limiting, LDH is added in excess to the reaction mixture and the PK activity is measured by the rate of fall of absorbance at 340 nm.

The reaction conditions are established in a 1-ml cuvette at 30°C by adding all the reagents shown in Table 10.6 except the substrate PEP to the cuvette and incubating them at 30°C for 10 min before starting the reaction by the addition of the PEP.

The amounts to be added for low-substrate conditions are also shown in Table 10.6. A commercial kit (Sigma–Aldrich) is also available.

Table 10.6 Reagents for Pyruvate kinase assay

Reagents	Assay (μl)	Blank (μl)	Low-S (μl)
Tris-HCl EDTA buffer, pH 8.0	100	100	100
KCl 1 mol/l	100	100	100
MgCl₂ 100 mmol/l	100	100	100
NADH 2 mmol/l	100	100	100
ADP, neutralized 30 mmol/l	50	–	20
LDH 60 μ/ml	100	100	100
1:20 haemolysate	20	20	20
Water	330	380	455
PEP 50 mmol/l	100	100	5

Low-S, low-substrate conditions.

The change in absorbance (A) is measured over the first 5 min and the activity of the enzyme in micromoles of NADH reduced/min/ml haemolysate is calculated as follows:

$$\frac{\Delta A/min}{6.22} \times 10$$

where 6.22 is the millimolar extinction coefficient of NADH at 340 nm.

Express results as for G6PD.

A blank assay should be carried out to be certain that the LDH is free of PK activity. Use the 2-mercapto-ethanol-EDTA stabilizing solution (p. 185) in place of haemolysate for both the blank and system mixtures. If no change in absorbance is observed, indicating that the LDH is free of contaminating PK, it is unnecessary to re-check on subsequent assays. Otherwise, the blank rate must be subtracted in computing the true enzyme activity each time.

Normal values
As with all enzyme assays, a normal range should be determined for each laboratory. Values should, however, not be widely different between laboratories if the ICSH methods are used. The normal range of PK activity at 30°C is 10.3 ± 2 eu/g Hb. At a low-substrate concentration, the normal activity is $15 \pm 3\%$ of that at the high-substrate concentration. Mean neonatal value is about 140% that of adults.[31]

Interpretation of results

PK, like G6PD, is a red cell age-dependent enzyme. But unlike G6PD deficiency, PK deficiency is usually associated with chronic haemolysis. Therefore, patients in whom PK deficiency is suspected almost invariably have a reticulocytosis, and if their PK level is below the normal range, they can be considered to be PK-deficient. Thus, once the technique and normal values are well established in a laboratory, and provided shipment controls are always included, the main problem is of underdiagnosis rather than of overdiagnosis of PK deficiency. One way to pick up abnormal variants has been included in the method recommended, i.e. the use of low-substrate concentrations. Even so, PK deficiency may be missed because marked reticulocytosis may increase PK activity quite markedly. This means that a PK activity in the normal range in the presence of a marked reticulocytosis is highly suspicious of inherited PK deficiency (because with reticulocytosis the activity ought to be *higher* than normal). In such cases, the importance of family studies cannot be overemphasized. Heterozygotes have about 50% of the normal PK activity, sometimes less; but they do not suffer from haemolysis. Therefore, the heterozygous parents of a patient may have a red cell PK activity lower than that of their homozygous PK-deficient offspring; this finding may clinch the diagnosis. In this context, assay of an alternative red cell age-dependent enzyme, e.g. G6PD or hexokinase, may be a useful aid to interpretation.

ESTIMATION OF REDUCED GLUTATHIONE[40]

The red cell has a high concentration of this sulphydryl-containing tripeptide. An important function of GSH in the red cell is the detoxification of low levels of hydrogen peroxide which may form spontaneously or as a result of drug administration. GSH may also function in maintaining the integrity of the red cell by reducing sulphydryl groups of haemoglobin, membrane proteins and enzymes which may have become oxidized. Maintenance of normal levels of GSH is a major preoccupation of the hexose monophosphate shunt. Reduction of GSSG (oxidized glutathione) back to the functional GSH is linked to the rate of reduction of $NADP^+$ in the initial step of the shunt.

Principle

The method described is based on the development of a yellow colour when 5,5'-dithiobis (2-nitrobenzoic acid) (Ellman's reagent, DTNB) is added to sulphydryl compounds. The colour which develops is fairly stable for about 10 min and the reaction is little affected by variation in temperature.

The reaction is read at 412 nm. GSH in red cells is relatively stable and venous blood samples anticoagulated with ACD maintain GSH levels for up to 3 weeks at 4°C. GSH is slowly oxidized in solution, so only fresh lysates should be used for the assay.

Reagents

Lysing solution. Disodium EDTA, 1 g/l.

Precipitating reagent. Metaphosphoric acid (sticks), 1.67 g; disodium EDTA, 0.2 g; NaCl, 30 g; water to 100 ml.

Solution is more rapid if the reagents are added to boiling water and the volume made up after cooling.

This solution is stable for at least 3 weeks at 4°C. If any EDTA remains undissolved, the clear supernatant should be used.

Disodium hydrogen phosphate, 300 mmol/l. $Na_2HPO_4.12H_2O$, 107.4 g/l, or $Na_2HPO_4.2H_2O$, 53.4 g/l or anhydrous Na_2HPO_4, 4.6 g/l.

DTNB reagent. Dissolve 20 mg of DTNB in 100 ml of buffer, pH 8.0. Trisodium citrate, 34 mmol/l (10 g/l) or Tris/HCl (p. 606), are suitable buffers.

The solution is stable for up to 3 months at 4°C.

Glutathione standards. When standard curves are constructed, suitable dilutions are made from a 1.62 mmol/l (50 mg/dl) stock solution of GSH.

The stock solution should be made freshly with degassed (boiled) water or saline for each run as GSH oxidizes slowly in solution.

Method

Add 0.2 ml of well-mixed, anticoagulated blood of which the PCV, red cell count and haemoglobin have been determined, to 1.8 ml of lysing solution and allow to stand at room temperature for no more than 5 min for lysis to be completed.

Add 3 ml of precipitating solution, mix the solution well and allow to stand for a further 5 min.

After remixing, filter through a single thickness Whatman No. 42 filter paper.

Add 1 ml of clear filtrate to 4 ml of freshly made Na_2HPO_4 solution. Record the absorbance at 412 nm (A_1). Then add 0.5 ml of the DTNB reagent, and mix well by inversion.

The colour develops rapidly and remains stable for about 10 min. Read its development at 412 nm in a spectrometer (A_2).

A reagent blank is made using saline or plasma instead of whole blood.

Standard curves. If assays are carried out frequently, it is not necessary to construct standard curves for each batch. They are, however, essential initially to calibrate the apparatus used and should be done regularly to check the suitability of the reagents. Suitable dilutions of GSH are achieved by substituting 5, 10, 20 and 40 µl of the 1.62 mmol/l stock solution, make up to 0.2 ml with lysing solution, for the blood in the reaction.

Calculation

Determination of extinction coefficient (ε). The molar extinction coefficient of the chromophore at 412 nm is 13 600. This only applies when a narrow band wavelength is available. When a broader waveband is used, the extinction coefficient is lower.

The system may be calibrated by comparing the extinction absorbance in the test system (D_2) with that obtained in a spectrometer with a narrow band at 412 nm (D_1). The derived correction factor, E_1, is given by D_1/D_2 and is constant for the test system.

Calculation of GSH concentration
The amount of GSH in the cuvette sample (GSH_c) is given by:

$$\Delta A^{412} \times \frac{E_1}{\varepsilon} \times 5.5 \ \mu mol$$

The concentration of GSH in the whole blood sample is:

$$\frac{GSH_c \times 5}{0.2} \ \mu mol/ml.$$

The unit is often expressed in terms of mg/dl of red cells. The molecular weight of GSH is 307. Thus, GSH in mg/dl packed red cells is given by:

$$\frac{GSH_c \times 5}{0.2} \times \frac{1}{PCV} \times 307 \times 100.$$

Normal range
The normal range may be expressed in a number of ways, e.g. 6.57 ± 1.04 µmol/g Hb or 223 ± 35 µmol (or 69 ± 11 mg)/dl packed red cells. Neonatal mean value is about 150% that of adults.[31]

Significance
Glutathione replenishment in mature red cells is accomplished through the consecutive action of two enzymes; γ-glutamylcysteine synthetase and glutathione synthetase. Although very rare, hereditary deficiency of either enzyme virtually abolishes the synthesis of GSH. The deficient cells are very prone to oxidative destruction and are short lived, resulting in a non-spherocytic haemolytic anaemia.

Increases in GSH have been described in various conditions such as dyserythropoiesis, myelofibrosis, P5N deficiency and other rare congenital haemolytic anaemias of unknown aetiology.

GLUTATHIONE STABILITY TEST

Principle
In normal subjects, incubation of red cells with the oxidizing drug acetylphenylhydrazine has little effect on the GSH content, since its oxidation is reversed by glutathione reductase, which in turn relies on G6PD for a supply to NADPH. Therefore, in G6PD-deficient subjects, the stability of GSH is significantly lowered.

Reagents
Acetylphenylhydrazine, 670 mmol/l. Dissolve 100 mg in 1 ml of acetone.

Transfer 0.05 ml volumes (containing 5 mg of acetylphenylhydrazine) by pipette to the bottom of 12×75 mm glass tubes.

Dry the contents of the tubes in an incubator at 37°C, stopper and store in the dark until used.

Method
Venous blood, anticoagulated with EDTA, heparin or ACD may be used; it may be freshly collected or previously stored at 4°C for up to 1 week.

Add 1 ml to a tube containing acetylphenyl-hydrazine and place a further 1 ml in a similar tube not containing the chemical. Invert the tubes several times and then incubate them at 37°C.

After 1 h, mix the contents of the tubes once more and incubate the tubes for a further 1 h. At the end of this time, determine and compare the GSH concentration in the test sample and in the control sample.

Interpretation

In normal adult subjects, red cell GSH is lowered by not more than 20% by incubation with acetylphenylhydrazine. In G6PD-deficient subjects, it is lowered by more than this: in heterozygotes (females), the fall may amount in about 50% whilst in hemizygotes (males) the fall is often much greater and almost all may be lost.

The test is not specific for G6PD deficiency and other rare defects of the pentose phosphate pathway may give abnormal results.

GSH and GSH stability in infants

During the first few days after birth, the red cells have a normal or high content of GSH. On the addition of acetylphenylhydrazine, the GSH is unstable in both normal and G6PD-deficient infants. In normal infants, however, the instability can be corrected by the addition of glucose and, by the time the normal infant is 3 to 4 days old, the cells behave like adult cells.[41,42]

2,3-DIPHOSPHOGLYCERATE

The importance of the high concentration of 2,3-diphosphoglycerate (DPG) in the red cells of man was recognized at about the same time by Chanutin & Curnish[43] and Benesch & Benesch.[44] DPG binds to a specific site in the β-chain of haemoglobin and it decreases its oxygen affinity by shifting the balance of the so-called T and R conformations of the molecule. The higher the concentration of DPG, the greater the partial pressure of oxygen (pO_2) needed to produce the same oxygen saturation of haemoglobin. This is reflected in a DPG-dependent shift in the oxygen dissociation curve.

Measurement of the concentration of DPG in red cells may also be useful in identifying the probable site of an enzyme deficiency in the metabolic pathway. In general, enzyme defects cause an increase in the concentration of metabolic intermediates above the level of the block and a decrease in concentration below the block. Thus DPG is increased in PK deficiency and decreased in hexokinase deficiency. In most other disorders of the glycolytic pathway, however, the DPG concentration is normal, because increased activity through the pentose phosphate pathway allows a normal flux of metabolites through the triose part of the glycolytic pathway.

MEASUREMENT OF RED CELL 2,3-DIPHOSPHOGLYCERATE

Various methods have been used to assay DPG. Krimsky[45] used the catalytic properties of DPG in the conversion of 3-phosphoglycerate (3PG) to 2-phosphoglycerate (2PG) by phosphoglycerate mutase (PGM). At very low concentrations of DPG, the rate of conversion is proportional to the concentration of DPG. This method is elegant and extremely sensitive but too cumbersome for routine use. A fluorimetric method was described by Lowry et al,[46] and this has been modified for spectrometry. Rose & Liebowitz[47] found that glycolate-2-phosphate increased the 2,3DPG phosphatase activity of PGM and a quantitative assay of the substrate, DPG, was evolved on this basis.

Principle

DPG is hydrolysed to 3PG by the phosphatase activity of PGM stimulated by glycolate-2-phosphate. This reaction is linked to the conversion of NADH to NAD by glyceral-dehyde-3-phosphate dehydrogenase (Ga3PD) and phosphoglycerate kinase (PGK):

$$2,3DPG \xrightarrow[\text{(glycolate-2-phosphate)}]{\text{2,3DPG phosphatase}} 3PG + Pi$$

$$3PG + ATP \xrightarrow{\text{PGK}} 1,3DPG + ADP$$

$$1,3DPG + NADH \xrightarrow{\text{Ga3PD}} Ga3P + Pi + NAD^+$$

The fall in absorbance at 340 nm, as NADH is oxidized, is measured.

Reagents

Triethanolamine buffer. 0.2 mol/l, pH 8.0. Dissolve 9.3 g of triethanolamine hydrochloride in *c* 200 ml of water; then add 0.5 g of disodium EDTA and 0.25 g of $MgSO_4.7H_2O$. Adjust the pH to 8.0 with 2 mol/l KOH (*c* 15 ml) and make up the volume to 250 ml with water.

ATP, sodium salt. 20 mg/ml. Dissolved in buffer, this is stable for several months when frozen.

NADH, sodium salt. 10 mg/ml. When dissolved in buffer, this is relatively unstable and should be made freshly each day.

Glyceraldehyde-3-phosphate dehydrogenase/Phosphoglycerate kinase. Mixed crystalline suspension in ammonium sulphate (Sigma No. 366–2).

Phosphoglycerate mutase. Crystalline suspension from rabbit muscle in ammonium sulphate (*c* 2500 u/ml).

Glycolate-2-phosphate. 2-Phosphoglycolic acid (Sigma), 10 mg/ml. When dissolved in water, this is stable for several months when frozen.

Method

Freshly drawn blood in EDTA or heparin may be used. If there is an unavoidable delay in starting the assay, blood (4 volumes) should be added to CPD anticoagulant (1 volume) and stored at 4°C. A control blood sample should be taken at the same time.

DPG levels are stable for 48 h if the blood is stored in this way. The haemoglobin, red cell count and PCV should be measured on part of the sample. It is not necessary to remove leucocytes or platelets.

Deproteinization. Add 1 ml of blood to 3 ml of ice-cold 80 g/l trichloracetic acid (TCA) in a 10-ml conical centrifuge tube.

Shake the tube vigorously, preferably on an automatic rotor mixer and then allow to stand for 5–10 min for complete deproteinization. The shaking is important; otherwise some of the precipitated protein will remain on the surface of the mixture.

Centrifuge at about 1200 *g* for 5–10 min at 4°C to obtain a clear supernatant. The DPG in the supernatant is stable for 2 to 3 weeks when stored at 4°C, and indefinitely if frozen.

Reaction

Deliver the reagents into a silica or high-quality glass cuvette, with a 1-cm light path. The following quantities are for a 4-ml cuvette:

	Test	Blank
Triethanolamine buffer	2.50 ml	2.50 ml
ATP	100 μl	100 μl
NADH	100 μl	100 μl
Deproteinized extract	250 μl	–
Ga-3-PD/PGK mixture	20 μl	20 μl
PGM	20 μl	20 μl
Water	–	250 μl
	3.00 ml	3.00 ml

Warm the mixtures at 30°C for 10 min and record the absorbance of both test and blank mixtures at 340 nm. Then start the reaction by the addition of 100 μl of glycolate-2-phosphate.

Re-measure the absorbance (at 35 min) of the test and blank mixtures on completion of the reaction.

Make further measurements after a further 5 min to make sure the reaction is complete.

Only one blank is required for each batch of test samples.

Calculation

DPG (μmol/ml blood)

$$= (\Delta A \text{ test} - \Delta A \text{ blank}) \times \frac{3.10}{6.22} \times 16$$
$$= (\Delta A \text{ test} - \Delta A \text{ blank}) \times 8 = D$$

where 3.10 = the volume of reaction mixture, 6.22 = mmolar extinction coefficient of NADH at 340 nm and 16 = dilution of original blood sample (1 ml in 3.0 ml of TCA, 0.25 ml added to cuvette).

The results of DPG assays are best expressed in terms of haemoglobin content or red cell volume. Thus, if the result of the above calculation is represented by D, then:

$$\frac{D \times 1000}{(Hb)} = \text{DPG in μmol/g Hb}$$

or

$$\frac{D \times 1000}{(Hb)} \times \frac{64}{1000} = \text{DPG in μmol/μmol Hb}$$

and

$$D \times \frac{1}{PCV} = \text{DPG in μmol/ml (packed) red cells,}$$

where Hb = haemoglobin in g/l of whole blood and 64 is the mol wt of haemoglobin $\times 10^{-3}$.

The molar ratio of DPG to haemoglobin in normal blood is about 0.75:1.

Normal range

4.5–5.1 µmol/ml packed red cells or 10.5–16.2 µmol/g haemoglobin. Neonatal values are about 20% lower than adult.[31]

Each laboratory should determine its own normal range.

Significance of DPG concentration

An increase in DPG concentration is found in most conditions in which the arterial blood is undersaturated with oxygen, as in congenital heart and chronic lung diseases; in most acquired anaemias; at high altitudes; in alkalosis, and in hyperphosphataemia. Decreased DPG levels occur in hypophosphataemic states and in acidosis.

Acidosis, which shifts the oxygen dissociation curve to the right, causes a fall in DPG, so that the oxygen dissociation curve of whole blood from patients with chronic acidosis (such as patients in diabetic coma or pre-coma) may have nearly normal dissociation curves. A rapid correction of the acidosis will lead to a major shift of the curve to the left, i.e. to a marked increase in the affinity of haemoglobin for oxygen, which may lead to tissue hypoxia. Caution should therefore be exercised in correcting acidosis.

From the diagnostic point of view, the main importance of DPG determination is (1) in haemolytic anaemias and (2) in the interpretation of changes in the oxygen affinity of blood.

1. As already mentioned, increased or decreased DPG may be associated with glycolytic enzyme defects, and increased DPG (up to 2 to 3 times normal) is particularly characteristic of most patients with PK deficiency. Although this finding certainly cannot be regarded as diagnostic, a normal or low DPG makes PK deficiency most unlikely.

2. Whenever a shift in the oxygen dissociation curve is observed, and an abnormal haemoglobin with altered oxygen affinity is suspected, determination of DPG is essential. Indeed, there is a simple correlation between DPG level and p_{50}, from which it is possible to work out whether any change in p_{50} is explained by an altered level of DPG.[48]

DPG levels are generally slightly lower than normal in HS and this probably accounts for the slight erythrocytosis which is sometimes seen after splenectomy. Extremely low red cell 2,3DPG concentration associated with erythrocytosis has been reported in a kindred with complete 2,3-diphosphoglycerate mutase deficiency.[49]

OXYGEN DISSOCIATION CURVE

The oxygen dissociation curve is the expression of the relationship between the partial pressure of oxygen and the saturation of haemoglobin with oxygen. Details of this relationship and the physiological importance of changes in this relationship were worked out in detail at the beginning of this century by the great physiologists Hüfner, Bohr, Barcroft, Henderson and many others. Their work was summarized by Peters & Van Slyke in *Quantitative Clinical Chemistry, Volume 1*.[50] The relevant chapters of this book have been reprinted and it would be difficult to better their description of the importance of the oxygen dissociation curve:

> The physiological value of haemoglobin as an oxygen carrier lies in the fact that its affinity for oxygen is so nicely balanced that in the lungs haemoglobin becomes 95–96% oxygenated, while in the tissues and capillaries it can give up as much of the gas as is demanded. If the affinity were much less, complete oxygenation in the lungs could not be approached: if it were greater, the tissues would have difficulty in removing from the blood the oxygen they need. Because the affinity is adjusted as it is, both oxyhaemoglobin and reduced haemoglobin exist in all parts of the circulation but in greatly varied proportions.

MEASURING THE OXYGEN DISSOCIATION CURVE

Determination of the oxygen dissociation curve depends upon two measurements: the partial pressure of oxygen (pO_2) with which the blood is equilibrated, and the proportion of haemoglobin which is saturated with oxygen. Methods for determining the dissociation curve fall into three main groups:

1. The pO_2 is set by the experimental conditions and the percentage saturation of haemoglobin is measured.
2. The percentage saturation is predetermined by mixing known proportions of oxygenated and deoxygenated blood and the pO_2 is measured.

3. The change in oxygen content of the blood is plotted continuously against pO_2 during oxygenation or deoxygenation and the percentage saturation calculated.

The multiplicity of methods available for measuring the oxygen dissociation curve suggests that no method is ideal. The advantages and disadvantages of the various techniques have been reviewed.[51,52] The standard method with which new methods are compared is the gasometric method of Van Slyke & Neill.[53] This method is slow and demands considerable expertise and is not suitable for most haematological laboratories. A method based on spectrometric measurement of reduced oxyhaemoglobin which uses a specially made tonometer-cuvette[54] was described in the 8th edition, page 242.

Commercial instruments are now available for performing the test and drawing the complete oxygen dissociation curve.* Such analysers are extremely quick and accurate and are therefore ideal for laboratories performing multiple determinations.

Interpretation

Figure 10.5 shows the sigmoid nature of the oxygen dissociation curve of Hb A and the effect of hydrogen ions on the position of the curve. A shift of the curve to the right indicates decreased affinity of the haemoglobin for oxygen and hence an increased tendency to give up oxygen to the tissues: a shift to the left indicates increased affinity and so an increased tendency for haemoglobin to take up and retain oxygen. Hydrogen ions, DPG and some other organic phosphates such as ATP shift the curve to the right. The amount by which the curve is shifted may be expressed by the $p_{50}O_2$, i.e. the partial pressure of oxygen at which the haemoglobin is 50% saturated.

The oxygen affinity, as represented by the $p_{50}O_2$, is related to compensation in haemolytic anaemias.[55] 1 g of haemoglobin can carry about 1.34 ml of O_2. Figure 10.6 shows the O_2 dissociation curves of Hb A and Hb S plotted according to the volume of oxygen contained in 1 litre of blood when the haemoglobin concentrations are 146 g/l and 80 g/l, respectively. The $p_{50}O_2$ of Hb A is given as 26.5 mmHg (3.5 kPa) and Hb S as 36.5 mmHg (4.8 kPa). It will be seen that in the change from

---

* e.g. Hemox-Analyzer, TCS Scientific Corporation.

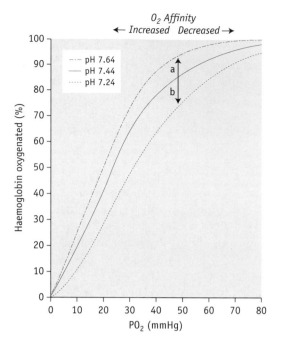

Fig. 10.5 The effect of pH upon the oxygen dissociation curve.

arterial to venous saturation, the same volume of oxygen is given up despite the difference in haemoglobin concentration. Patients with a high $p_{50}O_2$ achieve a stable haemoglobin at a lower level than normal and this should be taken into account when planning transfusion for these patients.

Bohr effect

Bohr et al described the effect of CO_2 on the oxygen dissociation curve.[56] An increase in CO_2 concentration produces a shift to the right, i.e. a decrease in oxygen affinity. It was soon realized that this effect was mainly due to changes in pH, although CO_2 itself has some direct effect. The Bohr effect is given a numerical value, $\Delta \log p_{50}O_2/\Delta pH$, where $\Delta \log p_{50}O_2$ is the change in $p_{50}O_2$ produced by a change in pH (ΔpH). The normal value of the Bohr effect at physiological pH and temperature is about 0.45.

Hill's constant

Hill thought that there was a constant ('n') which represented the number of molecules of oxygen which would combine with 1 molecule of haemoglobin.[57] Experiment showed that the value was 2.6 rather than the expected 4. The explanation

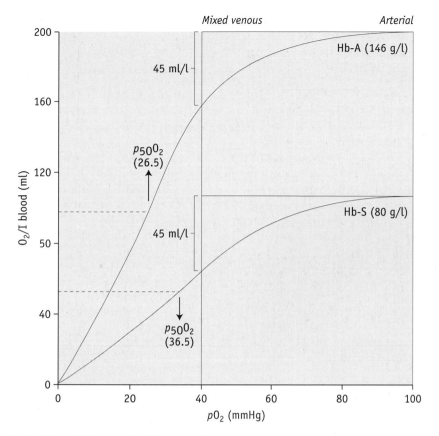

Fig. 10.6 The effect of O_2 affinity on O_2 delivery to tissues.

for this lies in the effect of binding 1 molecule of oxygen by haemoglobin on the affinity for binding further oxygen molecules by haemoglobin, the so-called allosteric effect of haem–haem interaction: 'n' is a measure of this effect and the calculation of the 'n' value helps in identifying abnormal haemoglobins, the molecular abnormality of which leads to abnormal haem–haem interaction.[58]

Abbreviations used in this chapter

ADP	Adenosine diphosphate	HE	Hereditary elliptocytosis
AGLT	Acidified glycerol lysis-time	Hi	Methaemoglobin
ATP	Adenosine triphosphate	HS	Hereditary spherocytosis
1,3DPG	1,3-Diphosphoglycerate	LDH	Lactate dehydrogenase
DPG	2,3-Diphosphoglycerate	MCF	Median corpuscular fragility
DTNB	5,5′-Dithiobis (2-nitrobenzoic) acid) (Ellman's reagent)	NAD	Nicotine adenine dinucleotide
		NADH	Reduced form of NAD
Ga3P	Glyceraldehyde-3-phosphate	NADP	Nicotine adenine dinucleotide phosphate
Ga3PD	Glyceraldehyde-3-phosphate dehydrogenase		
		NADPH	Reduced form of NADP
GLT	Glycerol lysis-time	OF	Osmotic fragility
G6P	Glucose-6-phosphate	PCA	Perchloric acid
G6PD	Glucose-6-phosphate dehydrogenase	PEP	Phosphoenolpyruvate
GSH	Reduced glutathione	6PG	6-Phosphogluconate
GSSG	Oxidized glutathione	6PGD	6-Phosphogluconate dehydrogenase

3PG, 2PG	3- (or 2-) Phosphoglycerate
PGK	Phosphoglycerate kinase
PGM	Phosphoglyceromutase
Pi	Inorganic phosphate

P5N	Pyrimidine-5′-nucleotidase
PK	Pyruvate kinase
Ru5P	Ribulose-5-phosphate
TCA	Trichloracetic acid

REFERENCES

1 Parpart AK, Lorenz PB, Parpart ER, et al 1947 The osmotic resistance (fragility) of human red cells. Journal of Clinical Investigation 26:636.

2 Murphy JR 1967 The influence of pH and temperature on some physical properties of normal erythrocytes and erythrocytes from patients with hereditary spherocytosis. Journal of Laboratory and Clinical Medicine 69:758.

3 Suess J, Limentani D, Dameshek W, et al 1948 A quantitative method for the determination and charting of the erythrocyte hypotonic fragility. Blood 3:1290.

4 Jacob HS, Jandl JH 1964 Increased cell membrane permeability in the pathogenesis of hereditary spherocytosis. Journal of Clinical Investigation 43:1704.

5 Cooper RA 1970 Lipids of human red cell membrane normal composition and variability in disease. Seminars in Hematology 7:296.

6 Dacie J 1985 The haemolytic anaemias, Vol. 1. The hereditary haemolytic anaemias, part 1. Churchill Livingstone, Edinburgh. (a) p 292, (b) p 146, (c) p 352.

7 Gunn RB, Silvers DN, Rosse WF 1972 Potassium permeability in β-thalassaemia minor red blood cells. Journal of Clinical Investigation 51:1043.

8 Gottfried EL, Robertson NA 1974 Glycerol lysis time as a screening test for erythrocyte disorders. Journal of Laboratory and Clinical Medicine 83:323.

9 Gottfried EL, Robertson NA 1974 Glycerol lysis time of incubated erythrocytes in the diagnosis of hereditary spherocytosis. Journal of Laboratory and Clinical Medicine 84:746.

10 Zanella A, Izzo C, Rebulla P, et al 1980 Acidified glycerol lysis test: a screening test for spherocytosis. British Journal of Haematology 45:481.

11 Streichman S, Gescheidt Y 1998 Cryohemolysis for the detection of hereditary spherocytosis: correlation studies with osmotic fragility and autohemolysis. American Journal of Hematology 58:206–210.

12 Selwyn JG, Dacie JV 1954 Autohemolysis and other changes resulting from the incubation in vitro of red cells from patients with congenital hemolytic anemia. Blood 9:414.

13 Morris LD, Pont A, Lewis SM 2001 Use of the HemoCue for measuring haemoglobin at low concentrations. Clinical and Laboratory Haematology 23:91–96.

14 de Gruchy GC, Santamaria JN, Parsons IC, et al 1960 Nonspherocytic congenital hemolytic anemia. Blood 16:1271.

15 Beutler E 1978 Why has the autohemolysis test not gone the way of the cephalin floculation test? Blood 51:109.

16 Palek J, Jarolim P 1993 Clinical expression and laboratory detection of red blood cell membrane protein mutations. Seminars in Hematology 30:249–283.

17 King M-J, Behrens J, Rogers C, et al 2000 Rapid flow cytometric test for the diagnosis of membrane cytoskeleton-associated haemolytic anemia. British Journal of Haematology 111:924–933.

18 Beutler E 1984 Red cell metabolism. A manual of biochemical methods, 2nd edn. Grune & Stratton, Orlando, FL

19 Beutler E, Blume KG, Kaplan JC, et al 1979 International Committee for Standardization in Haematology. Recommended screening test for glucose-6-phosphate dehydrogenase (G-6-PD) deficiency. British Journal of Haematology 43:465.

20 World Health Organization Scientific Group 1967 Standardization of procedures for the study of glucose-6-phosphate dehydrogenase. Technical Report Series, No. 366. WHO, Geneva.

21 Beutler E, Mitchell M 1968 Special modification of the fluorescent screening method for glucose-6-phosphate dehydrogenase deficiency. Blood 32:816.

22 Brewer GJ, Tarlov AR, Alving AS 1962 The methemoglobin reduction test for primaquine-type sensitivity of erythrocytes. A simplified procedure for detecting a specific hypersusceptibility to drug hemolysis. Journal of the American Medical Association 180:386.

23 Fujii H, Takahashi K, Miwa S 1984 A new simple screening method for glucose-6-phosphate dehydrogenase deficiency. Acta Haematologica Japonica 47:185–188.

24 Lyon MF 1961 Gene action in the X-chromosomes of the mouse (*Mus musculus* L.). Nature (London) 190:372.

25 Gall JC, Brewer GJ, Dern RJ 1965 Studies of glucose-6-phosphate dehydrogenase activity of

individual erythrocytes: the methemoglobin-elution test for identification of females heterozygous for G6PD deficiency. American Journal of Human Genetics 17:359.

26 Valentine WN, Fink K, Paglia DE, et al 1974 Hereditary haemolytic anaemia with human erythrocyte pyrimidine 5′-nucleotidase deficiency. Journal of Clinical Investigation 54:866.

27 Torrance J, West C, Beutler E 1977 A simple radiometric assay for pyrimidine 5′-nucleotidase. Journal of Laboratory and Clinical Medicine 90:563.

28 International Committee for Standardization in Haematology 1989 Recommended screening test for pyrimidine 5′-nucleotidase deficiency. Clinical and Laboratory Haematology 11:55.

29 International Committee for Standardization in Haematology 1977 Recommended methods for red-cell enzyme analysis. British Journal of Haematology 35:331.

30 Konrad PN, Valentine WN, Paglia DE 1972 Enzymatic activities and glutathione content of erythrocytes in the newborn. Comparison with red cells of older normal subjects and those with comparable reticulocytosis. Acta Haematologica 48:193.

31 Oski FA 1969 Red cell metabolism in the newborn infant: V. Glycolytic intermediates and glycolytic enzymes. Pediatrics 44:84–91.

32 Luzzatto L, Mehta A 1989 Glucose-6-phosphate dehydrogenase deficiency. In: Scriver CR, Beaudet A, Sly WS, Valle D (eds) The metabolic basis of inherited disease. McGraw-Hill, New York, pp. 2237–2265.

33 Yoshida A, Beutler E, Motulsky AG 1971 Human glucose-6-phosphate dehydrogenase variants. Bulletin of the World Health Organization 45:243.

34 World Health Organization Scientific Group on Glucose-6-Phosphate Dehydrogenase 1990 Bulletin of the World Health Organization, 67:601.

35 Vulliamy TJ, D'urso M, Battistuzzi G et al 1988 Diverse point mutations in the human glucose-6-phosphate dehydrogenase gene cause enzyme deficiency and mild or severe hemolytic anemia. Proceedings of the National Academy of Sciences of the USA 85:5171.

36 Beutler E 1989 Glucose-6-phosphate dehydrogenase: new perspectives. Blood 73:1397.

37 Miwa S, Fujii H, Takegawa S, et al 1980 Seven pyruvate kinase variants characterised by the ICSH recommended methods. British Journal of Haematology 45:575.

38 Miwa S, Nakashima K, Ariyoshi K et al 1975 Four new pyruvate kinase (PK) variants and a classical PK deficiency. British Journal of Haematology 29:157.

39 International Committee for Standardization in Haematology 1979 Recommended methods for the characterisation of red cell pyruvate kinase variants. British Journal of Haematology 43:275.

40 Beutler E, Duron O, Kelly B 1963 Improved method for the determination of blood glutathione. Journal of Laboratory and Clinical Medicine 61:882.

41 Lubin BH, Oski FA 1967 An evaluation of screening procedures for red cell glucose-6-phosphate dehydrogenase deficiency in the newborn infant. Journal of Pediatrics 70:788.

42 Zinkham WH 1959 An in-vitro abnormality of glutathione metabolism in erythrocytes from normal newborns: mechanism and clinical significance. Pediatrics 23:18.

43 Chanutin A, Curnish RR 1967 Effect of organic and inorganic phosphates on the oxygen equilibrium of human erythrocytes. Archives of Biochemistry and Biophysics 121:96.

44 Benesch R, Benesch RE 1967 The effect of organic phosphates from the human erythrocyte on the allosteric properties of haemoglobin. Biochemical and Biophysical Research Communications 26:162.

45 Krimsky I 1965 D-2,3-diphosphoglycerate. In: Bergmeyer HU (ed) Methods of enzymatic analysis. Academic Press, New York, p 238.

46 Lowry OH, Passonneau JV, Hasselberger FX, et al 1964 Effect of ischemia on known substrates and cofactors of the glycolytic pathway in brain. Journal of Biological Chemistry 239:18.

47 Rose ZB, Liebowitz J 1970 Direct determination of 2,3-diphosphoglycerate. Annals of Biochemistry and Experimental Medicine 35:177.

48 Duhm J 1971 Effects of 2,3-diphosphoglycerate and other organic phosphate compounds on oxygen affinity and intracellular pH of human erythrocytes. Pflügers Archiv für die gesampte Physiologie des Menschen und der Tiere 326:341.

49 Rosa R, Prehu MO, Beuzard Y, et al 1978 The first case of a complete deficiency of diphosphoglycerate mutase in human erythrocytes. Journal of Clinical Investigation 62:907.

50 Peters JP, Van Slyke DD 1931 Hemoglobin and oxygen. In: Quantitative clinical chemistry, vol. 1. Interpretations. Williams & Wilkins, Baltimore, p 525.

51 Bellingham AJ, Lenfant C 1971 Hb affinity for O_2 determined by O_2-Hb dissociation analyser and mixing technique. Journal of Applied Physiology 30:903.

52 Torrance JD, Lenfant C 1969–70 Methods for determination of O_2 dissociation curves, including Bohr effect. Respiration Physiology 8:127.

53 Van Slyke DD, Neill JM 1924 The determination of gases in blood and other solutions by vacuum extraction and manometric measurement. Journal of Biological Chemistry 61:523.

54 Rossi-Fanelli A, Antonini E 1958 Studies on the oxygen and carbon monoxide equilibria of human myoglobin. Archives of Biochemistry and Biophysics 77:478.

55 Bellingham AJ, Huehns ER 1968 Compensation in haemolytic anaemias caused by abnormal haemoglobins. Nature (London) 218:924.

56 Bohr C, Hasselbach K, Krogh A 1904 Ueber einen in biologischer Beziehung wichtigen Einfluss, den die Kohlensäurespannung des Blutes auf dessen Sauerstoffbindungübt. Skandinavisches Archiv für Physiologie 16:402.

57 Hill AV 1910 The possible effect of the aggregation of the molecules of haemoglobin on its dissociation curves. Journal of Physiology 40:4.

58 Bellingham AJ 1972 The physiological significance of the Hill parameter 'n'. Scandinavian Journal of Haematology 9:552.

11

Acquired haemolytic anaemias
F. Regan, M. Newlands & Barbara J. Bain

ASSESSING THE LIKELIHOOD OF ACQUIRED HAEMOLYTIC ANAEMIA

Haemolytic anaemia may be suspected from either clinical or laboratory abnormalities. Suggestive clinical features include anaemia, jaundice and splenomegaly. Other relevant clinical features that should be sought are a history of auto-immune disease, recent blood transfusion, recent infection, exposure to drugs or toxins, the presence of a cardiac prosthesis and risk of malaria.

The basic laboratory investigations when a haemolytic anaemia is suspected are listed in chapter 9 (p. 150). In this chapter tests are described that are more specific for the diagnosis of acquired haemolytic anaemia.

ASSESSMENT OF THE BLOOD FILM AND COUNT IN SUSPECTED ACQUIRED HAEMOLYTIC ANAEMIA

If haemolytic anaemia is suspected, a full blood count, reticulocyte count and blood film should always be performed. The blood count shows a reduced Hb and, usually, an increased MCV. The raised MCV is attributable to the fact that reticulocytes, which may constitute a significant proportion of total red cells, are larger than mature red cells. The abnormalities that may be detected in the blood film and their possible significance in acquired haemolytic anaemia are

Table 11.1 Abnormalities that may be detected on blood film examination and their possible significance

Morphological abnormality observed on blood film examination	Type of acquired haemolytic anaemia suggested
Schistocytes	Fragmentation syndromes including microangiopathic haemolytic anaemia and mechanical haemolytic anaemia
Spherocytes	Auto-immune, allo-immune or drug-induced immune haemolytic anaemia, burns, paroxysmal cold haemoglobinuria, *Clostridium welchii* sepsis
Microspherocytes	Burns, fragmentation syndromes
Irregularly contracted cells	Oxidant damage, Zieve's syndrome
Marked red cell agglutination	Cold-antibody-induced haemolytic anaemia
Minor red cell agglutination	Warm auto-immune haemolytic anaemia, paroxysmal cold haemoglobinuria
Hypochromia, microcytosis and basophilic stippling	Lead poisoning
Atypical lymphocytes	Cold-antibody-induced haemolytic anaemia associated with infectious mononucleosis or, less often, other infections
Lymphocytosis with mature small lymphocytes and smear cells	Auto-immune haemolytic anaemia associated with chronic lymphocytic leukaemia
Thrombocytopenia	Auto-immune haemolytic anaemia, thrombotic thrombocytopenic purpura, microangiopathic haemolytic anaemia associated with disseminated intravascular coagulation, paroxysmal nocturnal haemoglobinuria
Neutropenia	Paroxysmal nocturnal haemoglobinuria
No specific features	Paroxysmal nocturnal haemoglobinuria

shown in Table 11.1. Abnormalities detected in the blood film will direct further investigations. For example, a Heinz body preparation would be relevant if irregularly contracted cells were present. Similarly, a direct antiglobulin test (DAT) would be indicated if the blood film showed spherocytes. Various inherited forms of haemolytic anaemia enter into the differential diagnosis of suspected acquired haemolytic anaemia. Thus spherocytes could be attributable to hereditary spherocytosis as well as to auto- or allo-immune haemolytic anaemia. Haemolysis with irregularly contracted cells could be attributable not only to oxidant exposure but also to an unstable haemoglobin, homozygosity for haemoglobin C or glucose-6-phosphate dehydrogenase deficiency.

IMMUNE HAEMOLYTIC ANAEMIA

Acquired immune-mediated haemolytic anaemias are due to auto-antibodies to a patient's own red cell antigens, allo-antibodies in a patient's circulation or present in the serum or sometimes completely bound to red cells (e.g. transfused or neonatal red cells). Allo-antibodies may be present in a patient's serum and react with antigens on transfused donor red cells to cause haemolysis. Allo-antibodies may also occur in maternal serum and cause haemolytic disease of the newborn. Auto-immune haemolytic anaemia (AIHA) may be 'idiopathic' or secondary, associated mainly with lymphoproliferative disorders and auto-immune diseases, particularly systemic lupus erythematosus (SLE). AIHA may also follow atypical (*Mycoplasma pneumoniae*) pneumonia or infectious mononucleosis and other viral infections. Paroxysmal cold haemoglobinuria (PCH) also belongs to this group of disorders. Occasionally, drugs may give rise to a haemolytic anaemia of immunological origin which closely mimics idiopathic AIHA both clinically and serologically. This was a relatively common occurrence with α-methyldopa, a drug that is now used infrequently, but it also occurs occasionally with other drugs. A larger range of drugs give rise to an antibody that is directed primarily against the drug and only secondarily involves the red cells. This is an uncommon occurrence. Such drugs include penicillin, phenacetin, quinidine, quinine, the sodium salt of *p*-aminosalicylic acid, salicylazosulphapyridine and cephalosporins.[1]

TYPES OF AUTO-ANTIBODY

The diagnosis of an AIHA requires evidence of anaemia, haemolysis and demonstration of auto-antibodies attached to the patient's red cells, i.e. a positive DAT (see p. 207). A positive DAT may also be caused by the presence of *allo*-antibodies, e.g. owing to a delayed haemolytic transfusion reaction, so details of any transfusion in the past three months must be sought.

Auto-antibodies can often be demonstrated free in the serum of a patient suffering from an AIHA. The ease with which the antibodies can be detected depends on how much antibody is being produced, its affinity for the corresponding antigen on the red cell surface and the effect that temperature has on the adsorption of the antibody, as well as on the technique used to detect it. The auto-antibodies associated with AIHA can be separated into two broad categories depending on how their interaction with antigen is affected by temperature, i.e. warm antibodies, which are able to combine with their corresponding red cell antigen readily at 37°C, and cold antibodies, which cannot combine with antigen at 37°C but form an increasingly stable combination with antigen as the temperature falls from 30–32°C to 2–4°C.

Cases of AIHA can similarly be separated into two broad categories according to the temperature characteristics of the associated auto-antibodies, i.e. warm-type AIHA and the less frequent cold-type AIHA. The relative frequency of the two categories is illustrated in Table 11.2.

WARM AUTO-ANTIBODIES

The commonest type of warm auto-antibody is an IgG immunoglobulin which behaves in vitro very similarly to an anti-Rh allo-antibody; indeed many IgG auto-antibodies have Rh specificity. IgA and IgM warm auto-antibodies are much less common, and when present they are usually formed in addition to an IgG auto-antibody (Table 11.3).

Quite frequently, patients with warm-type AIHA have complement adsorbed onto their red cells, i.e. the cells are agglutinated by antisera specific for complement or a complement component such as C3d (see Table 11.3). In these cases, the complement is probably not being bound by an IgG antibody but is on the cell surface as the result of the action of small and otherwise undetected amounts of IgM auto-antibody. (IgA auto-antibodies are thought not to cause the binding of complement.)

Sometimes, patients with warm-type AIHA appear to have only complement on the red cell surface. This is more difficult to interpret, as weak reactions of this type are not uncommon in patients with a variety of disorders in whom there is little evidence of increased red cell destruction. In some patients, this may be due to the binding to the red cells of circulating immune complexes.

Warm auto-antibodies free in the patient's serum are best detected by means of the indirect antiglobulin test (IAT) or by the use of enzyme-treated, e.g. trypsinized or papainized, red cells. (Antibodies that agglutinate unmodified cells directly in vitro are seldom present.) Not infrequently, antibodies that agglutinate enzyme-treated cells, sometimes at high titres, are present in the sera of patients in whom the IAT using unmodified cells is negative (see Table 11.4). Occasionally, too, they are present in the sera of patients in whom the DAT is negative.

Antibodies in serum that can be shown to lyse (rather than simply agglutinate) unmodified red cells at 37°C in the presence of complement (warm haemolysins) are rarely demonstrable.[4a] If present, the patient is likely to suffer from extremely severe haemolysis. Antibodies in serum that lyse as well as agglutinate enzyme-treated cells but do not affect unmodified cells are, on the other hand, quite common. Their specificity is uncertain – they are not anti-Rh – and their presence is not necessarily associated with increased haemolysis.

Table 11.2 Relative incidence of different types of autoimmune haemolytic anaemia[2]

	Males	Females	Total
Warm antibodies			
'Idiopathic'	46	65	111
Associated with drugs (mostly α-methyldopa)	1	10	11*
Secondary			
Associated with:			
Lymphomas	14	23	37
Systemic lupus erythematosus (SLE)	1	15	16
Other possible or probable auto-immune disorders	8	13	21
Infections and miscellaneous	9	4	13
Ovarian teratoma	0	1	1
Totals	79	131	210
Cold antibodies			
'Idiopathic' (CHAD)**	16	22	38
Secondary			
Associated with:			
Atypical or *Mycoplasma pneumonia* infection	5	18	23
Infectious mononucleosis	1	1	2
Lymphoma	3	4	7
Paroxysmal cold haemoglobinuria			
'Idiopathic'	7	1	8
Secondary	4	3	7
Totals	**36**	**49**	**85**

* It should be noted that since this study was done the use of α-methyldopa has declined and this is now a rare cause of haemolytic anaemia.

**(CHAD) = chronic cold haemagglutinin disease. Although is often regarded as 'idiopathic', it is actually consequent on an occult lymphoproliferative disorder which leads to production of a cold agglutinin by a clone of neoplastic cells.

Table 11.3 Direct antiglobulin test in warm-antibody autoimmune haemolytic anaemia: incidence of different reactions to specific antiglobulin sera[3]

Anti-IgG	Anti-IgA	Anti-IgM	Anti-C	No. of patients	%
+	–	–	–	43	36
–	+	–	–	3	2
+	+	–	–	4	3
+	–	–	+	52	43
+	–	+	+	6	5
–	–	–	+	13	11
				121	100

COLD AUTO-ANTIBODIES

Cold auto-antibodies are nearly always IgM in type. In vivo, the majority do not cause haemolysis, although a minority can cause chronic intravascular haemolysis, the intensity of which is characteristically influenced by the ambient temperature. The resultant clinical picture is generally referred to as the cold haemagglutinin syndrome or disease (CHAD). Haemolysis is due to destruction of the red cells by complement which is bound to the red cell surface by the antigen–antibody reaction which takes place in the blood vessels of the exposed skin where the temperature is 28–32°C or less. The cold auto-antibody in CHAD is monoclonal, this syndrome being the result of a low-grade lymphoproliferative disorder.

Table 11.4 Results of testing for free auto-antibodies in the sera of 210 patients with warm-antibody auto-immune haemolytic anaemia[2]

Indirect antiglobulin test (IAT)	Agglutination of enzyme-treated red cells at 37°C	Lysis of enzyme-treated red cells at 37°C	Agglutination of normal red cells at 20°C	No. and percentage of patients in group	
+	+	+	+	4	
+	+	+	−	16	
+	+	−	−	64	41%
+	−	−	−	2	
+	−	−	+	1	
−	+	+	+	16	
−	+	+	−	31	
−	+	−	−	29	40%
−	+	−	+	7	
−	−	−	−	39	19%

Notes
1. In 41% of the patients, the IAT was positive and in 80% of the patients, the tests with enzyme-treated cells were positive (in half of these patients, the IAT was negative).
2. In 19% of the patients, all tests were negative.
3. In 13% of the patients, normal red cells were agglutinated at 20°C, probably by cold agglutinins.

The red cells of patients suffering from CHAD characteristically give positive antiglobulin reactions only with anti-complement (anti-C) sera. This is because of red cells which have irreversibly adsorbed sublytic amounts of complement; it is a sign, therefore, of an antigen–antibody reaction which has taken place at a temperature below 37°C. The complement component responsible for the reaction with anti-complement sera is the C3dg derivative of C3 (see p. 441).

In vitro, a cold-type auto-antibody will often lyse normal red cells at 20–30°C in the presence of fresh human complement, especially if the cell-serum mixture is acidified to pH 6.5–7.0; it will usually lyse enzyme-treated red cells readily in unacidified serum, and agglutination and lysis of these cells may still occur at 37°C. Most of these cold-type auto-antibodies have anti-I specificity, i.e. they react strongly with the vast majority of adult red cells and only weakly with cord-blood red cells. A minority are anti-i and react strongly with cord-blood cells and weakly with adult red cells.[5] Rarely, the antibodies have anti-Pr or anti-M specificity and react with antigens on the red cell surface that are destroyed by enzyme treatment.

Another quite distinct, but rarely met with, type of cold antibody is the Donath–Landsteiner (D–L) antibody. This is an IgG globulin and has anti-P specificity. The clinical syndrome the antibody produces is referred to as paroxysmal cold haemoglobinuria (PCH).

Some of the characteristics of IgG, IgM and IgA antibodies are listed in Table 11.5.

The clinical, haematological and serological aspects of the AIHAs have been summarized by Dacie[4] and others.[6–10]

METHODS OF INVESTIGATION

Many of the methods used in the investigation of a patient suspected of suffering from AIHA are described in Chapter 19. Detailed description is given here of precautions to be taken when collecting blood samples from patients and of methods of particular value in the investigations.

COLLECTION OF SAMPLES OF BLOOD AND SERUM

To determine the true thermal amplitude or titre of cold agglutinins requires that the blood sample is collected and maintained strictly at 37°C until serum and cells are separated. This can be achieved by collecting venous (clotted and EDTA sample) blood and keeping it warmed at 37°C – ideally in an insulated thermos, but usually in practice, by placing the sample tube in a beaker containing water at 37°C.

Table 11.5 Main characteristics of IgG, IgM and IgA auto-antibodies

	IgG	IgM	IgA
Mol wt (daltons)	146 000	970 000	160 000
Sedimentation constant (s)	7	19	7
No. of heavy-chain subclasses	4	1	2
Cross placenta	Yes	No	No
Cause activation of complement	Yes	Yes	No
Cause monocyte/macrophage attachment	Yes	No	No
No. of antigen-binding sites	2	5 or 10	2
Types of AIHA produced	Warm; PCH	Usually cold	Warm

AIHA, auto-immune haemolytic anaemia; PCH, paroxysmal cold haemoglobinuria.

Defibrination of a single non-anticoagulated blood sample (at 37°C) before centrifugation may sometimes be useful as it allows large volumes of red cells to be collected as well as serum. The red cells are available for antibody elution and the serum can be examined for free antibody or other abnormalities. The clotted sample should then be centrifuged to separate the serum at 37°C, e.g. in an ordinary centrifuge into the buckets of which water warmed to 37–40°C has been placed. The EDTA sample is used for the DAT and other tests involving the patient's red cells. If the auto-antibody in a particular case is known to be warm in type, the blood may be separated at room temperature; otherwise, as already indicated, this should be carried out at 37°C. When samples are sent by post, it is best to send separately: (a) serum (separated at 37°C) and (b) whole blood added to ACD or CPD solution. Sterility must be maintained.

STORAGE OF SAMPLES

Samples of patient's blood, while keeping quite well in ACD or CPD at 4°C, are more difficult to preserve than normal red cells. In particular, if marked spherocytosis is present, considerable lysis develops on storage. However, satisfactory eluates can be made from washed red cells frozen at –20°C for weeks or months.

The patient's serum should be stored at –20°C or below in small (1–2 ml) volumes. If complement is to be titrated and the titration is not performed immediately, the serum should be frozen as soon as practicable at –70° or below.

SCHEME FOR THE SEROLOGICAL INVESTIGATION OF HAEMOLYTIC ANAEMIA SUSPECTED TO BE OF IMMUNOLOGICAL ORIGIN

It is important to consider which are the most useful tests to carry out and the order in which they should be done. A suggested scheme it has been set out in the form of answers to questions. Whilst some information may be helpful in classifying the type of AIHA, the single most important practical consideration is to determine whether, in addition to an auto-antibody, there is any underlying allo-antibody present. This should be identified before transfusion is undertaken, in order to avoid a delayed haemolytic transfusion reaction which would compound existing haemolysis.

1. **Are the patient's red cells 'coated' by immunoglobulins or complement (indicating an antigen–antibody reaction)?**

   Perform a direct antiglobulin test (DAT) using a polyspecific 'broad-spectrum' reagent, which contains both anti-IgG and anti-complement. (If the DAT is negative, it is unlikely, although not impossible, that the diagnosis is AIHA. See DAT-negative AIHA, p. 208.)

2. **If the DAT is positive, are immunoglobulins or complement adsorbed to the red cells?**

   Repeat the DAT using monospecific sera (p. 449), i.e. anti-IgG and anti-C3d (if using gel technique cards, monospecific anti-IgA and anti-IgM are also included).

3. **If immunoglobulins are present on the red cells, is there antibody specificity?**

Prepare eluates from the patient's red cells. Test these later (see 6).

4. **What is the patient's blood group?**

Determine the patient's ABO and Rh D and Kell type. The Rh phenotype is particularly important in warm-type AIHA; other antigens must be determined if allo-antibodies are to be differentiated from auto-antibodies (see p. 439).

5. **Is there free antibody in the serum? How does it react, at what temperatures and by what methods can it be demonstrated? Is there any underlying allo-antibody present?**

Screen the serum with two or three red cell suspensions suitable for routine pre-transfusion antibody screening (see p. 478) looking for agglutination and lysis at 37°C by the IAT (p. 450). If positive, identify the antibody using an antibody identification panel.

(i) If an allo-antibody is identified, blood lacking the corresponding antigen must be selected for transfusion.

(ii) If no allo-antibody is identified in the serum or plasma, it is safe to assume there is no allo-antibody present, unless the patient has been transfused in the last month: in the latter case, a red cell eluate is required, as an allo-antibody may be bound to the recently transfused cells and there may not be free antibody detectable in the serum/plasma.

(iii) If the auto-antibody is pan-reacting, i.e. is reacting against all panel cells, antibody adsorption tests are needed, to remove the auto-antibody, in order to identify any underlying allo-antibody. If the patient has not been transfused within the last 3 months, a ZZAP auto-adsorption test is appropriate (see later). If the patient has been transfused within the last 3 months, differential allo-adsorption tests are needed. However, if the patient has been transfused within the last month an eluate is required, irrespective of results of adsorption tests.

6. **If there is a warm auto-antibody, what is the specificity of the auto-antibody?**

Test the serum also at 20°C against antibody-screening cells, to show whether cold or warm antibodies are present in the serum or a mixture of the two.

Test the eluate against the antibody identification panel of red cells by IAT and by using enzyme-treated red cells (p. 445). Titration of auto-antibody may be useful in the presence of a strong allo-antibody.

Titrate the serum/plasma by the methods that have given positive results in the screening test using the same panel of red cells – see 5(i).

7. **If there is a cold antibody:**
   a. **Has the antibody any specificity? Is it an auto-antibody or an allo-antibody? What is its titre?**
   b. **What is the thermal range of the antibody?**

Test the serum/plasma against a panel of O cells at 20°C, including A1, A2, B, cord and patient's own cells. If an auto-antibody is found, titrate at 4°C with ABO-compatible adult (I) cells, cord-blood (i) cells, the patient's cells and adult (i) cells (if possible):

(i) Determine the highest temperature at which auto-agglutination of the patient's whole blood takes place (p. 214).

(ii) Titrate the patient's serum/plasma at 20°C, 30°C and 37°C with pooled O adult cells O cord cells and patient's own cells. The panel of cells listed under 5(i). If there was any agglutination or lysis at 37°C in the screening test (5(i)), titrate with the appropriate cells at this temperature.

Paroxysmal noctural haemoglubinuria (PNH) red cells, if available, can be used as a valuable and sensitive reagent for detecting lytic activity by both warm and cold antibodies, in a difficult case.

(iii) If PCH is suspected, carry out the direct and indirect Donath–Landsteiner tests (p. 214).

8. **Is a drug suspected as the cause of the haemolytic anaemia?**

(i) If a penicillin-induced haemolytic anaemia is suspected, test for antibodies using cells pre-incubated with the appropriate drug (p. 216).

(ii) If haemolysis induced by other drugs is suspected, add the drug in solution to a mixture of the patient's serum, normal cells and fresh normal serum (p. 217). Look for agglutination of normal and enzyme-treated cells and use the IAT.

9. Are there any other serological abnormalities?

Consider carrying out the following tests: serum protein electrophoresis and quantitative estimation of immunoglobulins; estimation of complement; tests for antinuclear factor (ANF); serological tests for syphilis; a screening test for heterophile antibodies (infectious mononucleosis screening test); mycoplasma antibodies.

The suggested scheme summarizes what may be done by way of serological investigation of a patient suspected of having AIHA. Close collaboration between clinician and laboratory helps in deciding what tests should be done in any particular case.

DETECTION OF INCOMPLETE ANTIBODIES BY MEANS OF THE DIRECT ANTIGLOBULIN (COOMBS) TEST (DAT)
Principle
As already described, the DAT involves testing the patient's cells without prior exposure to antibody in vitro. For the investigation of cases of AIHA, antiglobulin reagents specific for IgG, IgM, IgA and C3d can be used.

Precautions
A blood sample in EDTA is preferred. (If a clotted sample is used, complement could be bound by normal incomplete cold antibody and give a false-positive result with anti-C3d.) Certain precautions are necessary when investigating a patient with possible AIHA. If a cold-reacting autoantibody is present, the patient's red cells should be washed four times in a large volume of saline* warmed to 37°C in order to wash off cold antibodies and obtain a smooth suspension of cells – there is no

risk of washing off adsorbed complement components. However, the washing process should be accomplished as quickly as possible and the test should be set up immediately afterwards, as, bound warm antibody occasionally elutes off the cells when they are washed and false-negative results may be obtained. If for any reason the washing process has to be interrupted once it has begun, the cell suspension should be placed at 4°C to slow down the dissociation of the antibody.

Method
A spin tube technique, as described on page 450, is recommended.

Make a 2–5% suspension of red cells which have been washed four times in saline. Add 1 volume (drop) of the cell suspension to 2 volumes (drops) of antiglobulin reagent. Centrifuge for 10–60 s (see p. 450). Refer to reagent manufacturer's instructions for specific details.

Examine for agglutination after gently resuspending the button of cells. A concave mirror and good light helps in macroscopic readings. If the result appears to be negative, confirm this microscopically.

Each DAT or batch of tests should be carefully controlled as previously described.

Check negative results with the polyspecific AHG or anti-IgG reagents by the addition of IgG-sensitized cells and anticomplement by the addition of complement-coated cells.

DAT using gel agglutination technology
A card of several microtubes enables multiple sample testing. The microtubes contain dextran acrylamide gel particles and the antiglobulin reagent to which donors' red cells are added. After centrifugation, unagglutinated cells pass to the tip of the tube, but agglutinates fail to pass through the gel, which acts as a 'sieve'. As the antiglobulin reagent is already present in the microtubes, no washing or addition of IgG-coated cells to negative tests is required. Refer to individual manufacturer's instructions for details of methods for performing the tests.

Reactions with IgG subclass antiglobulin reagents
This is not carried out routinely, but may occasionally be useful. The majority of IgG red cell

---

* Throughout this chapter, 'saline' refers to 9 g/l NaCl buffered to pH 7.0.

auto-antibodies are IgG1, sometimes in combination with IgG2 or IgG3. The formation of IgG3 (either alone or with IgG1) appears to be associated with active disease and marked haemolysis. Patients with IgG1 only on the red cell surface may or may not have marked haemolysis, whilst IgG2 and IgG4 do not appear to be associated with any haemolysis.[11] Thus it may be of value to know whether IgG3 is present since its presence indicates the likelihood of aggressive disease. The subclass reagents are available commercially.*

Significance of positive direct antiglobulin test[12]

A positive DAT does not necessarily mean that the patient has auto-immune haemolytic anaemia.[2] The causes of a positive test include the following:

1. An auto-antibody on the red cell surface with or without haemolytic anaemia.
2. An allo-antibody on the red cell surface, as for example in haemolytic disease of the newborn or after an incompatible transfusion.
3. Antibodies provoked by drugs adsorbed to the red cell (p. 216).
4. Normal globulins adsorbed to the red cell surface as the result of damage by drugs, e.g. some cephalosporins.
5. Adsorption of immune complexes to the red cell surface. This may be the mechanism of the (usually weak) reactions that are found in approximately 8% of hospital patients suffering from a wide variety of disorders (see below).
6. Sensitization in vitro if a sample other than EDTA is used. If, for instance, clotted or defibrinated normal blood is allowed to stand in a refrigerator at 4°C, or even at room temperature, and the antiglobulin test is subsequently carried out, the reaction may be positive because of the adsorption of incomplete cold antibodies and complement from normal sera.[4e] Samples of blood taken into EDTA or ACD and subsequently chilled do not give this type of false-positive result as the anticoagulant inhibits the complement reaction.
7. False-positive agglutination may also occur with a silica gel derived from glass.[13] It is also

not unknown for the DAT to be positive with the blood of apparently perfectly healthy individuals, e.g. blood donors. Such occurrences are rare and have not been satisfactorily explained (see below).

Positive DATs in normal subjects

The occurrence of a clearly positive DAT in an apparently healthy subject is a rare but well-known phenomenon. Worlledge[12] had reported an incidence in blood donors of approximately 1 in 9000. In a later report, Gorst et al[14] estimated that the incidence was approximately 1 in 14 000 with an increasing likelihood of a positive test with increasing age. Their report, and other subsequent reports,[15,16] suggest that the finding of a positive DAT, using an anti-IgG serum, in an apparently healthy person is usually of little clinical significance and that, although overt AIHA may subsequently develop, this is quite infrequent. In some patients the DAT eventually becomes negative.

Positive DATs in hospital patients

In contrast to the rarity of positive DATs in strictly healthy people, positive tests are much more frequent in hospital patients. Worlledge[12] reported that the red cells of 40 out of 489 blood samples (8.9%) submitted for routine tests were agglutinated by anti-complement sera. Only one sample was agglutinated by an anti-IgG serum and this had been obtained from a patient being treated with α-methyldopa. Freedman[17] reported a similar incidence – 7.8% positive tests with anti-complement sera. Lau et al[18] used anti-IgG sera only. The tests were seldom positive (0.9% positive out of 4664 tests). The probable explanation for the relatively high incidence of positive tests with anti-complement sera is that the reaction is between anti-complement antibodies and immune complexes adsorbed to the red cells.

Hypergammaglobulinaemia

Another possible explanation for positive DATs in hospital patients is hypergammaglobulinaemia. Szymanski et al[16] employed an AutoAnalyser and used Ficoll and PVP to enhance agglutination by an anti-IgG serum highly diluted (usually to 1 in 5000) in 0.5% bovine serum albumin. In this sensitive system, the strength of agglutination was positively correlated with the serum γ-globulin

---

* e.g. from the Central Laboratory of the Netherlands Red Cross Blood Transfusion Service, Amsterdam.

concentration, being subnormal in hypogamma-globulinaemia and supranormal in hypergamma-globulinaemia.

Typically, in hypergammaglobulinaemic patients in whom the DAT is positive attempts to demonstrate antibodies in eluates fail, i.e. eluates are non-reactive.[19,20]

False-negative antiglobulin tests

There are several causes:

1. Failure to wash the red cells properly – the antisera may then be neutralized by immunoglobulins or complement in the surrounding serum or plasma (p. 451).
2. Excessive agitation at the reading stage – this may break up agglutinates leading to a false-negative result.
3. The use of impotent antisera so that weakly sensitized cells are not detected.
4. The use of antisera lacking the antibody corresponding to the subclass of immunoglobulin responsible for the red cell sensitization.
5. The presence of an antibody that is readily dissociable and is eluted in the washing process.

DAT-NEGATIVE AUTO-IMMUNE HAEMOLYTIC ANAEMIA

In approximately 2–6% of patients who present with the clinical and haematological features of AIHA, the DAT is negative on repeated testing.[12,21,22]

In some of these patients, auto-antibodies are being formed but they are of such a nature (e.g. IgA) or present in such small amounts that routine testing fails to detect them. In such patients, evidence for auto-antibody formation can often be obtained by careful screening of an eluate made from the patient's red cells or by the manual Polybrene test (see below).

More complex techniques have also been used successfully to demonstrate low levels of immunoglobulin on the red cell surface in patients with a provisional diagnosis of DAT-negative AIHA. These methods include radioimmunoassay,[23] the use of the agglutination enhancers Polybrene and PVP in automated tests,[24,25] the complement-fixing antibody consumption (CFAC) test[26], enzyme-linked immunosorbent assays (ELISA) and enzyme-linked antiglobulin tests (ELAT).[9,27]

PREPARATION AND TESTING A CONCENTRATED ELUATE

This technique concentrates low levels of immunoglobulin present on the red cell surface so that antibody may then be detected by screening the eluate with group-O red cells by the IAT. Elution techniques reverse or neutralize the binding forces which exist between the red cell antigens and the antibody coating the cells. This may be achieved by several techniques, e.g. heat, alterations to the pH, use of organic solvents.

Manual direct polybrene test

The following method[28] is modified from that described by Petz & Branch[29] who based their technique on that of Lalezari & Jiang.[30] Polybrene is a polyvalent cationic molecule, hexadimethrine bromide, which can overcome the electrostatic repulsive forces between adjacent red cells, bringing the cells closer together. When low levels of IgG are present on the red cell surface, antibody linkage of adjacent red cells is enhanced. The Polybrene is then neutralized using a negatively charged molecule such as trisodium citrate. Sensitized red cells remain agglutinated after neutralization of the Polybrene. Unsensitized red cells will disaggregate after neutralization.

Reagents

Polybrene stock. 10% Polybrene in 9 g/l NaCl, pH 6.9 (saline).

Working Polybrene solution. Dilute the stock Polybrene solution 1 in 250 in saline.

Resuspending solution. 60 ml of 0.2 mol/l trisodium citrate added to 40 ml of 50 g/l dextrose.

Washing solution. 50 ml of 0.2 mol/l trisodium citrate in 950 ml of saline.

Low ionic medium (LIM). 50 g/l dextrose containing 2 g/l disodium ethylenediamine tetra-acetate. Adjust the pH of half the batch to 6.4. Store the remainder at the original pH (approx. 4.9); use this to repeat tests that are negative using LIM at pH 6.4.

Method

Ensure that all reagents are at room temperature.

Positive control

Dilute an IgG anti-D in normal group-AB serum. Find a dilution which gives a positive result with papainized cells but is negative by the IAT on standard testing with group-O, D-positive red cells (a dilution of 1 in 10 000 is often suitable).

Negative control

Normal group-AB serum which fails to agglutinate papainized group-O, Rh D-positive red cells.

1. Wash the cells four times in saline and make 3–5% suspensions of test and normal group-O Rh (D) red cells in saline.
2. Set up three 75×10 mm tubes as shown in Table 11.6. Leave at room temperature for 1 min.
3. Add 1 drop of working Polybrene solution to each tube and mix gently. Leave for 15 s at room temperature.
4. Centrifuge for 10 s at 1000 g. Decant, taking care to remove all the supernatant.
5. Leave for 3–5 min at room temperature before adding 2 drops of resuspending solution and mixing gently. Within 10 s aggregates will dissociate leaving true agglutination in the positive tubes.
6. Read macroscopically after 10–60 s. Check all negative results microscopically and compare with the negative control.
7. Repeat negative tests using LIM at the lower pH (c. 4.9).

If the direct Polybrene test is negative, a supplementary antiglobulin test may be performed by washing the cells twice in the washing solution, and testing with an anti-IgG antiglobulin reagent.

DETERMINATION OF THE BLOOD GROUP OF A PATIENT WITH AIHA

ABO grouping

No difficulty should be encountered in ABO grouping patients with warm-type AIHA using monoclonal reagents, but the presence of cold agglutinins may cause difficulties. The cells should in all cases be washed in warm (37°C) saline. They should then be groupable without trouble; the reactions must, however, be controlled with normal AB serum. Reverse grouping should be performed strictly at 37°C. Warm the known A_1, B and O cells to 37°C before adding them to the patient's serum at 37°C. Read the results macroscopically.

Rh D grouping

When the DAT is positive, monoclonal anti-D reagents should be used; if cold agglutinins are present, perform test at 37°C. Appropriate controls should be included (see p. 475).

DEMONSTRATION OF FREE ANTIBODIES IN SERUM

The sera of patients suffering from AIHA often contain free auto-antibodies. However, free auto-antibody is also often found with no haemolysis. As a result of improved reagent sensitivity, any clinically significant IgG complement-binding antibodies will be detected by current antibody screening methods.

IDENTIFICATION BY ABSORPTION TECHNIQUES OF CO-EXISTING ALLO-ANTIBODIES IN THE PRESENCE OF WARM AUTO-ANTIBODIES

Absorption techniques for the detection of allo-antibodies present in the sera or eluates of patients with suspected or proved AIHA can be helpful in the following situations:

1. In screening for co-existing serum allo-antibodies in patients with AIHA who have been pregnant or previously transfused and are found to have a pan-reactive antibody in their serum.
2. In differentiating between auto- and allo-antibodies in the eluate of recently transfused patients with AIHA.

Table 11.6 Setting up a direct manual Polybrene test

	Test	Positive control	Negative control
AB serum*	2	0	2
Dilute anti-D in AB serum*	0	2	0
2–3% test cells*	1	0	0
2–5% normal O Rh (D) cells*	0	1	1
LIM	0.6 ml	0.6 ml	0.6 ml

* Drops. LIM, Low ionic medium.

3. In investigating haemolytic transfusion reactions owing to red cell allo-antibodies in patients with AIHA.

In some cases of AIHA, an underlying allo-antibody may be detected by titrating the patient's serum and eluate against a panel of phenotyped reagent red cells. However, a high-titre auto-antibody may mask the allo-antibody; hence the need for absorption techniques, especially in the situations outlined above. The techniques described are based on those of Petz & Branch.[29]

Use of ZZAP reagent in auto-absorption techniques

'ZZAP' reagent[29] is a mixture of dithiothreitol and papain. It dissociates an auto-antibody already coating the patient's red cells and enzyme-treats them, thus increasing the amount of auto-antibody that can subsequently be adsorbed onto the patient's cells in vitro.

Reagents

Dithiothreitol (DTT), 0.2 mol/l.

Papain, 1%.

Phosphate buffered saline (PBS), pH 6.8–7.2.

Prepare a suitable volume of ZZAP by making up the reagents in the following ratio: 0.2 mol/l DTT 5 volumes; 1% papain 1 volume.

Check the pH and adjust to pH 6.0–6.5 using one drop at a time of 0.2 mol/l HCl or 0.2 mol/l NaOH.

Method

1. Add 2 volumes of ZZAP to 1 volume of four-times-washed packed red cells. Incubate at 37°C for 30 min mixing occasionally.
2. After incubation, wash the cells four times in saline, packing hard after the last wash.
3. Divide the cells into two equal volumes. To one volume, add an equal volume of the serum to be absorbed. Incubate at 37°C for 1 h.
4. Centrifuge at 1000 *g*. Remove the serum and add to the remaining volume of cells.
5. Repeat the absorption procedure.
6. Remove the absorbed serum and store at −20°C or below for allo-antibody screening or cross-matching, which may be performed by standard techniques.

Notes

The auto-absorption techniques should only be used in the following circumstances:

1. When the patient has not been transfused in the previous 3 months, as the presence of transfused red cells may allow the absorption of allo-antibody as well as auto-antibody.
2. When at least 2–3 ml of packed red cells are available from the patient.
3. When the auto-antibodies present react well with enzyme-treated red cells. If they do not, heat elution should be substituted for ZZAP treatment. Heat elution may be performed by shaking the washed cells for 5 min in a 56°C water-bath and then washing the cells.

Allo-absorption using papainized R₁R₁, R₂R₂ and rr cells

This method may be used when auto-absorption is not appropriate – for instance when the patient has been transfused in the previous 3 months or when at least 2–3 ml of the patient's red cells are not available.

1. Select three group-O antibody screening cells, which individually lack some of the blood-group antigens which commonly stimulate the production of clinically significant antibodies, e.g. C, E, K, Fyᵃ, Fyᵇ, Jkᵃ, Jkᵇ, S, s (Table 11.7).
2. Papainize 2 ml of packed cells from each sample after washing the cells in saline four times.
3. Add to 1 ml of each sample of washed, packed, papainized cells 1 ml of the patient's serum. Incubate for 1 h at 37°C.
4. Centrifuge to pack the cells. Remove the supernatant serum and add it to the second 1 ml volume of papainized cells. Incubate for 1 h at 37°C.
5. Centrifuge again to pack the cells. Remove the supernatant and store at −20°C or below for further testing, e.g. allo-antibody screening and cross-matching.

Method for testing allo-absorbed sera

Allo-antibody screening. Each absorbed serum is tested against a panel of phenotyped red cells by the IAT.

Cross-matching. Each absorbed serum must be tested separately against the donor red cells by the IAT, using undiluted serum.

Table 11.7 Testing an allo-absorbed serum against a phenotyped panel of red cells

No.	Rh	M	N	S	s	P$_1$	Lu^a	Le^a	Le^b	K	Kp^a	Fy^a	Fy^b	Jk^a	Jk^b	Serum A	Serum B	Serum C
1.	R$_1$R$_1$	+	+	+	+	+	−	−	−	+	−	+	+	+	+	1+	1+	−
2.	R$_1$R$_1$	+	−	−	+	−	+	−	+	−	−	+	+	+	+	1+	3+	−
3.	R$_2$R$_2$	+	+	+	+	+	+	+	−	−	−	−	+	−	+	1+	−	3+
4.	R$_1$R$_2$	+	+	+	−	+	−	−	+	−	−	−	+	+	−	1+	4+	1+
5.	r′r	+	−	+	+	+	−	−	+	−	−	+	+	−	+	−	−	−
6.	r″r	+	+	+	−	+	−	−	+	−	−	+	−	+	+	2+	2+	2+
7.	rr	+	+	−	+	+	−	−	−	+	−	+	+	+	−	2+	2+	−
8.	rr	+	−	+	+	+	−	+	−	−	−	+	−	+	−	1+	2+	(+)
9.	rr	−	+	−	+	+	−	+	−	−	+	+	+	+	+	2+	2+	−
10.	R$_1$R$_2$	−	+	+	+	−	−	−	+	+	−	−	+	+	−	1+	3+	2+

Phenotype of cells selected for absorption of serum / Absorbed serum

1. R$_1$R$_1$, C^w+, K−, Fy(a + b −), Jk(a − b +), M +, N −, s − — Serum A
2. R$_2$R$_2$, C^w−, K−, Fy(a − b +), Jk(a − b +), M +, N +, s + — Serum B
3. rr, C^w, K+, Fy(a + b −), Jk(a + b −), M +, N −, s − — Serum C

Example of allo-antibody detection using the allo-absorption technique in a recently transfused patient with AIHA

The patient's serum when first tested against a panel of group-O phenotyped red cells revealed only pan-reactive antibodies. In contrast, three absorbed sera, A, B and C, obtained by absorbing the patient's serum with three selected phenotyped samples of group-O cells, were shown to contain anti-E and anti-Jk^a when tested against a panel of phenotyped group-O cells using the IAT. The results of testing the absorbed sera, A, B and C are shown in Table 11.7. The patient's red cell phenotype was R$_1$r Jk (a–b–).

Explanation of the results of testing allo-absorbed sera, A, B and C

1. As the R$_1$R$_1$-absorbing cells were negative for the E and Jk^a antigens, absorbed serum A could contain anti-E and anti-Jk^a. Testing the absorbed serum A against the panel of cells suggested that this was so.
2. As the R$_2$R$_2$-absorbing cells were positive for the E antigen but negative for the Jk^a antigen, absorbed serum B could contain anti-Jk^a but not anti-E. Testing absorbed serum B against the panel of cells confirmed the presence of anti-Jk^a.
3. As the rr-absorbing cells were negative for the E antigen but positive for the Jk^a antigen, absorbed serum C could contain anti-E but not anti-Jk^a. Testing absorbed serum C against the panel of cells confirmed the presence of anti-E.
4. As the phenotype of the patient's own red cells was R$_1$r, Jk (a– b–), the anti-E and anti-Jk^a detected in the allo-absorbed sera must be allo-antibodies. Blood for transfusion should be E-negative, Jk^a-negative.

Additional notes on absorption techniques

1. If the patient has been transfused in the past month, an eluate must also be tested as allo-antibody may be present on red cells but not in serum/plasma.
2. If the patient's serum contains a haemolytic antibody, EDTA should be added to prevent the uptake of complement and subsequent lysis of the cells used for absorption. Add 1 volume of neutral EDTA (potassium salt) (see p. 604) to 9 volumes of serum. More commonly, a plasma sample is used.

3. It is often useful to allo-adsorb both serum and eluate to differentiate between auto- and allo-antibodies, particularly if the auto-antibody is the mimicking type described by Issitt.[10]

4. If the auto-antibody does not react with papainized cells, do *not* papainize the cells for absorption.

ELUTION OF ANTIBODIES FROM RED CELLS

The selection of any elution technique is often based on personal choice and the availability of the necessary reagents and equipment. However, heat elution techniques are best used for the elution of primary cold reactive (IgM) antibodies such as anti-A, anti-N, anti-M, anti-I and IgG anti-A and B antibodies associated with ABO HDN. The Lui freeze and thaw may also be used for ABO HDN investigations. Warm-reactive allo- or auto-antibodies are best eluted with organic solvents such as xylene or chloroform. Commercially prepared kits which alter the pH of the red blood cells are equally effective and circumvent the hazards of using organic solvents. Refer to the manufacturer's instructions for details. Methods for heat elution and Lui's elution techniques are given below. Commercial kits are now widely available.

Notes

1. A large volume of red blood cells is required to obtain enough eluate for testing.

2. The red blood cells must be washed at least six times and the last wash kept for testing to ensure removal of all free antibody.

3. Depending on the elution technique used, the prepared eluate may be frozen, if testing is not possible immediately after preparation.

4. All elution techniques which use organic solvents must be performed with glass test tubes and pipettes.

Heat elution (Landsteiner & Miller)[31]

Mix equal volumes of washed packed cells and saline or 6% BSA. Incubate at 56°C for 5 min. Agitate periodically. Centrifuge to pack the red cells. Remove the supernatant (the eluate) which may be haemoglobin stained. Test the eluate by appropriate techniques in parallel with the last wash from the red cells.

Freeze and thaw elution (Lui)[32]

Mix 0.5 ml of washed packed red cells with 3 drops of PBS or AB serum. Stopper the tube and rotate to coat the glass surface with red cells. Place at −30°C for 10 min. Thaw the red cells rapidly under warm running tap water or in the 37°C water-bath. Remove the stopper and centrifuge to sediment red cell stroma. Remove the supernatant and test in parallel with the last wash from the red cells by appropriate techniques.

Screening eluates

The eluate and the saline of the last wash (control) are first screened against two or three samples of washed normal group-O cells to see if they contain any antibodies using the IAT. If anti-A or anti-B is suspected, include A_1 and B cells. To 4–6 drops of eluate and control, add 2 drops of a 2% suspension by NISS technique of antibody screening cells. Incubate for $1–1\frac{1}{2}$ h at 37°C. Wash four times and, using optimal dilutions of anti-IgG, carry out the IAT by the tube method.

If the control preparation (the supernatant saline from the last washing) gives positive reactions, the possibility that an eluate contains serum antibody has to be considered.

DETERMINATION OF THE SPECIFICITY OF WARM AUTO-ANTIBODIES IN ELUATES AND SERA

When tested against a phenotyped panel, about two-thirds of auto-antibodies appear to have Rh specificity and in about half these cases specificity against a particular antigen can be demonstrated.[2,7,10] Within the Rh system, anti-e is the commonest specificity. −D− and RhNull cells are an advantage.

The other one-third of auto-antibodies may show specificity against other very high incidence antigens, e.g. Wr^b and En^a, and rarely other blood-group specificities are involved. It is essential to differentiate between auto- and allo-antibodies, especially if transfusion is being considered. The presence of allo-antibodies in addition to auto-antibodies is suggested by any discrepancy between the serum and eluate results.

As already mentioned, the presence of allo-antibodies in a serum complicates the determination of the specificity of an auto-antibody, and it can be argued that it would be better to test only the eluted auto-antibody and to leave the serum strictly alone. However, only a small volume of an eluate may be available, especially in anaemic patients, and it is generally wise to test both serum and eluate. The procedure is the same for both.

Titration of warm antibodies in eluates or sera
The methods used are those described in Chapter 19. The exact technique chosen, and the red cells used, should be those which have given the clearest results in the screening tests. Titration of the eluate can be useful in the presence of a pan-reacting auto-antibody to exclude an underlying allo-antibody.

In investigating cold auto-antibodies, the following tests may sometimes provide clinically useful information:

DETERMINATION OF THE SPECIFICITY OF COLD AUTO-ANTIBODIES
High-titre cold auto-antibodies have a well-defined blood-group specificity which is almost invariably within the I/i system.[10,33,34] Since the I antigen is poorly developed in cord-blood red cells, whilst the i antigen is well developed, group-O cord-blood red cells should be included in the panel used to test for I/i specificity. Adult cells almost always have the I antigen well expressed but the strength of the antigen varies and it is of considerable advantage to have available adult cells known to possess strong I antigen. (The rare adult i cells, if available, may be used.)

Titration of cold antibodies
If the screening test is positive for cold autoagglutinins, titrate as follows.

Prepare doubling dilutions of the serum in saline ranging from 1 in 1 to 1 in 512 and add 1 drop of each serum dilution into three series of (12 × 75 mm) glass tubes so that three replicate titrations can be made. Add 1 drop of a 2% suspension of pooled saline-washed adult group-O (I) cells to the first row, 1 drop of cord-blood group-O (i) cells to the second row and 1 drop of the patient's own cells to the third row. Mix and leave for several hours at 4°C. Before reading, place pipettes and a tray of slides at 4°C. Read macroscopically at room temperature using the chilled slides.

Normal range. Using sera from normal adult Caucasians and normal adult I red cells, the cold-agglutinin titre at 4°C is 1 to 32; and with cord-blood (i) cells the titre is 0 to 8. In chronic CHAD, the end-point may not have been reached at a dilution of 1 in 512; if so, further dilutions should be prepared and tested.

If a cold agglutinin is present at a raised titre, the presence of a cold allo-antibody has to be excluded. In this case, the patient's own red cells will be found to react *much* less strongly than do normal adult I red cells. It should be noted that in CHAD the patient's cells commonly react rather less strongly than do normal adult I cells (see Table 11.8).

Cold agglutinin titration patterns
The presence of high-titre cold agglutinins in a patient's serum will be indicated by the screening procedure described above. To demonstrate that the agglutinins are auto-antibodies, it is necessary

Table 11.8 Agglutination titres using various types of cold auto-antibodies and normal adult and normal cord red cells, the patient's red cells and enzyme-treated (papanized) normal adult red cells

Patient	Agglutination titre (4°C)			
	Adult (I) cells	**Cord (i) cells**	**Patient's cells**	**Papainized adult (I) cells**
A.G.	4000	512	2000	8000
F.B.	512	32000	128	8000
A.R.	2000	2000	2000	16

A.G. This patient had chronic cold haemagglutinin disease. The antibody was of the common anti-I type.
F.B. This patient had haemolytic anaemia associated with a lymphoma. The antibody was of the anti-i type.
A.R. This patient had chronic cold haemagglutinin disease. The antibody was of the rare anti-Pr type.

to show that the patient's own cells are also agglutinated. The titre using the patient's cells is usually less (one-half or one-quarter) than that of control normal adult red cells (Table 11.8).

In CHAD, whether 'idiopathic' or secondary to mycoplasma pneumonia or lymphoma, the auto-antibodies usually have anti-I specificity (Patient A.G. in Table 11.8).

In rare cases of haemolytic anaemia associated with infectious mononucleosis, an auto-antibody of anti-i specificity has been demonstrated (Patient F.B. in Table 11.8), and this specificity, too, has been found in certain patients with lymphoma. Rarely, in CHAD, the antibody has been shown to have anti-Pr or anti-M specificity: if enzyme-treated red cells are used, then in either type of case the antigen is destroyed by enzyme treatment (Patient A.R. in Table 11.8).

Determination of the thermal range of cold agglutinins

From a series of master doubling dilutions of serum in saline, place 1 drop of serum or serum dilution into three rows of (12×75 mm) tubes. Set them up at 30°C and at room temperature (20–25°C); to each tube add 1 drop of a 2% saline suspension of the following cells:

1. Pooled normal adult group-O (I) red cells.
2. Pooled cord-blood group-O (i) red cells.
3. Patient's red cells.

Titration should also be carried out at 37°C, if there had been agglutination at this temperature in the screening tests. After incubation at the appropriate temperature for 1 h, determine the presence or absence of agglutination macroscopically, over a light.

DETECTION AND TITRATION OF THE DONATH–LANDSTEINER ANTIBODY

The Donath–Landsteiner (D–L) antibody of PCH differs from the high-titre cold antibodies referred to previously in that it is an IgG antibody and has a quite different specificity. It is also far more lytic to normal cells in relation to its titre than are anti-I or anti-i antibodies. The lysis titre of a D–L antibody may be the same or greater than its agglutination titre. Almost maximal lysis develops in unacidified serum.

Direct Donath–Landsteiner test

Collect two samples of venous blood into glass tubes containing no anticoagulant, previously warmed at 37°C. Incubate the first sample at 37°C for $1\frac{1}{2}$ h. Put the second sample in a beaker packed with ice and allow to stand for 1 h; then place this tube at 37°C for a further 20 min. Centrifuge both tubes at 37°C and examine the supernatant serum for lysis. A positive test is indicated by lysis in the sample which had been chilled. If positive, investigate the antibody specificity (as below). If negative, proceed to an indirect D–L test.

Indirect Donath–Landsteiner test

Serum obtained from the patient's blood which has been allowed to clot at 37°C is used for this test. Add 1 volume of a 50% suspension of washed normal group-O, P-positive red cells to 9 volumes of patient's unacidified serum in a glass tube. Chill the suspension in crushed ice at 0°C for 1 h, then place the tube at 37°C for 30 min. Centrifuge at 37°C and examine for lysis. Three controls should be set up at the same time:

1. A duplicate of the test cell-serum suspension, but kept strictly at 37°C for the duration of the test.
2. A duplicate of the test cell-serum suspension, except that an equal volume of ABO-compatible fresh normal serum is first added to the patient's serum as a source of complement. One volume of the 50% cell suspension is added and the suspension is chilled and subsequently warmed in the same way as the test suspension. (This control excludes false-negative results owing to the patient's serum being deficient in complement.)
3. A duplicate of the test cell-serum suspension, except that fresh normal serum is used in place of the patient's serum. This control also is chilled and subsequently warmed.

A positive test will be indicated by lysis in the test suspension and in control No. 2. If ABO compatible *pp* cells are available they should be used in a duplicate set of tubes. No lysis will develop – confirming the P specificity of the antibody.

Titration of a Donath–Landsteiner antibody

Prepare doubling or fourfold dilutions of the patient's serum in fresh normal human serum. To each tube, add a one-tenth volume of a 50%

suspension of washed group-O, P-positive red cells and immerse each of the tubes in crushed ice at 0°C. After 1 h place at 37°C and incubate for a further 30 min. Then centrifuge and inspect for lysis.

Detection of a Donath–Landsteiner antibody by the indirect antiglobulin test

Since the D–L antibody is an IgG antibody, it can be detected by the IAT using an anti-IgG serum if the cells which have been exposed to the antibody in the cold are washed in cold (4°C) saline. At this temperature, the antibody will not be eluted during washing. It should be noted, however, that exposing normal red cells at 4°C to many fresh normal sera results in a positive IAT with broad-spectrum antiglobulin sera because of the adsorption of incomplete anti-H (a normally occurring cold antibody) on to the red cells. At a low temperature, complement is bound, too, and it is its adsorption which gives rise to the positive tests with broad-spectrum sera. The adsorption of complement can be prevented by adding an anti-coagulant such as EDTA to the serum.

Method

Add a one-tenth volume of EDTA, buffered to pH 7.0 (see p. 604) to the patient's serum. Prepare doubling dilutions in saline from 1 in 1 to 1 in 28.

Add 1 volume (drop) of a 50% suspension of group-O, P-positive red cells to 10 volumes (drops) of each dilution. Mix and chill at 4°C (preferably in a cold room).

After 1 h, wash the red cells four times in a large volume of cold (4°C) saline. Then carry out an antiglobulin test using an anti-IgG reagent, as described on page 450, but keeping the red cell-antiglobulin serum suspension at 4°C.

As controls, set up a series of tests using a serum known to contain a D–L antibody (if available) and a normal serum, respectively.

This technique is the most sensitive way of detecting, especially in stored sera, the presence of D–L antibody in an amount insufficient to bring about actual lysis.

Thermal range of Donath–Landsteiner antibody

The highest temperature at which D–L antibodies are usually adsorbed to red cells is about 18°C. Hence little or no lysis can be expected unless the cell-serum suspension is cooled below this temper-ature. Chilling in crushed ice results in maximum adsorption of the antibody and leads to the binding of complement which brings about lysis when the cell suspension is subsequently warmed at 37°C. Hence the 'cold-warm' biphasic proce-dure necessary for lysis to be demonstrated by a typical D–L antibody.

Specificity of the Donath–Landsteiner antibody

The D–L antibody appears to have a well-defined specificity within the P blood-group system, namely, anti-P. However, in practice, almost all samples of red cells are acted upon, for the cells that will not react (P^k and pp) are extremely rare.[35,36] Cord-blood cells are lysed to about the same extent as are adult P_1 and P_2 cells.

TREATMENT OF SERUM WITH 2-MERCAPTOETHANOL (2-ME) OR DITHIOTHREITOL (DTT)

Weak solutions of 2-mercaptoethanol or DTT destroy the inter-chain sulphydryl bonds of gammaglobulins. IgM antibodies treated in this way lose their ability to agglutinate red cells while IgG antibodies do not.[10,26] IgA antibodies may or may not be inhibited depending upon whether or not they are made up of polymers of IgA. Since almost all auto-antibodies are either IgM or IgG, treatment of serum or an eluate with 2-ME or DTT gives a reliable indication of the Ig class of auto-antibody under investigation.[10,37]

Method

a 2-mercaptoethanol

To 1 volume of undiluted serum add 1 volume of 0.1 mol/l 2-ME in phosphate buffer, pH 7.2 (see p. 605).

As a control, add a volume of the serum to the phosphate buffer alone. Incubate both at 37°C for 2 h.

Then titrate the treated serum and its control with the appropriate red cells.

If IgG antibody is present, the antibody titra-tion in the control serum will be the same as that of the treated serum. However, if the antibody is IgM, the treated serum will fail to agglutinate the test cells or will agglutinate them to a much lower titre compared with the control untreated serum.

The control must remain active to show that the absence of agglutination is due to reduction of IgM antibody and not due to dilution.

b. Dithiothreitol

0.01 mol/l DTT can be used in place of 0.1 mol/l 2-ME in the above method.

DRUG-INDUCED HAEMOLYTIC ANAEMIAS OF IMMUNOLOGICAL ORIGIN

As already mentioned, acquired haemolytic anaemias may develop as the result of immunological reactions consequent on the administration of certain drugs.[7,38,39] Clinically, they often closely mimic AIHA of 'idiopathic' origin and for this reason a careful enquiry into the taking of drugs is a necessary part of the interrogation of any patient suspected of having an acquired haemolytic anaemia.

Two immunological mechanisms leading to a drug-induced haemolytic anaemia are recognized. These mechanisms can be referred to as 'drug-dependent immune' and 'drug-induced auto-immune'. Both types of antibody may be present in some patients.[40–42] In a unifying concept, the target orientation of these antibodies covers a spectrum in which the primary immune response is initiated by an interaction between the drug or its metabolites and a component of the blood cell membrane to create a neoantigen.[43] Drug-dependent antibodies bind to both the drug and the cell membrane, but not to either separately. If the drug is withdrawn, the immune reaction subsides. It has been postulated that in the case of the auto-antibodies, the greater part of the neoantigen is sufficiently similar to the normal cell membrane to allow binding without the drug being present. Similar mechanisms have been described for drug-induced immune thrombocytopenia and neutropenia of immunological origin (p. 457).

Drug-dependent immune haemolytic anaemia

In these cases, the drug is required in the in-vitro system for the antibodies to be detected. The red cells become damaged by one of two mechanisms:

1. *Complement lysis.* A typical history is for haemolysis, which may be severe and intravascular, to follow the re-administration of a drug with which the patient has previously been treated, and for the haemolysis to subside when the offending drug is withdrawn. The DAT is likely to become strongly positive during the haemolytic phase, the patient's red cells being agglutinated by anti-C and sometimes by anti-IgG.

   Drugs which have been shown to cause haemolysis by the above mechanism include quinine, quinidine and rifampicin, as well as chlorpropamide, hydrochlorothiazide, nomifensine, phenacetin, salicylazosulphapyridine, the sodium salt of *p*-aminosalicylic acid and stibophen. Petz & Branch[39] listed 25 drugs reported to have brought about haemolysis by this mechanism.

2. *Extravascular haemolysis.* This is brought about by IgG antibodies that usually do not activate complement, or if they do, not beyond C3. The DAT will be positive with anti-IgG, and sometimes also with anti-C.

   The haemolytic anaemia associated with prolonged high-dose penicillin therapy is caused by the above mechanism, and other penicillin derivatives, as well as cephalosporins and tetracycline, may cause haemolysis in a similar fashion. Haemolysis ceases when the offending drug has been identified and withdrawn.

   Cephalosporins, in addition to causing the formation of specific antibodies, may alter the red cell surface so as to cause non-specific adherence of complement and immunoglobulins. This may lead to a positive DAT but is seldom associated with increased haemolysis, though where it occurs it can be very severe.

Drug-induced auto-immune haemolytic anaemias

In these cases, the antibody reacts with the red cell in the absence of the drug (these are sometimes referred to as 'drug-independent antibodies'). The anti-red cell auto-antibodies seem to be serologically identical to those of 'idiopathic' warm-type AIHA. The great majority of cases followed the use of the anti-hypertension drug α-methyldopa. The red cells are coated with IgG and the serum contains auto-antibodies which characteristically have Rh specificity.

Other drugs that have been reported to act in a similar fashion to α-methyldopa include L-dopa, chlordiazepoxide, mefenamic acid, flufenamic acid and indomethicin.[2]

Typical serological features of the different types of drug-induced haemolytic anaemia of immunological origin are summarized in Table 11.9.

Table 11.9 Serological features of the different types of drug-induced haemolytic anaemia of immunological origin

Mechanism	Prototype drug	DAT	IAT		
			No drug	Serum + drug	Eluate + drug
Drug-dependent antibody:					
(a) C-activation	Quin(id)ine	C*	Neg	C*	Neg
(b) No C-activation	Penicillin	IgG	Neg	IgG	IgG
Auto-antibody	α-Methyldopa	IgG	IgG		

* Occasionally also IgG.

Detection of anti-penicillin antibodies

The characteristic features of penicillin-induced haemolytic anaemia are:

1. Haemolysis occurs only in patients receiving large doses of a penicillin for long periods (e.g. weeks).
2. The DAT is strongly positive with anti-IgG reagents.
3. The patient's serum and antibody eluted from the patient's red cells react *only* with penicillin-treated red cells – they do not react with normal untreated red cells.

Reagents

Barbitone buffer. 0.14 mol/l, pH 9.5 (see p 601).

Penicillin solution. 0.4 g of penicillin G dissolved in 6 ml of barbitone buffer.

Penicillin-coated normal red cells

Wash group-O reagent red cells three times in saline and make *c* 15% suspension in saline to which a one-tenth volume of barbitone buffer has been added. Add 2 ml of the red cell suspension to 6 ml of penicillin solution and incubate at 37°C for 1 h. Then wash four times in saline and make 2% red cell suspensions in saline (for tube tests).

Control normal red cells

These should be treated in exactly the same way as the penicillin-coated red cells except that the 6 ml of penicillin solution is replaced by 6 ml of barbitone buffer.

Method

Anti-penicillin antibodies can be detected by the IAT in the usual way using the penicillin-coated red cells in place of normal unmodified cells. However, three extra controls are necessary.

1. Red cells which have not been exposed to penicillin should be added to the patient's serum.
2. Penicillin-treated red cells should be added to two normal sera known not to contain anti-penicillin antibodies (*negative controls*).
3. Penicillin-treated red cells should be added to a serum (if one is available) known to contain anti-penicillin antibodies (*positive control*).

Cephalosporin can be used in a similar way to sensitize red cells. Control (2) is particularly important when drugs such as cephalosporins are used, since over-exposure in vitro to these drugs can lead to positive results with normal sera.

Note

Some drugs do not dissolve easily; incubation at 37°C, crushing tablets with a pestle and mortar and vigorous shaking of the solution may help.

High-titre IgG anti-penicillin antibodies often cause direct agglutination of penicillin-treated red cells in low dilutions of serum. The antibodies can be differentiated from IgM-agglutinating antibodies by treatment with 2-ME or DTT (p. 215).

Detection of antibodies against drugs other than penicillin

In a patient with an immune haemolytic anaemia whose serum and red cell eluate does *not* react with normal red cells and who is receiving a drug or drugs other than penicillin or a penicillin derivative, antibodies which react with red cells only in the presence of the suspect drugs or drugs should be looked for in the following way.

The patient's serum and red cell eluates should be tested with normal and enzyme-treated group-O red cells, carrying out the tests with and without the drug that the patient is receiving. The approach is essentially empirical. A saturated solution of the drug or its metabolite should be prepared in saline and the pH adjusted to 6.5–7.0.

Set up six tubes containing the patient's serum and the drug solution in the proportions shown in Table 11.10 and add one drop of a 50% saline suspension of group-O cells to each tube. Incubate at 37°C for 1 h and examine for agglutination and lysis. Wash the red cells four times in saline and carry out an IAT using anti-IgG and anti-C separately.

Interpretation

Tubes 1 and 2 test the patient's serum (? drug-dependent antibody) and normal red cells in the presence of the drug (Tube 1) and without the drug (Tube 2).

Table 11.10 Investigation of a suspected drug-induced immune haemolytic anaemia

	Tube no.					
	1	2	3	4	5	6
Patient's serum volumes (drops)	10	10	5	5	0	0
Fresh normal serum volumes (drops)	0	0	5	5	10	10
Drug solution volumes (drops)	2	0	2	0	2	0
Saline volumes (drops)	0	2	0	2	0	2
50% normal group-O cells volumes (drops)	1	1	1	1	1	1

Tubes 3 and 4 test the effect of added complement on the above reactions.

Tubes 5 and 6 without the patient's serum act as controls for tubes 3 and 4.

OXIDANT-INDUCED HAEMOLYTIC ANAEMIA

Oxidant-induced haemolytic anaemia should be suspected when the blood film of a patient exposed to an oxidant drug or chemical shows irregularly contracted cells. A Heinz-body test (see p. 273) is confirmatory. The oxidant may also cause methaemoglobinaemia or sulphaemoglobinaemia, both of which can be confirmed by spectroscopy (see p. 163) or co-oximetry. The differential diagnosis of haemolysis induced by an exogenous oxidant includes other causes of haemolysis with irregularly contracted cells, e.g. Zieve's syndrome, G6PD deficiency and the presence of an unstable haemoglobin. In Zieve's syndrome (haemolysis associated with alcohol excess, fatty liver and hyperlipidaemia), the plasma may be visibly lipaemic; if this syndrome is suspected, further investigations should include liver function test and serum lipid measurements.

MICROANGIOPATHIC AND MECHANICAL HAEMOLYTIC ANAEMIAS

Microangiopathic or mechanical haemolytic anaemia should be suspected when a blood film shows red cell fragments. Examination of the blood film is, in fact, the most important laboratory procedure in making this diagnosis. Since haemolysis is intravascular, useful confirmatory tests include serum haptoglobin estimation (see p. 153) and, when the condition is chronic, a Perls' stain of urinary sediment to detect the presence of haemosiderin (p. 157). As a microangiopathic haemolytic anaemia is often part of a more generalized syndrome consequent on microvascular damage, other tests are also indicated in unexplained cases. They include tests of renal function, a platelet count and a coagulation screen including tests for D-dimer or fibrin degradation products (p. 386). Tests for verotoxin-secreting *E. coli* are indicated in cases of microangiopathic haemolytic anaemia with renal failure.

PAROXYSMAL NOCTURNAL HAEMOGLOBINURIA

PNH is an acquired clonal disorder of haemopoiesis in which the patient's red cells are abnormally sensitive to lysis by normal constituents of plasma. In its classical form, it is characterized by haemoglobinuria during sleep (nocturnal haemoglobinuria), jaundice and haemosiderinuria. Not uncommonly, however, PNH presents as an obscure anaemia without obvious evidence of intravascular haemolysis or it develops in a patient suffering from aplastic anaemia or more rarely from myelofibrosis or myeloid leukaemia.[44-46]

PNH red cells are unusually susceptible to lysis by complement.[47,48] This can be demonstrated in vitro by a variety of tests, e.g. the acidified-serum (Ham),[49,50] sucrose,[49,50] thrombin,[52] cold-antibody lysis,[53] inulin[54] and cobra-venom[53] tests. In the acidified-serum, inulin and cobra-venom tests, complement is activated via the alternative pathway, while in the cold-antibody test, and probably in the thrombin test, complement is activated by the classical sequence initiated through antigen–antibody interaction. In the sucrose lysis test, a low ionic strength is thought to lead to the binding of IgG molecules non-specifically to the cell membrane and to the subsequent activation of complement via the classical sequence. In addition, the alternative pathway appears to be activated.[56] In each test, PNH cells undergo lysis because of their greatly increased sensitivity to lysis by complement.

Minor degrees of lysis may be observed in the cold-antibody lysis and sucrose tests with the red cells from a variety of dyserythropoietic anaemias, e.g. aplastic anaemia, megaloblastic anaemia and myelofibrosis.[57,58] Weak positive results in these tests have thus to be interpreted with care. PNH red cells, however, almost always undergo considerable lysis in these tests.

A characteristic feature of a positive test for PNH is that not all the patient's cells undergo lysis, even if the conditions of the test are made optimal for lysis (Fig. 11.1). This is because only a proportion of any patient's PNH red cell population is hypersensitive to lysis by complement. This population varies from patient to patient, and there is a direct relationship between the proportion of red cells that can be lysed (in any of the diagnostic tests) and the severity of in-vivo haemolysis.

The phenomenon of some red cells being sensitive to complement lysis and some insensitive was studied quantitatively by Rosse & Dacie who obtained two-component complement sensitivity curves in a series of PNH patient.[48] Later, Rosse and his coworkers reported that in some cases three populations of red cells could be demonstrated.[59-61]

1. Very sensitive (Type III) cells, 10–15 times more sensitive than normal cells.
2. Cells of medium sensitivity (Type II), 3–5 times more sensitive than normal cells.
3. Cells of normal sensitivity (Type I).

In vivo, the proportion of Type III cells parallels the severity of the patient's haemolysis.

PNH is an acquired clonal disorder[60] resulting from a somatic mutation occurring in a haemopoietic stem cell. It has been demonstrated that a proportion of granulocytes, platelets and lymphocytes are also part of the PNH clone.[63,64] The characteristic feature of cells belonging to the PNH clone is that they are deficient in several cell-membrane bound proteins including red cell acetylcholinesterase,[65-68] neutrophil alkaline phosphatase,[69-71] CD55 (decay accelerating factor or DAF),[72-73] homologous restriction factor

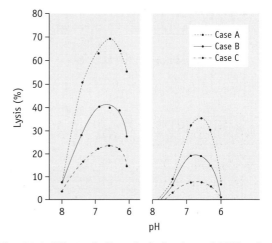

Fig. 11.1 Effect of pH on lysis in vitro of PNH red cells by human sera. The red cells of three patients of different sensitivity were used, and two fresh normal sera, one serum being more potent than the other.

(HRF)[47,74] and CD59 (membrane inhibitor of reactive lysis or MIRL),[75–77] amongst others. CD55, CD59 and HRF all have roles in the protection of the cell against complement-mediated attack. CD59 inhibits the formation of the terminal complex of complement, and it has been established that the deficiency of CD59 is largely responsible for the complement sensitivity of PNH red cells. PNH type III red cells have a complete deficiency of CD59 whereas PNH Type II red cells have only a partial deficiency and it is this difference which accounts for their variable sensitivities to complement.[78,79] The analysis of these deficient proteins on PNH cells by flow cytometry, particularly of the red cells and neutrophils, has recently become a useful research and diagnostic tool, but is only applicable in centres with a significant number of patients requiring investigation for PNH. By comparing the proportion of cells with deficient CD59 to the percentage lysis in the Ham test, it has been possible to assess the sensitivity of the Ham test. The standard Ham test is reasonably good at estimating the proportion of PNH red cells as long as they are PNH Type III cells and comprise less than 20% of the total. In cases in which the PNH cells are Type II and more than 20% are present, the standard Ham test significantly underestimates the proportion of PNH red cells. The standard Ham test can be negative when there are less than 5% PNH Type III cells or less than 20% PNH Type II cells. When the Ham test is supplemented with magnesium, to optimize the activation of complement, the percentage lysis gives a more accurate estimation of the proportion of PNH cells (Fig. 11.2).[80]

Certain chemicals, in particular sulphydryl compounds, can act on normal red cells in vitro so as to increase their complement sensitivity. In this way, PNH-like red cells can be created in the laboratory and can be used as useful reagents (p. 225).

ACIDIFIED-SERUM LYSIS TEST (HAM TEST)

Principle

The patient's red cells are exposed at 37°C to the action of normal or the patient's own serum suitably acidified to the optimum pH for lysis (pH 6.5–7.0) (Table 11.11).

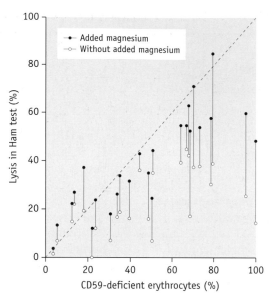

Fig. 11.2 Comparison of the proportion of CD59-deficient red cells with the lysis in the Ham test. The percentage lysis in the Ham test with added magnesium (●) and without added magnesium (○) is plotted against the proportion of CD59-deficient red cells in the same samples from 25 patients with PNH (with thanks to P. Hillmen, M. Bessler, D. Roper and L. Luzzatto, unpublished observation).

The patient's red cells can be obtained from defibrinated, heparinized, oxalated, citrated or EDTA blood, and the test can be satisfactorily carried out even on cells which have been stored at 4°C for up to 2 to 3 weeks in ACD or Alsever's solution, if kept sterile. The patient's serum is best obtained by defibrination, since in PNH if it is obtained from blood allowed to clot in the ordinary way at 37°C or at room temperature, it will almost certainly be markedly lysed. Normal serum should similarly be obtained by defibrination, although serum derived from blood allowed to clot spontaneously at room temperature or at 37°C can be used. Normal serum known to be strongly lytic to PNH red cells is to be preferred to patient's serum, the lytic potentiality of which is unknown. However, if the test is positive using normal serum, it is important, particularly if the patient appears not to be suffering from overt intravascular haemolysis, to obtain a positive result using the patient's serum, in order to exclude hereditary erythroblastic multinuclearity associated with a positive acidified-serum test (HEMPAS) (see p. 223).

Table 11.11   The acidified-serum lysis test with added magnesium

	Test (ml)			Controls (ml)		
Reagent	1	2	3	4	5	6
Fresh normal serum	0.5	0.5	0	0.5	0.5	0
Heat-inactivated normal serum	0	0	0.5	0	0	0.5
0.2 mol/l HCl	0	0.05	0.05	0	0.05	0.05
50% patient's red cells	0.05	0.05	0.05	0	0	0
50% normal red cells	0	0	0	0.05	0.05	0.05
* Magnesium chloride (250 mmol/l; 23.7 g/l)	0.01	0.01	0.01	0.01	0.01	0.01
Lysis (in a positive modified test)	Trace (2%)	+++ (30%)	–	–	–	–

* only for modified test

The variability between the sera of individuals in their capacity to lyse PNH red cells is shown in Figure 11.3. The activity of a single individual's serum also varies from time to time[79] and it is always important to include in any test, as a positive control, a sample of known PNH cells or artificially created 'PNH-like' cells (see p. 225).

The sera should be used within a few hours of collection. Their lytic potency is retained for several months at −70°C, but at 4°C, and even at −20°C, this deteriorates within a few days.

Method (Table 11.11)

Deliver 0.5 ml samples of fresh normal serum, group AB or ABO-compatible with the patient's blood, into six (three pairs) of 75 × 12 mm glass tubes. Place two tubes at 56°C for 10–30 min to inactivate complement. Keep the other two pairs of tubes at room temperature and add to the serum in two of the tubes one-tenth volumes (0.05 ml) of 0.2 mol/l HCl. Add similar volumes of acid to the inactivated serum samples. Then place all the tubes in a 37°C water-bath.

While the serum samples are being dealt with, wash samples of the patient's red cells and of control normal red cells (compatible with the normal serum) twice in saline and prepare 50% suspensions in the saline. Then add one-tenth volumes of each of these cell suspensions (0.05 ml) to one of the tubes containing unacidified fresh serum, acidified fresh serum and acidified inactivated serum, respec-

tively. Mix the contents carefully and leave the tubes at 37°C. Centrifuge them after about 1 h.

Add 0.05 ml of each cell suspension to 0.55 ml of water so as to prepare a standard for subsequent quantitative measurement of lysis and retain 0.5 ml of serum for use as a blank. For the measurement of lysis, deliver 0.3 ml volumes of the supernatants of the test and control series of cell-serum suspensions, and of the blank serum and of the lysed cell suspension equivalent to 0% and 100% lysis, respectively, into 5 ml of 0.4 ml/l ammonia or Drabkin's reagent. Measure the lysis in a photoelectric colorimeter using a yellow-green (e.g. Ilford 625) filter or in a spectrometer at a wavelength of 540 nm.

If the test cells are from a patient with PNH, they will undergo definite, although, as already mentioned, incomplete lysis in the acidified serum. Very much less lysis, or even no lysis at all, will be visible in the unacidified serum. No lysis will be brought about by the acidified inactivated serum. The normal control sample of cells should not undergo lysis in any of the three tubes.

In PNH, 10–50% lysis is usually obtained, when lysis is measured as liberated haemoglobin. Exceptionally, there may be as much as 80% lysis or as little as 5%.

The red cells of a patient who has been transfused will undergo less lysis than before the transfusion, because the normal transfused cells do not have increased sensitivity to lysis. In PNH, it is

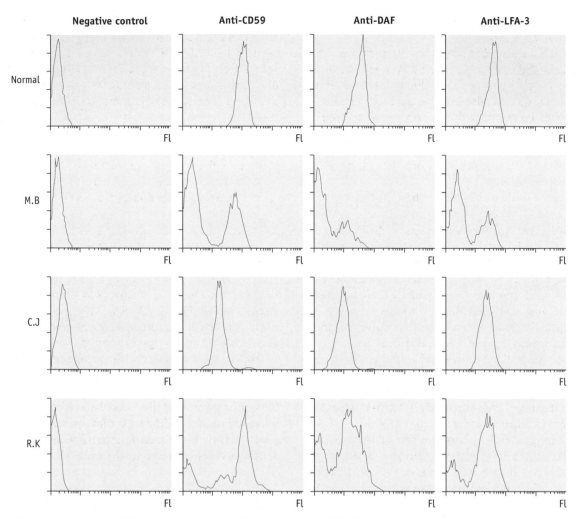

Fig. 11.3 Expression of GPI-linked proteins on the red cells in PNH. Flow cytometry of the erythrocytes from a normal control and 3 patients with PNH stained with a negative control antibody and antibodies to several GPI-linked proteins. M.B: 2 populations; normal and absent GPI-linked proteins. C.J: Mainly reduced GPI-linked proteins, but there is also a very small normal component present. R.K: 3 populations; normal, reduced and absent GPI-linked proteins. FI: fluorescence intensity.

characteristic that a young cell (reticulocyte-rich) population, such as the upper red cell layer obtained by centrifugation, undergoes more lysis than the red cells derived from mixed whole blood.

ACIDIFIED-SERUM TEST LYSIS WITH ADDITIONAL MAGNESIUM (MODIFIED HAM TEST)

Principle
The sensitivity of the Ham test can be improved by the addition of magnesium to the test to enhance the activation of complement.

Method
The method is identical to that for the standard Ham test (see above) with the addition of 10 μl of 250 mmol magnesium chloride (final concentration = 4 mmol) to each tube prior to the incubation (Table 11.11).

SIGNIFICANCE OF THE ACIDIFIED-SERUM LYSIS TEST
A positive acidified-serum test, carried out with proper controls, denotes the PNH abnormality, and PNH cannot be diagnosed unless the acidified-serum test is positive. The addition of magnesium

chloride increases the sensitivity of the acidified-serum test

When the acidified-serum test is positive, a direct antiglobulin test (p. 448) should also be carried out. If this is positive, it could be due to a lytic antibody which has given a false-positive acidified-serum test. This can be confirmed by appropriate serological studies. In such complex cases flow cytometry after reaction of the red cells with anti-CD59 is recommended since it is a more definitive test for PNH (see below).

The only disorder other than PNH that may appear to give a clear-cut positive test is a rare congenital dyserythropoietic anaemia, CDA Type II or HEMPAS.[82,83] In contrast to PNH, however, HEMPAS red cells undergo lysis in only a proportion (about 30%) of normal sera; moreover, they do not undergo lysis in the patient's own acidified serum and the sucrose lysis test is negative. In HEMPAS, the expression of glycosylphosphatidylinositol (GPI)-linked proteins, such as CD55 and CD59, is normal. Lysis in HEMPAS appears to be due to the presence on the red cells of an unusual antigen which reacts with a complement-fixing IgM antibody ('anti-HEMPAS') present in many, but not in all, normal sera.[83]

Heating at 56°C inactivates the lytic system and, if there is lysis in inactivated serum, the test cannot be considered positive. Markedly spherocytic red cells or effete normal red cells may lyse in acidified serum, probably owing to the lowered pH, and such cells may also lyse in acidified inactivated serum.

PNH red cells are not unduly sensitive to lysis by a lowered pH per se. The addition of the acid adjusts the pH of the serum-cell mixture to the optimum for the activity of the lytic system. As is shown in Figure 11.1, it is possible to construct pH-lysis curves, if different concentrations of acid are used. The optimum pH for lysis is between pH 6.5 and 7.0 (measurements made after the addition of the red cells to the serum).

SUCROSE LYSIS TEST[50,51,54]

An iso-osmotic solution of sucrose (92.4 g/l) is required. This can be stored at 4°C for up to 2 to 3 weeks.

For the test, set up two tubes, one containing 0.05 ml of fresh normal group AB or ABO-compatible serum diluted in 0.85 ml of sucrose solution and the other containing 0.05 ml of serum diluted in 0.85 ml of saline. Add to each tube, 0.1 ml of a 50% suspension of washed red cells. After incubation at 37°C for 30 min, centrifuge the tubes and examine for lysis. If lysis is visible in the sucrose-containing tube, measure this in a photoelectric colorimeter or a spectrometer as described above, using the tube containing serum diluted in saline as a blank and a tube containing 0.1 ml of the red cells suspension in 0.9 ml of 0.4 ml/l ammonia in place of the sucrose–serum mixture as a standard for 100% lysis.

Interpretation

The sucrose lysis test is based on the fact that red cells absorb complement components from serum at low ionic concentrations.[81,85] PNH cells, because of their great sensitivity will undergo lysis but normal red cells do not. The red cells from some cases of leukaemia[57] or myelofibrosis[86] may undergo a small amount of lysis, almost always <10%; in such cases, the acidified-serum test is usually negative and PNH should not be diagnosed. In PNH, lysis usually varies from 10% to 80%, but exceptionally may be as little as 5%. Sucrose lysis and acidified-serum lysis of PNH red cells are fairly closely correlated. The sucrose lysis test is typically negative in HEMPAS.

FLOW-CYTOMETRY ANALYSIS OF THE GPI-LINKED PROTEINS ON RED CELLS

Principle

The patient's red cells are stained with a fluorescein-labelled antibody which is specific for one of several GPI-linked proteins, e.g. CD55, CD59 or LFA-3, which are deficient in PNH red cells. The stained cells are then analysed with a flow cytometer. In some laboratories, where facilities are available, flow cytometry has replaced the Ham test as the primary method for the diagnosis of PNH.

The patient's red cells can be obtained in any of the anticoagulants described for the Ham test. The cells, if taken into ACD, can be stored for 2 to 3 weeks prior to analysis. Fluorescein-conjugated anti-CD59* gives excellent results when used for red cell analysis. It is important to use the conjugated antibody, as staining with unconjugated anti-CD59

---

* (MEM 43, Cymbus Bioscience Ltd, Southampton, UK)

followed by a fluorescein-conjugated second layer antibody may result in artefact, probably owing to red cell agglutination. There is no suitable anti-DAF antibody commercially available at present. Anti-LFA-3* gives reproducible results for red cell analysis, but the level of LFA-3 expression on PNH Type-II cells is higher than that of many other GPI-linked proteins and thus studying LFA-3 expression is useful but not ideal.[87]

Method
Chill 1×10^6 cells in 50 μl of PBS on ice with 50 μl of monoclonal antibody for 30 min. Wash twice in PBS + azide (200 mg/l), and then chill with fluorescein-labelled goat anti-mouse antibody on ice in the dark for 30 min. Wash twice in PBS + azide, and then fix with approximately 0.5 ml of 1% formaldehyde in Isoton II (Coulter). Analysis is performed using a flow cytometer. A negative control antibody should always be used to assess the fluorescence of cells lacking the antigen. The cells from a normal subject should be stained as an additional control to verify that negative cells in the test sample are true PNH cells and not artefactual.

OTHER IMMUNOLOGICAL TECHNIQUES
The GPI-linked proteins such as CD59 can also be studied by a modification of the gel technology used for blood grouping.

FLOW CYTOMETRY ANALYSIS OF THE GPI-LINKED PROTEINS ON NEUTROPHILS

Principle
A proportion of the patient's neutrophils have been demonstrated to be part of the PNH clone in all patients with PNH. GPI-linked proteins which are suitable for analysis include CD16, CD24, CD55, CD59 and CD67.[88,89] There are available numerous fluorescein-conjugated antibodies to CD16 which are suitable for use in this analysis, e.g. fluorescein-conjugated anti-Leu-11a (Becton Dickinson) or fluorescein-conjugated anti-CD59 (Cymbus Biosciences).

Method
The patient's neutrophils are obtained by collecting blood, anticoagulating with preservative-free

* (BRIC5, Bioproducts Laboratories, UK, used at 20 μg/ml)

heparin (10 iu/ml) and obtaining a buffy coat. The formation of a buffy coat can be accelerated by adding 1 ml of 6% hetastarch in 0.9% sodium chloride (Hespan, DuPont) to 10 ml of blood. $1–2 \times 10^6$ cells are analysed. It is important that all the subsequent staining and washing are performed at 4°C to minimize non-specific staining. Chill the cells in 50 μl of PBS on ice with 50 μl of monoclonal antibody (MoAb) for 30 min. Wash twice in PBS + 0.1% bovine serum albumin (PBS + BSA), and then chill with fluorescein-labelled goat anti-mouse antibody on ice in the dark for 30 min. Wash twice in PBS + BSA, and then fix with approximately 0.5 ml of 1% formaldehyde in Isoton II. For conjugated antibodies, a single incubation step only is required followed by a wash and then fixing prior to analysis. Analysis is performed using a flow cytometer. Appropriate normal controls and negative controls should always be tested in parallel to the patient's samples.

A negative control antibody should always be used to assess the fluorescence of cells lacking the antigen. The cells from a normal subject should be stained as an additional control to verify that negative cells in the test sample are true PNH cells and not an artefact.

Significance of flow cytometric analysis
The presence of a population of cells with a deficiency of more than one GPI-linked protein is diagnostic of PNH (Fig. 11.3). It is important to analyse more than one protein because there are extremely rare cases in which an inherited deficiency of one protein has been described (i.e. the Inab-phenotype[90–92] – a deficiency of CD55 owing to a defect of the structural gene encoding this protein; inherited deficiency of CD59[93] owing to a defect in the gene encoding CD59). Analysis of the expression of CD59 on erythrocytes allows the identification of PNH Type II as well as PNH Type III red cells. This is important because although patients with only PNH Type II red cells do not usually suffer from significant haemolysis, they may suffer some of the complications of PNH, such as thrombosis. The analysis of neutrophils for GPI-linked proteins is more difficult than red cell analysis. It is, however, probably more sensitive as the proportion of abnormal neutrophils is usually higher than the proportion of PNH red cells because of the reduced survival of PNH red

cells compared to normal and because of the effect of transfusions. Thus flow cytometry applied to neutrophils is a more sensitive method for the diagnosis of PNH than methods relying on the complement sensitivity of PNH red cells.

PNH-LIKE RED CELLS

By treating normal red cells with certain chemicals, it is possible to increase their complement sensitivity so that they take on many of the characteristics of PNH cells.[94] The chemicals include sulphydryl compounds such as L-cysteine, reduced glutathione (GSH), 2-aminoethyl-*iso*-thiouronium bromide (AET) and 2-mercaptobenzoic acid (MBA).[95] AET and MBA cells can be used conveniently as a positive control for in-vitro lysis tests for PNH.[96]

PREPARATION OF AET CELLS[97]
Prepare an 8 g/l solution of AET and adjust its pH to 8.0 with 5 mol/l NaOH. Collect normal blood into ACD and wash it twice in 9 g/l NaCl. Add 1 volume of the packed cells to 4 volumes of the AET solution in a 75×12 mm glass tube which is then stoppered. Mix the contents gently and place the tube at 37°C for 10–20 min. (The optimal time of incubation varies from red cell sample to red cell sample.[50]) Then wash the cells repeatedly with large volumes of saline until the supernatant is colourless. The red cells are now ready to use.

SUMMARY OF THE TEST FOR PNH

The Ham test remains the main diagnostic test for PNH. If carried out with additional magnesium chloride, and performed with the necessary controls, it is more sensitive and remains specific for the diagnosis of PNH. The inclusion of a further test, such as the sucrose lysis test, is optional. The use of flow cytometry gives a better estimate of the size of the PNH clone and identifies the type of red cell abnormality. However, more experience and expensive equipment are required to perform flow cytometry reliably than to perform a Ham test. Flow cytometry is a useful diagnostic test in certain circumstances, especially when the patient is heavily transfused, and it becomes necessary to analyze neurophils or when following a patient after bone marrow transplantation. Flow cytometry may also

be useful in the follow-up of groups of patients with aplastic anaemia as clonal evolution into PNH may be detected at an earlier stage. For laboratories already using gel technology for blood grouping and antibody screening this provides a simple method for screening red cells for deficiency of GPI-linked protein.

REFERENCES

1 Garratty G 1999 Serology of antibodies to second and third generation cephalosporins associated with immune hemolytic anaemia and/or positive direct antiglobulin tests. Transfusion 39:1239.
2 Dacie JV, Worlledge SM 1969 Auto-immune hemolytic anaemias. Progress in Hematology 6:82.
3 Dacie JV 1975 Auto-immune hemolytic anemias. Archives of Internal Medicine 135:1293.
4 Dacie J 1992 The haemolytic anaemias, vol. 3. The auto-immune haemolytic anaemias, 3rd edn. Churchill Livingstone, Edinburgh, (a) p 136, (b) p 139, (c) p 275, (d) p 228, (e) p 276.
5 Marsh WL, Jenkins WJ 1960 Anti-i: a new cold antibody. Nature (London) 188:753.
6 Pirofsky B 1969 Autoimmunization and the autoimmune hemolytic anemias. Williams & Wilkins, Baltimore.
7 Petz LD, Garratty G 1980 Acquired immune hemolytic anemias. Churchill Livingstone, New York.
8 Sokol RJ, Hewitt S 1985 Autoimmune hemolysis: a critical review. CRC Critical Reviews in Oncology/Hematology 4:125.
9 Sokol RJ, Hewitt S, Booker DJ et al 1985 Enzyme linked direct antiglobulin tests in patients with autoimmune haemolysis. Journal of Clinical Pathology 38:912.
10 Issitt PD 1985 Serological diagnosis and characterization of the causative autoantibodies. Methods in Hematology 12:1.
11 Engelfriet CP, von dem Borne AEG, Beckers D et al 1974 Auto-immune haemolytic anaemia: serological and immunochemical characteristics of the auto-antibodies: mechanisms of cell destruction. Series Haematologica VII:328.
12 Worlledge SM 1978 The interpretation of a positive direct antiglobulin test. British Journal of Haematology 39:157 (Annotation).
13 Stratton F, Renton PH 1955 Effect of crystalloid solutions prepared in glass bottles on human red cells. Nature (London) 175:727.
14 Gorst DW, Rawlinson VI, Merry AH, et al 1980 Positive direct antiglobulin test in normal individuals. Vox Sanguinis 38:99.

15 Bareford D, Longster G, Gilks L et al 1985 Follow-up of normal individuals with a positive antiglobulin test. Scandinavian Journal of Haematology 35:348.

16 Szymanski IO, Odgren PR, Fortier NL et al 1980 Red blood cell associated IgG in normal and pathologic states. Blood 55:48.

17 Freedman J 1979 False-positive antiglobulin tests in healthy subjects. Journal of Clinical Pathology 32:1014.

18 Lau P, Haesler WE, Wurzel HA 1976 Positive direct antiglobulin reaction in a patient population. American Journal of Clinical Pathology 65:368.

19 Heddle NM, Kelton JG, Turchyn KL et al 1988 Hypergammaglobulinemia can be associated with a positive direct antiglobulin test, a nonreactive eluate, and no evidence of hemolysis. Transfusion 28:29.

20 Huh YO, Liu FJ, Rogge K, et al 1988 Positive direct antiglobulin test and high serum immunoglobulin G levels. American Journal of Clinical Pathology 90:197.

21 Chaplin H Jr 1973 Clinical usefulness of specific antiglobulin reagents in autoimmune hemolytic anemia. Progress in Hematology 8:25.

22 Worlledge SM, Blajchman MA 1972 The autoimmune haemolytic anaemias. British Journal of Haematology 23 (Suppl): 61.

23 Schmitz N, Djibey T, Kretschmer V, et al 1981 Assessment of red cell autoantibodies in autoimmune hemolytic anemia of warm type by radioactive anti-IgG test. Vox Sanguinis 41:224.

24 Hsu TCS, Rosenfield RE, Burkart P, et al 1974 Instrumental PVP augmented antiglobulin tests. II. Evaluation of acquired hemolytic anemia. Vox Sanguinis 26:305.

25 Lalezari P, Oberhardt B 1971 Temperature gradient dissociation of the red cell antigen-antibody complexes in the Polybrene technique. British Journal of Haematology 21:131.

26 Gilliland BC, Baxter E, Evans RS 1971 Red-cell antibodies in acquired hemolytic anemia with negative antiglobulin serum test. New England Journal of Medicine 285:252.

27 Bodensteiner D, Brown P, Skikne B, et al 1983 The enzyme-linked immunosorbent assay: accurate detection of red blood cell antibodies in autoimmune hemolytic anemia. American Journal of Clinical Pathology 79:182.

28 Owen I, Hows J 1990 Evaluation of the manual Polybrene technique in the investigation of autoimmune hemolytic anemia. Transfusion 30:814.

29 Branch DR, Petz LD 1999 Detecting calloantibodies in patients with autoantibodies. Transfusion 39:6–10.

30 Lalezari P, Jiang AC 1980 The manual Polybrene test: a simple and rapid procedure for detection of red cell antibodies. Transfusion 20:206.

31 Landsteiner K, Miller CP Jr 1925 Serological studies on the blood of primates. II. The blood groups in anthropoid apes. Journal of Experimental Medicine 42:853.

32 Eicher CA, Wallace ME, Frank S et al 1978. The Lui elution: a simple method of antibody elution. Transfusion 18: 647.

33 Roelcke D 1989 Cold agglutination. Transfusion Medicine Review 3:140.

34 Wiener AS, Unger LJ, Cohen L, et al 1956 Type-specific cold auto-antibodies as a cause of acquired hemolytic anemia and hemolytic transfusion reactions: biologic test with bovine red cells. Annals of Internal Medicine 44:221.

35 Levine P, Celano MJ, Falkowski F 1963 The specificity of the antibody in paroxymal cold hemoglobinuria (P. C. H.). Transfusion 3:278.

36 Worlledge SM, Rousso C 1965 Studies on the serology of paroxysmal cold haemoglubinuria (P. C. H.) with special reference to a relationship with the P blood group system. Vox Sanguinis 10:293.

37 Freedman J, Masters CA, Newlands M et al 1976. Optimal conditions fo the use of suphydryl compounds in dissociating red cell antibodies. Vox sarguinis, 30, 231.

38 Habibi B 1987 Drug-induced immune haemolytic anaemias. Baillières Clinical Immunology and Allergy 1:343.

39 Petz LD, Branch DR 1985 Drug-induced immune hemolytic anemias. Methods in Hematology 12:47.

40 Habibi B 1985 Drug induced red blood cell autoantibodies co-developed with drug specific antibodies causing haemolytic anaemias. British Journal of Haematology 61:139.

41 Salama A, Göttsche B, Mueller-Eckhardt C 1991 Autoantibodies and drug- or metabolite-dependent antibodies in patients with diclofenac-induced immune haemolysis. British Journal of Haematology 77:546.

42 Salama C, Mueller-Eckhardt C 1987 Cianidanol and its metabolites bind tightly to red cells and are responsible for the production of auto- and/or drug-dependent antibodies against these cells. British Journal of Haematology 66:263.

43 Salama A, Mueller-Eckhardt C 1992 Immune-mediated blood dyscrasias related to drugs. Seminars in Hematology 29:54.

44 Dacie JV, Lewis SM 1972 Paroxysmal nocturnal haemoglobinuria: clinical manifestations, haematology and nature of the disease. Series Haematologica 5:3.

45 Hansen NE, Killman S-A 1969 Paroxysmal nocturnal haemoglobinuria. A clinical study. Acta Medica Scandinavica 184:525.

46 Sirchia G, Lewis SM 1975 Paroxysmal nocturnal haemoglobinuria. Clinics in Haematology 4:199.

47 Hansch GM, Schonermark S, Roeicke D 1987 Paroxysmal nocturnal hemoglobinuria type III: lack of an erythrocyte membrane protein restricting the lysis by C5b-9. Journal of Clinical Investigation 80:7.

48 Rosse WF, Dacie JV 1966 Immune lysis of normal human and paroxysmal nocturnal hemoglobinuria (PNH) red blood cells. 1. The sensitivity of PNH red cells to lysis by complement and specific antibody. Journal of Clinical Investigation 45:736.

49 Ham TH, Dingle JH 1939 Studies on destruction of red blood cells. II. Chronic hemolytic anemia with paroxysmal nocturnal hemoglobinuria: certain immunological aspects of the hemolytic mechanism with special reference to serum complement. Journal of Clinical Investigation 18:657.

50 Jenkins DE Jr 1979 Paroxysmal nocturnal hemoglobinuria hemolytic systems. In: A seminar on laboratory management of hemolysis. American Association of Blood Banks, Washington, p 45–49.

51 Hartmann RC, Jenkins DE Jr, Arnold AB 1970 Diagnostic specificity of sucrose hemolysis test for paroxysmal nocturnal hemoglobinuria. Blood 35:462.

52 Crosby WH 1950 Paroxysmal nocturnal hemoglobinuria. A specific test for the disease based on the ability of thrombin to activate the hemolytic factor. Blood 5:843.

53 Dacie JV, Lewis SM, Tills D 1960 Comparative sensitivity of the erythrocytes in paroxysmal nocturnal haemoglobinuria to haemolysis by acidified normal serum and by a high-titre cold antibody. British Journal of Haematology 6:362.

54 Brubaker LH, Schaberg DR, Jefferson DH, et al 1973 A potential rapid screening test for paroxysmal nocturnal hemoglobinuria. New England Journal of Medicine 288:1059.

55 Kabakci T, Rosse WF, Logue GL 1972 The lysis of paroxysmal nocturnal haemoglobinuria red cells by serum and cobra factor. British Journal of Haematology 23:693.

56 Logue GL, Rossi WF, Adams JP 1973 Mechanisms of immune lysis of red blood cells in vitro. I. Paroxysmal nocturnal hemoglobinuria cells. Journal of Clinical Investigation 52:1129.

57 Catovsky D, Lewis SM, Sherman D 1971 Erythrocyte sensitivity to in-vitro lysis in leukaemia. British Journal of Haematology 21:541.

58 Lewis SM, Dacie JV, Tills D 1961 Comparison of the sensitivity to agglutination and haemolysis by a high-titre cold antibody of the erythrocytes of normal subjects and of patients with a variety of blood diseases including paroxysmal nocturnal haemoglobinuria. British Journal of Haematology 7:64.

59 Rosse WF 1972 The complement sensitivity of PNH cells. Series Haematologica 5:101.

60 Rosse WF 1973 Variations in the red cells in paroxysmal nocturnal haemoglobinuria. British Journal of Haematology 24:327.

61 Rosse WF, Adams JP, Thorpe AM 1974 The population of cells in paroxysmal nocturnal haemoglobinuria of intermediate sensitivity to complement lysis: significance and mechanism of increased immune lysis. British Journal of Haematology 28:281.

62 Oni SB, Osunkoya BO, Luzzatto L 1970 Paroxysmal nocturnal hemoglobinuria: evidence for monoclonal origin of abnormal red cells. Blood 36:145.

63 Kinoshita T, Medof ME, Silber R et al 1985 Distribution of decay-accelerating factor in the peripheral blood of normal individuals and patients with paroxysmal nocturnal hemoglobinuria. Journal of Experimental Medicine 162:75.

64 Nicholson-Weller A, Spicier DB, Austen KF 1985 Deficiency of the complement regulating protein 'decay accelerating factor' on membranes of granulocytes, monocytes, and platelets in paroxysmal nocturnal hemoglobinuria. New England Journal of Medicine 312:1091.

65 Auditore JV, Hartmann RC 1959 Paroxysmal nocturnal hemoglobinuria: II. Erythrocyte acetylcholinesterase defect. American Journal of Medicine 27:401.

66 Chow F-L, Telen MJ, Rosse WF 1985 The acetylcholinesterase defect in paroxysmal nocturnal hemoglobinuria: evidence that the enzyme is absent from the cell membrane. Blood 66:940.

67 De Sandre G, Ghiotto G, Mastella G 1956 L'acetilcolinesterasi eritrocitaria. II. Rapporti con le malattie emolitiche. Acta Medica Patavina 16:310.

68 De Sandre G, Ghiotto G 1960 An enzymic disorder in the erythrocytes of paroxysmal nocturnal haemoglobinuria: a deficiency in acetylcholinesterase activity. British Journal of Haematology 6:39.

69 Beck WS, Valentine WN 1965 Biochemical studies on leucocytes. II. Phosphatase activity in chronic lymphatic leucemia, acute leucemia and miscellaneous hematologic conditions. Journal of Laboratory and Clinical Medicine 38:245.

70 Hartmann RC, Auditore JV 1959 Paroxysmal nocturnal hemoglobinuria I. Clinical studies. American Journal of Medicine 27:389.

71 Lewis SM, Dacie JV 1965 Neutrophil (leucocyte) alkaline phosphatase in paroxysmal nocturnal haemoglobinuria. British Journal of Haematology 11:549.

72 Nicholson-Webber A, March JP, Rosenfield SI et al 1983 Affected erythrocytes of patients with paroxysmal nocturnal hemoglobinuria are deficient in the complement regulatory protein, decay accelerating factor. Proceedings of the National Academy of Sciences of the U.S.A. 80:5066.

73 Pangburn MK, Schreiber RD, Müller-Eberhard HF 1983 Deficiency of an erythrocyte membrane protein with complement regulatory activity in paroxysmal nocturnal hemoglobinuria. Proceedings of the National Academy of Sciences U.S.A. 80:5430.

74 Zalman LS, Wood LM, Frank MM et al 1987 Deficiency of the homologous restriction factor in paroxysmal nocturnal hemoglobinuria. Journal of Experimental Medicine 165:572.

75 Davies A, Simmons DL, Hale G et al 1989 CD59 and LY-6-like protein expressed in human lymphoid cells, regulates the action of the complement membrane attack complex on homologous cells. Journal of Experimental Medicine 170:637.

76 Holguin MH, Wilcox LA, Bernshaw NJ, et al 1989 Relationship between the membrane inhibitor of reactive lysis and the erythrocyte phenotypes of paroxysmal nocturnal hemoglobinuria. Journal of Clinical Investigation 84:1387.

77 Holguin MH, Fredrick NJ, Bernshaw LA, et al 1989 Isolation and characterization of a membrane protein from normal human erythrocytes that inhibits reactive lysis of the erythrocytes of paroxysmal nocturnal hemoglobinuria. Journal of Clinical Investigation 84:7.

78 Rosse WF, Hoffman S, Campbell M, et al 1991 The erythrocytes in paroxysmal nocturnal haemoglobinuria of intermediate sensitivity to complement lysis. British Journal of Haematology 79:99.

79 Shichishima T, Terasawa T, Hashimoto C, et al. 1991 Heterogenous expression of decay accelerating factor and CD59/membrane attack complex inhibition factor on paroxysmal nocturnal haemoglobinuria (PNH) erythrocytes. British Journal of Haematology 78:545.

80 May JE, Rosse WF, Frank MM 1973 Paroxysmal nocturnal hemoglobinuria: alternative-complement-pathway-mediated lysis induced by magnesium. New England Journal of Medicine 289:705.

81 Packman CH, Rosenfeld SI, Jenkins DE Jr, et al 1979 Complement lysis of human erythrocytes. Differing susceptibility of two types of paroxysmal nocturnal hemoglobinuria cells to C5b-9. Journal of Clinical Investigation 64:428.

82 Crookston JH, Crookston MC, Burnie KL, et al 1969 Hereditary erythroblastic multinuclearity associated with a positive acidified-serum test: a type of congenital dyserythropoietic anaemia. British Journal of Haematology 17:11.

83 Verwilghen RL, Lewis SM, Dacie JV 1973 HEMPAS: congenital dyserythropoietic anaemia (type II). Quarterly Journal of Medicine 42:257.

84 Hartmann RC, Jenkins DE Jr 1966 The 'sugar water' test for paroxysmal nocturnal hemoglobinuria. New England Journal of Medicine 275:155.

85 Mollison PL, Polley MJ 1964 Uptake of γ-globulin and complement by red cells exposed to serum at low ionic strength. Nature (London) 203:535.

86 Stratton F, Evans DIK 1967 Lysis of PNH cells in solutions of low ionic strength. British Journal of Haematology 13:862.

87 Hillmen P, Hows JM, Luzzatto L 1992 Two distinct patterns of glycosylphosphatidylinositol (GPI) linked protein deficiency in the red cells of patients with paroxysmal nocturnal haemoglobinuria. British Journal of Haematology 80:399.

88 Plesner T, Hansen NE, Carlsen K 1990 Estimation of PI-bound proteins on blood cells from PNH patients by quantitative flow cytometry. British Journal of Haematology 75:585.

89 van der Schoot CE, Huizinga TWJ, van't Veer-Korthof ET, et al 1990 Deficiency of glycosyl-phosphatidylinositol-linked membrane glycoproteins of leukocytes in paroxysmal nocturnal hemoglobinuria, description of a new diagnostic cytofluorometric assay. Blood 76:1853.

90 Merry AH, Rawlinson VI, Uchikawa M, et al 1989 Studies on the sensitivity to complement-mediated lysis of erythrocytes (Inab phenotype) with a deficiency of DAF (decay accelerating factor). British Journal of Haematology 73:248.

91 Merry AH, Rawlinson VI, Uchikawa M, et al 1989 Lack of abnormal sensitivity to complement-mediated lysis in erythrocytes deficient only in decay accelerating factor. Biochemical Society Transactions 17:514.

92 Telen MJ, Green AM 1989 The Inab phenotype: characterization of the membrane protein and complement regulatory defect. Blood 74:437.

93 Yamashina M, Ueda E, Kinoshita T, et al 1990 Inherited complete deficiency of 20-kilodalton homologous restriction factor (CD59) as a cause of

paroxysmal nocturnal hemoglobinuria. New England Journal of Medicine 323:1184.

94 Sirchia G, Ferrone S 1972 The laboratory substitutes of the red cell of paroxysmal nocturnal haemoglobinuria (PNH): PNH-like red cells. Series Haematologica 5:137.

95 Francis DA 1983 Production of PNH-like red cells using 2-mercaptobenzoic acid. Medical Laboratory Sciences 40:33.

96 Sirchia G, Marubini E, Mercuriali F, et al 1973 Study of two in vitro diagnostic tests for paroxysmal nocturnal haemoglobinuria. British Journal of Haematology 24:751.

97 Sirchia G, Ferrone S, Mercuriali F 1965 The action of two sulfhydryl compounds on normal human red cells. Relationship to red cells of paroxysmal nocturnal hemoglobinuria. Blood 25:502.

12

Investigation of abnormal haemoglobins and thalassaemia

Barbara J. Wild & Barbara J. Bain

THE HAEMOGLOBIN MOLECULE

Human haemoglobin is formed from two pairs of globin chains each with a haem group attached. Seven different globin chains are synthesized in normal subjects: four are transient embryonic haemoglobins referred to as Hb Gower 1, Hb Gower 2, Hb Portland 1 and Hb Portland 2. Hb F is the predominant haemoglobin of fetal life and comprises the major proportion of haemoglobin found at birth. Hb A is the major haemoglobin found in adults and children. Hb A₂ and Hb F are found in small quantities in adult life (approximately 2–3.3% and 0.2–1.0% respectively). The adult proportions of Hbs A, A₂ and F are usually attained by 6 to 12 months of age.

The individual chains synthesized in postnatal life are designated α, β, γ and δ. Hb A has two α chains and two β chains ($\alpha_2\beta_2$); Hb F has two α chains and two γ chains ($\alpha_2\gamma_2$), and Hb A₂ has two α chains and two δ chains ($\alpha_2\delta_2$). The α chain is thus common to all three types of haemoglobin molecule.

α-chain synthesis is directed by two α genes, $\alpha 1$ and $\alpha 2$, on chromosome 16, and β- and δ-chain synthesis by single β and δ genes on chromosome

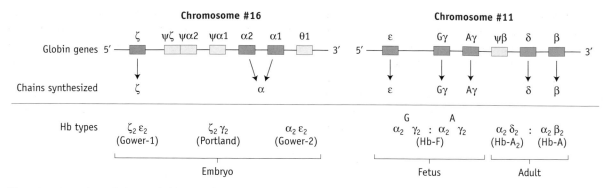

Fig. 12.1 Location of the α-globin gene cluster on chromosome 16 and that of the β-globin gene cluster on chromosome 11. The black boxes represent functional genes. The α- and γ-globin genes are duplicated; the two α-globin genes have the same product while the products of the two γ-globin genes are slightly different ($^{G}\gamma$ = γ136 Gly; $^{A}\gamma$ = γ136 Ala).

11. γ-chain synthesis is directed by two genes, $^{G}\gamma$ and $^{A}\gamma$, also on chromosome 11. The globin genes are shown diagrammatically in Figure 12.1.

The four chains are associated in the form of a tetramer: the $\alpha_1\beta_1$ (and equivalent $\alpha_2\beta_2$) contact is the strongest and involves many amino acids with many interlocking side chains; the $\alpha_1\beta_2$ (and equivalent $\alpha_2\beta_1$) contact is less extensive, and the contacts between like chains are relatively weak. The binding of a haem group into the haem pocket in each chain is vital for the oxygen-carrying capacity of the molecule and stabilizes the whole molecule. If the haem attachment is weakened, the globin chains dissociate into dimers and monomers.

There are many naturally occurring, genetically determined variants of human haemoglobin (over 750)[1] and although many are harmless, some have serious clinical effects. Collectively, the clinical syndromes resulting from disorders of haemoglobin synthesis are referred to as 'haemoglobinopathies'. They can be grouped into three main categories:

1. Those owing to structural variants of haemoglobin, such as Hb S.
2. Those owing to failure to synthesize one or more of the globin chains of haemoglobin at a normal rate, as in the thalassaemias.
3. Those owing to failure to complete the normal neonatal switch from fetal haemoglobin (Hb F) to adult haemoglobin (Hb A). These comprise a group of disorders referred to as hereditary persistence of fetal haemoglobin (HPFH).

An individual can also have a combination of more than one of these abnormalities.

STRUCTURAL VARIANTS OF HAEMOGLOBIN

Alterations in the structure of haemoglobin are usually brought about by point mutations affecting one or, in some cases, two or more bases, coding for amino acids of the globin chains. An example of such a point mutation is Hb S caused by the substitution of valine for glutamic acid in position 6 of the β-globin chain ($\beta^{6Glu\rightarrow Val}$). Less commonly, structural change is caused by shortening or lengthening of the globin chain. For example, five amino acids are deleted in the β chain of Hb Gun Hill whereas in Hb Constant Spring 31 amino acids are added to the α chain. Mutations associated with a frame shift can also lead to synthesis of a structurally abnormal haemoglobin which may be either shorter or longer than normal. There may also be combinations of segments of β and δ or γ chains resulting in hybrid haemoglobins: the β and δ combinations are known as the Lepore and anti-Lepore haemoglobins.

Many variant haemoglobins are haematologically and clinically silent, because the underlying mutation causes no alteration in the function, solubility or stability of the haemoglobin molecule. Many of these variants are separated using electrophoresis or chromatography, but some are not and remain undetected. Some structural variants are associated with severe clinical phenotypes in the homozygous or even heterozygous state; these mutations affect the physical or chemical properties of the haemoglobin molecule resulting in changes in haemoglobin solubility, stability or oxygen-binding properties. Some of these variants separate on electrophoresis or chromatography whereas others do not. Fortuitously, the common haemoglobin variants which have clinical significance or genetic significance, e.g. Hbs S, C, D^{Punjab}, E and O^{Arab} are readily detectable by electrophoretic and chromatographic techniques.

HAEMOGLOBINS WITH REDUCED SOLUBILITY

Hb S

By far the most common haemoglobin variant in this group is sickle haemoglobin or Hb S. As a result of the replacement of glutamic acid by valine in position 6 of the β chain, Hb S has poor solubility in the deoxygenated state and can polymerize within the red cells. The red cell shows a characteristic shape change because of polymer formation and becomes distorted and rigid, the so-called sickle cell (p. 89 Fig. 5.72). In addition, intracellular polymers lead to red cell membrane changes, generation of oxidant substances and abnormal adherence of red cells to vascular endothelium.

Clinical syndromes associated with common structural variants and those owing to their interaction with β thalassaemia are shown in Table 12.1.

Sickle cell disease[2]

Sickle cell disease (occasionally called disorder) is a collective name for a group of conditions causing clinical symptoms which are characterized by the formation of sickle red cells. It is common in people originating from Africa, but is also found in considerable numbers of people of Indian, Arabic and Greek descent.

The homozygous state or sickle-cell anaemia (β genotype SS) causes moderate to severe haemolytic anaemia. The main clinical disability arises from repeated episodes of vascular occlusion by sickled red cells resulting in acute crises and eventually in end-organ damage. The clinical severity of sickle-cell anaemia is extremely variable. This is partly due to the effects of inherited modifying factors, such as interaction with β thalassaemia or increased synthesis of Hb F, and partly to

Table 12.1 Clinical syndromes encountered with structural variants

Hb	Genotype	Name	Clinical problems
S	β^A/β^S	Sickle cell trait	None
	β^S/β^S	Sickle cell anaemia	Severe haemolytic anaemia, vaso-occlusive episodes
C	β^A/β^C	C trait	None
	β^C/β^C	C disease	Occasional mild anaemia
D^{Punjab}	β^A/β^D	D trait	None
	β^D/β^D	D disease	Occasional mild anaemia
O^{Arab}	$\beta^A/\beta^{O\ Arab}$	O trait	None
	$\beta^{O\ Arab}/\beta^{O\ Arab}$	O disease	Haemolytic anaemia
Interactions	β^S/β^C	SC disease	Mild anaemia, vaso-occlusive problems
	$\beta^S/\beta^{D\ Punjab}$	SD disease	As for sickle cell anaemia
	$\beta^S/\beta^{O\ Arab}$	SO disease	As for sickle cell anaemia
	β^{Othal}/β^S	Sickle-β^0 thal	As for sickle cell anaemia
	β^{+thal}/β^S	Sickle-β^+ thal	Mild sickle cell disease
	β^{thal}/β^C	C/βthal	Mild haemolytic anaemia
	β^{thal}/β^D	D/βthal	Mild haemolytic anaemia
	$\beta^{thal}/\beta^{O\ Arab}$	O/βthal	Thalassaemia intermedia

socio-economic conditions and other factors that influence general health.[2]

Sickle cell trait (β genotype AS), the heterozygous state, is very common, affecting millions of people worldwide. There are no associated haematological abnormalities. In vivo sickling occurs only at very high altitudes and at low oxygen pressures. Spontaneous haematuria, owing to sickling in the renal papillae, is found in about 1% of people with sickle cell trait.

Other forms of sickle cell disease

Sickle cell/Hb C disease is a compound heterozygous state for Hbs S and C. The abbreviation 'SC disease' is ambiguous and should be avoided; however, the term Hb SC disease is acceptable. This compound heterozygous state usually results in a milder form of sickle cell disease. *Sickle β/thalassaemia* arises as a result of inheritance of one Hb S and one β thalassaemia gene. Africans and Afro-Caribbeans with this condition are often heterozygous for a mild $β^+$ thalassaemia allele resulting in the production of about 20% of Hb A. This gives rise to a mild sickling disorder. Inheritance of Hb S and $β^0$ thalassaemia trait is associated with severe sickle-cell disease. Interaction of Hb S with haemoglobin D^{Punjab} (Hb D$^{Los Angeles}$) or with Hb O^{Arab} gives rise to severe sickle cell disease.[2]

Hb C

Hb C is the second most common structural haemoglobin variant in people of African descent. The substitution of glutamic acid in position 6 of the β chain by lysine results in a haemoglobin molecule with a highly positive charge, decreased solubility and tendency to crystallize. However, Hb C does not give a positive sickle solubility test. Heterozygotes are asymptomatic but target cells and irregularly contracted cells may be present in blood films. Homozygotes may have mild anaemia with numerous target cells and irregularly contracted cells (p. 76 Fig. 5.32). Interaction with $β^0$ and $β^+$ thalassaemia trait results in mild or moderate haemolytic anaemia.

Other sickling haemoglobins

In addition to Hb S, there are six haemoglobins (Hb S^{Antilles}, HbC^{Ziquinchor}, Hb C^{Harlem}, Hb S^{Providence}, Hb S^{Oman}, Hb S^{Travis}) which have both the β6 glutamic acid to valine mutation and an additional single point mutation in the β globin chain. These haemoglobins also have a positive solubility test since they have a reduced solubility but generally exhibit different electrophoretic and chromatographic properties from Hb S. These haemoglobins have potentially the same clinical significance as Hb S.

UNSTABLE HAEMOGLOBINS[3,4]

Amino-acid substitutions close to the haem group, or at the points of contact between globin chains, can affect protein stability and result in intracellular precipitation of globin chains. The precipitated globin chains attach to the red cell membrane giving rise to Heinz bodies and the associated clinical syndromes were originally called the *Congenital Heinz Body Haemolytic Anaemias*. Changes in membrane properties may lead to haemolysis, often aggravated by oxidant drugs. There is considerable heterogeneity in the haematological and clinical effects of unstable haemoglobins. Many are almost silent and are detected only by specific tests, whereas others are severe, causing haemolytic anaemia in the heterozygous state. Hb Köln is the most common variant in this rare group of disorders.

HAEMOGLOBINS WITH ALTERED OXYGEN AFFINITY[5]

Haemoglobin variants with altered oxygen affinity are a rare group of variants which result in increased or reduced oxygen affinity. Mutations which *increase* oxygen affinity are generally associated with benign life-long erythrocytosis. This may be confused with polycythaemia vera and inappropriately treated with cytotoxic drugs or P^{32}.

Haemoglobin variants with *decreased* oxygen affinity are even less common and are usually associated with mild anaemia and cyanosis. However, owing to the reduced oxygen affinity, these patients are not functionally anaemic despite the reduced Hb.

THE Hb Ms[6]

Hb Ms are another rare group of variants. Such haemoglobins have a propensity to form methaemoglobin, generated by the oxidation of ferrous iron in haem to ferric iron, which is incapable of binding oxygen. Despite marked cyanosis, there are few clinical problems. Most are associated with substitutions which disrupt the normal six-ligand state of haem iron.

Methaemoglobinaemia is also found in congenital NADH methaemoglobin reductase deficiency, as well as after exposure to oxidant drugs and chemicals (nitrates, nitrites, quinones, chlorates, phenacetin, dapsone and many others).

THALASSAEMIA SYNDROMES[7]

The thalassaemia syndromes are a heterogeneous group of inherited conditions characterized by defects in the synthesis of one or more of the globin chains that form the haemoglobin tetramer. The clinical syndromes associated with thalassaemia arise from the combined consequences of inadequate haemoglobin production and of unbalanced accumulation of one type of globin chain. The former causes anaemia with hypochromia and microcytosis; the latter leads to ineffective erythropoiesis and haemolysis. Clinical manifestations range from completely asymptomatic microcytosis to profound anaemia which is incompatible with life and can cause death in utero (see Table 12.2). This clinical heterogeneity arises as a result of the variable severity of the primary genetic defect in haemoglobin synthesis and the co-inheritance of modulating factors, such as the capacity to synthesize increased amounts of Hb F.

Thalassaemias are inherited as alleles of one or more of the globin genes located on either chromosome 11 (for β, γ and δ chains) or on chromosome 16 (for α chains). They are encountered in every population in the world but are most common in the Mediterranean littoral and near equatorial regions of Africa and Asia. Gene frequencies for the α- and β thalassaemias on a global basis range from 1–80% in areas where malaria is endemic.[8]

β THALASSAEMIA SYNDROMES[9]

Many different mutations cause β thalassaemia and its related disorders. These mutations can affect every step in the pathway of globin gene expression: transcription; processing of the mRNA precursor; translation of mature mRNA; and preservation of post-translational integrity of the β chain. Almost 200 mutations have been described.[10] Most types of β thalassaemia are due to point mutations affecting the globin gene, but some large deletions are also known. Certain mutations are particularly common in some communities. This helps to simplify prenatal diagnosis which is carried out by detection or exclusion of a particular mutation in fetal DNA.

The effect of different mutations varies greatly. At one end of the spectrum are a group of rare mutations, mainly involving exon 3 of the β globin gene, which are so severe that they can produce

Table 12.2 Clinical syndromes of thalassaemia

Clinically asymptomatic
Silent carriers
  α^+ thalassaemia trait (some cases)
  Rare forms of β thalassaemia trait
Thalassaemia minor (low MCH and MCV, with or without mild anaemia)
  (α^+ thalassaemia trait (some cases)
  α^0 thalassaemia trait
  α^+/α^+ homozygotes
  β^0 thalassaemia trait
  β^+ thalassaemia trait
  δ/β thalassaemia trait

Thalassaemia intermedia (transfusion independent)
Some β^+/β^+ thalassaemia homozygotes
Interaction of β^0/β^0 or β^+/β^+ with α thalassaemia
Interaction of β^0/β or β^+/β with triple α thalassaemia
Hb H disease
α^0/Hb Constant Spring thalassaemia
$\beta^0/\delta\beta$ or $\beta^+/\delta\beta$ thalassaemia compound heterozygotes
$\delta\beta/\delta\beta$ thalassaemia
Some cases of Hb E/β thalassaemia and Hb Lepore/β thalassaemia
Rare cases of heterozygotes for β thalassaemia mutation, particularly involving exon 3

Thalassaemia major (transfusion dependent)
β^0/β^0 thalassaemia
β^+/β^+ thalassaemia
β^0/β^+ thalassaemia
β^0/Hb Lepore, β^+/Hb Lepore thalassaemia
β^0/Hb E. β^+/Hb E thalassaemia

the clinical syndrome of thalassaemia intermedia in the heterozygous state. At the other end are mild alleles which produce thalassaemia intermedia in the homozygous or compound heterozygous state, and some which are so mild that they are completely haematologically silent, with normal MCV and Hb A_2 in the heterozygous state. In between are the great majority of β^+ and β^0 alleles which cause β thalassaemia major in the homozygous or compound heterozygous state, and in the heterozygous state give rise to a mild anaemia (or Hb at the low end of the normal range), with microcytic, hypochromic indices, and raised Hb A_2.[11]

β-*Thalassaemia major* is a severe, transfusion-dependent inherited anaemia. There is a profound defect of β-chain production. Excess α chains accumulate and precipitate in the red cell precursors in the bone marrow resulting in ineffective erythropoiesis. The few cells which leave the marrow are laden with precipitated α chains and are rapidly removed by the reticulo-endothelial system. The constant erythropoietic drive causes massive expansion of bone marrow and extramedullary erythropoiesis. 80% of untreated children with β thalassaemia major die within the first 5 years of life.

Heterozygotes for β thalassaemia alleles usually have a mild microcytic hypochromic anaemia with elevated Hb A_2 which may be accompanied by an elevated Hb F. Laboratory features of various β thalassaemia syndromes are shown in Table 12.3.

α THALASSAEMIA SYNDROMES[12]

There are four syndromes of α thalassaemia: α^+ thalassaemia trait where one of the two globin genes on a single chromosome fails to function, α^0 thalassaemia trait where two genes on a single chromosome fail to function, Hb H disease with three genes affected and Hb Bart's hydrops fetalis where all four are defective. These syndromes are usually due to deletions of one or more genes although approximately 20% of the mutations described are non-deletional. α^+ thalassaemia is particularly common in Africa, and α^0 thalassaemia in South-East Asia. The laboratory features are shown in Table 12.3.

Hb Bart's hydrops fetalis occurs mainly in people from South-East Asia but is also occasionally observed in people from Greece, Turkey and Cyprus. Affected fetuses are stillborn or die shortly after birth. Severe anaemia and oedema are the hallmarks of this condition. Women carrying a hydropic fetus have a high incidence of complications of pregnancy. Ideally prenatal diagnosis should be offered for women at risk of having a fetus with Hb Bart's hydrops fetalis.

Hb H disease gives rise to haemolytic anaemia; patients rarely require transfusion or splenectomy.

Table 12.3 Laboratory findings in thalassaemia

Phenotype	Genotype	Usual MCV	Usual MCH	Hb A_2	Hb H inclusions
α Thalassaemia					
α thalassaemia trait	$-\alpha/\alpha\alpha$ (α^+/α)	N	N	N or ↓	–
α thalassaemia trait	$-\alpha/-\alpha$ or $--/\alpha\alpha$ (α^+/α^+ or α^0/α)	N or ↓	N or ↓	N or ↓	+
Hb H disease:					
mild	$--/-\alpha$ (α^0/α^+)	↓	↓	N or ↓	+++
severe	$--/\alpha\alpha^T$ (α^0/α^T)	↓	↓	N or ↓	+++
Hb Bart's hydrops (α Thalassaemia major)	$--/--$ (α^0/α^0)	↓	↓	–	–
β Thalassaemia					
β thalassaemia trait	β^0/β or β^+/β	↓	↓	↑	–
δβ thalassaemia trait	$\delta\beta^0/\beta$	↓	↓	N or ↓	–
β thalassaemia trait with normal Hb A_2	β^+/β	↓	↓	N	–
Hb Lepore trait	Hb Lepore/β	↓	↓	N ↓	–
β thalassaemia intermedia	Heterogeneous	↓	↓	↑, N or ↓	–
β thalassaemia major	β^0/β^0, β^0/β^+. β^+/β^+	↓	↓	↑, N or ↓	–

α^0 thalassaemia *trait* is characterized by microcytic, hypochromic indices. The haemoglobin level may be normal or slightly reduced. α^+ *thalassaemia trait* can be completely silent with only borderline microcytosis and slightly reduced or normal MCH. Haematologically, homozygosity for α^+ thalassaemia trait resembles heterozygosity for α^0 thalassaemia trait but the genetic implications are very different. Both α^+ thalassaemia trait and α^0 thalassaemia trait are more difficult to diagnose than β thalassaemia trait because there is no characteristic elevation in Hb A_2 and Hb H bodies are frequently not demonstrated. Definitive diagnosis of the α thalassaemia traits is more reliably made with the use of DNA techniques or globin chain biosynthesis studies.

Thalassaemic structural variants

These are abnormal haemoglobins characterized by both a biosynthetic defect and an abnormal structure, such as the Lepore haemoglobins (see Table 12.4).

INCREASED Hb F IN ADULT LIFE[13]

Haemoglobin production in humans is characterized by two major switches in the haemoglobin composition of the red cells. During the first 3 months of gestation, human red cells contain embryonic haemoglobins (see p. 232), whereas during the last 6 months of gestation, red cells contain predominantly fetal haemoglobin. The major transition from fetal to adult haemoglobin synthesis occurs in the perinatal period and by the end of the first year of life red cells have a haemoglobin composition that usually remains constant throughout adult life. The major haemoglobin is then Hb A, but there are small amounts of Hb A_2 and Hb F. Only 0.2–1% of total haemoglobin in human red cells is Hb F and it is restricted to a few cells called 'F' cells. Both the number of F cells and the amount of Hb F per cell can be increased in various conditions, particularly if there is rapid bone marrow regeneration.

The general organization of human globin gene clusters is shown in Figure 12.1. The products of two γ genes differ in only one amino acid: $^G\gamma$ has glycine in position 136, whereas $^A\gamma$ has alanine. In fetal red cells, the ratio of $^G\gamma$ to $^A\gamma$ is approximately 3:1; in adult red cells, it is approximately 2:3.

In recent years, these has been much interest in the attempts to manipulate the fetal switch pharmacologically. If it were possible to reactivate Hb F synthesis reliably beyond the perinatal period, both β thalassaemia major and sickle-cell disease would be ameliorated.

Inherited abnormalities which increase Hb F concentration[13,14]

More than 50 mutations which increase Hb F synthesis have been described. They result in one of two phenotypes, hereditary persistence of Hb F (HPFH) or $\delta\beta$ thalassaemia; differentiation between these two types is not always simple but has clinical relevance. In general, HPFH has a higher percentage of Hb F and much more balanced chain synthesis. The most common, the African type of HPFH, is associated with a high concentration of

Table 12.4 Thalassaemic structural variants*

Haemoglobin	Structure	When heterozygous	When homozygous	In combination with other haemoglobinopathies
Lepore	Combination of δ and β chains owing to unequal crossover	Microcytosis, mild anaemia	Thalassaemia major or intermedia	With β thalassaemia gives thalassaemia major or intermedia
E**	$\beta^{26Glu\rightarrow Lys}$ resulting in abnormal mRNA	Microcytosis, mild anaemia	Microcytosis, mild anaemia	With β thalassaemia gives thalassaemia major or intermedia
Constant Spring	Elongated α chain owing to incorporation of 31 extra amino acids	Microcytosis, mild anaemia	Microcytosis, mild anaemia	With α^0 gives Hb H disease

* Many other thalassaemic structural variants have been described but are much rarer than the three shown in this table.

** 13–30% frequency in Cambodia, Thailand, Vietnam and some parts of China.

Hb F (15–45%), pancellular distribution of Hb F on Kleihauer staining and normal red cell indices. Mutations causing increased synthesis of Hb F are mostly deletions, but some non-deletion mutations have also been described. In contrast, subjects with δβ thalassaemia have lower levels of Hb F accompanied by microcytic, hypochromic indices. The major clinical significance of these abnormalities is their interaction with β thalassaemia and Hb S. Compound heterozygotes for either of these conditions and HPFH have much milder clinical syndromes than the homozygotes. Compound heterozygotes for either of these conditions and δβ thalassaemia have a condition much closer in severity to the homozygous states.

Increased Hb F is also found in many other haematological conditions, including congenital red cell aplasia and congenital aplastic anaemia (Blackfan–Diamond and Fanconi's anaemia respectively), in juvenile chronic myelomonocytic leukaemia (previously designated juvenile chronic myeloid leukaemia) and in some myelodysplastic syndromes. A small but significant increase in Hb F may occur in the presence of erythropoietic stress (haemolysis, bleeding, recovery from acute bone marrow failure) and in pregnancy.

INVESTIGATION OF PATIENTS WITH A SUSPECTED HAEMOGLOBINOPATHY

Investigation of persons at risk of a haemoglobinopathy encompasses the confirmation or exclusion of the presence of a structural variant and/or thalassaemia trait. If a structural haemoglobin variant is present, it is necessary to ascertain the clinical significance of the particular variant in order that the patient is appropriately managed. If it is confirmed that thalassaemia trait is present, it is not usually necessary to determine the precise genotype of the mutation since the clinical significance is usually negligible. The exception to this is an antenatal patient whose partner has also been found to have thalassaemia trait. If prenatal diagnosis is being considered, it may be necessary to undertake mutation analysis in order to accurately predict fetal risk and to facilitate prenatal diagnosis (see p. 275).

Since the inheritance of a haemoglobinopathy per se has genetic implications, it is important that genetic counselling is available for these patients.

In the majority of patients, the presence of a haemoglobinopathy can be diagnosed with sufficient accuracy for clinical purposes from knowledge of the patient's ethnic origin and clinical history (including family history) and the results of physical examination combined with relatively simple haematological tests. Initial investigations should include determination of haemoglobin concentration and red cell indices. A detailed examination of a well-stained blood film should be carried out. In some instances, a reticulocyte count and a search for red cell inclusions give valuable information. Assessment of iron status by estimation of serum iron and total iron-binding capacity and/or serum ferritin is sometimes necessary to exclude iron deficiency. Other important basic tests are haemoglobin electrophoresis or chromatography, a sickle solubility test and measurement of Hb A_2 and HbF percentage. In cases of common haemoglobin variants and classical β thalassaemia trait, accurate data from these tests will facilitate a reliable diagnosis without the need for more sophisticated investigations. However, definitive diagnosis of some thalassaemia syndromes can only be obtained using DNA technology (see pages 266 and 507). Similarly, in particular situations, haemoglobin variants will require unequivocal identification by the use of DNA technology or protein analysis by mass spectrometry. Individuals or families who require such investigation must be carefully selected on the basis of family history and on the results of the basic investigations described below. Large-scale screening programmes are increasingly being undertaken in some countries where individual case histories and the results of other laboratory tests are not usually available. The problems of such programmes are discussed on page 252.

The majority of errors occurring in the detection and identification of a haemoglobinopathy are due to either failure to obtain correct laboratory data or failure to interpret data correctly. In this chapter, a sequence of investigations is proposed based on procedures which should be available in any hospital laboratory. Automated high performance liquid chromatography (HPLC) is increasingly replacing haemoglobin electrophoresis as the initial investigative procedure in laboratories analyzing large numbers of samples. Isoelectric focusing (IEF) continues to be used selectively, mainly for neonatal screening or in specialist laboratories and is only briefly described. Investigation of globin chain synthesis was described in the 6th edition of this book.

Laboratory investigation of a suspected haemoglobinopathy should follow a defined protocol which has been devised to suit individual laboratory requirements. The data obtained from the clinical findings, blood picture and electrophoresis or HPLC will usually indicate in which direction to proceed. The investigation for a structural variant is described in the first section and that for a suspected thalassaemia syndrome in the second section of this chapter.

LABORATORY DETECTION OF HAEMOGLOBIN VARIANTS

A proposed scheme of investigation is shown in Figure 12.2 and a list of procedures given below.

1. Blood count and film examination (p. 240).
2. Collection of blood and preparation of haemolysates (p. 240).
3. Cellulose acetate electrophoresis, Tris buffer, pII 8.5 (p. 241).
4. Citrate agar or acid agarose gel electrophoresis, pH 6.2 (p. 243).
5. Automated High Performance Liquid Chromatography (p. 244).

6. Isoelectric focusing (p. 246).
7. Globin chain electrophoresis, pH 8.0 and 6.3 (p. 246).
8. Tests for Hb S (p. 250).
9. Detection of unstable haemoglobins (p. 253).
10. Detection of Hb Ms (p. 254).
11. Detection of altered affinity haemoglobins (p. 255).
12. Differentiation of common structural variants (p. 255).
13. Neonatal screening (p. 252).

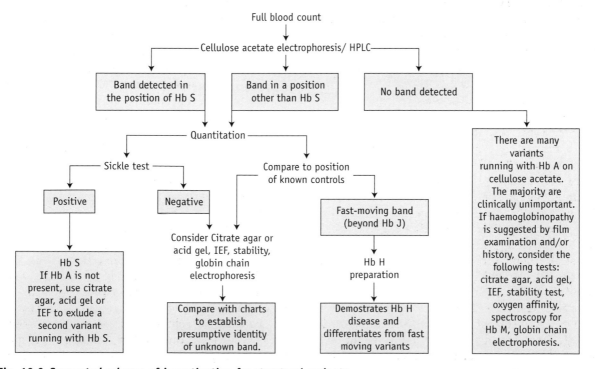

Fig. 12.2 Suggested scheme of investigation for structural variants.

BLOOD COUNT AND FILM

The blood count, including Hb and red cell indices, provides valuable information useful in the diagnosis of both α and β thalassaemia interactions with structural variants (see Ch. 3). A film examination may reveal characteristic red cell changes such as target cells in Hb C trait and sickle cells in sickle cell disease (see Ch. 5).

COLLECTION OF BLOOD AND PREPARATION OF HAEMOLYSATES

Ethylenediaminetetra-acetic acid (EDTA) is the most convenient anticoagulant as this is used for the initial full blood count and film, although samples taken into any anticoagulant are satisfactory. Cells freed from clotted blood can also be used if necessary.

Preparation of haemolysate for qualitative haemoglobin electrophoresis
See individual methods.

Preparation of haemolysate for the quantification of haemoglobins and stability tests
This can be used for qualitative electrophoresis, and is necessary for quantitation of Hb A_2 and F or variant haemoglobins by elution. It is also essential for reliable stability tests and globin electrophoresis. See individual methods for details.

Lyse 2 volumes of washed packed cells in 1 volume of distilled water then add 1 volume of carbon tetrachloride (CCl_4). Alternatively, lyse by freezing and thawing, then add 2 volumes of CCl_4. Shake the tubes vigorously for approximately 1 min, then centrifuge at $1200\,g$ (3000 rev/min) for 30 min at 4°C. Transfer the supernatant to a clean sample container and adjust the Hb to 100 ± 10 g/l with water. If an unstable Hb is suspected, organic solvents should be avoided.

Note: Whole blood samples are best stored as washed, packed cells frozen as droplets in liquid nitrogen and subsequently stored at –20°C, –70°C or over liquid nitrogen. Alternatively, haemolysates may be frozen at –20°C, –70°C or over liquid nitrogen.

CONTROL SAMPLES

Interpretation of migration patterns of test samples is undertaken by comparison to migration and separation of known abnormal haemoglobins used as control materials. Ideally, a mixture of Hbs A, F, S and C should be included on each electrophoretic separation. This material can be prepared as follows:

1. The control can be made from either the combination of a sickle cell trait (Hb A + Hb S) sample combined with a Hb C trait sample and normal cord blood (Hb F + Hb A) or the combination of normal cord blood with a sample from a person with Hb SC disease (Hb S + Hb C).
2. Prepare lysates by the method given for a purified haemolysate.
3. Mix equal volumes of the lysates together and add a few drops of 0.3 mol/l KCN (20 g/l).
4. Analyze samples by electrophoresis to assess quality.
5. Aliquot and store frozen.

Note: Repeated freezing and thawing should be avoided.

Lyophilized controls are stable for considerably longer than liquid, and can be purchased from commercial sources.

QUALITY ASSURANCE[15]

Since the haemoglobinopathies are inherited conditions, some of which carry considerable clinical and genetic implications, precise documentation and record keeping are of paramount importance. The use of cumulative records when reviewing patient's data is very useful as it of itself constitutes an aspect of quality assurance. In some situations, repeat sampling and/or family studies may be required to elucidate the nature of the abnormality in an individual.

In-house standard operating procedures should be followed carefully, particularly in this field of haematology where a small difference in technique can make a significant difference in the results obtained and can lead to misdiagnosis. Many of the techniques described have attention drawn to specific technical details which are important for ensuring valid results.

It is necessary to use reference standards and control materials in each of the analyses undertaken, and in some cases to use duplicate analysis to demonstrate precision. There are international standards for HbF and HbA_2 (see p. 607) whilst in some countries national reference preparations are also available from National Standards Institutions. These are extremely valuable since the target values have been established by collaborative studies. Control materials can be prepared in-house or obtained commercially. Samples stored as whole blood at 4°C can be used reliably for several weeks. All laboratories should confirm the normal range for their particular methods and the normal range obtained should not differ significantly from published data.

All laboratories undertaking haemoglobin analysis should participate in an appropriate proficiency testing programme. In the UK, the National External Quality Assessment Scheme (NEQAS) provides samples for detection and quantitation of variant haemoglobins as well as for quantitation of Hbs A_2, F and S.

National and international guidelines have been published for all aspects of the investigations given here.[11,16–21]

CELLULOSE ACETATE ELECTROPHORESIS AT ALKALINE pH[18,20,21]

Haemoglobin electrophoresis at pH 8.4–8.6 using cellulose acetate membrane is simple, reliable and rapid. It is satisfactory for the detection of most common clinically important haemoglobin variants.

Principle
At alkaline pH, haemoglobin is a negatively charged protein and when subjected to electrophoresis will migrate towards the anode (+). Structural variants which have a change in the charge on the surface of the molecule at alkaline pH will separate from Hb A. Haemoglobin variants which have an amino acid substitution which is internally sited may not separate and those which have an amino acid substitution which has no effect on overall charge will not separate by electrophoresis.

Equipment
Electrophoresis tank and power pack. Any horizontal electrophoresis tank which will allow a bridge gap of 7 cm. A direct current power supply capable of delivering 350 V at 50 mA is suitable for both cellulose acetate and citrate agar electrophoresis.

Wicks of filter or chromatography paper.

Blotting paper.

Applicators. These are available from most manufactures of electrophoresis equipment, but fine microcapillaries are also satisfactory.

Cellulose acetate membranes. Plastic-backed membranes (7.6 × 6.0 cm) are recommended for ease of use and storage.

Staining equipment.

Reagents

Electrophoresis buffer. Tris/EDTA/borate (TEB) pH 8.5. Tris-(hydroxymethyl)aminomethane (Tris), 10.2 g, EDTA (disodium salt), 0.6 g, boric acid, 3.2 g, water to 1 litre. The buffer should be stored at 4°C and can be used up to 10 times without deterioration.

Wetting agent, such as Zip-prep solution (Helena Laboratories). 1 drop Zip-prep in 100 ml water.

Fixative/stain solution. Ponceau S, 5 g, trichloroacetic acid, 7.5 g, water to 1 litre.

Destaining solution. 3% (v/v) acetic acid, 30 ml, water to 1 litre.

Haemolyzing reagent. 0.5% (v/v) Triton X-100 in 100 mg/l potassium cyanide.

Method

1. Centrifuge samples at 1200 *g* for 5 min. Dilute 20 µl of the packed red cells with 150 µl of the haemolyzing reagent. Mix gently and leave for at least 5 min. If purified haemolysates are used, dilute 40 µl of 10 g/dl haemolysate with 150 µl of lysing reagent.

2. *With the power supply disconnected*, prepare the electrophoresis tank by placing equal amounts of TEB buffer in each of the outer buffer compartments. Wet two chamber wicks in the buffer and place one along each divider/bridge support ensuring that they make good contact with the buffer.

3. Soak the cellulose acetate by lowering it slowly into a reservoir of buffer. Leave the cellulose acetate to soak for at least 5 min before use.

4. Fill the sample well plate with 5 µl of each diluted sample or control and cover with a

50 mm coverslip or a 'short' glass slide to prevent evaporation. Load a second sample well plate with Zip-prep solution.

5. Clean the applicator tips immediately prior to use by loading with Zip-prep solution and then applying them to a blotter.

6. Remove the cellulose acetate strip from the buffer and blot twice between two layers of clean blotting paper. Do not allow the cellulose acetate to dry.

7. Load the applicator by depressing the tips into the sample wells twice and apply this first loading onto some clean blotting paper. Reload the applicator and apply the samples to the cellulose acetate.

8. Place the cellulose acetate plates across the bridges, with the plastic side uppermost. Place two glass slides across the strip to maintain good contact. Electrophorese at 350 V for 25 min.

9. After 25 min electrophoresis, immediately transfer the cellulose acetate to Ponceau S and fix and stain for 5 min.

10. Remove excess stain by washing for 5 min in the first acetic acid reservoir and for 10 min in each of the remaining two. Blot once, using clean blotting paper and leave to dry.

11. Label the membranes and store in a protective plastic envelope.

Interpretation and comments

Figure 12.3 shows the relative electrophoretic mobilities of some common haemoglobin variants at pH 8.5 on cellulose acetate. Satisfactory separation of Hbs C, S, F, A, and J is obtained (Fig. 12.4). In general Hbs S, D and G migrate closely together as do Hbs C, E and O^{Arab}. Differentiation between these haemoglobins can be obtained by using acid agarose gels, citrate agar electrophoresis, HPLC or IEF. However, there are slight differences in mobility between Hbs S, Lepore and D^{Punjab}, and also between Hbs C and E, and optimization of the technique will facilitate detection of the difference.

All samples showing a single band in either the S or C position should be analyzed further using acid agarose or citrate agar gel electrophoresis, HPLC or IEF to exclude the possibility of a compound heterozygote such as SD, SG, CE or CO^{Arab}.

The quality of separation resulting from this procedure is affected primarily by both the

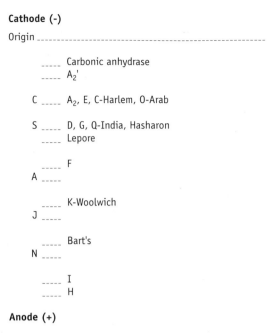

Fig. 12.3 **Schematic representation of relative mobilities of some abnormal haemoglobins.** Cellulose acetate pH 8.5.

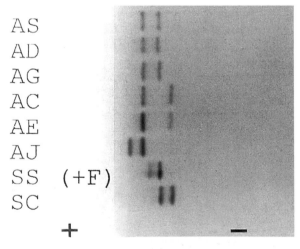

Fig. 12.4 **Relative mobilities of some abnormal haemoglobins.** Cellulose acetate pH 8.5.

amount of haemoglobin applied and the positioning of the origin. Also, delays between application of the sample and commencement of the electrophoresis, delay in staining after electrophoresis or inadequate blotting of the acetate prior to application will cause poor results. This technique is

Table 12.5 Results of laboratory investigations in interactions of Hb S and α or β thalassaemia in adults

	MCV	% S	% A	% A$_2$	% F
AS	N	35–38	62–65	<3.5	<1
SS	N	88–93	0	<3.5	5–10
S/β^0 Thalassaemia	L	88–93	0	>3.5	5–10
S/β^+ Thalassaemia	L	50–93	3–30	>3.5	1–10
S/HPFH	N	65–80	0	<3.5	20–35
AS/α^+ Thalassaemia	N/L	28–35	62–70	<3.5	<1
AS/α^0 Thalassaemia	L	20–30	68–78	<3.5	<1
SS/α Thalassaemia	N/L	88–93	0	<3.5	1–10

sensitive enough to separate Hb F from Hb A and to detect Hb A$_2$ variants.

If an abnormal haemoglobin is present, the detection of a Hb A$_2$ variant band in conjunction with the abnormal fraction is evidence that the variant is an α- chain variant. Globin electrophoresis at both acid and alkaline pH is also useful in elucidating which globin chain is affected. However, with the more ready availability of HPLC, it is less often needed.

When an abnormal haemoglobin is found, it may be of diagnostic importance to measure the percentage of the variant; this can be done by the electrophoresis with elution procedure for Hb A$_2$ estimation given on page 256. Quantitation of Hb S is often clinically useful, either in sickle-cell disease patients who are being treated by transfusion or for the conditions in which Hb S is co-inherited with α and β thalassaemia, as outlined in Table 12.5. Quantitation of Hb S can also be done by the same procedure or by microcolumn chromatography (p. 260).

CITRATE AGAR ELECTROPHORESIS AT pH 6.0[22,23]

Equipment

Electrophoresis tank and power pack. Any horizontal electrophoresis tank which will allow a bridge gap of 7 cm. A direct current power supply capable of delivering 350 V at 50 mA is suitable for both cellulose acetate and citrate agar electrophoresis.

Cooling bars (Helena Laboratories).

Perspex trays, 80 × 100 × 2 mm.

Wicks of sponge, filter paper or chromatography paper.

Applicators. These are available from most manufacturers of electrophoresis equipment, but fine microcapillaries are also satisfactory.

Reagents

Difco Bacto-agar.

Lysing reagent. 0.5% (v/v) Triton X-100 in 100 mg/l potassium cyanide.

Buffer

Stock buffer. Trisodium citrate dihydrate, 73.5 g; 0.5 mol/l citric acid, 34.0 ml; water to 1 litre.

Working buffer. Dilute stock buffer 1 in 5 with water. Prepare on day of use.

5 g/dl potassium cyanide. Potassium cyanide, 0.5 g, distilled water to 100 ml.

Dianisidine stain. 3% Hydrogen peroxide (10 vol), 1.0 ml; 1% Sodium nitroprusside (nitroferricyanide), 1.0 ml; 3% acetic acid, 10.0 ml; 0.2% o-dianisidine in methanol, 5.0 ml. Prepare mixture just before use.

Wetting agent, such as Zip-prep solution (Helena Laboratories). 1 drop in 100 ml water.

3% Acetic acid. 120 ml glacial acetic acid made up to 4 litres with water.

Gel-Bond or similar support.

Method

1. Centrifuge sample (1200 g for 5 min). Dilute 20 µl of packed red cells with 300 µl of haemolyzing reagent. Mix gently and leave for at least 5 min. For cord blood samples, dilute 20 µl of packed red cells with 150 µl of the lysing reagent. For purified haemolysates, dilute 20 µl of 10 g/dl haemolysate with 150 µl of lysing reagent.

2. *With the power supply disconnected*, place equal volumes working buffer in each of the outer buffer compartments. Wet two sponge wicks in the buffer and place one in each compartment against the divider. Place two frozen cooling sticks in each central chamber. If cooling bars or ice packs are not available, run the electrophoresis at 4°C.

3. Add 0.5 g agar to 50 ml working buffer. Heat to approximately 95°C, stirring gently until the agar has dissolved. Allow to cool to 60°C, add 0.5 ml of 5 g/dl potassium cyanide. Pipette approximately 10 ml into each of four perspex trays ($80 \times 100 \times 2$ mm) and allow to stand for about 15 min at room temperature until set. These gels may be kept for 1 week at 4°C in a sealed plastic bag. Allow gels to come to room temperature before use.

4. Fill the sample well plate with 5 µl of each sample and cover with a 6 cm coverslip or glass slide. Load a second sample well plate with Zip-prep solution. Clean the applicator tips by loading with Zip-prep solution and then applying them to blotting paper. Load the applicator and apply this first loading onto some clean blotting paper. Reload the applicator and apply the samples to the agar gel.

5. Place gel plate in an inverted position in the electrophoresis tank so that the gel is in contact with sponge wicks and run at a constant voltage of 50 V for 60 min.

6. After 60 min, disconnect from power supply, remove gel and apply the stain solution by layering onto the agar using a pasteur pipette. Allow to stain for 10 min at room temperature.

7. Wash in three changes of 3% acetic acid, float gels onto the hydrophilic side of a piece of Gel Bond and leave to dry. These mounted gels may then be kept indefinitely.

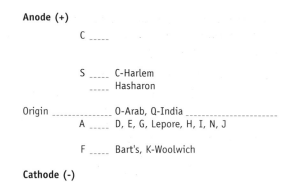

Fig. 12.5 Schematic representation of relative mobilities of some abnormal haemoglobins. Citrate agar pH 6.0.

Interpretation and comments
Figure 12.5 shows the relative electrophoretic mobilities of some common haemoglobin variants at pH 6.0 on citrate agar.

AGAROSE GEL ELECTROPHORESIS

Agarose gels are commercially available as substitutes for both alkaline and acid separation systems. They are simple to use and are useful in laboratories which process small numbers of samples.

Reagents and method
The manufacturer's method should be followed.

Interpretation
With acid agarose systems, the principle of the test is the same as that of citrate agar electrophoresis at the same pH but it should be noted that there are significant differences in mobility of some variant haemoglobins. With alkaline systems, in general the same separation patterns are obtained, but where individual application notes are available these should be used for reference. Since not all kits provide these, laboratories may need to build up their own data on known variants.

AUTOMATED HIGH PERFORMANCE LIQUID CHROMATOGRAPHY[24]

Automated cation-exchange HPLC is being used increasingly as the initial diagnostic method in haemoglobinopathy laboratories with a high workload.[25] Both capital and consumable costs are higher than with haemoglobin electrophoresis but labour costs are less, overall costs may be similar.[26] In comparison with haemoglobin electrophoresis, HPLC has four advantages:

1. The analyzers are automated and thus utilize less staff time and permit processing of large batches.
2. Very small samples (5 μl) are sufficient for analysis – this is especially useful in paediatric work.
3. Quantification of normal and variant haemoglobins is available on every sample.
4. A provisional identification of a larger proportion of variant haemoglobins can be made.

Principle

HPLC depends on the interchange of charged groups on the ion exchange material with charged groups on the haemoglobin molecule. A typical column packing is 5 μm spherical silica gel. The surface of the support is modified by carboxyl groups to have a weakly cationic charge, which allows the separation of haemoglobin molecules with different charges by ion exchange. When a haemolysate containing a mixture of haemoglobins is adsorbed onto the resin, the rate of elution of different haemoglobins is determined by the pH and ionic strength of any buffer applied to the column. With automated systems now in use, elution of the charged molecules is achieved by a continually changing salt gradient; fractions are detected as they pass through an ultraviolet/ visible light detector, and are recorded on an integrating computer system. Analysis of the area under these absorption peaks gives the percentage of the fraction detected. The rate of elution (retention time) of any normal or variant haemoglobin present is compared with that of known haemoglobins, providing quantification of both normal haemoglobins (A, F and A_2) and many variants.

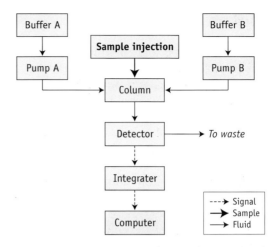

Fig. 12.6 Diagramatic representation of HPLC showing the flow of sample and buffers.

Figure 12.6 shows a schematic representation of an HPLC system and Figure 12.7 shows a chromatogram of a mixture of different haemoglobins. Systems are available from various manufacturers.

Method

The manufacturer's procedure should be followed. To prolong the life of the column it is important to follow the manufacturer's instructions with regard to the concentration of haemoglobin in the sample to be injected.

Interpretation and comments

Results are accurate and reproducible, but as with every method of haemoglobin analysis, controls should be run with every batch. If the system is being used for the detection of haemoglobin variants, elution times can be compared with those of known controls; actual times however are affected

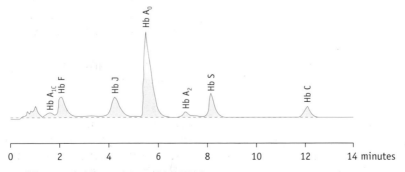

Fig. 12.7 A mixture of haemoglobins separated by HPLC.

by the batch of buffer and column, the age of the column, and the laboratory temperature. A better comparison can be obtained using the relative elution time which is calculated by dividing the elution time of the variant with that of the main Hb A fraction. It should be noted that Hb A is separated into its component fractions of A_0, A_1, and the A_1 fraction frequently subdivides into several peaks. Skill is required in interpretation of the results since various normal and abnormal haemoglobins may have the same retention time and a glycosylated variant haemoglobin will have a different retention time from the non-glycosylated form. HPLC usually separates Hbs A, A_2, F, S, C, D^{Punjab} and $G^{Philadelphia}$ from each other.[25,27] However, both Hb E and Hb Lepore co-elute with haemoglobin A_2 (as other haemoglobins co-elute with A, S and F). The retention time of glycosylated and other derivatives of Hb S can be the same as those of Hb A_0 and A_2. For these reasons, and because there are more than 750 variants identified, HPLC can never definitively identify any haemoglobin. It is important to analyze variants found using second-line techniques, such as sickle solubility, alkaline and acid electrophoresis or IEF.

HPLC is also applicable for the quantification of Hb A_{1c} for the monitoring of diabetes mellitus; in order to make optimal use of staff and equipment, this procedure is sometimes carried out in haematology laboratories.

ISOELECTRIC FOCUSING

Principle[28,29]

IEF utilizes a matrix containing carrier ampholytes of low molecular weight and varying isoelectric points (pI). These molecules migrate to their respective pIs when a current is applied, resulting in a pH gradient being formed; for haemoglobin analysis, a pH gradient of 6–8 is usually employed. Haemoglobin molecules migrate through the gel until they reach the point at which their individual pIs equal the corresponding pH on the gel. At this point, the charge on the haemoglobin is neutral, and migration ceases. The pH gradient counteracts diffusion, and the haemoglobin variant forms a discrete narrow band.

Method

Pre-prepared plates of either polyacrylamide or agarose gel can be obtained from various manufacturers. For the exact method, the manufacturer's instructions should be followed.

Interpretation and comments

IEF is satisfactory for analysis of haemolysates, whole blood samples or dried blood spots. The use of dried blood spots is suitable for samples which have to be transported long distances and where only a few drops of blood can be obtained. Whilst IEF has the advantage that it separates more variants than cellulose acetate, it also has the disadvantage that it separates haemoglobin into its post-translational derivatives. For instance, Hb F separates into F_1 (acetylated F) and F_{11}; Hb A can produce five bands (A_0, A_1, A(αmet), A(βmet) and A($\alpha\beta$met)) and similarly for other haemoglobins. This makes interpretation more difficult. Identification of variants is still only provisional using IEF and second-line methods should be used for further analysis.

Figure 12.8 shows the relative isoelectric points of some common haemoglobin variants and Figure 12.9 shows the separation obtained.

GLOBIN CHAIN ELECTROPHORESIS[30,31]

Principle

Electrophoresis of globin chains is employed to establish which chain is affected, i.e. α or β (or γ). This information is useful in further predicting the nature of the variant and possible interactions.

ALKALINE GLOBIN CHAIN ELECTROPHORESIS, pH 8.0
Reagents

Acid acetone. Add 2 ml concentrated hydrochloric acid to 98 ml of acetone which has been cooled to −20°C. The reagent should be prepared just before use.

Buffer

Stock buffer. Diethyl barbituric acid, 36.8 g, 1 mol/l sodium hydroxide solution, 120 ml. Dissolve the diethyl barbituric acid in 1500 ml of boiling distilled water. Allow to cool to room temperature and adjust pH to 8.0 with 1 mol/l NaOH. Make up to a final volume of 2 litres. Store at room temperature.

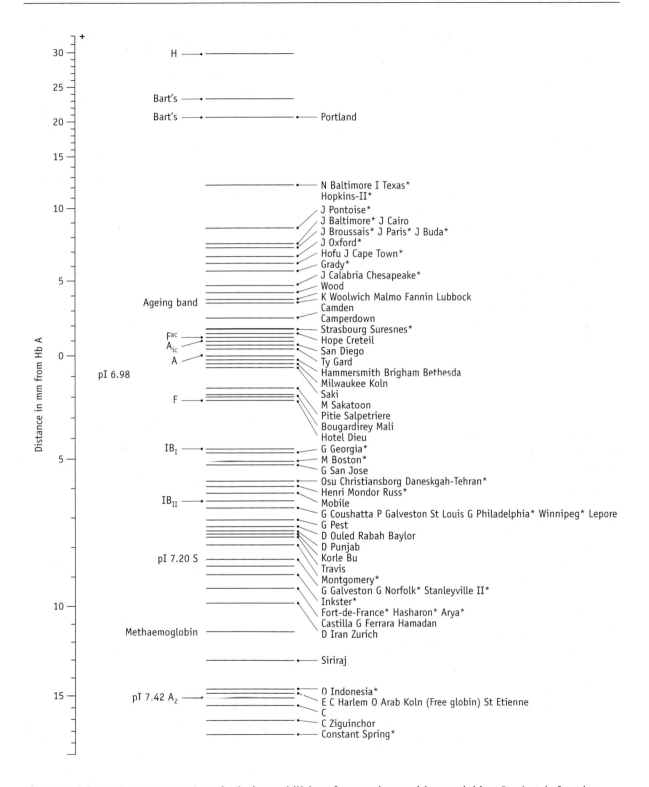

Fig. 12.8 Schematic representation of relative mobilities of some abnormal haemoglobins. Isoelectric focusing. Note the presence of two bands for haemoglobin Bart's. The scale in mm is not linear. *Indicates α-chain mutations. (Reproduced with permission from Basset et al.[29])

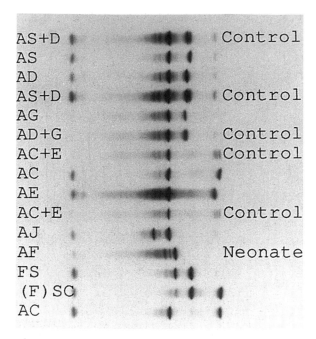

Fig. 12.9 Relative mobilities of some abnormal haemoglobins. Isoelectric focusing. The controls are mixtures of various haemoglobins.

Working buffer. Stock buffer, 600 ml, urea, 360 g, DL-dithiothreitol (DTT), 60 mg. Prepare on day of use.

Stain solvent. Glacial acetic acid, 400 ml, methanol, 1800 ml, distilled water, 1800 ml.

Amido black stain. Stain solvent, 1 litre, amido black (Naphthol black), 0.4 g.

Diethyl ether.

Equipment

Electrophoresis tank and power pack. Any horizontal electrophoresis tank which will allow a bridge gap of 7 cm. A direct current power supply capable of delivering 350 V at 50 mA is suitable for both cellulose acetate and citrate agar electrophoresis.

Wicks of filter or chromatography paper.

Blotting paper.

Applicators. These are available from most manufacturers of electrophoresis equipment, but fine microcapillaries are also satisfactory.

Cellulose acetate membranes. Plastic backed membranes (7.6 × 6.0 cm) are recommended for ease of use and storage.

Staining equipment.

Glass centrifuge tubes.

Method

1. With a whole blood sample, wash the cells twice in 9 g/l NaCl and lyse by adding an equal volume of water to the washed, packed cells. Purified haemolysates are also suitable.
2. Add 20 ml of the haemolysate to 10 ml of cold acid-acetone in a glass centrifuge tube, dispersing the haemoglobin rapidly by flushing with the pipette.
3. Centrifuge at 700 g for 10 min in a refrigerated centrifuge.
4. With a Venturi pump, remove all but a small amount of the supernatant acid acetone. Avoid contamination of the pipette by the globin pellet. Resuspend the globin pellet by means of a vortex mixer.
5. Add 10 ml of cold acetone forcefully to thoroughly disperse the globin.
6. Centrifuge at 700 g for 5 min in a refrigerated centrifuge.
7. Repeat steps 4 to 6.
8. Remove the acetone and resuspend the globin. Add 10 ml of diethyl ether and agitate forcefully to disperse the globin.
9. Centrifuge at 700 g for 5 min in a refrigerated centrifuge.
10. Dry the globin to a cream-coloured pellet by sucking air over the globin with a pasteur pipette attached to a Venturi pump. The globin can be stored at −20°C until tested. Dissolve each of the globin pellets in 200 ml of working buffer before use.
11. *With the power supply disconnected*, prepare the electrophoresis tank by placing 100 ml of working buffer in each of the outer buffer compartments. Soak two paper wicks and place one along each of the dividers.
12. Carefully lower cellulose acetate plate(s) into a reservoir of working buffer. Allow to soak for at least 1 h before use.
13. Place 5 µl of the patient and control globin samples in a sample well plate.
14. Remove the cellulose acetate from the working buffer and blot between two layers of clean blotting paper until nearly dry.

15. Load the sample applicator and apply onto clean blotting paper, reload and apply onto the cellulose acetate in the central position.
16. Place the cellulose acetate plate in the electrophoresis tank with two microscope slides across each plate to maintain contact with the wicks.
17. Electrophorese at 200 V for 1 h.
18. On completion of the electrophoresis, place the plate into the amido black stain solution and leave to fix and stain for 10 min.
19. Destain the plates in stain solvent, leaving for 5–10 min in each reservoir until the background is clear.
20. Remove the plates from the solvent and allow to dry between two clean sheets of blotting paper.

Interpretation and comments

Normal α chains migrate towards the cathode and normal β chains towards the anode. The relative migration of globins from the test samples are compared to both the known controls and the mobilities of the test samples on cellulose acetate electrophoresis. The relative mobilities of some abnormal α and β chains are shown in Figure 12.10.

ACID GLOBIN CHAIN ELECTROPHORESIS, pH 6.3
Reagents

Lysing solution. 40% w/v tetrasodium EDTA stock, 0.25 ml, 10 g/dl potassium cyanide (KCN) stock, 1.0 ml, water to 100 ml.

30% citric acid. Citric acid, 30 g, make up to 100 ml with water.

Buffers

Stock Tris-EDTA-borate (TEB) buffer, pH 8.5. Tris, 10.2 g, EDTA, 0.6 g, boric acid, 3.2 g.

TEB-Urea soaking buffer, pH 6.3. Stock TEB buffer, 138 ml, distilled water, 282 ml, urea, 216 g. Dissolve the urea in the diluted TEB buffer, then adjust the pH to 6.3 with 30% citric acid. Prepare on day of use.

TEB-Urea-merceptoethanol working buffer, pH 6.3. Stock TEB buffer, 490 ml, urea, 250 g. Dissolve the urea in the TEB buffer, then adjust the pH to 6.3 with 30% citric acid. **It is essential that TRIS-sensitive electrodes are used in the pH adjustment.** Save 2 ml of this buffer to use later as sample diluent, then add 5.6 ml of 2-mercaptoethanol to the remainder of the buffer, while stirring. Prepare on day of use.

Cathode (—)

TEB-Urea-Citrate pH 6.3	TEB-Urea pH 8.0
_____ α G-Philadelphia	
_____ α A	
	_____ α G-Philadelphia
	_____ α A
_____ α I	_____ β C
_____ β E	_____ β E, δ A$_2$
_____ β C	_____ β O-Arab
_____ δ A$_2$	_____ α I
_____ β S, O-Arab	_____ β S
_____ β D-Punjab, G-Coushatta	_____ β D-Punjab, G-Coushatta
_____ β A	
	_____ β A, γ F
_____ γ F	_____ β K-Woolwich
_____ β K-Woolwich, J-Baltimore	_____ β J-Baltimore
	_____ β N-Seattle
_____ β N-Seattle	

Origin _____ Origin

Anode (+)

Fig. 12.10 Schematic representation of relative mobilities of some globin chains.

Ponceau S (0.5% in 7.5% TCA). Ponceau S, 20 g, trichloroacetic acid, 300 ml, water to 4 litres. Store at room temperature

3% acetic acid. Glacial acetic acid, 120 ml, water to 4 litres. Store at room temperature.

9 g/l NaCl.

Equipment

Electrophoresis tank and power pack. Any horizontal electrophoresis tank which will allow a bridge gap of 7 cm. A direct current power supply capable of delivering 350 V at 50 mA is suitable for both cellulose acetate and citrate agar electrophoresis.

Wicks of filter or chromatography paper.

Blotting paper.

Applicators. These are available from most manufacturers of electrophoresis equipment, but fine microcapillaries are also satisfactory.

Cellulose acetate membranes. Plastic-backed membranes (7.6×6.0 cm) are recommended for ease of use and storage.

Staining equipment.

Method

1. Wash at least 40 μl of packed red cells twice in 9 g/l NaCl. Add 20 μl of washed, packed cells to 60 μl of lysing solution, mix gently and leave for 5 min. Transfer 20 μl of this lysate to a tube containing 20 μl of fresh TEB-urea working buffer, then add 4 ml 2-mercaptoethanol immediately before use. Purified haemolysates may also be used.

2. *With the power supply disconnected*, prepare the electrophoresis tank by placing 50 ml of TEB-urea-mercaptoethanol working buffer in each of the outer buffer compartments. Soak and position a paper wick along each divider.

3. Soak the cellulose acetate membrane plate(s) overnight in TEB-urea soaking buffer.

4. Blot the plate(s) and transfer to 600 ml of TEB-urea-mercaptoethanol working buffer. Leave to soak for between 30 min and 1 h.

5. Place 5 μl of the patient and control samples in a sample well plate.

6. Remove the cellulose acetate from the working buffer and blot between two sheets of clean blotting paper until nearly dry.

7. Load the sample applicator and apply onto clean blotting paper, reload and apply the samples onto the cellulose acetate in the central position.

8. Place the cellulose acetate plate in the electrophoresis tank with the cellulose acetate in contact with the anode and cathode wicks. Place two microscope slides onto the back of the plate to maintain contact with the wicks.

9. Electrophorese at 150 V for 2 h.

10. Prepare the staining equipment by filling the first reservoir with Ponceau S solution and three more reservoirs with 3% acetic acid.

11. On completion of the electrophoresis, place the plate into the Ponceau S stain solution and leave to fix and stain for 5 min.

12. Remove excess stain by immersing the plates into 3% acetic acid, leaving for 5–10 min in each reservoir until the background is clear. Do not agitate the plate in the acetic acid as the cellulose acetate becomes very fragile and easily peels off the backing plastic.

13. Remove the plates from the acetic acid and allow to dry between two clean sheets of blotting paper.

Results

Normal α chains migrate towards the cathode and normal β chains towards the anode. The relative migration of globins from the test samples are compared to both the known controls and the mobilities of the test samples on cellulose acetate electrophoresis. The relative mobilities of some abnormal α and β chains are shown in Figure 12.10.

TESTS FOR Hb S

Tests to detect the presence of Hb S depend on the decreased solubility of this haemoglobin at low oxygen tensions.

SICKLING IN WHOLE BLOOD

The sickling phenomenon may be demonstrated in a thin wet film of blood (sealed with a petroleum jelly/paraffin wax mixture or with nail varnish). If Hb S is present, the red cells lose their smooth, round shape and become sickled. This process may take up to 12 h in Hb S trait, whereas changes are apparent in homozygotes and compound hetero-zygotes after 1 h at 37°C. These changes can be hastened by the addition of a reducing agent such as sodium dithionite as follows:

Reagents

A. Disodium hydrogen phosphate (Na$_2$HPO$_4$). 0.114 mol/l (16.2 g/l).

B. Sodium dithionite (Na$_2$S$_2$O$_4$). 0.114 mol/l (19.85 g/l). Prepare freshly just before use.

Working solution. Mix 3 vol of A with 2 vol of B to obtain a pH of 6.8 in the resultant solution. Use immediately.

Method

Add 5 drops of the freshly prepared reagent to 1 drop of anticoagulated blood on a slide. Seal between slide and cover-glass with a petroleum jelly/paraffin wax mixture, or with nail varnish. Sickling takes place almost immediately in sickle-cell anaemia and should be obvious in sickle-cell trait within 1 h (Fig. 12.11). A positive control of Hb AS must be included.

Hb S SOLUBILITY TEST[32]

Principle

Sickle-cell haemoglobin is insoluble in the deoxy-genated state in a high molarity phosphate buffer. The crystals that form refract light and cause the solution to be turbid.

Reagents

Phosphate buffer. Anhydrous dipotassium hydro-gen phosphate, 215 g, anhydrous potassium dihy-drogen phosphate, 169 g, sodium dithionite, 5 g, saponin, 1 g, water to 1 litre.

Note: Dissolve the K$_2$HPO$_4$ in water before adding the KH$_2$PO$_4$, then add the dithionite and finally the saponin. This solution is stable for 7 days. Store refrigerated.

Method

1. Pipette 2 ml of reagent into three 12 × 75 mm test tubes.

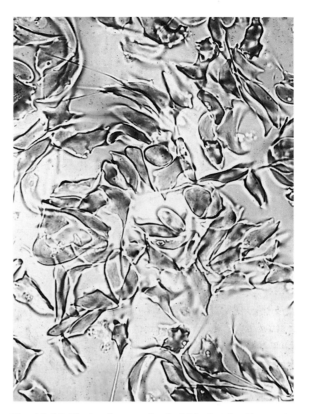

Fig. 12.11 Photomicrograph of sickled red cells. Sickle-cell anaemia. Sealed preparation of blood. Fully sickled filamentous forms predominate.

2. Allow the reagent to warm to room temperature.
3. Add 10 μl of packed cells (from EDTA-antico-agulated blood) to one tube, 10 μl of packed cells from a known sickle-cell trait subject as a positive control to the second tube and 10 μl packed cells from a normal subject as a negative control to the final tube.
4. Mix well and leave to stand for 5 min*.
5. Hold tube 2.5 cm in front of a white card with narrow black lines and read for turbidity, in comparison with the positive and negative control samples.
6. If the test appears to be positive, centrifuge at 1200 *g* for 5 min. A positive test will show a dark red band at the top while the solution below will be pink or colourless.

---

* The blood reagent mixture should be light pink or red. A light orange colour indicates that the reagent has deteriorated.

Interpretation and comments

A positive solubility or sickling test indicates the presence of Hb S and as such is useful in the differential diagnosis of Hbs D and G which migrate with Hb S.

Positive results are also obtained on samples containing the rare haemoglobins which have both the Hb S mutation and an additional mutation in the β chain. A positive solubility test merely indicates the presence of a sickling haemoglobin and does not differentiate between homozygotes, compound heterozygotes and heterozygotes. In an emergency, it may be necessary to decide if an individual suffers from sickle cell disease before the haemoglobin electrophoresis results are available. In these circumstances, if the solubility test is positive, a provisional diagnosis of sickle cell trait can be made if the red cell morphology is normal on the blood film. If the blood film shows any sickle or target cells, irrespective of the Hb, a provisional diagnosis of sickle-cell disease should be made; many patients with sickle cell/Hb C compound heterozygosity will have a normal Hb. Remember that the sickle test is likely to be negative in infants with sickle cell disease (see below).

False-positive results have been reported in severe leucocytosis, in hyperproteinaemia (such as myeloma), and in the presence of an unstable haemoglobin, especially after splenectomy. The use of packed cells, as described in this method, minimizes the problem of false-positive results caused by hyperproteinaemia and hyperlipidaemia.

False-negative results can occur in patients with a low Hb, and the use of packed cells will overcome this problem. False-negative results may also occur if old or outdated reagents are used, and if the dithionite/buffer mixture is not freshly made. They are likely to be found in infants under the age of 6 months, and in other situations, e.g. post-transfusion, when the Hb S level is under 20%.

All sickle tests, whether positive or negative, must be confirmed by electrophoresis or HPLC at the earliest opportunity.

DETECTION OF Hb S USING MONOCLONAL ANTIBODIES

Monoclonal antibodies have now been developed against several haemoglobin variants and can be used in ELISA assays; such a test for Hb S is marketed in kit form as HemoCard A plus S*. This kit contains both anti-Hb S and anti-Hb A. Thus with this test it is possible to differentiate homozygotes from heterozygotes. The antibodies are murine monoclonals that bind specifically to the amino acid at position 6 of the β chain. The antibodies are absorbed onto suspended metal sol particles, which form a red complex with their specific haemoglobin molecule. This complex binds to the reaction vessel surface and remains whilst unbound antibody is washed away. This bound complex is indicative of a positive test.

The limit of detectability for Hb S is much lower than in the solubility test; the method is therefore suitable for infants. Very low (<7.5 g/dl) and very high (>22.5 g/dl) levels of Hb may give erroneous results; the samples under test should be adjusted accordingly. Samples containing Hb E with Hb S give a false-positive result for Hb A. An equivalent kit, HemoCard C, permits the provisional diagnosis of Hb S/Hb C compound heterozygosity.

All tests, whether positive or negative, should be checked by electrophoresis or HPLC at the earliest opportunity. There have been some problems in availability and reliability of some of these kits. They may have a role in confirming the nature of a variant haemoglobin detected during adult or neonatal screening.

NEONATAL SCREENING

Cord blood or a heel-prick sample from all babies at risk of sickle-cell disease or β thalassaemia major, i.e. where the mother has a gene for Hb S, C, D^{Punjab}, E, O^{Arab}, Lepore, β or δβ thalassaemia trait should be tested. In areas where the frequency of haemoglobinopathies is high, universal neonatal screening should be undertaken where possible.

If a cord blood specimen is used, it is important that the sample is collected by venepuncture of the cleaned umbilical vein to avoid contamination with maternal blood. Small quantities of maternal

---

* Isolab Inc., Akron, Ohio, USA.

blood can cause a case of sickle cell disease to be misdiagnosed as sickle cell trait.

Umbilical cord blood samples can be examined using haemoglobin electrophoresis utilizing cellulose acetate at alkaline pH or citrate agar at acid pH.[18] Alternatively, samples can be analyzed by HPLC or IEF. If any abnormality is detected, a confirmatory technique, such as citrate agar or agarose gel electrophoresis at acid pH, should also be undertaken. If a large number of babies are to be tested or the samples are sent to the laboratory as dried blood spots on filter paper, IEF or HPLC may be the preferred technique.

Babies provisionally diagnosed as having Hbs SS, SC, SD[Punjab], SO[Arab] or Sβ thalassaemia should be retested within 6 to 8 weeks of birth. After confirmation of the diagnosis, they should be followed in a paediatric clinic, immediately started on prophylactic penicillin to prevent pneumococcal infections and appropriately managed in the long term.[3] Babies with β thalassaemia major will also be detected by the routine screening protocol; no Hb A is detected either at birth or when the babies are retested. The diagnosis of β thalassaemia trait cannot be reliably made until 12 months of age unless DNA techniques are used.

DETECTION OF AN UNSTABLE HAEMOGLOBIN[33]

Haemoglobin variants exhibit a wide variety of instability but the clinically unstable haemoglobins can be detected by both the heat stability test and the isopropanol test. However, minor degrees of instability which have little or no clinical significance may need other techniques. The unstable haemoglobins are frequently silent using electrophoretic or chromatographic techniques, and tests for haemoglobin instability are essential in the detection or exclusion of an unstable haemoglobin.

Several methods are available for the demonstration of haemoglobin instability. Samples analyzed should be as fresh as possible and certainly less than 1 week old. Controls should be of the same age as the test sample; a normal cord blood sample can be used as a positive control. The isopropanol test utilizes chemically prepared controls.

HEAT STABILITY TEST[34,35]

Principle
When haemoglobin in solution is heated, the hydrophobic van der Waals bonds are weakened and the stability of the molecule is decreased. Under controlled conditions, unstable haemoglobins precipitate while stable haemoglobins remain in solution.

Reagent
Tris-HCl buffer, pH 7.4, 0.05M. Tris, 6.05 g, water to 1 litre. Adjust the pH to 7.4 with concentrated HCl. See note on page 251 on Tris-sensitive electrodes.

Method
1. Add 0.2 ml of lysate, freshly prepared by the purified haemolysate method given on page 240, to a tube containing 1.8 ml of buffer. The negative control is obtained from a fresh normal sample.
2. Place the tubes in a water-bath at 50°C for 120 min. Examine the tubes at 60, 90 and 120 min for precipitation.

Interpretation and comments
A major unstable haemoglobin will have undergone marked precipitation at 60 min and profuse flocculation at 120 min. The normal control may show some (fine) precipitation at 60 min, but this should be minimal.

ISOPROPANOL STABILITY TEST[36]

Principle
When haemoglobin is dissolved in a solvent such as isopropanol, which is more non-polar than water, the hydrophobic van der Waals bonds are weakened and the stability of the molecule is decreased. Under controlled conditions, unstable haemoglobins precipitate while stable haemoglobins remain in solution. This method has the advantage that it does not require a 37°C water-bath, and positive controls can be made by modification of the reagent buffer.

Reagents
Tris-HCl buffer, pH 7.4, 0.1 mol/l. Tris, 12.11 g, water to 1 litre. Adjust the pH to 7.4 with

concentrated HCl. See note on p. 249 on Tris-sensitive electrodes.

Isopropanol buffer, 17%. 17 volumes of iso-propanol are made up to 100 volumes with tris-HCl buffer. The 17% isopropanol buffer solution may be stored in a tightly stoppered glass bottle for 3 months at 4°C.

Positive controls. These are buffers produced by adding small amounts of zinc to the standard 17% isopropanol buffer. For the strongest positive control, 5+, add 0.6 mmol/l zinc acetate and for the weaker positive control, 1+, add 0.1 mmol/l zinc acetate to the buffer.

Method

1. Prepare oxyhaemoglobin haemolysates from test and normal control samples as given on page 240.
2. Pipette 2.0 ml of the standard isopropanol buffer into two tubes, followed by 2.0 ml of the 1+ and 5+ control solutions respectively into two further tubes.
3. Add 0.2 ml of test sample to the first tube. Add 0.2 ml normal control sample into the three remaining tubes.
4. Place the tubes in a water-bath at 37°C for 30 min. Examine the tubes at 5, 20 and 30 min for turbidity and fine flocculation.

Interpretation and comments

A normal sample will remain clear until 30 min, when a slight cloudiness may appear. Some unstable haemoglobins will show clearly observable precipitation even after 5 min incubation, whereas milder variants will not show precipitation until 20 min.

Positive results may be given by samples containing as little as 10% Hb F or by samples containing increased methaemoglobin as a result of prolonged storage. If the normal sample undergoes premature precipitation, check the temperature of the water-bath, as it is likely to be over 37°C.

False-negative results should be avoided by continuing the incubation until the normal control undergoes precipitation.

DETECTION OF Hb Ms

Methaemoglobin (Hi) has iron present in the ferric form. Inherited variants of haemoglobin which undergo oxidation to methaemoglobin more readily than Hb A are referred to as Hb Ms. This is one of the causes of a very rare condition, congenital methaemoglobinaemia. The other cause of inherited methaemoglobinaemia is methaemoglobin reductase deficiency (see p. 164). Methaemoglobin levels vary, but may be as high as 40% of the total haemoglobin. Methaemoglobinaemia per se may also be caused by oxidant chemicals.

Methaemoglobin variants may be detected by haemoglobin electrophoresis at pH 7, but almost all can be distinguished from methaemoglobin A (Hi A) by their absorption spectra. Each methaemoglobin has its own distinct absorption spectrum. Hi A has two absorption peaks at 502 nm and 632 nm, whilst the peak absorbance for the variant Hb Ms are at different wavelengths (Fig. 12.12).

Reagent

Potassium ferricyanide, 0.1 mol/l.

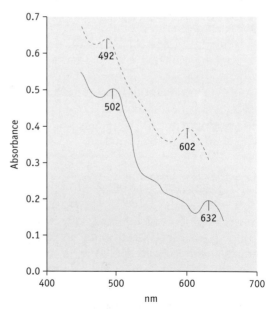

Fig. 12.12 Absorption maxima of methaemoglobins in the range 450–650 nm. —— Normal methaemoglobin; – – – – Hb M Saskatoon. (Reproduced with permission from Lehmann H, Huntsman KG, 1974 Man's haemoglobins, 2nd edn. North-Holland, Amsterdam, p 214.)

Method

1. Lyse washed red cells from a blood sample of known Hb A and of the test sample with water to give a haemoglobin concentration of about 1 g/l.
2. Convert the haemoglobin to Hi by the addition of 5 µl of potassium ferricyanide solution to each ml of haemolysate.
3. Leave for 10 min at room temperature.
4. Record the spectrum of Hi A using an automatic scanning spectrometer.
5. Compare to the spectrum of Hi in the test sample.

DETECTION OF ALTERED AFFINITY HAEMOGLOBINS

Electrophoretic and chromatographic techniques are frequently unsuccessful in separating these abnormal haemoglobins and cannot be relied upon for detection, since the amino acid substitution often does not involve a change in charge.

The most informative investigation is the measurement of the oxygen dissociation curve (p. 193). The most significant finding is a decreased Hill's constant ('n' value), since this can only come about by a change in the structure of the haemoglobin. The p_{50} may be either increased (low affinity haemoglobin) or decreased (high affinity haemoglobin). High affinity haemoglobins result in an increase in Hb level whereas low affinity haemoglobins result in a decrease in Hb level. The p_{50} alone may be affected by other factors such as the high concentration of 2,3-DPG in pyruvate kinase deficiency. Aspects of this are discussed in Chapter 10.

DIFFERENTIAL DIAGNOSIS OF COMMON HAEMOGLOBIN VARIANTS

Suggested methods are given in Table 12.6. Figure 12.13 gives a comparison of some common variants using different techniques.

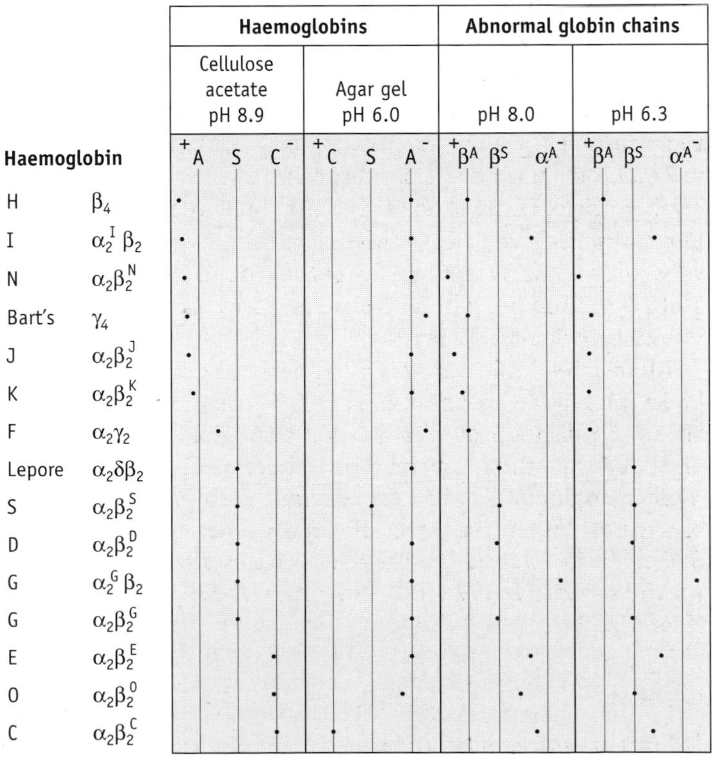

Haemoglobin		Haemoglobins Cellulose acetate pH 8.9			Haemoglobins Agar gel pH 6.0			Abnormal globin chains pH 8.0			Abnormal globin chains pH 6.3		
		$^+$A	S	C$^-$	$^+$C	S	A$^-$	$^+\beta^A$	β^S	α^{A-}	$^+\beta^A$	β^S	α^{A-}
H	β_4	•											
I	$\alpha_2^I \beta_2$	•											
N	$\alpha_2\beta_2^N$	•											
Bart's	γ_4	•											
J	$\alpha_2\beta_2^J$	•											
K	$\alpha_2\beta_2^K$	•											
F	$\alpha_2\gamma_2$		•										
Lepore	$\alpha_2\delta\beta_2$		•										
S	$\alpha_2\beta_2^S$		•										
D	$\alpha_2\beta_2^D$		•										
G	$\alpha_2^G \beta_2$		•										
G	$\alpha_2\beta_2^G$		•										
E	$\alpha_2\beta_2^E$			•									
O	$\alpha_2\beta_2^O$			•									
C	$\alpha_2\beta_2^C$			•									

Fig. 12.13 Comparison of the relative mobilities of some abnormal haemoglobins by different methods. The position of Hbs A, S and C and their corresponding chains are indicated by the vertical lines. (Adapted from ICSH[20].)

Table 12.6 Methods helpful in the differential diagnosis of common structural variants

Initial finding on cellulose acetate electrophoresis	Most likely variant	Differentiation
Band in position of Hb S	Hb S, D, G-Philadelphia, Lepore	Blood count, quantitation, solubility test, citrate agar/acid gel electrophoresis, IEF, HPLC
Band in position of Hb C	Hb C, E, O-Arab	Quantitation, citrate agar/acid gel electrophoresis, IEF
Very fast band	Hb I, H	H bodies

INVESTIGATION OF SUSPECTED THALASSAEMIA

A suggested scheme of investigations is shown in Figure 12.14 and the methods used are listed below.

1. Estimates of Hb A_2 between 3.3% and 3.8% need careful assessment and should be repeated using a second method.
2. Hb A_2 values in α thalassaemia trait are usually below 2.5%. Some types of β thalassaemia trait have normal Hb A_2 values.

METHODS FOR INVESTIGATION OF THALASSAEMIA

1. Full blood count with red cell indices.
2. Hb A_2 measurement by cellulose acetate electrophoresis with elution (p. 256).
3. Hb A_2 measurement of microcolumn chromatography (p. 258).
4. Automated High Performance Liquid Chromatography (HPLC) (p. 260).
5. Quantitation of Hb F (p. 261 or HPLC).
6. Assessment of the distribution of Hb F (p. 263).
7. Assessment of iron status (p. 265).
8. Demonstration of red cell inclusion bodies (p. 265).
9. DNA analysis (p. 266).

Blood count

The blood count, including haemoglobin and red cell indices, provides valuable information useful in the diagnosis of both α- and β thalassaemia. In classical cases, there will be an elevation in the red cell count, accompanied by a decrease in MCV and MCH.

QUANTITATION OF Hb A_2

A raised Hb A_2 level is characteristic of heterozygous β thalassaemia, and its accurate measurement is required for the diagnosis or exclusion of β thalassaemia trait. Estimations may be made by elution after cellulose acetate electrophoresis or by chromatography, either microcolumn or HPLC.

MEASUREMENT OF Hb A_2 BY ELUTION FROM CELLULOSE ACETATE[37,38]

Principle
Haemolysate is separated into its component fractions by alkaline electrophoresis on cellulose acetate membrane. The relative proportions of the separated fractions are quantitated by spectrometry of the eluates of the separated fractions.

Equipment
Electrophoresis tank and power pack. See page 241.

Wicks of double filter paper or chromatography paper.

Cellulose acetate membranes (78 × 150 mm).

Reagent
Tris-EDTA-borate (TEB) buffer, pH 8.5. Tris(hydroxymethyl) methylamine, 40.8 g; disodium disodium EDTA, 2.4 g; orthoboric acid, 12.8 g; water to 4 litres.

Method

1. Prepare a purified haemolysate from washed red cells as described on page 240. The haemolysate may be kept at 4°C for up to 1 week before analysis.

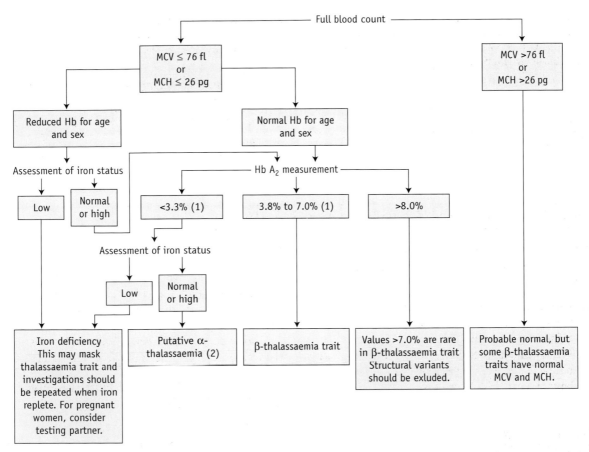

Fig. 12.14 Suggested scheme of investigation for thalassaemia.

(1) Values between 3.3% and 3.8% need careful assessment and should be repeated using a second method.
(2) A_2 values in α-thalassaemia are usually below 2.5%. some types of β-thalassamia trait have normal Hb A_2 values

2. *With the power supply disconnected*, pour equal amounts of TEB buffer into both the anode and the cathode chambers. Cut lengths of filter or chromatography paper, soak them in the buffer chamber and place them along the bridge supports as wicks. Set the bridge gap to 7 cm.

3. Soak the cellulose acetate by carefully floating the cellulose acetate sheet onto the surface of the buffer, making sure that no air bubbles are trapped underneath it. When the sheet has absorbed the buffer, submerge the sheet. Leave for at least 5 min, remove and blot carefully between two sheets of blotting paper.

4. Position the cellulose acetate across the bridge supports so that the long end of the sheet is on the anodal side. Using a ruler as a guideline, apply 30 μl of lysate to each sheet 1 cm from the cathode in a single line. Leave 1 cm margin at each end of the application line.

5. Run at a constant voltage of 250 V until separation is complete. This will take approximately 60 min and there should be at least a 1 cm gap between the A and A_2 bands at the end of the run. Check the separation at 40 min, ensuring that the Hb A (or variant such as Hb J or Hb N) does not travel onto the wicks. Check again at 5–10 min thereafter. Samples with a variant band between the A and A_2 bands will take up to 30 min longer to obtain satisfactory separation.

6. Remove the sheet, holding it carefully at the anodal wick contact; do not place on a work surface. Cut off and discard the cellulose acetate which has been in contact with the cathodal wick. Cut a 'blank' strip of approximately 2 cm wide from the cathodal end of one sheet (do

not use cellulose acetate that includes the application line). Cut out the Hb A_2 section, cutting the band into pieces approximately 1 cm square directly into a clean universal container. Cut out any variant band in the same way and finally cut out the Hb A band.

7. Add 4 ml of distilled water to both the blank and Hb A_2 containers, and 16 ml water to the Hb A container. Variant bands are usually eluted in 8 ml of water, although this may vary.

8. Mix the eluates for 20 min, and mix again by inversion just before measuring the absorbance.

9. Read the absorbance of the blank against water at 415 nm. This reading should be less than 0.005. Read the absorbances of the haemoglobin solutions at 415 nm against the cellulose acetate blank.

Calculation

$$\% \text{ Hb } A_2 = \frac{\text{Absorbance of Hb } A_2 \times 100}{\text{Absorbance of Hb } A_2 + \\ (\text{Absorbance of Hb } A \times 4)}$$

Interpretation and comments

For interpretation of results and normal ranges, see page 260. Duplicate values obtained should be within 0.2%. This method is inappropriate in the presence of Hb C, Hb E and Hb O^{Arab} since they do not separate from Hb A_2.

The procedure is useful for the measurement of haemoglobin variants – in these cases, the volume of water used for elution should be adjusted to the apparent quantity of the variant as judged on electrophoresis. Particular care must be taken when cutting strips on which a variant of haemoglobin, e.g. Hb S, is present, as the separation between Hb S and Hb A_2 is diminished.

In order to obtain accurate and precise results, use the same cuvette when reading the blank, Hb A_2 and Hb A absorbance of each sample. Read the blank, Hb A_2 and Hb A in that order to minimize the effects of carry over. Some types of cellulose acetate are unsuitable for elution – this can be detected by a very high blank reading. The haemoglobin concentration of the haemolysate is important: the absorbance reading of the haemoglobin A_2 must be at least 0.1 absorbance unit, since low values will give inaccurately low Hb A_2 results.

MEASUREMENT OF Hb A_2 BY MICROCOLUMN CHROMATOGRAPHY

Principle

Microcolumn chromatography depends on the interchange of charged groups on the ion exchange cellulose with charged groups on the haemoglobin molecule. When a mixture of haemoglobins is adsorbed onto the cellulose, a particular haemoglobin component may be eluted from the column using a buffer (developer) with a specific pH and/or ionic strength, while other components (either a single haemoglobin or a mixture of haemoglobins) may be eluted by changing the pH or ionic strength of the developer. The separation of haemoglobin components depends on the pH and/or ionic strength of the developers used for the equilibration of the column and for the elution, the type of cellulose, the volume of the sample added, the size of the column, the gradient, flow rates and temperature. The methods described below use the anion exchanger diethylaminoethyl (DEAE) cellulose (Whatman DE-52 microgranular pre-swollen), with Tris-HCl developers[39] or glycine-KCN developers.[40]

MEASUREMENT OF Hb A_2 BY MICROCOLUMN CHROMATOGRAPHY WITH TRIS-HCl BUFFERS[39]

Reagents

DE-52 ion exchange cellulose (Whatman).

Stock buffer 1.0 mol/l Tris. Tris, 121.1 g; water to 1 litre. See note on p. 249 on tris-sensitive electrodes

Working buffer 1. KCN, 200 mg; stock buffer, 100 ml; water to 2 litres; adjust to pH 8.5 with concentrated HCl.

Working buffer 2. KCN, 200 mg; stock buffer, 100 ml; water to 2 litres; adjust to pH 8.3 with concentrated HCl.

Working buffer 3. KCN, 200 mg; stock buffer, 100 ml; water to 2 litres; adjust to pH 7.0 with concentrated HCl.

Important: If the buffers are stored at 4°C, they must be allowed to come to room temperature before use.

Method

1. Prepare the slurry by adding 10 g of DE-52 to 200 ml of buffer 1. Mix gently, and allow the

cellulose to settle. Decant the supernatant and add a further 200 ml of buffer 1, mix gently for 10 min, then adjust the pH of the thoroughly suspended cellulose to 8.5 with concentrated HCl. Allow the cellulose to settle, remove the supernatant and resuspend in a further 200 ml of buffer 1. Mix gently for 10 min and ensure the pH is 8.5. Allow to settle and remove enough buffer so that the settled cellulose constitutes about half the total volume.

2. Secure short-form pipettes vertically in a support rack. Place either a 3 mm glass bead or a small piece of cotton wool in the tapered part of the pipette to act as a support for the slurry.
3. Fill the pipettes with thoroughly suspended cellulose slurry and allow the column to pack to a height of 5–6 cm.
4. Dilute 1 drop of haemolysate (100 g/l) with 5 drops of buffer 1.
5. When the excess buffer has drained from the column, gently apply the diluted lysate to the top of the column and allow it to be adsorbed onto the resin. Do not allow the surface of the column to dry out.
6. Apply 8 ml buffer 2 gently to the column with a 10–15 cm length of polythene tubing attached to the top of the pipette acting as a reservoir. Collect the elute in a 10 ml flask and make the volume up to 10 ml with buffer 2.
7. Elute the remaining Hb A, using 10 ml of buffer 3; collect the eluate and make the volume up to 25 ml with the remaining buffer 3.
8. Read the absorbance of the eluted haemoglobins at 415 nm in a spectrometer, using water as a blank.

Calculate the Hb A_2 as follows:

$$\% \ \text{Hb} \ A_2 = \frac{A^{415} \ \text{Hb} \ A_2 \times 100}{A^{415} \ \text{Hb} \ A_2 + (2.5 \times A^{415} \ \text{Hb} \ A)}$$

Interpretation and comments

For interpretation and normal ranges, see page 260. The technique is inappropriate in the presence of haemoglobin variants (see below). Factors affecting quality assurance include the concentration of haemoglobin applied to the column – excess haemoglobin will cause contamination of the Hb A_2 fraction with Hb A. An inadequate amount of haemoglobin will result in an eluate with an absorbance too low for accurate measurement.

The flow rate of the column may be adjusted by altering the height of the reservoir above the column. A flow rate of 10–20 ml/h is satisfactory. Raising the reservoir increases the flow rate but broadens the Hb A_2 band on the column which will not affect quantitation providing there is adequate separation. 8 ml of buffer 2 should be used to elute the Hb A_2 band, the greater part of which should elute between 4 and 6 ml.

MEASUREMENT OF Hb A_2 BY MICROCOLUMN CHROMATOGRAPHY WITH GLYCINE–POTASSIUM CYANIDE DEVELOPERS[40]

The method described below is suitable for samples containing variants such as Hb S. The elution of Hb A_2 is dependent on the pH of the ion exchanger and on the molarity of the developer.

Reagents

Developer A. Glycine, 15.0 g, KCN, 0.1 g, water to 1 litre.

Developer B. NaCl, 9.0 g, water to 1 litre.

DE-52 ion exchange cellulose (Whatman).

Method

1. Prepare the slurry by adding 50 g of DE-52 to 250 ml of developer. Mix gently, then allow to settle and remove the supernatant. Repeat this process at least twice, then adjust the pH of the thoroughly suspended cellulose to 7.6 with 0.1 mol/l HCl.
   If the slurry is made too acidic, it should be discarded since any attempt to readjust it would increase the total ionic concentration and therefore alter the elution pattern. The slurry may be stored for up to 3 to 4 weeks but the pH should be checked and if necessary, readjusted before use.
2. Secure short-form pipettes vertically in a support rack. Place either a 3 mm glass bead or a small piece of cotton wool in the tapered part of the pipette to act as a support for the slurry.
3. Fill the pipette with thoroughly suspended DE-52 slurry and allow the column to pack under gravity to a height of about 6 cm.
4. Check each batch of columns with a Hb AS haemolysate. The Hb A_2 should elute in the

first 3–4 ml and the Hb S in the next 15–20 ml of the developer.

5. Dilute 1 drop of lysate (100 g/l) with 6 drops of water.

6. When all the excess buffer has drained from the column, gently apply the diluted lysate to the top of the column, and allow it to be adsorbed onto the resin. Do not allow the surface of the column to dry out.

7. Apply developer A gently to the column with a piece of polythene tubing attached to the top of the pipette acting as a reservoir. About 3–4 ml of developer should be used to elute the Hb A$_2$ band. Collect the eluate in a 5 ml flask and make the volume up to 5 ml with developer A.

8. Elute the remaining Hb A, or Hb S + Hb A, using 15–20 ml of developer B; collect the eluate and make the volume up to 25 ml with developer B. If, at any stage, the flow through the column stops, it should be discarded.

9. Read the absorbance of the eluted haemoglobins at 415 nm in a spectrometer, using water as a blank.

Calculate the Hb A$_2$ as follows:

$$\% \text{ Hb A}_2 = \frac{A^{415} \text{ Hb A}_2 \times 100}{A^{415} \text{ Hb A}_2 + (5 \times A^{415} \text{ Hb A})}$$

Modification for the measurement of Hb S

To estimate the percentage of Hb S and the remaining haemoglobin as well as that of Hb A$_2$, Hb A$_2$ is eluted in the first 3–4 ml with developer A; Hb S is eluted in the next 15–20 ml of the same developer A, and the remaining haemoglobin with developer B. The eluate containing Hb A$_2$ is diluted to 5 ml and the eluates containing Hb S and the remaining haemoglobin diluted to 25 ml. To ensure elution of all the Hb A$_2$ in the first 3–4 ml, and all the Hb S in the next 15–20 ml, the pH of the ion exchanger may need adjustment following a test chromatogram.[40]

Interpretation and comments

Hb A$_2$ percentages tend to be very slightly lower using the Tris buffer system, but with either procedure there should be a distinction between normal and classical β thalassaemia trait subjects.[39] An advantage of the glycine–KCN method is less sensitivity to minor changes in the pH of the developer; also it may be used for samples containing Hb S.

It should be noted that measurement of Hb A$_2$ in the presence of Hb S is not usually a very useful test. It is not necessary in order to distinguish sickle-cell trait from sickle cell/β$^+$ thalassaemia and is not always reliable in distinguishing sickle-cell anaemia from sickle cell/β^0 thalassaemia, since there is often interaction with α thalassaemia trait. In these circumstances, family studies can be extremely helpful.

MEASUREMENT OF Hb A$_2$ BY HIGH PERFORMANCE LIQUID CHROMATOGRAPHY

The principle of HPLC has been explained on page 245. When this technology is used as the primary method for detecting variant haemoglobins, simultaneous quantitation of Hb A$_2$ and Hb F means that it can replace three separate traditional methods: haemoglobin electrophoresis, and quantitation of Hb A$_2$ and Hb F in the investigation of suspected β thalassaemia trait. Each laboratory should establish its own reference range for the quantitation of Hb A$_2$ by this method which should be similar to the published range. Because the quantitation of Hb A$_2$ may be inaccurate in the presence of certain variant haemoglobins, such as Hb E, Hb Lepore and Hb S, each chromatogram should always be inspected. If the quantity of a haemoglobin with the retention time of Hb A$_2$ is higher than expected, an alternative technique should be applied to confirm its identity, since a peak labelled as Hb A$_2$ can be Hb E or another haemoglobin which elutes with Hb A$_2$.

INTERPRETATION OF Hb A$_2$ VALUES[11,41–44]

Hb A$_2$ values should be interpreted in relation to a reference range established in each individual laboratory using blood samples from the local population with a normal Hb and red cell indices. The standard operating procedure for the relevant method should be strictly followed and 95% reference ranges should be determined. Ranges may differ slightly between methods and between laboratories. For example, in one of our laboratories the range determined for microcolumn chromatography was 2.2–3.3% whereas in another it was 2.3–3.5%. Technical variables affecting the range may include the use of packed cells rather than whole blood. Results obtained by HPLC analysis may be 0.1–0.2% higher than the results obtained by electrophoresis with elution. Once a reference range is determined, there is still a practical problem with borderline results, given that repeat estimates may vary by 0.1–0.2%. We rec-ommend that Hb A_2 levels of 3.4–3.7% be regarded as borderline and that the assay should be repeated both on the same sample and on a fresh sample. When assays are being performed for genetic counselling, it can be useful to investi-gate the partner whenever borderline results are obtained.

The Hb A_2 percentage should be interpreted with a knowledge of the Hb and red cell indices.

Hb A_2 range (%)	Interpretation
>7.0	Hb A_2 values of >7.0% are extremely rare. Exclude a structural variant. Repeat Hb A_2 estimation. Rare β thalassaemia mutations
3.8–7.0	β thalassaemia trait, unstable haemoglobin.
3.4–3.7	Severe iron deficiency in β thalassaemia trait. Additional δ-chain variant with β thalassaemia trait. (Total A_2 must be measured.) Interaction of α- and β thalassaemia. Rare β thalassaemia mutations Presence of Hb S, making accurate measurement difficult. Interaction of α thalassaemia and Hb S. Analytical error. Repeat analysis.
2.0–3.3	Normal. δβ thalassaemia (if Hb F elevated). Rare cases of β thalassaemia trait, including co-existing β- and δ thalassaemia and co-existing β and α thalassaemia. α thalassaemia trait.
<2.0	δβ thalassaemia (if Hb F elevated). α thalassaemia trait. Hb H disease. Additional δ-chain variant present (total Hb A_2 must be measured.)

QUANTITATION OF Hb F[45]

Hb F may be estimated by several methods based on its resistance to denaturation at alkaline pH, by HPLC or by an immunological method. Of the alkaline denaturation methods that of Betke et al[46] is reliable for small amounts (below 10–15%) of Hb F, whilst for levels over 50%, and in cord blood, the method of Jonxis & Visser[47] is preferable; however, this method is not reliable at levels below 10%.

Recently, immunological methods have been devised to measure Hb F by immunodiffusion[48] – there are commercially available kits* – and by enzyme-linked immunoassay (ELISA).[49]

---

* Helena Laboratories, Beaumont, Texas, USA.

MODIFIED BETKE METHOD FOR THE ESTIMATION OF Hb F[46]

Principle

To measure the percentage of Hb F in a mixture of haemoglobins, sodium hydroxide is added to a lysate and, after a set time, denaturation is stopped by adding saturated ammonium sulphate. The ammo-nium sulphate lowers the pH and precipitates the denatured haemoglobin. After filtration, the quan-tity of undenatured (unprecipitated) haemoglobin is measured. The proportion of alkali-resistant (fetal) haemoglobin is then calculated as a percentage of the total amount of haemoglobin present.

Equipment

Filter paper. Whatman no. 42.

Vortex mixer.

Glass tubes.

Reagents

Cyanide solution. Potassium cyanide, 25 mg; potassium ferricyanide, 100 mg. Dissolve in 500 ml distilled water. Store in a dark bottle.

Saturated ammonium sulphate solution. Bring 1 litre of water to the boil and add ammonium sulphate until the solution is saturated. Cool and equilibrate at 20°C before use.

1.2 mol/l Sodium hydroxide. Sodium hydroxide 4.8 g; distilled water to 100 ml. Prepare monthly. Equilibrate at 20°C before use.

Method

1. Prepare a lysate as described on page 242. The lysate may be stored at 4°C for up to 1 week before use.
2. Add 0.25 ml lysate to 4.75 ml cyanide solution to make a solution of haemiglobincyanide (HiCN).
3. Transfer 2.8 ml of the haemiglobincyanide solution to a glass test tube and allow to equilibrate at 20°C.
4. Blow in 0.2 ml of 1.2 mol/l of NaOH and mix on a vortex mixer for 2–3 s.
5. After exactly 2 min, blow in 2 ml saturated ammonium sulphate solution and mix on a vortex mixer. Leave tubes to stand for 5–10 min at 20°C.
6. Filter twice through the **same** Whatman No. 42 filter paper, using a clean test tube to collect the filtrate each time. If the filtrate is not completely clear, re-filter again through the same paper. This filtrate contains the alkali-resistant haemoglobin.
7. To measure the total haemoglobin, transfer 0.4 ml of the haemiglobincyanide solution from step 2 into another tube and add 13.9 ml of water.
8. Read the absorbance of the alkali-resistant and total haemoglobin at 420 nm against a water blank.
9. Calculate the percentage alkali-resistant haemoglobin as follows:

$$\% \text{ Alkali-resistant haemoglobin} = \frac{A^{420} \text{ alkali-resistant Hb}}{A^{420} \text{ total Hb} \times 20} \times 100$$

Interpretation and comments

Elevation of Hb F is due to a variety of causes (see p. 264). In very exceptional situations, other abnormal haemoglobins will also exhibit resistance to alkali, giving high results. It is imperative that haemoglobin electrophoresis or HPLC is done on these samples tested for Hb F to exclude the possibility of an unusual variant being present.

A normal and a raised Hb F control should be tested with every batch of samples. The raised Hb F control should ideally contain between 5 and 15% Hb F, and this can be prepared from a mixture of cord and adult blood. Each laboratory must verify its own normal range which should not differ significantly from published values; for adults the range is 0.2–1.0%.

Zago et al[50] reported variability in the capacity of different batches of filter paper to absorb haemoglobin from the filtrate which caused low results. It is necessary to equilibrate the temperature of the reagents to 20°C, and to control the reaction temperature to 20°C to obtain accurate and reproducible results.

METHOD OF JONXIS AND VISSER[47]

Principle

The increased resistance of Hb F to denaturation by alkali is detected by recording the change in absorption at 576 nm each min caused by the addition of ammonium hydroxide. At this wavelength, the absorption of oxyhaemoglobin differs from that of the alkali haemochromogen which is formed on denaturation.

When the logarithm of the percentage of haemoglobin remaining undenatured is plotted against time, a straight line is obtained. By extrapolation to time zero, the percentage of Hb F in the original sample can be calculated.

Reagents

Ammonium hydroxide solution. NH_4OH, 100 g, water to 1 litre.

Sodium hydroxide solution 0.06 mol/l. Sodium hydroxide, 2.4 g, water to 1 litre.

Method

1. All reagents should be allowed to reach room temperature before use. Add 0.1 ml of blood or lysate (100 g/l) to 10 ml of water and mix.
2. Add 2 drops of ammonium hydroxide solution and mix.
3. Measure the absorbance in a spectrophotometer at 576 nm (A_B).
4. Add 0.1 ml of the same blood or lysate to 10 ml of sodium hydroxide solution; then add 2 drops of ammonium hydroxide solution and mix thoroughly.
5. Measure the absorbance in a spectrometer at 576 nm every min for 15 min (A_T); then incubate the solution at 37°C for 15 min, cool to room temperature and measure the absorbance (A_E). The ratio A_B:A_E should be constant.
6. Calculate the percentage of undenatured haemoglobin at each min as follows:

$$\frac{A_T{}^{576} - A_E{}^{576}}{A_B{}^{576} - A_E{}^{576}} \; (\times\, 100)$$

7. Plot the percentage on the logarithmic scale of semi-logarithmic paper against time. This should produce a straight line from which the original amount of Hb F at time zero can be found by extrapolation.

Interpretation and comments

Comments regarding controls and normal ranges given for the Betke method are also applicable to this method. In addition, the Jonxis & Visser method requires an accurate spectrometer, as the maximum absorption peak at 576 nm is very narrow and the difference in extinction between oxyhaemoglobin and alkali haemochromogen is relatively small.

For interpretation of results, see page 264.

RADIAL IMMUNODIFFUSION[48]

The radial immunodiffusion (RID) procedure can be used for the quantitation of Hb F. The principle is based on an antibody–antigen reaction; the anti-Hb F is incorporated into the gel support medium resulting in the formation of a visible opaque precipitin ring.

The square of the diameter of this ring is directly proportional to the concentration of Hb F. A standard curve must be prepared from samples containing known levels of Hb F plotted against their haemoglobin concentrations. Helena Laboratories market a kit providing prepared plates, a microdispenser and a measuring device.

The RID method is simple but the formation of the precipitin rings requires at least 18 h incubation at room temperature. For this reason, rapid diagnostic work is not possible. Care must be taken with sample application as damage to the plate wells results in asymmetrical precipitin rings and erroneous measurements.

ASSESSMENT OF THE INTRACELLULAR DISTRIBUTION OF Hb F

Differences in the intracellular distribution of Hb F are used to differentiate between heterozygotes for δβ thalassaemia and the African type of HPFH. In the former, it can be shown that not all red cells contain Hb F (heterocellular distribution), whilst in the latter every cell contains Hb F (pancellular distribution), although there is some variability in content from cell to cell. It has been suggested that a heterocellular distribution may be more apparent than real and merely reflects that high levels of Hb F tend to give a more pancellular distribution than lower levels. For this reason, results should be treated with caution and not used to make a diagnosis in isolation.

Two techniques have been widely used for demonstrating intracellular Hb F distribution. The most frequently used is the acid elution test of Kleihauer[51] which was originally developed for the detection of fetal red cells in the maternal circulation following transplacental haemorrhage. This method is described on page 275. Less frequently used is the more sensitive immunofluorescent technique described below.

IMMUNOFLUORESCENT METHOD[14]

Principle

Anti-Hb F antibody binds specifically and quantitatively to Hb F in fixed red cells. These cells can be identified after treatment with a second fluorescent labelled antibody directed against the anti-Hb F.

Equipment

Glass slides.

Coplin jars.

Microscope. Equipped with accessories for UV fluorescence.

Moist chamber. Made from a Petri dish with moistened filter paper in the bottom.

Reagents

Phosphate buffered saline (PBS), pH 7.1. See page 605.

Rabbit anti-human Hb F serum. Dilute the antiserum 1 in 64 in PBS; store in small aliquots at −20°C. Stable for several months.

Sheep (or goat) anti-rabbit immunoglobulin labelled with fluorescein isothiocyanate. Dilute 1 in 32 in PBS; store in small aliquots at −20°C. Stable for several months.

Fixative. Acetone, 90 ml, methanol, 10 ml.

Method

1. Prepare thin blood films and allow to dry overnight.
2. Fix for 5 min at room temperature, shake off excess fixative and rinse immediately in PBS. If the films are too thick, they will peel off at this stage.
3. Rinse the slides in water and allow to dry.
4. Layer 5 μl of the anti-Hb F antisera onto the slide.
5. Incubate in the moist chamber at 37°C for 30 min or at room temperature for 60 min.
6. Rinse the slides thoroughly in PBS to remove any unbound antiserum.
7. Rinse the slides in water and allow to dry.
8. Layer 5 μl of the anti-rabbit antisera onto the slide.
9. Incubate in the moist chamber at 37°C for 30 min or at room temperature for 60 min.
10. Rinse the slides thoroughly in PBS to remove any unbound antiserum.
11. Rinse the slides in water and allow to dry.
12. Examine microscopically using a ×40 objective and filters suitable for use with fluorescein isothiocyanate. To quantitate the number of Hb F-containing cells, count the total number of cells in a field under white light using an eyepiece grid, then the number of stained cells under the UV light. If the level of Hb F is less than 10%, at least 2000 cells should be counted.

Comments

In normal adults, from 0.1–7.0% of cells show detectable fluorescence. The proportion of positive cells correlates well with the percentage of Hb F as measured by alkali denaturation at levels between 0.5 and 5.0%. As little as 1 pg of Hb F per cell can be detected, giving much greater sensitivity than the acid elution method. This increased sensitivity, however, may make a heterocellular distribution appear pancellular if the proportion of Hb F if greater than 10%.[45]

INTERPRETATION OF Hb F VALUES[11,14]

Hb F range (%)	Interpretation
0.2–1.0	Normal results.
1.0–5.0	In approx. 30% of β thalassaemia traits. Some heterozygotes for a variant haemoglobin. Some homozygotes for a variant haemoglobin. Some compound heterozygotes for a variant haemoglobin and β thalassaemia. Some individuals with haematological disorders (aplastic anaemia, myelodysplastic syndromes, etc.). Some pregnant women (second trimester). Sporadically in the general population, particularly in Afro-Caribbeans (representing heterozygosity for non-deletional HPFH).
5.0–20.0	Occasional cases of β thalassaemia trait. Some homozygotes for a variant haemoglobin. Some compound heterozygotes for a variant haemoglobin and β thalassaemia. Some types of heterozygous HPFH. δβ thalassaemia.
15.0–45.0	Heterozygous HPFH – African type (usually above 20%). Some cases of β thalassaemia intermedia.
>45.0	β thalassaemia major. Some cases of β thalassaemia intermedia. Neonates.
>95.0	Homozygous African type (deletional) HPFH. Some neonates (particularly if premature).

ASSESSMENT OF IRON STATUS IN THALASSAEMIA

Concurrent iron deficiency makes the diagnosis of thalassaemia trait more difficult as it masks the typical blood picture and can reduce Hb A_2 synthesis.[41,42,44] In β thalassaemia trait, dependent on the severity of the anaemia, the Hb A_2 value may be reduced to borderline, or even to normal levels (3.0–3.5%). However, in many patients with β thalassaemia trait and iron deficiency, the Hb A_2 will still be raised.

Whenever possible, individuals should not be investigated for the presence of thalassaemia trait if they are iron deficient. Iron stores are usually replete after 3 to 4 months of treatment with iron. However, if a pregnant woman is suspected of having a thalassaemia trait, it is not possible to wait for the correction of iron deficiency to establish the diagnosis. The woman and her partner should be tested without delay and globin chain synthesis or preferably DNA analysis of globin genes carried out if both are suspected of having thalassaemia trait (see Ch. 21).

In addition to traditional methods for iron assessment, such as serum iron and total iron-binding capacity and ferritin measurement, estimation of zinc protoporphyrin (ZPP) is of potential value in haematology. It can be carried out on an EDTA sample and is a measure of iron incorporation at the cellular level.

MEASUREMENT OF ZINC PROTOPORPHYRIN IN RED CELLS

Principle
Haem is formed in the developing red cell by insertion of iron into a preformed porphyrin ring.

In the event of an insufficient supply of iron, or impaired iron utilization, zinc is substituted for iron into protoporphyrin IX. The ZPP formed in the chelation process is stable and remains in the red cell throughout its life-span. Thus the level of ZPP in the red cell is a functional indicator of iron utilization at the time of cell maturation. ZPP can be measured in whole blood using a front face fluorimeter*.

Method
The manufacturer's instructions on method of use should be followed.

Interpretation and comments
Samples should be washed before analysis to remove possible contaminants such as bilirubin. Severely haemolyzed samples are not suitable for analysis.

A normal and iron-deficient control should be tested with every batch of samples and each laboratory must establish its own normal range. This method does not detect iron overload. High values are found in iron deficiency, lead poisoning and in the anaemia of chronic disorders in which iron release from the reticulo-endothelial system is blocked. However, it should be noted that although levels are higher in iron deficiency than in thalassaemia trait, some patients with thalassaemia trait have been reported to have an elevated level. A formula which relates MCV (in fl) to ZPP (in mmol/mol Hb) has been reported to discriminate correctly between iron deficiency and thalassaemia in 95% of cases.[52]

RED CELL INCLUSIONS

The most important red cell inclusions found in the haemoglobinopathies are Hb H inclusion bodies (precipitated β-chain tetramers) found in α thalassaemia,[53] β-chain inclusions found in β thalassaemia major,[7,54] and Heinz bodies found in unstable haemoglobin diseases.[35,55]

Precipitated α-chains are found in the cytoplasm of nucleated red cell precursors of patients with β thalassaemia major; they can be demonstrated by supravital staining of the bone marrow with methyl violet (as can Heinz bodies) and appear as irregularly shaped bodies close to the nucleus of normoblasts. After splenectomy they may also be found in the peripheral blood normoblasts and reticulocytes. Heinz bodies (insoluble denatured globin chains) form as a result of

* Helena Laboratories, Beaumont, Texas, USA.

exposure to oxidant drugs or chemicals, and develop spontaneously in G6PD deficiency and in the unstable haemoglobin diseases. They are usually only seen in the peripheral blood after splenectomy. When caused by the presence of an unstable haemoglobin, they may be demonstrated in the peripheral blood of patients with an intact spleen if their blood is kept at 37°C for 24–48 h. The use of methyl violet and of brilliant cresyl blue in the demonstration of precipitated α-chain and Heinz bodies is described in Chapter 13.

DEMONSTRATION OF Hb H INCLUSION BODIES

Reagent

Staining solution. 1.0% brilliant cresyl blue or New methylene blue. New batches of stain must be tested with a known positive control, as the redox action of the dyes may vary from batch to batch.

Method

1. Mix 2 vol of fresh blood (within 24 h of collection) with 1 vol of staining solution.

2. Incubate at 37°C for 2 h, or at room temperature for 4 h.
3. Resuspend the cells and spread a thin blood film.
4. Examine the film as for a reticulocyte count. The inclusion bodies appear as multiple greenish-blue dots, like the pitted pattern on a golf ball (p. 274).

They can be readily distinguished from reticulocytes which exhibit uneven reticular material.

Interpretation and comments

In α^+ thalassaemia trait, only a very occasional H body (1:1000 to 1:10 000) is usually seen; they are more numerous in α^0 thalassaemia but the number of cells developing inclusions is not reliable in differentiating the various gene deletion patterns seen in α thalassaemia and the absence of demonstrable inclusions does not preclude a diagnosis of α thalassaemia trait. This test is most useful in Hb H disease, where inclusions are usually found in more than 30% of red cells.

FETAL DIAGNOSIS OF GLOBIN GENE DISORDERS[17]

Prenatal diagnosis is carried out if the fetus is at-risk of thalassaemia major or a severe form of sickle cell disease such as sickle cell anaemia. Two approaches to fetal diagnosis are available: globin chain synthesis (used if the putative father is not available) and DNA analysis. DNA can be obtained from a chorionic villus sample or from amniotic fluid. Methods used for DNA analysis are described in Chapter 21.

When a potentially at-risk couple is detected, they will require counselling and if a fetal diagnosis is requested, it is necessary to confirm the parental haemoglobin phenotype. The family or parental blood samples are sent to the diagnostic centre and the timing of fetal sampling is arranged.

Sample requirements

Blood samples for globin chain synthesis have to be fresh (received within a few hours of collection) and transported at 4°C. Blood samples for DNA analysis can be sent by overnight delivery without refrigeration but must be processed, at the latest, within 3 days of collection. 10 ml of blood in EDTA or heparin are required from each parent. If restriction fragment length polymorphism (RFLP) linkage analysis is required, the following additional samples are needed: blood from either a homozygous normal or affected child, or from a heterozygous child and one set of grandparents, or if no child is available, blood from both sets of grandparents. The samples must be carefully and clearly labelled and the family tree drawn. Particulars of all haematological tests must be given.

Chorionic villus samples must be dissected free of any maternal tissue and sent by overnight delivery in tissue culture medium or, preferably, in a special buffer obtainable from the DNA diagnostic laboratory. Amniotic fluid samples (15–20 ml are needed) must be received within 24 h of collection. If a longer transit time is unavoidable, the amniocytes should be resuspended in tissue culture medium.

It is essential that follow-up data are obtained on all cases that have undergone fetal diagnosis. This should include tests on cord blood or heel prick sample at birth and a test at 6 months to confirm the carrier state. Whenever possible, DNA analysis of the child's globin genes should be carried out.

REFERENCES

1 Huisman THJ, Carver MFM, Efremov GD 1998 Human hemoglobin variants, 2nd edn. Sickle Cell Anemia Foundation, Augusta, Georgia.

2 Serjeant GR 1992 Sickle cell disease, 2nd edn. Oxford University Press, Oxford.

3 Dacie JV 1988 The haemolytic anaemias, vol 2: The hereditary haemolytic anaemias, 3rd edn. Churchill Livingstone, Edinburgh, part 2, p 322.

4 White JM 1974 The unstable haemoglobin disorders. Clinics in Haematology 3:333.

5 Stephens AD 1977 Annotation: Polycythaemia and high affinity haemoglobins British Journal of Haematology 36:153–159.

6 Kiese M 1974 Methemoglobinemia: A complete treatise. CRC Press, Cleveland, Ohio.

7 Weatherall DJ, Clegg JB 1981 The thalassaemia syndromes, 3rd edn. Blackwell Scientific, Oxford.

8 Flint J, Harding RM, Boyce AJ, et al 1993. In: The haemoglobinopathies. Baillière's Clinical Haematology, vol. 6. Baillière Tindall, London, p 215–262.

9 Thein SL 1993 β- thalassaemia. In: Higgs DR, Weatherall DJ (eds). The haemoglobinopathies. Baillière's Clinical Haematology, vol 6. Baillière Tindall, London, p 151.

10 Thein SL 2000 β thalassaemia. Fifth congress of the European Haematology Association. Educational Book (Ed AR Green), Birmingham, p. 132–137

11 British Committee for Standards in Haematology 1994 Guidelines for the investigation of the α and β thalassaemia traits. Journal of Clinical Pathology 47:289.

12 Higgs DR 1993 α-Thalassaemia. In: Higgs DR, Weatherall DJ (eds) The haemoglobinopathies. Baillière's Clinical Haematology, vol 6. Baillière Tindall, London, p 117.

13 Wood WG 1993 Increased Hb F in adult life. In: Higgs DR, Weatherall DJ (eds) The haemoglobinopathies. Baillière's Clinical Haematology, vol 6. Baillière Tindall, London, p 177.

14 Wood WG, Stamatoyannopoulos G, Lim G, et al 1975 F cells in the adult: normal values and levels in individuals with hereditary and acquired elevations of Hb F. Blood 46:671.

15 Stephens AD, Wild BJ 1990 Quality control in haemoglobinopathy investigations. Methods in Hematology, 22:72–85.

16 British Committee for Standards in Haematology 1988 Guidelines for haemoglobinopathy screening. Clinical and Laboratory Haematology 10:87–94.

17 British Committee for Standards in Haematology 1994 Guidelines for fetal diagnosis of globin gene disorders. Journal of Clinical Pathology 47:199.

18 International Committee for Standardization in Haematology 1988 Recommendations for neonatal screening for haemoglobinopathies. Journal of Clinical and Laboratory Haematology 10:335.

19 British Committee for Standards in Haematology Working Party of the General Haematology Task Force 1998 The laboratory diagnosis of haemoglobinopathies. British Journal of Haematology 101:783–792.

20 International Committee for Standardization in Haematology 1978 Simple electrophoretic system for presumptive identification of abnormal hemoglobins. Blood 52:1058.

21 International Committee for Standardization in Haematology 1978 Recommendations for a system for identifying abnormal hemoglobins. Blood 52:1065.

22 Schneider RG 1974 Identification of hemoglobin by electrophoresis. In: Schmidt RM, Huisman THJ, Lehmann H (eds) The detection of hemoglobinopathies. CRC Press, Cleveland, Ohio, p 11.

23 Marder VJ, Conley CL 1959 Electrophoresis of hemoglobin on agar gel. Frequency of hemoglobin D in a Negro population. Bulletin of the Johns Hopkins Hospital 105:77.

24 Schroeder WA, Skelton JB, Skelton JR 1980 Separation of hemoglobin peptides by high performance liquid chromatography HPLC. Hemoglobin 4:551.

25 Wild BJ, Stephens AD 1997 The use of automated HPLC to detect and quantitate haemoglobins. Clinical and Laboratory Haematology 19:171–176.

26 Phelan L, Bain BJ, Roper D, et al 1999 An analysis of relative costs and potential benefits of different policies for antenatal screening for β thalassaemia trait and variant haemoglobins. Journal of Clinical Pathology 52:697–700.

27 Riou J, Godart CM, Hurtrel D, et al 1997 Cation-exchange HPLC evaluated for presumptive identification of hemoglobin variants. Clinical Chemistry 43:34–39.

28 Righetti PG, Gianazza E, Bianchi-Bosisio A, et al 1986 The hemoglobinopathies: conventional isoelectric focusing and immobilized pH gradients for hemoglobin separation and identification. Methods in Hematology 15:47.

29 Bassett P, Beuzard Y, Garel MC, et al 1978 Isoelectric focusing of human hemoglobins: its

application to screening to characterization of 70 variants and to study of modified fractions of normal hemoglobins. Blood 51:971.

30 Neda S, Schneider RG 1969. Rapid identification of polypeptide chains of hemoglobin by cellulose acetate electrophoresis of hemolysates. Blood 34:230.

31 Schneider RG 1974 Differentiation of electrophoretically similar hemoglobins – such as S, D, G and P or A_2, C, E and O by electrophoresis of the globin chains. Clinical Chemistry 20:1111.

32 Evatt BL, Gibbs WN, Lewis SM, et al 1992 Fundamental diagnostic hematology: Anemia, 2nd edn. U.S. Department of Health and Human Services, Atlanta and World Health Organization, Geneva.

33 Carrell RW 1986 The hemoglobinopathies: methods of determining hemoglobin instability (unstable hemoglobins). Methods in Haematology 15:109.

34 Grimes AJ, Meisler A 1962 Possible cause of Heinz bodies in congenital Heinz body anaemia. Nature 194:190.

35 Grimes AJ, Meisler A, Dacie JV 1964 Congenital Heinz-body anaemia: further evidence on the cause of Heinz-body production in red cells. British Journal of Haematology 10:21.

36 Carrell RW, Kay R 1972 A simple method for the detection of unstable haemoglobins. British Journal of Haematology 23:615.

37 Marengo-Rowe AJ 1965 Rapid electrophoresis and quantitation of hemoglobins on cellulose acetate. Journal of Clinical Pathology 18:790.

38 International Committee for Standardization in Haematology 1978 Recommendations for selected methods for quantitative estimation of Hb A2 and for Hb A2 reference preparation. British Journal of Haematology 38:73.

39 Efremov GD, Huisman THJ, Bowman K, et al 1974 Microchromatography of hemoglobins: II A rapid method for the determination of Hb A_2. Journal of Laboratory and Clinical Medicine 83:657.

40 Huisman THJ, Schroeder WA, Brodie AR, et al 1975 Microchromatography of hemoglobins III. A simplified procedure for the determination of hemoglobin A_2. Journal of Laboratory and Clinical Medicine 86:700.

41 Kattamis C, Panayotis L, Metaxotou-Mavromati A, et al 1972 Serum iron and unsaturated iron binding capacity in β thalassaemia trait: their

relation to the levels of Hb A, A_2 and F. Medical Genetics 9:154.

42 Alperin JB, Dow PA, Peteway MB 1977 Hemoglobin A_2 levels in health and various hematological disorders. American Journal of Clinical Pathology 67:219.

43 Efremov GD 1986 The hemoglobinopathies: quantitation of hemoglobins by microchromatography. Methods in Hematology 15:72.

44 Wasi P, Na-Nakorn S, Pootrakul S, et al 1969 Alpha- and beta-thalassemia in Thailand. Annals of New York Academy of Sciences 165:60.

45 Felice AE 1986. The hemoglobinopathies: quantitation of fetal hemoglobin. Methods in Hematology 15:91.

46 Betke K, Marti HR, Schlicht L 1959 Estimation of small percentage of foetal haemoglobin. Nature 184:1877.

47 Jonxis JHP, Visser HKA 1956 Determination of low percentages of fetal hemoglobin in blood of normal children. American Journal of Diseases of Children 92:588.

48 Chudwin DS, Rucknagel DL 1974 Immunological quantification of hemoglobins F and A_2. Clinica Chimica Acta 50:413.

49 Makler MT, Pesce AJ 1980 ELISA assay for measurement of hemoglobin A and hemoglobin F. American Journal of Clinical Pathology 74:673.

50 Zago MA, Wood WG, Clegg JB, et al 1979. Genetic control of F-cells in human adults. Blood 53:977.

51 Kleihauer E 1974 Determination of fetal hemoglobin: elution technique. In: Schmidt RM, Huisman THJ, Lehmann H (eds) The detection of hemoglobinopathies. CRC Press Cleveland, Ohio, p 20.

52 Harthoon-Lasthuizen EJ, Lindemans J, Langenhuizsen MMAC 1998 Combined use of erythrocyte zinc protoporphyrin and mean corpuscular volume in differentiation of thalassemia from iron deficiency anemia. European Journal of Haematology 60:245–251.

53 Weatherall DJ 1983 The thalassemias: haematologic methods. Methods in Haematology 6:27.

54 Fessas P 1963 Inclusions of hemoglobin in erythroblasts and erythrocytes of thalassemia. Blood 21:21.

55 White JM, Dacie JV 1971 The unstable hemoglobins – molecular and clinical features. Progress in Hematology 7:69.

13

Erythrocyte and leucocyte cytochemistry – leukaemia classification

D. Swirsky & Barbara J. Bain

ERYTHROCYTE CYTOCHEMISTRY

SIDEROCYTES AND SIDEROBLASTS

Siderocytes are red cells containing granules of non-haem iron; they were originally described by Grüneberg[1] in small numbers in the blood of normal rat, mouse and human embryos, and in large numbers in mice with a congenital anaemia. The granules are formed of a water-insoluble complex of ferric iron, lipid, protein and carbohydrate. This siderotic material (or haemosiderin) reacts with potassium ferrocyanide to form a blue coloured compound, ferriferrocyanide; this reaction is the basis of a positive Prussian blue (Perls') reaction. The material also stains by Romanowsky dyes and then appears as basophilic granules which have been referred to as 'Pappenheimer bodies' (Fig. 13.1).[2] By contrast, ferritin, which is a water-soluble non-haem compound of iron with the protein apoferritin, is not detectable by Perls' reaction. Ferritin is normally present in all cells in the body, whereas in health haemosiderin is mainly found in macrophages in the bone marrow, liver (Küpffer cells) and spleen; when the body is overloaded with iron, as in haemochromatosis or transfusional haemosiderosis, excess iron is also found in other tissues.

Iron is transported in plasma attached to a β-globulin, transferrin, and passes selectively to the bone marrow, where the iron-transferrin complex binds to transferrin receptors on the surface of the erythroblast; the iron is released from transferrin and enters the cell. Most of the iron is rapidly converted to haem in the mitochondria. The non-haem residue is in the form of ferritin. Degradation of the ferritin turns some of it into haemosiderin which can be visualized under the light microscope as golden-yellow refractile particles in phagocytic cells; when stained by Perls' reaction, haemosiderin is blue.

In health, siderotic granules can normally be seen, in preparations stained by Perls' reaction, in

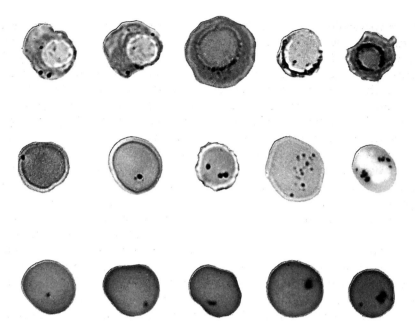

Fig 13.1 Siderotic granules and 'Pappenheimer bodies'. Photomicrographs of normoblasts and red cells stained by the acid-ferrocyanide method to show siderotic granules (top two rows) and stained by Jenner–Giemsa's stain to demonstrate 'Pappenheimer bodies' (bottom row).

the cytoplasm of many of the normoblasts of human bone marrow and in marrow reticulocytes.[3] However, they are not normally seen in human peripheral blood red cells. After splenectomy, however, siderocytes can always be found in the peripheral blood, often in large numbers. The reason for this is probably because reticulocytes, after delivery from the marrow, are normally sequestered for a time in the spleen and there complete haem synthesis and utilize, for this purpose, the iron stored in their cytoplasm within the siderotic granules. After splenectomy, this stage of reticulocyte maturation has to take place in the bloodstream, with the result that even in an otherwise healthy person a small percentage of siderocytes can then be found in the peripheral blood. The spleen is also probably able to remove large siderotic granules – as may be found in disease – from red cells by a process of pitting,[4] and in its absence such granules persist in the red cells throughout their life-span.

Method of staining siderotic granules

Air-dry films of peripheral blood or bone marrow and fix with methanol for 10–20 min. When dry, place the slides in a solution of 10 g/l potassium ferrocyanide in 0.1 mol/l HCl made by mixing equal volumes of 47 mmol/l (20 g/l) potassium ferrocyanide and 0.2 mol/l HCl immediately before use.

Leave the slides in the solution for about 10 min at c 20°C. Wash well in running tap water for 20 min, rinse thoroughly in distilled water and then counterstain with 1 g/l aqueous neutral red or eosin for 10–15 s. Care must be taken to avoid contamination by iron which may have been present on the slides or in staining dishes. Prepare the glassware by soaking in 3 mol/l HCl before washing (see p. 609). For quality control, a positive bone marrow film should always be stained together with the test films.

Prussian-blue staining can be applied to films which have previously been stained by Romanowsky dyes, even after years of storage. It is advisable to let the films stand in methanol overnight to remove most of the Romanowsky stain. The film can be checked, before carrying out Perls' reaction, to ensure that there is no residual blue staining that could obscure Prussian-blue staining. Sundberg & Bromann described a technique whereby films were stained first by a Romanowsky dye (Wright's stain) and then overstained by the acid-ferrocyanide method.[5] This can give beautiful pictures but the small blue-stained iron-containing granules tend to be masked in young erythroblasts by the general basophilia of the cell cytoplasm. Hayhoe & Quaglino described a method for combined PAS and iron staining.[6] This may be helpful in the investigation of abnormal erythropoiesis where the erythroblasts give a positive periodic acid-schiff (PAS) reaction (see p. 282). A rapid method has been described for demonstrating siderotic granules by staining with 1% bromochlorphenol blue for 1 min.[7] Iron-containing granules stain dark purple.

Significance of siderocytes

Siderocytes contain one or two (rarely many) small iron-containing unevenly distributed granules which stain a Prussian-blue colour. In about 40% of polychromatic erythroblasts there are normally a few very small scattered siderotic granules.[3] They stain faintly and may be difficult to see by light microscopy. The percentage of erythroblasts recognizable as sideroblasts is increased in haemolytic anaemias and megaloblastic anaemias and in haemochromatosis and haemosiderosis, in proportion to the degree of saturation of transferrin, i.e. to the amount of iron available. A disproportionate increase in the percentage of erythroblasts that are sideroblasts occurs when the synthesis of haemoglobin is impaired, in which case the siderotic granules are both more numerous and larger than normal (Fig. 13.2). When there is a defect in haem synthesis, the granules are deposited in mitochondria and frequently appear to be arranged in a collar around the nucleus (Fig. 13.3) giving the 'ring sideroblasts' characteristic of sideroblastic anaemias. In contrast, the distribution of the granules within the cell tends to be mainly normal in conditions in which globin synthesis alone is affected, e.g. in thalassaemia, or when there is iron overload.

There are several types of sideroblastic anaemia. These include the congenital (hereditary) type, pyridoxine (vitamin B_6) deficiency (rarely), sideroblastic anaemia caused by B_6 antagonists, e.g. drugs used in anti-tuberculosis therapy, and secondary sideroblastic anaemia in alcoholism and lead poisoning. The presence of ring sideroblasts is a defining feature of refractory anaemia with ring sideroblasts (also known as primary acquired sideroblastic anaemia) which is one of the myelodysplastic syndromes.[8] Ring sideroblasts are not uncommon in other haematological neoplasms including other myelodysplastic syndromes, idiopathic myelosclerosis and acute myeloid leukaemia (AML), particularly erythroleukaemia (FAB category M6 AML) and the WHO categories of

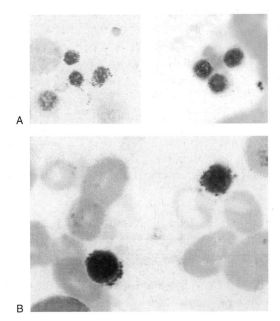

A

B

Fig 13.3 Pathological sideroblasts. Sideroblastic anaemias. Accumulation of iron-containing granules in normoblasts, arranged characteristically around the nucleus. (A) Hereditary type; (B) myelodysplastic syndrome. Perls' reaction.

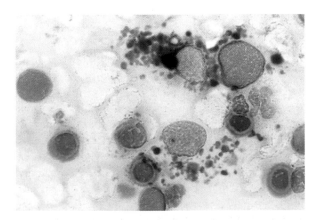

Fig 13.2 Pathological sideroblasts. Thalassaemia. There is massive accumulation of iron-containing granules in normoblasts and phagocytic cells. Perls' reaction.

therapy-related AML and AML with trilineage myelodysplasia.

In sideroblastic anaemia as a feature of a haematological neoplasm, erythroblasts at all stages of maturity may be loaded with siderotic granules whereas in the secondary sideroblastic anaemias and in the hereditary types, the more mature cells seem most affected.

In addition to the siderotic granules within erythroblasts, haemosiderin can normally be seen in marrow films as accumulations of small granules, lying free or in macrophages in marrow fragments.[9] The amount of haemosiderin will be markedly increased in patients with increased iron stores whereas haemosiderin is absent in iron-deficiency anaemia (Fig. 13.4). In chronic infections, and in other examples of 'anaemia of chronic disease', the iron stores may be increased, with much siderotic material in macrophages but little or none visible in erythroblasts. Markedly

excessive iron in macrophages is also a feature of thalassaemia intermedia and major and some dyserythropoietic anaemias. Conversely, absence of iron is diagnostic of iron depletion or deficiency and may be found before anaemia becomes evident. In practice, staining to demonstrate iron stores in marrow fragments and siderotic granules in erythroblasts is a simple and valuable diagnostic procedure and should be applied to marrow films as a routine.

There is no cytochemical method of demonstrating ferritin. Methods of assay are described in Chapter 7.

HAEMOGLOBIN DERIVATIVES

HEINZ BODIES IN RED CELLS

Heinz, in 1890, was the first to describe in detail inclusions in red cells developing as the result of the action of acetylphenylhydrazine on the

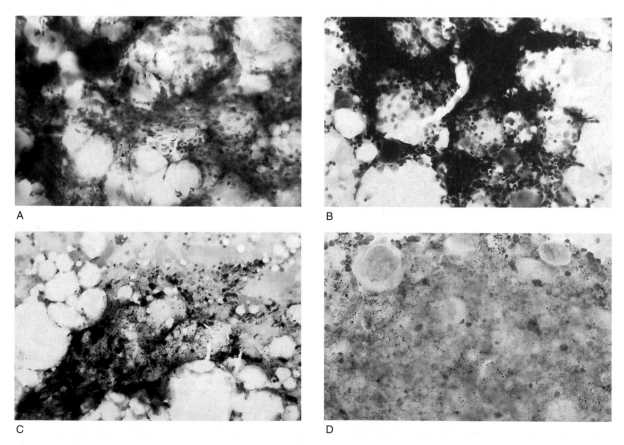

Fig 13.4 Prussian-blue staining (Perls' reaction) on aspirated bone marrow particles to demonstrate iron stores.
(A) normal, (B) absent, (C) increased, (D) grossly increased.

blood.[10] It is now known that 'Heinz' bodies can be produced by the action on red cells of a wide range of aromatic nitro- and amino-compounds, as well as by inorganic oxidizing agents such as potassium chlorate. They also occur when one or other of the globin chains of haemoglobin is unstable. In man, the finding of Heinz bodies is a sign of either chemical poisoning, drug intoxication, glucose-6-phosphate dehydrogenase (G6PD) deficiency or the presence of an unstable haemoglobin, e.g. Hb Köln. When of chemical or drug origin, Heinz bodies are likely to be visible in red cells only if the patient has been splenectomized previously or when massive doses of the chemical or drug have been taken. When owing to an unstable haemoglobin they are rarely visible in freshly withdrawn red cells except after splenectomy. They may nevertheless develop in vitro in pre-splenectomy blood if it is incubated for 24–48 h.[11] Heinz bodies are a late sign of oxidative damage, and represent an end-product of the degradation of haemoglobin. Reviews dealing with Heinz bodies include those by Jacob[12] and by White.[13]

DEMONSTRATION OF HEINZ BODIES
Unstained preparations
Heinz bodies may be seen as refractile objects in dry unstained films, if the illumination is cut down by lowering the microscope condenser, and they can be seen by dark-ground illumination or phase-contrast microscopy. However, it is preferable to look for them in stained preparations (see below). In size they vary from 1 to 3 μm. One or more may be present in a single cell. They are usually close to the cell membrane and may cause a protrusion of the membrane; in wet preparations, they may move around within the cells in a slow Brownian movement.

The degradation product of an unstable haemoglobin, e.g. haemoglobin Köln, exhibits green fluorescence when excited by blue light at 370 nm in a fluorescence microscope.[14]

Stained preparations
Methyl violet stains Heinz bodies excellently.

Dissolve c 0.5 g of methyl violet in 100 ml of 9 g/l NaCl and filter. Add 1 volume of blood (in any anticoagulant) to 4 volumes of the methyl violet solution and allow the suspension to stand for c 10 min at room temperature. Then prepare

films and allow them to dry or view the suspension of cells between slide and cover-glass. The Heinz bodies stain an intense purple (Figs 13.5, 13.6).

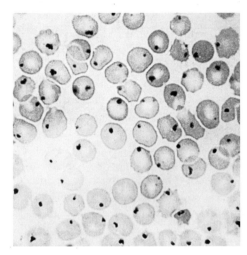

Fig 13.5 Unstable haemoglobin disease. Hb Köln (after splenectomy). Many of the cells contain large Heinz bodies. Stained supravitally by methyl violet.

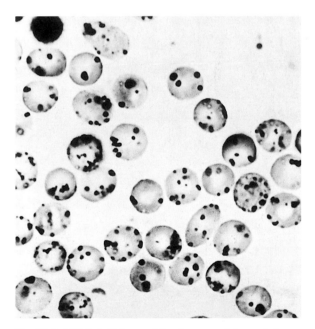

Fig 13.6 G6PD deficiency. Blood exposed to acetyl phenylhydrazine. The majority of the cells contain several Heinz bodies. Stained supravitally by methyl violet. (Reproduced with kind permission from Beutler E, Dern RJ, Alving AS 1955 The hemolytic effects of primaquine. VI. An in vitro test for sensitivity of erythrocytes to primaquine. Journal of Laboratory and Clinical Medicine 45:40.)

Heinz bodies also stain with other basic dyes. Brilliant green stains them well and none of the stain is taken up by the remainder of the red cell.[15] Rhodanile blue (5 g/l solution in 10 g/l NaCl) stains them rapidly,[16] i.e. within 2 min, at which time reticulocytes are only weakly stained. Compared with methyl violet, Heinz bodies stain less intensely with brilliant cresyl blue or New methylene blue. Nevertheless, they may be readily seen as pale blue bodies in a well-stained reticulocyte preparation, if the preparation is not counterstained.

If permanent preparations are required, fix the vitally stained films by exposure to formalin vapour for 5–10 min. Then counterstain the fixed films with 1 g/l eosin or neutral red, after thoroughly washing in water. If films are fixed in methanol, Heinz bodies are decolourized.

In β-thalassaemia major, methyl violet staining of the bone marrow will demonstrate precipitated α chains. These appear as large irregular inclusions in late normoblasts, usually single and closely adhering to the nucleus. If such patients are splenectomized, inclusions are also found in reticulocytes and mature red blood cells.

DEMONSTRATION OF HAEMOGLOBIN H INCLUSIONS

Patients with α-thalassaemia, who form haemoglobin H (β₄), have red cells in which multiple blue-green spherical inclusions develop on exposure to brilliant cresyl blue or New methylene blue as in reticulocyte preparations[17] (Fig. 13.7). This is mainly a feature of haemoglobin H disease but small numbers of similar cells may be seen in α thalassaemia trait, particularly, but not only, α⁰ thalassaemia trait.

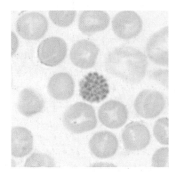

Fig 13.7 Denaturation of Hb H by brilliant cresyl blue. The round bodies consist of precipitated Hb H.

Method

Mix together in a small tube as for staining reticulocytes (p. 27) equal volumes of fresh blood or blood collected into EDTA and 10 g/l brilliant cresyl blue or 20 g/l New methylene blue in iso-osmotic phosphate buffer pH 7.4. Leave the preparation at 37°C for 1–3 h, and make films at intervals during this time. Allow the films to dry and examine without counterstaining. Haemoglobin H precipitates as multiple pale-staining greenish-blue, almost spherical, bodies of varying size (Fig. 13.8) which can be clearly differentiated from the darker-staining reticulofilamentous material of reticulocytes (Fig. 13.9).

The number of cells containing inclusions varies according to the type of α-thalassaemia. In α⁰-thalassaemia trait only 0.01–1% of the red cells contain inclusions, but this finding provides a significant clue to diagnosis. In haemoglobin H disease (e.g. resulting from α⁰-thalassaemia/α⁺-thalassaemia compound heterozygosity, --/-α), as a rule at least 10% of the cells develop inclusions and, in some cases, the percentage is considerably greater.

When few cells are affected, they will be easier to detect in an enriched preparation.[18] Fill 2 to 3 capillary tubes with the blood and centrifuge for 5 min in a microhaematocrit centrifuge. Then score the tubes just below the buffy coat layer and also *c* 1 cm further down; break them at the score marks and carefully transfer the broken-off

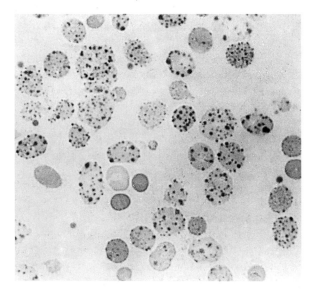

Fig 13.8 Hb H disease. Almost every erythrocyte is affected. Compare with Figure 13.9.

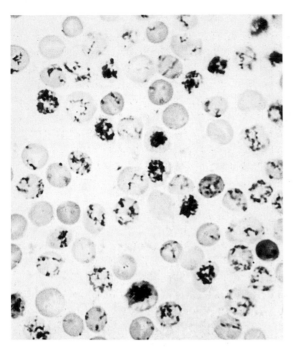

Fig 13.9 Film of blood from patient with pyruvate kinase deficiency. Postsplenectomy. Almost every erythrocyte is a reticulocyte. Stained supravitally by brilliant cresyl blue. Compare with Figure 13.8.

segments into a small tube. Add one drop of stain and incubate at 37°C for 3 h before making a film.

It should be noted that a haemoglobin H preparation is not recommended when precise diagnosis of the type of α thalassaemia trait is required, e.g. in antenatal diagnosis. DNA analysis is then indicated (see p. 498).

CARBOXYHAEMOGLOBIN AND METHAEMOGLOBIN

Carboxyhaemoglobin and methaemoglobin-containing cells can be demonstrated cytochemically.[19] These methods now have little practical value.

FETAL HAEMOGLOBIN

An acid-elution cytochemical method was introduced by Kleihauer et al in 1957.[20] It is a sensitive procedure which identifies individual cells containing haemoglobin F even when few are present, and their detection in the maternal circulation has provided valuable information on the pathogenesis of haemolytic disease of the newborn.

The identification of cells containing haemoglobin F depends upon the fact that they resist acid-elution to a greater extent than do normal cells; thus, in the technique described below, they appear as isolated darkly-stained cells amongst a background of palely-staining ghost cells. The occasional cells which stain to an intermediate degree are less easy to evaluate; some may be reticulocytes as these also resist acid-elution to some extent. The following method in which elution is carried out at pH 1.5 is recommended.[21]

Reagents

Fixative. 80% ethanol.

Elution solution. Solution A: 7.5 g/l haematoxylin in 90% ethanol. Solution B: $FeCl_3$, 24 g; 2.5 mol/l HCl, 20 ml; doubly-distilled water to 1 litre.

For use, mix well 5 volumes of A and 1 volume of B. The pH is approximately 1.5. The solution can be used for *c* 4 weeks: if a precipitate forms, the solution should be filtered.

Counterstain. 1 g/l aqueous erythrosin or 2.5 g/l aqueous eosin.

Method

Prepare fresh air-dried films. Immediately after drying, fix the films for 5 min in 80% ethanol in a Coplin jar. Then rinse the slides rapidly in water and stand vertically on blotting paper for about 10 min to dry. Next, place the slides for 20 s in a Coplin jar containing the elution solution. Then wash the slides throughly in water and finally place them in the counterstain for 2 min. Rinse in tap water and allow them to dry in the air. Fetal cells stain red and adult ghost-cells stain pale pink (Fig. 13.10). Films prepared from cord blood and from normal adult blood should be stained alongside the test films as positive and negative controls, respectively.

A number of modifications of the Kleihauer method have been proposed. In one, New methylene blue is incorporated in the buffer solution, the reaction time is prolonged and buffer is used for washing the films.[22] The advantage of this technique is that reticulocytes stain blue, whilst cells containing haemoglobin F stain pink.

An immunofluorescent staining method has been developed based on the use of a specific antibody against haemoglobin F which does not react with haemoglobin A.[23] By using a double-labelling procedure with rhodamine-labelled antibody

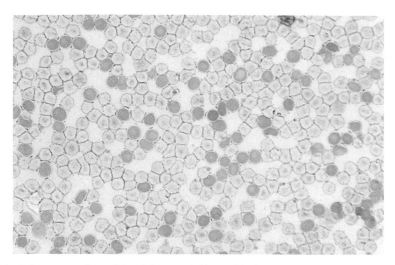

Fig 13.10 Cytochemical demonstration of fetal haemoglobin. Acid elution method. The preparation consists of a mixture of cord and normal adult blood. The darkly staining cells are fetal cells.

against γ globin and a fluorescein-labelled antibody against β globin, it is possible to detect the presence of haemoglobin F and haemoglobin A in the same cell.[24]

HAEMOGLOBIN S AND OTHER HAEMOGLOBIN VARIANTS

Immunodiffusion with specific antibody has been used for the identification of haemoglobin S, haemoglobin A_2 and haemoglobin F in red cells.[25,26] An alternative method is by fluorescent microscopy (flow cytometry) after labelling the cells with fluorescein isothiocyanate (FITC).[25] By a double-labelling method similar to that described above, it is possible to identify haemoglobin S as well as another haemoglobin in individual cells.

CYTOCHEMICAL TESTS FOR DEMONSTRATING DEFECTS OF RED CELL METABOLISM

Chemical tests for the recognition of defects of red cell metabolism are described in Chapter 10. Cytochemical methods have been developed by means of which some of these defects are demonstrable in individual cells. Thus tests have been described for demonstrating red cells deficient in G6PD.[27–29] The principle on which the methods are based is that red cells are treated with sodium nitrite to convert their oxyhaemoglobin (HbO_2) to methaemoglobin (Hi). In the presence of G6PD,

Hi reconverts to HbO_2, but in G6PD deficiency, Hi persists. The blood is then incubated with a soluble tetrazolium compound (MTT) which will be reduced by HbO_2 (but not by Hi) to an insoluble formazan form.[29] Alternatively, the presence of Hi can be demonstrated by converting it to HiCN with potassium cyanide and then adding hydrogen peroxide which elutes HiCN but not HbO_2.[28] The cells are then stained, e.g. with eosin, and the HbO_2-containing cells can be readily distinguished from unstained ghosts, which had contained the Hi and which do not stain.

Attempts have been made to improve the reliability of the test for detecting heterozygotes, e.g. by controlled slight fixation of the red cells and accelerating the reaction with an exogenous electron carrier (1-methoxyphenazine metho-sulphate).[30] These cytochemical procedures are not more sensitive in the demonstration of G6PD deficiency than are the simple screening tests described on page 179. They may, however, be useful in genetic studies and when assessing G6PD activity in women;[31] they may be the only way to detect deficiency in the heterozygous state.

DEMONSTRATION OF G6PD DEFICIENT CELLS

Reagents

Sodium nitrite. 0.18 mol/l (12.5 g/l). The solution must be stored in a dark bottle and made up monthly.

Incubation medium. 9 g/l NaCl, 4 ml; 50 g/l glucose, 1.0 ml; 0.3 mol/l phosphate buffer pH 7.0, 2.0 ml; 0.11 g/l Nile blue sulphate, 1.0 ml; water, 2.0 ml.

MTT tetrazolium. 5 g/l of 3-(4,5-dimethyl-thiazolyl-1–2)-2, 5-diphenyltetrazolium bromide in 9 g/l NaCl.

Hypotonic saline. 6 g/l NaCl.

Method[27]

Venous blood collected into ACD should be used. The test should be carried out within 8 h of collection and the blood should be kept at 4°C until it is tested. Centrifuge the blood at 4°C for 20 min at 1200–1500 g. Discard the supernatant and add 0.5 ml of the packed red cells to 9 ml of 9 g/l NaCl and 0.5 ml of sodium nitrite solution contained in a 15-ml glass centrifuge tube. Incubate at 37°C for 20 min. Centrifuge at 4°C for 15 min at c 500 g, then discard the supernatant fluid without disturbing the buffy coat and uppermost layer of red cells. Wash the cells three times in cold saline. After the last washing, remove the buffy coat, mix the packed cells well and transfer 50 µl to a glass tube containing 1 ml of the incubation medium. Incubate the suspension undisturbed at 37°C for 30 min. Then add 0.2 ml of MTT solution, shake gently and incubate at 37°C for 1 h. Resuspend the cells thoroughly. Place one drop adjacent to one drop of

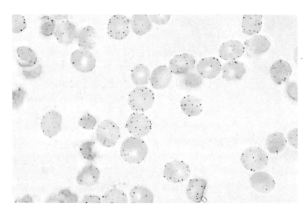

Fig 13.11 Cytochemical demonstration of G6PD. Normal blood; positive reaction with formazan granules in the red cells.

hypotonic saline on a glass slide, mix the drops thoroughly and cover with a cover-glass.

Examine the red cells with an oil-immersion objective, noting the presence of formazan granules (Fig. 13.11).

Another satisfactory method is described on p. 182

Interpretation

When G6PD activity is normal, all the red cells are stained. In G6PD hemizygotes, the majority of the red cells are unstained. In heterozygotes, mosaicism is usually easily seen, a proportion of cells appearing normal and the remainder being devoid or almost devoid of stainable material.

LEUCOCYTE CYTOCHEMISTRY

Leucocyte cytochemistry encompasses the techniques used to identify diagnostically useful enzymes or other substances in the cytoplasm of haemopoietic cells. These technique are particularly useful for the characterization of immature cells in the acute myeloid leukaemias, and the identification of maturation abnormalities in the myelodysplastic syndromes and myeloproliferative disorders. There are many variations in the staining techniques, as discussed in the recommendations of an Expert Panel of the International Committee for Standardization in Haematology.[32,33] Detailed reference works discussing the theoretical and practical aspects of cytochemistry are available.[34] The use of cytochemistry to characterize lymphoproliferative

disorders has been largely superseded by immunological techniques (see Ch. 14). The results of cytochemical tests should always be interpreted in relation to Romanowsky stains and immunological techniques. Control blood or marrow slides should always be stained in parallel to assure the quality of the staining. The principal uses of cytochemistry are:

1. To characterize the blast cells in acute leukaemias as myeloid.
2. To identify granulocytic and monocytic components of acute myeloid leukaemia.
3. To indentify unusual lineages occasionally involved in clonal myeloid disorders, e.g. basophils and mast cells.

4. To detect of cytoplasmic abnormalities and enzyme deficiencies in myeloid disorders, e.g. myeloperoxidase-deficient neutrophils in myelodysplasia or acute leukaemia, neutrophil alkaline phosphatase-deficient neutrophils in chronic myeloid leukaemia (CML).

MYELOPEROXIDASE

Myeloperoxidase (MPO) is located in the primary and secondary granules of granulocytes and their precursors, in eosinophil granules and in the azurophil granules of monocytes. The MPO in eosinophil granules is cyanide resistant, whereas that in neutrophils and monocytes is cyanide sensitive. MPO splits H_2O_2, and in the presence of a chromogenic electron donor forms an insoluble reaction product. Various benzidine substitutes have been used, of which 3,3'-diaminobenzidine (DAB) is the preferred chromogen.[35,36] The reaction product is stable, insoluble and non-diffusible. Staining can be enhanced by immersing the slides in copper sulphate or nitrate, but this is generally not required in normal diagnostic practice. Alternative non-benzidine based techniques employ 4-chloro-1-naphthol (4CN)[37] or 3-amino-9-ethylcarbazole.[38] The former gives very crisp staining, but is soluble in some mounting media and immersion oil, the latter shows some diffusibility and does not stain as strongly as DAB.

METHOD WITH 3,3'-DIAMINOBENZIDINE
Method and reagents
Reagents

Fixative. Buffered formal acetone (BFA) (p. 606).

Substrate. 3,3'-diaminobenzidine (Sigma D-8001).

Buffer. Sorensen's phosphate buffer pH 7.3 (p. 606).

Hydrogen peroxide (H_2O_2, 100 vol).

Counterstain. Aqueous haematoxylin.

Method

1. Fix air-dried smears for 30 s in cold BFA.
2. Rinse thoroughly in gently running tap water and air-dry.
3. Incubate for 10 min in working substrate solution:

Thoroughly mix 30 mg DAB in 60 ml buffer, add 120 µl H_2O_2, mix well.
4. Counterstain with haematoxylin for 1–5 min, rinse in running tap water and air-dry.

Technical considerations
MPO is not inhibited by heparin, oxalate or EDTA anticoagulants. Films should be made within 12 h of blood collection. Staining is satisfactory on slides kept at room temperature for at least week. The DAB should be stored frozen at −20°C in 1-ml aliquots of 30 mg in 1 ml of buffer. For optimum results, it is essential to dissolve the DAB thoroughly in the buffer, and make sure the reagents in the incubation mixture are well mixed. The stain is robust and not strictly pH dependent, with identical results being obtained when using buffers ranging in pH from 7.0 to 9.0. The counterstaining time should be adjusted to the minimum time to give clear nuclear detail. Methyl green is an alternative counterstain, giving excellent contrast with the DAB reaction product, but nuclear detail is more difficult to discern.

Results and interpretation
The reaction product is brown and granular (Fig. 13.12a). Red cells and erythroid precursors show diffuse brown cytoplasmic staining. The most primitive myeloblasts are negative, with granular positivity appearing progressively as they mature towards the promyelocyte stage. The positivity may be localized to the Golgi region. Promyelocytes and myelocytes are the most strongly staining cells in the granulocyte series, with positive (primary) granules packing the cytoplasm. Metamyelocytes and neutrophils have progressively fewer positive (secondary) granules. Eosinophil granules stain strongly, and the large specific eosinophil granules are easily distinguished from neutrophil granules. Eosinophil granule peroxidase is distinct biochemically and immunologically from neutrophil peroxidase. Monoblasts and monocytes may be negative or positive. When positive, the granules are smaller than in neutrophils and diffusely scattered throughout the cytoplasm. MPO activity is present in basophil granules but is not demonstrable in mature basophils by the DAB reaction given above.

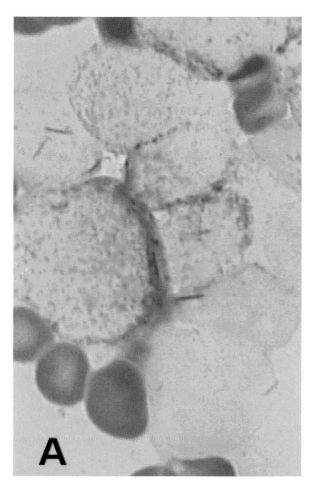 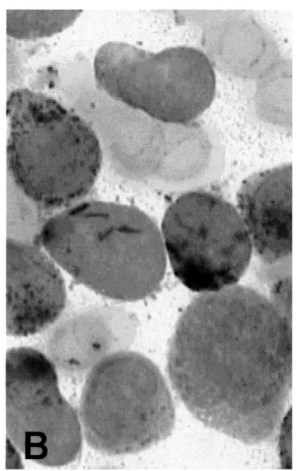

Fig 13.12 (A) Myeloperoxidase (MPO) and (B) Sudan black B (SBB). Bone marrow in acute myeloid leukaemia (FAB M1). MPO staining shows over rods and cytoplasmic granular staining, whilst with SBB localised positive reaction in the blast cells is more definite and Auer rods are prominent.

Pathological variations

Rare individuals have congenital deficiency of neutrophil MPO. All stages of granulocytes from the myeloblast onwards are negative. In these individuals, the eosinophils stain normally. Dysplastic neutrophils may be negative. Auer rods stain well with DAB, and are more frequently on MPO staining than on Romanowsky-stained films.

SUDAN BLACK B

Sudan black B is a lipophilic dye that binds irreversibly to an undefined granule component in granulocytes, eosinophils and some monocytes. It cannot be extracted from the stained granules by organic dye solvents, and gives comparable information to that of MPO staining.[39] The currently used staining solution is essentially that described by Sheehan & Storey in 1974.[40]

Method and reagents

Reagents

Fixative. 40% formaldehyde solution.

Stain. Sudan black B (Sigma No. S 2380) 0.3 g in 100 ml absolute ethanol

Phenol buffer. Dissolve 16 g crystalline phenol in 30 ml absolute ethanol. Add to 100 ml distilled water in which 0.3 g $Na_2HPO_4.12H_2O_2$ has been dissolved.

Working stain solution. Add 40 ml buffer to 60 ml Sudan black B solution.

Counterstain. May–Grünwald–Giesma or Leishman stain (see p. 51).

Method

1. Fix air-dried smears in formalin vapour as follows: Place a small square of filter paper in the bottom of a Coplin jar. Add 2 drops of 40% formalin, put on the lid and leave for 15 min to allow vaporization. Place the slides in the Coplin jar and replace the lid. After 5–10 min, remove the slides and stand on end for 15 min to 'air-wash'.
2. Immerse the slides in the working stain solution for 1 h in a Coplin jar with a lid on.
3. Transfer slides to a staining rack and immediately flood with 70% alcohol. After 30 s, tip the 70% alcohol off and flood again for 30 s. Repeat three times in total.
4. Rinse in gently running tap water and air-dry.
5. Counterstain without further fixation with Leishman stain or May–Grünwald– Giemsa.

Technical considerations

Buffered formol acetone fixation for 30 s is a satisfactory alternative to formalin vapour. The working stain solution should be replaced after 4 weeks. Bone marrow smears with fatty spicules containing lipid-soluble Sudan black B benefit from a 5-second swirl in xylene followed by rinsing in running tap water and air-drying prior to counterstaining. The Romanowsky counterstain gives excellent cytological detail of all cells present.

Results and interpretation

The reaction product is black and granular. The results are essentially similar to those seen with MPO staining, both in normal and leukaemic cells (Fig. 13.12 and 13.16B). MPO-negative neutrophils are also Sudan black B negative. The only notable difference is in eosinophil granules, which have a clear core when stained with Sudan black B. Rare cases of acute lymphoblastic leukaemia (1–2%) show non-granular smudgy positivity not seen with MPO staining.[41] Basophils are generally not positive, but may show bright red/purple metachromatic staining of the granules.

NEUTROPHIL ALKALINE PHOSPHATASE (NAP)

Alkaline phosphatase activity is found predominantly in mature neutrophils, with some activity in metamyelocytes. Although demonstrated as a granular reaction product in the cytoplasm, enzyme activity is associated with a poorly characterized intracytoplasmic membranous component distinct from primary or secondary granules.[42] Other leucocytes are generally negative, but rare cases of lymphoid malignancies show cytochemically demonstrable activity.[43] Bone marrow macrophages are positive. Early methods of demonstrating alkaline phosphatase relied on the use of glycerophosphate or other phosphomonoesters as the substrate at alkaline pH, with a final black reaction product of lead sulphide.[44] Azo-dye techniques are simpler, giving equally good results. These methods use substituted naphthols as the substrate, and it is the liberated naphthol rather than phosphate that is utilized to combine with the azo-dye to give the final reaction product.[45–47]

Method and reagents
Reagents

Fixative. 4% formalin methanol. Add 10 ml 40% formalin to 90 ml methanol. Keep at –20°C or in the freezer compartment of a refrigerator. Discard after 2 weeks.

Substrate. Naphthol AS phosphate (Sigma N-5625). Store in freezer.

Buffer. 0.2 mol/l Tris buffer pH 9.0 (see p. 606)

Stock substrate solution. Dissolve 30 mg naphthol AS phosphate in 0.5 ml N,N-dimethylformamide (Sigma D-4254). Add 100 ml 0.2 mol/l Tris buffer, pH 9.1. Store in a refrigerator at 2–4°C. The solution is stable for several months.

Coupling azo-dye. Fast Blue BB salt (Sigma F-0250). Store in freezer.

Counterstain. Neutral red, 0.02% aqueous solution.

Method

1. Fix freshly made air-dried blood films for 30 s in cold 4% formalin methanol.
2. Rinse with tap water and air-dry.

3. Prepare working substrate solution by allowing 40 ml of stock substrate solution to warm to room temperature. Add 24 mg of Fast Blue BB and mix thoroughly until dissolved. Incubate slides for 15 min.
4. Wash in tap water and air-dry.
5. Counterstain for 3 min in 0.02% aqueous Neutral Red, rinse briefly and air-dry.

Technical considerations

N,N-dimethylformamide may dissolve some types of plastic, therefore a glass tube should be used to dissolve the substrate. Blood films should be made soon after blood collection, preferably within 30 min, as NAP activity decreases rapidly in EDTA anticoagulated blood. Once spread, the blood film should be stained within 6 h. Control films with a predictably high score (see below), e.g. from a patient with reactive neutrophilia or a pregnant woman, should be made if possible, also from fresh blood samples. The technical aspects of blood film preparation and the effects of fixation on NAP activity are discussed by Kaplow.[48] The normal range for healthy adults should be established in individual laboratories using a standard staining technique and consistent scoring criteria (see below).

Results and interpretation

The reaction product is blue and granular. The intensity of reaction product in neutrophils varies from negative to strongly positive, with coarse granules filling the cytoplasm and overlying the nucleus (Fig. 13.13). An overall score is obtained by assessing the stain intensity in 100 consecutive neutrophils, with each neutrophil scored on a scale of 1–4 as follows:

0 Negative, no granules
1 Occasional granules scattered in the cytoplasm
2 Moderate numbers of granules
3 Numerous granules
4 Heavy positivity with numerous coarse granules crowding the cytoplasm, frequently overlying the nucleus

The overall possible score will range between 0 and 400. Reported normal ranges show some variations, owing possibly in part to variations in scoring criteria and methodology.

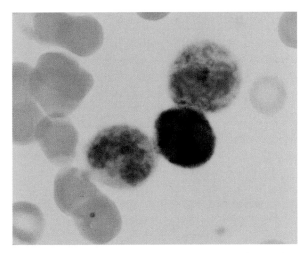

Fig 13.13 Neutrophil alkaline phosphatase. A strongly positive (4+) and moderately positive (3+ and 2+) intensity of reaction are shown.

Published normal ranges illustrate the need for establishing a normal range in any one laboratory:

Hayhoe & Quaglino[49]	14–100 (mean 46)
Kaplow[45]	13–160 (mean 61)
Rutenberg et al[50]	37–98 (mean 68)
Bendix-Hansen & Helleberg-Rasmussen[51]	11–134 (mean 48)

The scoring system described by Bendix-Hansen & Helleberg-Rasmussen differs slightly in emphasis from the others, but gives similar results.

In normal individuals, it is rare to find neutrophils with scores of 3, and scores of 4 should not be present. There is some physiological variation in NAP scores. Newborn babies, children and pregnant women have high scores, and premenopausal women have, on average, scores one-third higher than men.[42] In pathological states, the most significant diagnostic use of the NAP score is in chronic myeloid leukaemia. In the chronic phase of the disease, the score is almost invariably low, usually zero. Transient rises may occur with intercurrent infection. In myeloid blast transformation or accelerated phase, the score rises. Low scores are also commonly found in paroxysmal nocturnal haemoglobinuria (PNH) and the very rare condition of hereditary hypophosphatasia. There are many causes of a raised NAP score, notably in the neutrophilia of infection, polycythaemia rubra vera, leukaemoid reactions and Hodgkin's disease. In aplastic anaemia, the NAP score is high, but falls if PNH supervenes.

ACID PHOSPHATASE REACTION

Cytochemically demonstrable acid phosphatase is ubiquitous in haemopoietic cells. The staining intensity of different cell types is somewhat variable according to the method employed. Its main diagnostic use is in the diagnosis of T-cell acute leukaemias and hairy cell leukaemia,[52] but these diseases are more reliably diagnosed and characterized by immunophenotyping when this is available (see Ch. 14), and the tartrate-resistant acid phosphatase stain using Fast Garnet GBC as coupler is of historical interest only.[32,53] The pararosaniline method given below, modified from Goldberg & Barka[54], is recommended for demonstrating positivity in T lymphoid cells.

Method and reagents
Reagents

Fixative. Methanol, 10 ml, acetone, 60 ml, water, 30 ml, citric acid, 0.63 g. Adjust to pH 5.4 with 1 mol/l NaOH before use.

Buffer pH 5.0. Sodium acetate trihydrate, 19.5 g, sodium barbiturate, 29.5 g, water to 1 litre (Michaeli's veronal acetate buffer).

Substrate solution. 25 mg naphthol AS-BI phosphate (Sigma N 2125) dissolved in 2.5 ml N,N-dimethylformamide.

Sodium nitrite. 4% $NaNO_2$ aqueous solution.

Coupling reagent.

(1) Stock pararosaniline. Dissolve 1 g pararosaniline (Sigma No. P-7632) in 25 ml warm 2 mol/l HCl. Filter when cool. Store at room temperature in the dark. Stable for 2 months.
(2) 4% sodium nitrite solution. Dissolve 200 mg sodium nitrite in 5 ml distilled water. Stable for 1 week at 4–10°C.
(3) Hexazotized pararosaniline. Mix equal volumes of pararosaniline and 4% sodium nitrite together 2 min before use.

Counterstain. 1% Aqueous methyl green or Aqueous haematoxylin.

Working solution. Mix 92.5 ml of buffer with 2.5 ml of substrate solution. Add 32.5 ml of distilled water and then add 4 ml of hexazotized pararosaniline. Mix well, adjust pH to 5.0 using 1 mol/l NaOH.

Method

1. Air-dry smears for several hours (24 h if possible).
2. Fix for 10 min in methanol/acetone/citric acid, rinse in tap water and air-dry
3. Incubate for 1 h at 37°C in the working solution.
4. Rinse in tap water and air-dry.
5. Counterstain in 1% aqueous methyl green or aqueous haematoxylin for 5 min.
6. Rinse in tap water and mount wet in warmed glycerin jelly.

Results and interpretation
The reaction product is red with a mixture of granular and diffuse positivity (Fig. 13.14). In T cells, acid phosphatase is an early differentiation feature. Almost all acute and chronic T-cell leukaemias show strong activity. In T-cell acute leukaemias, the activity is usually highly localized (polar). Granulocytes are strongly positive. Monocytes, eosinophils and platelets show variable positivity. In the bone marrow, macrophages, plasma cells and megakaryocytes are strongly positive.

PERIODIC ACID-SCHIFF (PAS) REACTION

Periodic acid specifically oxidizes 1–2 glycol groups to produce stable dialdehydes. These dialdehydes give a red reaction product when exposed to Schiff's reagent (leucobasic fuchsin). Positive reactions occur with carbohydrates, principally glycogen, but also monosaccharides, polysaccharides, glycoproteins, mucoproteins, phosphorylated

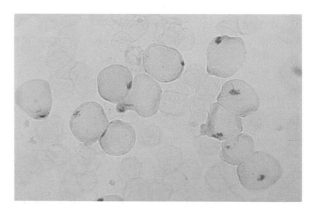

Fig 13.14 Acid phosphatase. T -cell acute leukaemia wih intense localised staining. *Courtesy Professor D. Catovsky.*

sugars, inositol derivatives and cerebrosides.[55] Glycogen can be distinguished from other positively reacting substances by its sensitivity to diastase digestion. In haemopoietic cells, the main source of positive reactions is glycogen.

Method and reagents

Reagents

Fixative. Methanol.

1% periodic acid. $HIO_{4.2}H_2O$, 10 g/l in distilled water.

Schiff's reagent. Dissolve 5 g basic fuchsin in 500 ml of hot distilled water. Filter when cool. Saturate with SO_2 gas by bubbling for 1–12 h in a fume cupboard. Shake vigorously with 2 g activated charcoal for 1 min in a conical flask in a fume cupboard and filter immediately through a large Whatman No. 1 filter into a dark bottle. The reagent is stable for 6 months at room temperature, stored in the dark.

Counterstain. Aqueous haematoxylin.

Method

1. Fix films for 15 min in methanol.
2. Rinse in gently running tap water and air-dry.
3. If required, expose fixed control films to digestion in diastase (100 mg in 100 ml of 0.9 g/l NaCl) for 20–60 min at room temperature.
4. Flood slides with 1% periodic acid for 10 min.
5. Rinse in running tap water for 10 min and air-dry.
6. Immerse in Schiff's reagent for 30 min in a Coplin jar with a lid (the Schiff's reagent can be returned to the stock bottle).
7. Rinse in running tap water for 10 min and air-dry.
8. Counterstain in aqueous haematoxylin for 5–10 min.

Technical considerations

Formalin vapour (5 min), formalin/ethanol (10 ml 40% formalin/90 ml ethanol) (10 min) or buffered formalin acetone (45 s) are satisfactory alternative fixatives. Previously fixed, iron-stained or Romanowsky-stained smears can be overstained with the PAS reaction satisfactorily. Romanowsky-stained smears can be partly decolourized by soaking in methanol for 1 h prior to step 4 above.

The intensity of the reaction product depends on the quality of the Schiff's reagent. Normal neutrophils should always stain intensely red, and deterioration of the Schiff's reagent can be detected by examination of control normal films. Some methods recommend rinsing in a dilute sodium metabisulphite HCl solution ('SO_2 water') after step 6 above, but this is not necessary with good quality Schiff's reagent.

Results and interpretation

The reaction product is red, with intensity ranging from pink to bright red (Figs 13.15 and 13.16C). Cytoplasmic positivity may be diffuse or granular. Granulocyte precursors show diffuse weak positivity, with neutrophils showing intense confluent granular positivity. Eosinophil granules are negative, with diffuse cytoplasmic positivity. Basophils may be negative but often show large irregular blocks of positive material not related to the granules. Monocytes and their precursors show variable diffuse positivity with superimposed fine granules, often at the periphery of the cytoplasm. Normal erythroid precursors and red cells are negative. Megakaryocytes and platelets show variable, usually intense, diffuse positivity with superimposed fine granules, coarse granules and large blocks. 10–40% of peripheral lymphocytes show granular positivity with negative background cytoplasm, with no detectable differences between T and B cells.[56,57]

ESTERASES

Leucocyte esterases are a group of enzymes that hydrolyse acyl or chloroacyl esters of α-naphthol or naphthol AS. Li et al[58] identified nine esterase isoenzymes using polyacrylamide gel electrophoresis of leucocyte extracts from normal and pathological cells. The gels were stained in parallel with cell smears. The isoenzymes fell into two groups: bands 1, 2, 7, 8, and 9 corresponded to the 'specific' esterase of granulocytes, staining specifically with naphthol AS-D chloroacetate esterase (chloroacetate esterase, CAE), while bands 3, 4, 5 and 6 corresponded to 'non-specific' esterase (NSE), staining with α-naphthyl acetate esterase (ANAE) and α-naphthyl butyrate esterase (butyrate esterase, BE). Band 4 was best demonstrated by BE and band 5 by ANAE. The non-specific esterases are inhibited by sodium fluoride

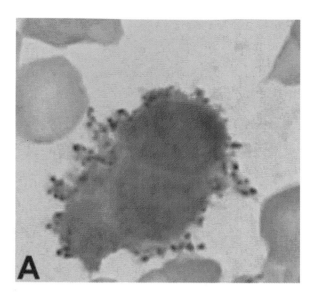

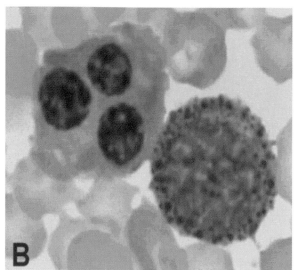

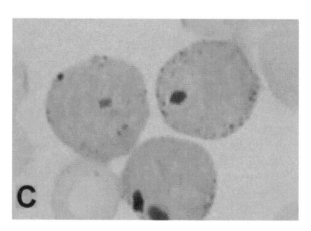

Fig 13.15 PAS stain. (A) Dysplastic micromegakaryocytes with diffuse cytoplasmic staining and some coarse granules; (B) dyserythropoiesis with diffuse staining in a trinucleate normoblast and coarse granular and diffuse staining in a pro-erythroblast; (C) acute lymphoblastic leukaemia with blasts showing block positivity.

(NaF). Naphthol AS acetate and naphthol AS-D acetate react with both specific and non-specific esterases, but only the reaction with the non-specific esterases is inhibited by NaF. The methods employing parallel slides with and without NaF are not generally used anymore, as it is generally more informative to perform a combination of chloroacetate esterase and one of the 'non-specific' esterase stains on a single slide. The combined methods have the advantage of demonstrating pathological double staining of individual cells. All the esterase stains can be performed using a variety of coupling reagents, each of which gives a different coloured reaction product. The methods outlined below have been chosen for their simplicity and reliability.

NAPHTHOL AS-D CHLOROACETATE ESTERASE[32]
Method and reagents
Reagents

Fixative. Buffered formalin acetone (p. 606).

Buffer. 66 mmol/l phosphate buffer pH 7.4 see p. 606.

Naphthol AS-D chloroacetate substrate solution. Dissolve 0.1 g of naphthol AS-D chloroacetate (Sigma N-0758) in 40 ml N,N-dimethylformamide (Sigma D-4254). Keep refrigerated.

Working substrate solution. Add 2 ml of naphthol AS-D chloroacetate stock solution to 38 ml 66 mmol/l phosphate buffer pH 7.4. Mix well.

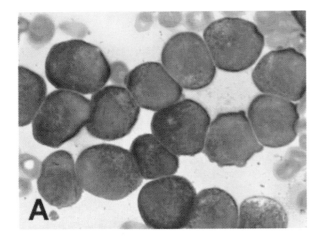
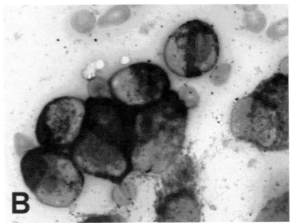
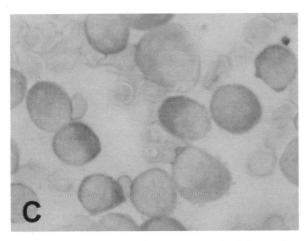
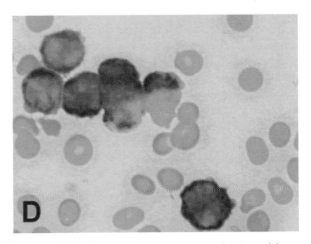

Fig 13.16 Acute promyelocytic leukaemia. (A) May-Grünwald-Giemsa stain shows hypergranular promyelocytes with scattered Auer rods; (B) Sudan black B with strongly stained cytoplasm; (C) PAS staining shows diffuse cytoplasmic blush; (D) Chloroacetate esterase gives strong cytoplasmic staining.

Add 0.4 ml of freshly prepared hexazotized New Fuchsin. Mix well.

Coupling reagent.

(1) Hexazotized New fuchsin. Dissolve 4 g of New fuchsin in 100 ml of 2N HCl.
(2) Sodium nitrite solution 0.3 mol/l. Dissolve 2.1 g of sodium nitrite ($NaNO_2$) in 100 ml of water.
(3) Immediately prior to using, add 0.2 ml New fuchsin to 0.4 ml sodium nitrite, mix well and leave for 1 min before adding to substrate solution.

Haematoxylin. Aqueous haematoxylin

Method

1. Fix air-dried smears in cold buffered formalin acetone for 30 s.
2. Rinse in gently running tap water and air-dry.
3. Immerse the slides in the working substrate solution in a Coplin jar for 5–10 min.
4. Rinse in running tap water and air-dry.
5. Counterstain in aqueous haematoxylin for 1 min.
6. 'Blue' in running tap water for 1 min and air-dry.

Technical considerations

The CAE stain is robust and reliable. 40 mg Fast blue BB is a satisfactory alternative to New Fuchsin, but requires thorough vigorous mixing with the substrate solution. The incubation time is important, as most haemopoietic cells show some scattered granular staining if the incubation is prolonged. Hydrolysis of the substrate is rapid, with staining virtually complete within 3–5 min.

Results and interpretation

The reaction product is bright red (Fig. 13.16D). It is confined to cells of the granulocyte series and mast cells. Cytoplasmic CAE activity appears as myeloblasts mature to promyelocytes. Positivity in myeloblasts is rare, but promyelocytes and myelocytes stain strongly, with reaction product filling the cytoplasm. Later granulocytes stain strongly but less intensely. It is therefore useful as a marker of cytoplasmic maturation in the granulocytic leukaemias. In acute promyelocytic leukaemia, the cells show heavy cytoplasmic staining. The characteristic multiple Auer rods stain positively, often with a hollow core. It is rare to see CAE-positive Auer rods in other forms of AML except cases with the t(8;21) translocation.[59]

α-NAPHTHYL BUTYRATE ESTERASE
Method and reagents
Reagents

Fixative. Buffered formalin acetone (see p. 606).

Buffer. 100 mmol/l Phosphate buffer (Sorensen's) pH 8.0.

Substrate stock solution. α-naphthyl butyrate (Sigma N-8125) 100 μl in 5 ml acetone. The solution should be stored at −20°C and is stable for at least 2 months.

Coupling reagent. Fast Garnet GBC (Sigma F 8761) 15 mg.

Counterstain. Aqueous haematoxylin.

Method

1. Fix air-dried smears in buffered formalin acetone for 30 s. Rinse in gently running tap water and air-dry.
2. Add the Fast garnet GBC to 50 ml buffer and mix well.
3. Add 0.5 ml of the α-naphthyl butyrate/acetone solution and mix well.
4. Pour the incubation medium into a Coplin jar containing the fixed slides and incubate for 20–40 min.

5. Rinse thoroughly by running tap water into the Coplin jar until clear.
6. Air-dry and counterstain in aqueous haematoxylin for 1–5 min.

Technical considerations

The reaction product is soluble in immersion oil and synthetic mounting media. If slides are to be looked at repeatedly, they should be mounted in an aqueous mounting medium, e.g. Apathy's or glycerin/gelatin. There may be batch-to-batch variation of the Fast Garnet GBC. Staining can be controlled by removing the control-slide from the incubation medium after 20 min and examining it wet under a low power (e.g. x20) objective, returning it to the incubation medium while still wet. When the monocytes show as dark brown, staining is complete. Hexazotized pararosaniline is an alternative coupling reagent, which gives an insoluble brown reaction product and is suitable for mounting in synthetic mounting media.[58]

Results and interpretation

The reaction product is brown and granular (Fig. 13.17). The majority of monocytes (>80%) stain

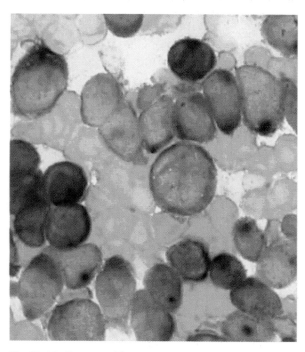

Fig 13.17 Non-specific esterase. Positive (brown) reaction in acute monocytic leukaemia (FAB M5).

strongly, the remainder showing some weak staining. Negative monocytes are rare. Neutrophils, eosinophils, basophils and platelets are negative. B lymphocytes are negative and T lymphocytes are unreliably stained. In the bone marrow, monocytes, their precursors and macrophages stain strongly. α-naphthyl butyrate is more specific for identifying a monocytic component in AML than α-naphthyl acetate (see below).

α-NAPHTHYL ACETATE ESTERASE
Method and reagents
Reagents

Fixative. Buffered formalin acetone.

Buffer. 66 mmol/l phosphate buffer pH 6.3.

Substrate solution. Dissolve 100 mg α-naphthyl acetate (Sigma N-8505) in 5 ml ethylene monomethyl ether. Store at 4–10°C.

Coupling reagent.

(1) Stock pararosaniline. Dissolve 1 g pararosaniline (Sigma No. P-7632) in 25 ml warm 2 mol/l HCl. Filter when cool. Store at room temperature in the dark. Stable for 2 months.
(2) 4% sodium nitrite solution. Dissolve 200 mg sodium nitrite in 5 ml distilled water. Stable for 1 week at 4–10°C
(3) Hexazotized pararosaniline. Mix equal volumes of pararosaniline and 4% sodium nitrite together 1 min before use

Incubation medium. Add 2 ml of the α-naphthyl acetate solution to 38 ml of the 66 mmol/l phosphate buffer pH 6.3 and mix well. Add 0.4 ml of freshly prepared hexazotized pararosaniline and mix well.

Counterstain. Aqueous haematoxylin.

Method

1. Fix air-dried smears in cold buffered formalin acetone for 30 s.
2. Rinse in running tap water and air-dry.
3. Immerse the slides for 30–60 min in the incubation medium in a Coplin jar.
4. Rinse in gently running tap water in the Coplin jar until clear and air-dry.
5. Counterstain in aqueous haematoxylin for 2–5 min.

Technical considerations
Fast Blue BB 80 mg can be substituted as coupling reagent. This gives a dark green/brown granular reaction product which is soluble in mounting media and immersion oil. The haematoxylin staining time should be adjusted to give clear nuclear detail without overstaining to obscure nucleoli and chromatin texture.

Results and interpretation
The reaction product is diffuse red/brown in colour. Normal and leukaemic monocytes stain strongly. Normal granulocytes are negative, but in myelodysplasia or AML may give positive reactions of varying intensity. Megakaryocytes stain strongly, and leukaemic megakaryoblasts may show focal or diffuse positivity. Most T lymphocytes and some T lymphoblasts show focal 'dot-like' positivity, but immunophenotyping has superseded cytochemistry for identifying and subcategorizing T cells. Leukaemic erythroblasts may show focal or diffuse positivity.

SEQUENTIAL COMBINED ESTERASE STAIN USING ANAE AND CAE
Method and reagents
Reagents
As above.

Method

1. Follow the method and steps 1–4 above for α-naphthyl acetate stain, rinse in tap water and air-dry.
2. Without further fixation, prepare the naphthol AS-D chloroacetate incubation medium as above, substituting 10 mg Fast Blue BB (Sigma No. F 0250) for hexazotized New Fuchsin, and incubate for 10 min.
3. Rinse in tap water and counterstain with aqueous haematoxylin for 1–3 min.

Technical considerations
Fast Blue BB is relatively insoluble, and the chloroacetate incubation medium should be mixed vigorously before use.

Results and interpretation
The ANAE gives a brown reaction product, the CAE a granular bright blue product (Fig. 13.18). Staining patterns are identical to those seen with

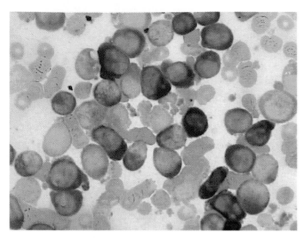

Fig 13.18 Combined esterase stain. Acute myelomonocytic leukaemia with almost equal numbers of chloroacetate esterase (blue) and non-specific esterase (brown) positive cells.

the two stains used separately. The double-staining technique avoids the need to compare results from separate slides, and shows up aberrant staining patterns. In myelomonocytic leukaemias, cells staining with both esterases may be present. In myelodysplasia and AML with dysplastic granulocytes, double staining of individual cells may be present. This may be helpful in the diagnosis of dubious cases of myelodysplasia, but the same abnormal pattern may be seen in non-clonal dysplastic states such as megaloblastic anaemia.

SINGLE INCUBATION DOUBLE ESTERASE[60] (NAPHTHOL AS-D CHLOROACETATE [CAE] AND α-NAPHTHYL BUTYRATE)
Method and reagents
Reagents

Fixative. Buffered formalin acetone.

Buffer. 100 mmol/l phosphate buffer pH 8.0 (Sorensen's).

Substrates.

(1) 2.5 mg naphthol AS-D chloroacetate (Sigma N-0758) in 1 ml acetone.
(2) 4 mg α-naphthyl butyrate (Sigma N-8000) in 1 ml acetone.

Coupling reagent. Fast Blue BB salt (Sigma No. F-0250).

Counterstain. Aqueous haematoxylin.

Method

1. Fix air-dried smears in buffered formalin acetone for 30 s.
2. Rinse in tap water and air-dry.
3. Dissolve 80 mg Fast Blue BB in 50 ml phosphate buffer by vigorous mixing.
4. Add naphthol AS-D chloroacetate and mix well.
5. Add α-naphthyl butyrate and mix well.
6. Incubate slides for 10–15 min in a Coplin jar in the dark.
7. Flush the Coplin jar with running tap water until clear.
8. Air-dry the slides.
9. Counterstain in aqueous haematoxylin for 1 min, rinse and air-dry.

Technical considerations
Steps 4 and 5 should be carried out rapidly. Staining can be extended to 30 min if necessary to ensure maximal ANB staining, but at longer incubation times some non-specific granular CAE staining may occur.

Results and interpretation
The CAE reaction product is bright blue (granulocytes); the ANB product is dark green/brown (monocytes). ANB does not stain megakaryocytes or T cells as strongly as α-naphthyl acetate. Lam et al suggest the use of hexazotized pararosaniline as coupling reagent in a single incubation combined esterase, which gives contrasting bright red and brown reaction products.[61]

In AML, the stain is useful for identifying monocytic and granulocytic components.

TOLUIDINE BLUE STAIN

Toluidine blue staining is useful for the enumeration of basophils and mast cells. It binds strongly to the granules in these cells, and is particularly useful in pathological states where the cells may not be easily identifiable on Romanowsky stains. In AML, CML and other myeloproliferative disorders, basophils may be dysplastic and poorly granular, as may the mast cells in some forms of acquired mastocytosis.

Method and reagents
Reagents

Toluidine blue 1% w/v in methanol. Add 1 g of toluidine blue (BDH 34077) to 100 ml methanol and mix for 24 h on a roller or with a magnetic flea. The stain is stable indefinitely at room temperature. Keep tightly stoppered.

Method

1. Place air-dried smears on a staining rack and flood with the toluidine blue solution.
2. Incubate for 5–10 min.
3. Rinse briefly in gently running tap water until clear and air-dry.

Results and interpretation
The granules of basophils and mast cells stain a bright red/purple, and are discrete and distinct (Fig. 13.19). Nuclei stain blue, and cells with abundant RNA may show a blue tint to the cytoplasm. Although toluidine blue is said to be specific for these granules, with >10-min incubations, the primary granules of promyelocytes are stained red/purple. However these are smaller and finer than the mast cell or basophil granules and easily distinguished.

CYTOCHEMICAL REACTIONS AND LEUKAEMIA CLASSIFICATION

MYELODYSPLASTIC SYNDROMES
The myelodysplastic syndromes are acquired clonal preleukaemic bone marrow disorders characterized

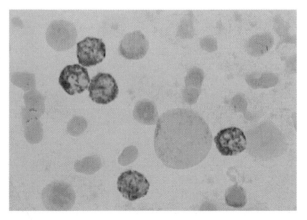

Fig 13.19 Toluidine blue. Chronic myeloid leukaemia in accelerated phase. There are five strongly positive basophils.

largely by cellular or hypercellular marrows, peripheral cytopenias and variable morphological abnormalities of the non-lymphoid haemopoietic cells. The classification system proposed by the French-American-British (FAB) co-operative group in 1982[62] has been generally accepted. It is based on the percentage of blast cells in the marrow (maximum 29%), the presence or absence of Auer rods in the blasts, the percentage of bone marrow ring sideroblasts and the circulating blast cell and monocyte count (Table 13.1), and recognizes five subtypes.

Cytochemistry is helpful in defining monocytic cells (ANAE and BE), the presence of Auer rods (Sudan black B and MPO) and the presence of dysplasia (double staining cells with chloroacetate and ANAE, and Sudan black B- or MPO-negative neutrophils).

ACUTE MYELOID LEUKAEMIA
FAB classification of AML
Since 1976, the classification of AML has by general acceptance been according to the criteria suggested by the FAB group, with subsequent modifications.[63–66] The FAB system utilizes immunophenotyping, morphology and cytochemistry only, although the link to cytogenetic abnormalities is clear in acute promyelocytic leukaemia (M3), and M4Eo.

Cytochemistry is essential in confirming the assessment made of the Romanowsky stained blood and marrow smears. Myeloblasts tend to have eccentric nuclei and show localized MPO and Sudan black B positivity. Auer rods are seen approximately twice as frequently on Suden black B and MPO staining as on the Romanowsky stains. Monoblasts are larger with a central nucleus and are frequently negative for Sudan black B and MPO, but reliably stain strongly with ANAE or BE. Care should be taken when diagnosing monoblastic leukaemias in the absence of positive esterase staining. CAE is helpful in defining the granulocytic component of acute myeloid leukaemias, reliably staining promyelocytes and more mature granulocytes. The PAS stain is useful for confirming dyserythropoiesis and the presence of abnormal megakaryocytes. Table 13.2 outlines the FAB classification of AML and the role of cytochemistry in defining the various subtypes

Table 13.1 FAB classification of myelodysplastic syndromes

Category	Peripheral blood		Bone marrow
Refractory anaemia (RA) Includes cases without anaemia but with neutropenia and thrombocytopenia	Anaemia/cytopenia Blasts <1% Monocytes <1 × 10⁹/l Mainly red cell abnormalities	and	Blasts <5% Ring sideroblasts <15% of erythroid precursors Mainly dyserythropoiesis
Refractory anaemia with ring sideroblasts (RARS)	Anaemia Anisopoikilocytosis Dimorphic red cells Other cytopenias infrequent	and	Blasts <5% Ring sideroblasts >15% of erythroid precursors Mainly dyserythropoiesis Poor haemoglobinization of late normoblasts
Refractory anaemia with excess blasts (RAEB)	Cytopenias of two or more major lineages Blasts <5% Morphological abnormalities prominent	and	Blasts 5–20% Ring sideroblasts may be present Dysgranulopoiesis, dyserythropoiesis and dysmegakaryopoiesis in varying degrees
Chronic myelomonocytic leukaemia (CMML)	Blasts <5% Monocytes > 1 × 10⁹/l Granulocytes often increased Leucocytosis may be marked	and	Blasts usually <5%, but may be up to 20% Monocytopoiesis may be prominent
Refractory anaemia with excess blasts in transformation (RAEB-T)	Blasts >5% or any blasts with unequivocal Auer rods	or	Blasts 20–29% or any blasts with unequivocal Auer rods Morphological abnormalities may be marked

World Health Organization proposals for the classification of AML

A clinical advisory committee of the World Health Organization (WHO) has proposed a new classification system for AML. This is based not only on morphological appearances, but takes account of recurrent translocations, multilineage dysplasia, preceding haematological disorders and preceding chemo/radiotherapy.[67] A major departure from the FAB classification is as lower percentage of bone marrow blasts required (20%), thus dispensing with the FAB category of refractory anaemia with excess blasts in transformation (RAEB-T). This is based on the short clinical course of RAEB-T which is similar to AML.[68] The WHO system recognizes four major categories of AML.

AML with recurrent translocations
This group includes four subcategories, namely all cases with t(8;21), t(15;17), inv/del/t(16) and cases with 11q23 (*MLL* gene) abnormalities. Evidence of these translocations from metaphase

cytogenetics, RT–PCR or fluorescence in-situ hybridization (FISH) is sufficient to make the diagnosis, and in a departure from all other types of AML, there is no lower blast cell threshold for diagnosis. This is particularly applicable to cases with t(8;21), which occurs in FAB category M2 (the majority of cases) but also M1, RAEB-T and rarely RAEB. The morphological, biological and clinical features of the first three subcategories are distinctive. These three subtypes have good response to treatment, even though they occur in a younger age group than AML as a whole.

AML with multilineage dysplasia
Dysplasia can only be identified with the light microscope. In the granulocyte series, giant pseudo-Chediak granules in promyelocytes, hypogranular late granulocytes and abnormal nuclear segmentation of neutrophils (mononuclear, bilobed or hypersegmentation) are the main abnormalities. Dysplastic neutrophils may be MPO or Sudan black B negative. Dyserythropoiesis is manifest as

Table 13.2 FAB classification of acute myeloid leukaemia (AML)

FAB category	Criteria for FAB typing	Cytochemistry
M0 (AML with minimal evidence of myeloid maturation)	• Morphologically undifferentiated blasts • Myeloid phenotype • Lymphoid markers negative	• <3% blasts positive for SBB or MPO • No Auer rods present on SBB or MPO • Esterases negative in the blast cells
M1 (AML without maturation)	• Blasts >90% of BM non-erythroid cells (NEC) • Maturing monocytic cells <10% • Maturing granulocytes <10%	• 3–100% blasts positive for SBB or MPO • Localized pattern of positivity • SBB- or MPO-positive Auer rods frequently present • Chloroacetate esterase-positive cells <10% • NSE- or BE-positive cells scanty or absent
M2 (AML with maturation)	• Blasts 30–89% of NEC • Maturing granulocytes >10% of NEC • Monocytic component <20%	• 3–100% blasts positive for SBB or MPO • SBB- or MPO-positive Auer rods frequently present • SBB- or MPO-negative neutrophils may be present if dysplastic • Chloroacetate esterase-positive cells >10% (maturing granulocytes) • NSE- or BE-positive cells scanty or absent
M3 (Hypergranular promyelocytic leukaemia) M3 variant (Hypogranular promyelocytic leukaemia)	• M3 shows marrow replacement by granular and hypergranular promyelocytes • M3 variant shows mainly agranular basophilic cells, bilobed nuclei	• SBB and MPO show characteristic heavy staining filling the cytoplasm • Multiple SBB- or MPO-positive Auer rods present, often obscured by heavy cytoplasmic staining • Majority of cells are chloroacetate esterase-positive • Auer rods are chloroacetate esterase-positive • Leukaemic promyelocytes show a deep pink cytoplasmic blush with PAS stain • t(15;17) demonstrable by cytogenetics, RT-PCR or FISH
M4 (Acute myelomonocytic leukaemia)	• Blasts >30% of NEC • Granulocyte component >20% of BM NEC • Monocytic component >20% of BM NEC	• Esterase stains show a mixture of chloroacetate- and NSE- or BE-positive cells, usually >20% of each • Some cells may show both types of esterase • 3–100% blasts positive for SBB- or MPO, localized pattern in the myeloblasts, scattered pattern in monoblasts/monocytes • SBB- or MPO-positive Auer rods common • SBB- or MPO-negative neutrophils if dysplasia present
M4Eo	• Typical large 'eosinobasophils' present which define presence of inv/del/t(16)	• Usually conforms to M4 by conventional criteria, but may occasionally be M2 by FAB criteria • inv/del/t(16) demonstrable by cytogenetics, RT-PCR or FISH
M5a and M5b (Acute monoblastic leukaemia without maturation [M5a] and with maturation [M5b])	• Blasts>30% of BM NEC • <80% monocytic component of BM NEC • M5a when monoblasts >80% of BM NEC • M5b when monoblasts <80% of BM NEC	• Usually >80% of BM cells show NSE or BE positivity • Chloroacetate esterase-positive cells usually rare, but always <20% • SBB and MPO may be negative in the blasts/monocytes • SBB- and MPO-positive Auer rods rare

Table 13.2 (contd.)

FAB category	Criteria for FAB typing	Cytochemistry
M6 (Erythroleukaemia)	• Erythroid cells (all stages) >50% of BM nucleated cells • Myeloid blasts <30% of BM NEC	• Some/many erythroid precursors positive on PAS stain, rarely all negative • Some myeloid blasts SBB- or MPO-positive • SBB- or MPO-positive Auer rods occasionally present
M7 (Acute megakaryoblastic leukaemia)	• Blasts mainly megakaryoblasts shown by immunological methods	• Immunological confirmation of megakaryocytic blasts required • Trephine biopsy may be helpful • Megakaryoblasts may show platelet-like granules on PAS stain • Focal NSE (but not BE) positivity may be present • Myeloid blasts may show SBB or MPO positivity and rarely Auer rods

BE, butyrate esterase; BM, bone marrow; FISH, fluorescence in situ hybridization; MPO, myeloperoxidase; NSE, non-specific esterase; PAS, periodic acid-Schiff; RT–PCR, reverse transcriptase–polymerase chain reaction; SBB, Sudan black B.

binucleated or multinucleated precursors, poor haemoglobinization of late normoblasts, sideroblastic change and/or the presence of PAS positive erythroid precursors. Abnormal megakaryocytes may be hyperlobated, hypolobated, show nuclear lobe separation or be present as micromegakaryocytes. Micromegakaryocytes characteristically have heavily condensed nuclear chromatin, scanty cytoplasm showing buds or blebs, and occasionally recognizable platelet granules. Brito-Babapulle and colleagues have shown the poor remission rate in patients with de novo AML and multilineage dysplasia.[69]

WHO recognizes two subcategories of AML with multilineage dysplasia. First, cases arising de novo, with a short clinical history, and, second those cases developing from myelodysplasia and myeloproliferative disorders, and much more rarely, those cases following aplastic anaemia or paroxysmal nocturnal haemoglobinuria. WHO suggests that cases showing definite dysplasia in two or more of the three major lineages (granulocyte/monocyte, erythroid or megakaryocyte) should be included in this category.

AML therapy related

This category includes two major subtypes. AML following alkylating agent treatment, and those following epipodophyllotoxin treatment. These cases generally have a poor prognosis. They often exhibit very marked dysplasia and may follow a period of myelodysplasia.

AML not otherwise categorized

Approximately 40–50% of cases of AML do not fall into the above categories, and are identified and classified by immunophenotyping and morphological criteria, and in general follow the patterns established by the FAB group. Two new categories of AML have been added, namely acute basophilic leukaemia and a category of acute panmyelosis with myelofibrosis. Details of these two categories are awaited. Abnormal basophils may be difficult to identify on Romanowsky stains, but, if suspected, can be confirmed by toluidine blue staining. It is assumed that confirmatory genetic tests for acute promyelocytic leukaemia and inv/del/t(16) cases are available, and there are no morphological categories for acute promyelocytic leukaemia or M4Eo in this section. The recognized categories are as follows, with the 'equivalent' FAB categories in brackets:

- AML minimally differentiated (FAB M0)
- AML without maturation (FAB M1)
- AML with maturation (FAB M2)
- Acute myelomonocytic leukaemia (FAB M4)
- Acute monocytic leukaemia (FAB M5a and M5b)
- Acute erythroid leukaemia (FAB M6)
- Acute megakaryoblastic leukaemia (FAB M7)
- Acute basophilic leukaemia
- Acute panmyelosis with myelofibrosis.

ACUTE LYMPHOBLASTIC LEUKAEMIA

The modern diagnosis and classification of all forms of acute lymphoblastic leukaemia (ALL) is by immunophenotyping (see Ch. 14), but the general diagnosis of lymphoblastic leukaemia may frequently be made on cytological and cytochemical criteria.[70] On Romanowsky staining, lymphoblasts may rarely contain fine azurophil granules. Auer rods are never seen. Lymphoblasts are MPO negative, both by cytochemical and immunocytochemical methods, but true biphenotypic leukaemias may show MPO positivity.[71] The PAS stain is helpful. Although not lineage specific, the pattern of PAS positivity, if present, is helpful.[34] 95% of cases of ALL show positive blocks or granules of bright red PAS-positive material. This may be present in very few blasts (<1%) or the majority. The critical difference from granular or block positivity in other leukaemic cells is the glass-clear background cytoplasm in lymphoblasts. Myeloblasts, monoblasts, leukaemic erythroblasts and megakaryoblasts all show some degree of diffuse cytoplasmic positivity. Acid phosphatase staining is more likely to give focal positivity in T-cell than B-cell acute leukaemias but the difference is not clear enough to be of diagnostic certainty. Esterase staining is generally unhelpful, but some T-cell cases show focal positivity with ANAE.

CHRONIC MYELOPROLIFERATIVE DISORDERS

Although low NAP scores are typical in chronic phase CML, and high scores are usually found in other myeloproliferative disorders, the finding of a high NAP score is too non-specific to be of diagnostic help.

CHRONIC LYMPHOPROLIFERATIVE DISORDERS

These are now characterized by immunophenotyping. The reactions for acid hydrolases (acid phosphatase, ANAE, β-glucuronidase and β-glucosaminidase) show focal positivity in most T-cell disorders, but are negative in B-cell disorders.

REFERENCES

1 Grüneberg H 1941 Siderocytes: a new kind of erythrocyte. Nature (London) 148:469.
2 Pappenheimer AM, Thompson KP, Parker DD, et al 1945 Anaemia associated with unidentified erythrocytic inclusions after splenectomy. Quarterly Journal of Medicine 14:75.
3 Kaplan E, Zuelzer WW, Mouriquand C 1954 Sideroblasts. A study of stainable nonhemoglobin iron in marrow normoblasts. Blood 9:203.
4 Crosby WH 1957 Siderocytes and the spleen. Blood 12:165.
5 Sundberg RD, Bromann H 1955 The application of the Prussian blue stain to previously stained films of blood and bone marrow. Blood 10:160.
6 Hayhoe FGJ, Quaglino D 1960 Refractory sideroblastic anaemia and erythraemic myelosis: possible relationship and cytochemical observations. British Journal of Haematology 6:381.
7 Kass L, Eickholt MM 1978 Rapid detection of ringed sideroblasts with bromchlorphenol blue. American Journal of Clinical Pathology 70:738.
8 Bennett JM 1986 Classification of the myelodysplastic syndromes. Clinics in Haematology 15:909.
9 Rath CE, Finch CA 1948 Sternal marrow hemosiderin: a method for the determination of available iron stores in man. Journal of Laboratory and Clinical Medicine 33:81.
10 Heinz R 1890 Morphologische Veränderungen der rother Blutkörperchen durche Gifte. Virchows Archiv 122:112.
11 Dacie JV, Grimes AJ, Meisler A, et al 1964 Hereditary Heinz-body anaemia. A report of studies on five patients with mild anaemia. British Journal of Haematology 10:388.
12 Jacob HS 1970 Mechanisms of Heinz body formation and attachment to red cell membrane. Seminars in Hematology 7:341.
13 White JM 1976 The unstable haemoglobins. British Medical Bulletin 32:219.
14 Eisenger J, Flores J, Tyson JA, et al 1985 Fluorescent cytoplasm and Heinz bodies of hemoglobin Köln erythrocytes: evidence for intracellular heme catabolism. Blood 65:886.
15 Schwab MLL, Lewis AE 1969 An improved stain for Heinz bodies. American Journal of Clinical Pathology 51:673.
16 Simpson CF, Carlisle JW, Mallard L 1970 Rhodanile blue: a rapid and selective stain for Heinz bodies. Stain Technology 45:221.
17 Gouttas A, Fessas Ph, Tsevrenis H, et al 1955 Description d'une nouvelle variété d'anémie hémolytique congénitale. Sang 26:911.
18 Lin CK, Gau JP, Hsu HC, et al 1990 Efficacy of a modified technique for detecting red cell haemoglobin H inclusions. Clinical and Laboratory Haematology 12: 409.
19 Van Noorden CJF, Vogels IMC 1985 A sensitive cytochemical staining method for glucose-6-phosphate dehydrogenase activity in individual erythrocytes. British Journal of Haematology 60:57.

20 Kleihauer E, Braun H, Betke K 1957 Demonstration von fetalem Hämoglobin in den Erythrocyten eines Blutausstrichs. Klinische Wochenschrift 35:637.

21 Nierhaus K, Betke K 1968 Eine vereinfachte Modifikation der säuren Elution für die cytologische Darstellung von fetalem Hämoglobin. Klinische Wochenschrift 46:47.

22 Clayton EM, Felhaus WD, Phython JM 1963 The demonstration of fetal erythrocytes in the presence of adult red blood cells. American Journal of Clinical Pathology 40:487.

23 Tomoda Y 1964 Demonstration of foetal erythrocytes by immunofluorescent staining. Nature (London) 202:910.

24 Thorpe SJ, Huehns EG 1983 A new approach for the antenatal diagnosis of β-thalassaemia: a double labelling immunofluorescence microscopy technique. British Journal of Haematology 53:103.

25 Headings V, Bhattacharya S, Shukla S, et al 1975 Identification of specific hemoglobins within individual erythrocytes. Blood 45:263.

26 Papayannopoulou Th, McGuire TC, Lim G, et al 1976 Identification of haemoglobin S in red cells and normoblasts using fluorescent anti-Hb antibodies. British Journal of Haematology 34:25.

27 Fairbanks VF, Lampe LT 1968 A tetrazolium-linked cytochemical method for estimation of glucose-6-phosphate dehydrogenase activity in individual erythrocytes: applications in the study of heterozygotes for glucose-6-phosphate dehydrogenase deficiency. Blood 31:589.

28 Gall JC, Brewer GJ, Dern RJ 1965 Studies of glucose-6-phosphate dehydrogenase activity of individual erythrocytes: the methaemoglobin-elution test for identification of females heterozygous for G6PD deficiency. American Journal of Human Genetics 17:359.

29 Tönz O, Rossi E 1964 Morphological demonstration of two red cell populations in human females heterozygous for glucose-6-phosphate dehydrogenase deficiency. Nature (London) 202:606.

30 Kleihauer E, Betke K 1963 Elution procedure for the demonstration of methaemoglobin in red cells of human blood smears. Nature (London) 199:1196.

31 Vogels IMC, Van Noorden CJF, Wolf BHM, et al 1986 Cytochemical determination of heterozygous glucose-6-phosphate dehydrogenase deficiency in erythrocytes. British Journal of Haematology 63:402.

32 Shibata A, Bennett JM, Castoldi GL, et al 1985 Recommended methods for cytological procedures in haematology. Clinical and Laboratory Haematology 7:55.

33 International Council for Standardization in Haematology 1993 Procedures for the classification of acute leukaemias. Leukemia and Lymphoma 11:37–48.

34 Hayhoe FGJ, Quaglino D 1988 Haematological cytochemistry, 2nd edn. Edinburgh: Churchill Livingstone.

35 Graham RC, Karnovsky MJ 1966 The early stages of absorption of injected horseradish peroxidase in the proximal tubules of mouse kidney: ultrastructural cytochemistry by a new technique. Journal of Histochemistry and Cytochemistry 14:291.

36 Novikoff AB, Goldfischer S 1969 Visualization of peroxisomes (microbodies and mitochondria with diaminobenzidine). Journal of Histochemistry and Cytochemistry 17:675.

37 Elias JM 1980 A rapid sensitive myeloperoxidase stain using 4-chloro-1-naphthol. American Journal of Clinical Pathology 73:797.

38 Graham RC, Lundholm U, Karnovsky MJ 1965 Cytochemical demonstration of peroxidase activity with 3-amino-9-ethylcarbazole. Journal of Histochemistry and Cytochemistry 13:150.

39 Lillie RD, Burtner HJ 1953 Stable sudanophilia of human neutrophil leucocytes in relation to peroxidase and oxidase. Journal of Histochemistry and Cytochemistry 1:8.

40 Sheehan HL, Storey GW 1974 An improved method of staining leucocyte granules with Sudan Black B. Journal of Pathology and Bacteriology 49:580.

41 Stass SA, Pui C-H, Mel Vin S, et al 1984 Sudan black B positive acute lymphoblastic leukaemia. British Journal of Haematology 57:413.

42 Rosner F, Lee SL 1965 Endocrine relationships of leukocyte alkaline phosphatase. Blood 25:356.

43 Poppema S, Elema JD, Halie MR 1981 Alkaline phosphatase positive lymphomas: A morphologic, immunologic and enzyme histochemical study. Cancer 47: 1303.

44 Gomori G 1952 Microscopic histochemistry. Principles and practice. Chicago: University of Chicago Press.

45 Kaplow LS 1955 A histochemical procedure for localizing and evaluating leucocyte alkaline phosphatase activity in smears of blood and marrow. Blood 10:1023.

46 Kaplow LS 1963 Cytochemistry of leukocyte alkaline phosphatase. Use of complex naphthol AS phosphates in azo-dye coupling technics. American Journal of Clinical Pathology 39:439.

47 Rustin GJS, Wilson PD, Peters TJ 1979 Studies on the subcellular localisation of human neutrophil alkaline phosphatase. Journal of Cell Science 36:401.

48 Kaplow LS 1968 Leukocyte alkaline phosphatase cytochemistry: applications and methods. Annals of the New York Academy of Sciences 155:911.

49 Hayhoe FGJ, Quaglino D 1958 Cytochemical demonstration and measurement of leucocyte alkaline phosphatase in normal and pathological states by modified azo-dye coupling technique. British Journal of Haematology 4:375.

50 Rutenberg AB, Rosales CL, Bennett JM 1965 An important histochemical method for the demonstration of leukocyte alkaline phosphatase activity: clinical applications. Journal of Laboratory and Clinical Medicine 65:698.

51 Bendix-Hansen K, Helleberg-Rasmussen I 1985 I. Evaluation of neutrophil alkaline phosphatase. Untreated myeloid leukaemia, lymphoid leukaemia and normal humans. Scandinavian Journal of Haematology 34:264.

52 Yam LT, Li CY, Lam KW 1971 Tartrate-resistant acid phosphatase isoenzyme in the reticulum cells of leukemic reticuloendotheliosis. New England Journal of Medicine 284:357.

53 Li Cy, Yam LT, Lam KW 1970 Acid phosphatase isoenzyme in human leucocytes in normal and pathologic conditions. Journal of Histochemistry and Cytochemistry 18:473.

54 Goldberg AF, Barka T 1962 Acid phosphatase activity in human blood cells. Nature 195:297.

55 Hotchkiss RD 1948 A microchemical reaction resulting in the staining of polysaccharide structures in fixed tissue preparations. Archives of Biochemistry 16:131.

56 Higgy KE, Burns GF, Hayhoe FGJ 1977 Discrimination of B, T and null lymphocytes by esterase cytochemistry. Scandinavian Journal of Haematology 18:437.

57 Quaglino D, Hayhoe FGJ 1959 Observations on the periodic acid-Schiff reaction in lymphoproliferative diseases. Journal of Pathology and Bacteriology 78:521.

58 Li CY, Yam LT, Lam KW 1973 Esterases in human leucocytes. Journal of Histochemistry and Cytochemistry 21:1.

59 Swirsky DM, Li YS, Matthews JG, et al 1983 8; 21 translocation in acute granulocytic leukaemia: cytological, cytochemical and clinical features. British Journal of Haematology 56:199.

60 Swirsky DM 1984 Single incubation double esterase cytochemical reaction using a single coupling reagent. Journal of Clinical Pathology 37:1187.

61 Lam KW, Li CY, Yam LT 1985 Simultaneous demonstration of non-specific esterase and chloro-acetate esterase in human blood cells. Stain Technology 60:169.

62 Bennett JM, Catovsky D, Daniel M-T, et al 1982 Proposals for the classification of the myelodysplastic syndromes. British Journal of Haematology 51:189.

63 Bennett JM, Catovsky D, Daniel M-T, et al 1976 Proposals for the classification of the acute leukaemias FAB cooperative group. British Journal of Haematology 33:451.

64 Bennett JM, Catovsky D, Daniel M-T, et al 1985 Proposed revised criteria for the classification of acute myeloid leukaemia. British Journal of Haematology 103:626.

65 Bennett JM, Catovsky D, Daniel M-T et al 1985 Criteria for the diagnosis of acute leukaemia of megakaryocytic lineage (M7) A report of the French-American-British cooperative group. Annals of Internal Medicine 103:460.

66 Bennett JM, Catovsky D, Daniel M-T, et al 1991 Proposal for the recognition of minimally differentiated acute myeloid leukaemia (AML-M British Journal of Haematology 78:325.

67 Harris NL, Jaffe ES, Diebold J, et al 1999 WHO classification of neoplastic disease of the hematopoietic and lymphoid tissue. Journal of Clinical Oncology 17:3835.

68 Greenberg P, Cox C, Lebeau MM, et al 1997 International scoring system for evaluating prognosis in myelodysplastic syndromes. Blood 89:2079.

69 Brito-Babapulle F, Catovsky D, Galton DA 1987 Clinical and laboratory features of de novo acute myeloid leukaemia with trilineage myelodysplasia. British Journal of Haematology 66:445.

70 Bennett JM, Catovsky D, Daniel M-T, et al 1981 The morphological classification of acute lymphoblastic leukaemia – concordance among observers and clinical correlations. British Journal of Haematology 47:553.

71 Matutes E, Morilla R, Farahat N, et al 1997 Definition of acute biphenotypic leukemia. Haematologica 82:64.

14

Immunophenotyping

E. Matutes, R. Morilla & D. Catovsky

INTRODUCTION

Since the development of the hybridoma technology in the 1970s, there have been major advances in the immunophenotypic characterization of haemopoietic malignancies and this, in turn, has resulted in a better understanding of normal haemopoietic differentiation. Prior to the availability of monoclonal antibodies (McAbs), it was possible to distinguish B from T lymphocytes and mature from early lymphoid precursor cells by the expression of surface or cytoplasmic immunoglobulins in B lymphocytes, the ability to form rosettes with sheep erythrocytes (E-rosettes) in T lymphocytes and the expression of the nuclear enzyme terminal deoxynucleotidyl transferase (TdT) in lymphoid precursors. Over the last two decades, the application of new technology has had a major impact on the diagnosis of acute and chronic leukaemias and has also provided clues to the pathogenesis of these disorders and useful information for monitoring the detection of small numbers of residual leukaemic cells.

In addition to the availability of a large number of McAbs that identify antigens in haemopoietic cells which are lineage specific and/or are restricted to particular levels of differentiation, a number of immunological techniques have been developed which permit:

1. detection of both membrane and cytoplasmic or nuclear antigens by flow cytometry in previously fixed and stabilized cells;
2. simultaneous double and triple immunostaining with directly labelled McAb with different fluorochromes;
3. analysis of whole blood or bone marrow specimens without requiring to separate mononuclear cells;
4. quantification of the number of molecules at a single cell level;
5. analysis of selected cell populations such as the estimation of CD34 stem cells by applying gating strategies to CD45-labelled cells.

Although the important diagnostic role of immunophenotyping is well recognized, results should always be interpreted in the light of morphology and other relevant laboratory data.

This chapter includes descriptions of:

1. techniques currently used for immunophenotyping;
2. panel of markers useful for the diagnosis of acute leukaemia and chronic lymphoproliferative disorders and the rationale for their selection;
3. immunophenotypic profiles that characterize the different types of acute leukaemias and chronic lymphoproliferative disorders;

4. use of new McAbs, e.g. against the tumour suppressor gene p53 and cyclin D1, which are relevant for prognosis and differential diagnosis;
5. strategies to detect minimal residual disease by immunophenotyping.

METHODS FOR THE STUDY OF IMMUNOLOGICAL MARKERS

There are several ways of testing cell markers:

1. flow cytometry to test suspensions of viable cells or fixed cells;
2. immunocytochemistry to examine cells on cytospin-made slides, or directly on blood or bone marrow films;
3. immunohistochemistry to study cells in frozen or paraffin-embedded sections from bone marrow biopsies or other haemopoietic tissues.

The first two methods are used in haematology laboratories dealing with analysis of leukaemic samples and the last is used, as a rule, in histopathology laboratories.

PREPARATION OF THE SPECIMENS AND CELL SEPARATION

Immunophenotyping can be performed on isolated mononuclear (MN) cells as described below or in whole blood specimens using adequate lysing solutions.

The MN cell fraction contains lymphocytes, monocytes, blasts and other MN cells (according to the sample). Methods for separating MN cells include density gradient centrifugation with Ficoll-Triosil, Hypaque or Lymphoprep. When necessary, platelets can also be excluded by defibrinating the blood before separation.

Lymphoprep method of separation (Nycomed)
Dilute 10 ml of anticoagulated (e.g. heparinized) blood with an equal volume of phosphate buffer saline, pH 7.3 (p. 606) or Hanks' solution. Add 10 ml of the diluted blood, drop by drop, to 7.5 ml of Lymphoprep and then centrifuge for 30 min at 2000 rpm*. There are three layers visible: upper plasma layer, a rim of MN cells in the middle and the bottom layer containing red cells and neutrophils. After removing the plasma, pipette the MN cell layer into another tube and wash three times with Hanks solution or tissue culture medium.

---

* Approximately 500 g (see p. 609)

Lysing method
Blood and bone marrow samples are treated with a hypotonic erythrocyte lysing solution of commercial NH_4Cl^- bases containing reagents. These are often supplied by the manufacturers of McAb, e.g. FACS lysing solution (Becton Dickinson). The samples are treated at the time of incubation with the McAb (see below) without loss of fractions of MN cells. The time of incubation with the lysing reagent is important as prolonged exposure may alter the forward and side light scatter (FSC/SSC) patterns while too short exposure leaves red cells intact, resulting in excess debris, making the results inaccurate.

Prior to incubation with the lysing solution, the white cell count of the blood or bone marrow specimen should be estimated and, if necessary, the sample should be diluted to a maximum white cell concentration of $25–30 \times 10^6$ cells/ml.

Flow cytometry methods
Immunophenotyping on cell suspensions is the method for detecting membrane antigens in viable cells and cytoplasmic and nuclear antigens in previously fixed and stabilized cells. If a flow cytometer is not available, reading can also be performed by fluorescence microscopy. Both flow cytometry or fluorescence microscopy permit simultaneous detection of membrane and nuclear or cytoplasmic antigens by means of double or triple immunostaining.

DETECTION OF MEMBRANE ANTIGENS

Direct immunofluorescence (double staining) (Fig. 14.1)
Label tubes with the name of the patient, type of specimen, laboratory number and the combination of fluorochrome-conjugated McAb including isotopic controls. The latter are mouse immunoglobulin (Ig) of the same isotope as the McAb but with no antigen specificity.

Pipette 100 µl of specimen (whole peripheral blood or bone marrow).

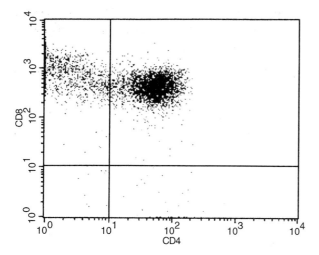

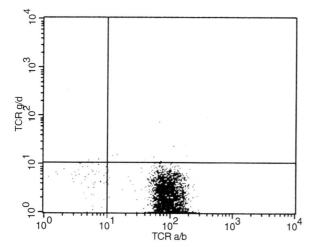

Fig. 14.1 Double direct immunofluorescence staining.
Upper: Dot plot showing the coexpression of CD4 and CD8 in cells from a case of T-cell prolymphocytic leukaemia.
Lower: Dot plot showing that the majority of lymphocytes express in the membrane the T-cell receptor (TCR) α/β complex and are negative with McAb against the TCR γ/δ complex.

Add the appropriate McAb combination labelled with fluorescein (FITC), phycoerythrin (PE) or tricolour. The volume of the McAb ranges between 5 and 20 μl according to the manufacturer's instructions.

Incubate at room temperature for 15 min.

Add 1 ml of lysing solution (commercially available from the McAb manufacturer) and leave for 10 min at room temperature. Centrifuge for 5 min at 2000 rpm and discard the supernatant.

Add 2 ml of phosphate buffered saline (PBS) (pH 7.3) containing 0.02% sodium azide, 0.02% bovine serum albumin (BSA) and 0.01% EDTA (PBS-azide-BSA). Centrifuge for 5 min at 2000 rpm and discard supernatant.

Add 2 ml of PBS-azide-BSA or Hanks solution, centrifuge for 5 min at 2000 rpm and discard the supernatant.

Resuspend the cells in 0.2–0.5 ml of sheath fluid solution (e.g. Isoton, Beckman Coulter).

Read on a flow cytometer or by fluorescence microscopy after mounting the cells on a slide.

Indirect immunofluorescence (single staining)

Label tubes with the name of the patient, type of specimen, laboratory number and the McAb.

Add 100 μl of specimen (whole blood or bone marrow).

Add the appropriate McAb (first layer non-labelled antibody). The volume ranges from 5 to 20 μl according to the manufacturer's instructions. Incubate at room temperature for 15 min.

Add 2 ml of PBS-azide-BSA or Hanks solution and centrifuge for 5 min at 2000 rpm.

Discard supernatant and repeat this step once more.

Following the manufacturer's instructions, add the appropriate volume and concentration of the second layer which is usually a goat or a rabbit anti-mouse Ig F(ab)2 fragment.

Incubate for 15 min at room temperature.

Add 1 ml of lysing solution (commercially available from the McAb manufacturer) for 10 min at room temperature. Centrifuge for 5 min at 2000 rpm and discard the supernatant.

Add 2 ml of PBS-azide-BSA, centrifuge for 5 min at 2000 rpm and discard the supernatant after centrifugation.

Resuspend the cells in 0.25 to 0.5 ml of sheath fluid solution (e.g. Isoton) provided by the manufacturer.

Read on a flow cytometer or by fluorescence microscopy.

DETECTION OF SURFACE IMMUNOGLOBULIN

Surface Ig heavy and light chains can be detected by means of double or triple immunostaining. The object is to demonstrate clonality of a B-cell population. Double staining uses double colour conjugated polyclonal anti-kappa and anti-lambda labelled with different fluorochromes in a single tube (Fig. 14.2) or combines a FITC-labelled B-cell marker, e.g. CD19, and a PE-labelled anti-light chain, either anti-kappa or anti-lambda. The triple colour immunostaining combines a FITC-conjugated anti-kappa, PE-conjugated anti-lambda and a B-cell marker, e.g. CD19, labelled with a third colour in a single tube.

The immunostaining of surface Ig differs from the method used to detect other surface antigens by McAb. The reason is that soluble serum Ig coats the surface of cells, mainly monocytes but also lymphocytes, and interferes with the detection of Ig, giving rise to misleading results, false positive or false negative. To overcome this problem, cells have to be washed with Hanks solution or PBS prior to incubating with the anti-kappa and anti-lambda reagents.

There are two methods suitable for detecting surface Ig in blood and bone marrow cells, according to whether a PBS wash or a lysing procedure is used as the first step.

Method 1 (PBS wash as first step, no lysing)
Label tubes with the name of the patient, type of specimen, laboratory number and the McAb.

Pipette 100 μl of the specimen (blood or bone marrow)

Add 2 ml of PBS-azide-BSA kept at 37°C and centrifuge for 5 min at 2000 rpm. Using a pipette, carefully discard the supernatant. Repeat the procedure and resuspend the specimen in 50 μl of PBS-azide-BSA.

Add the appropriate McAb combination, e.g. anti-kappa and anti-lambda or CD19 and anti-kappa. The volume of the McAb is usually between 5 and 20 μl according to the manufacturer's instructions.

Incubate at room temperature for 15 min.

Add 1 ml of lysing solution (commercially available from most McAb manufacturers) and incubate for 10 min at room temperature.

Add 1 ml of PBS-azide-BSA or Hanks solution, centrifuge for 5 min at 2000 rpm, and discard the supernatant. Repeat this step again.

Resuspend cells in 0.2–0.5 ml of sheath fluid solution (e.g. Isoton).

Read on a flow cytometer or by fluorescence microscopy.

Method 2 (lysing as first step)
Label tubes with the name of the patient, type of specimen, laboratory number and the McAb.

Pipette 100 μl of the specimen (whole blood or bone marrow).

Add 2 ml of lysing solution, incubate for 10 min at room temperature and wash twice in PBS-azide-BSA.

Add the appropriate volume of McAb combination according to the manufacturer's recommendations.

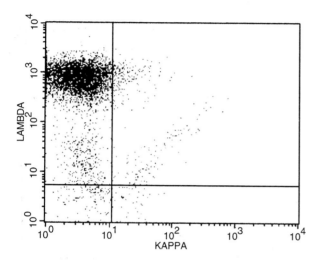

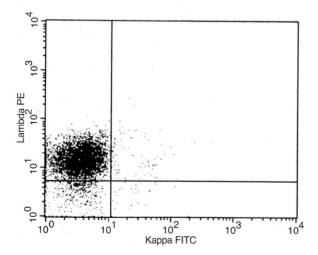

Fig. 14.2 Surface immunoglobulin light chain staining.
Upper: Dot plot showing strong expression of lambda light chain in a case of follicular lymphoma.
Lower: By contrast to the upper case, weak/dim expression of lambda light chain in a case of chronic lymphocytic leukaemia. Cells are negative with anti-kappa in both cases.

Incubate for 15 min at 40°C.

Add 2 ml of PBS-azide-BSA or Hanks solution, centrifuge for 5 min at 2000 rpm and discard the supernatant. Repeat this step.

Resuspend cells in 0.2–0.5 ml of sheath fluid (e.g. Isoton) and read on a flow cytometer.

DETECTION OF INTRACELLULAR ANTIGENS

There are several commercially available kits containing solutions to fix and stabilize cells in order to detect cytoplasmic and/or nuclear antigens. Overall, these reagents have little or no effect on the light scatter pattern although their reliability and consistency for detecting particular nuclear and cytoplasmic antigens may vary.[1,2]

The kits contain two solutions: solution A is the fixing agent based in a paraformaldehyde solution and solution B is a stabilizing agent based on a combination of a lysing solution and a detergent.

The methods follow the manufacturer's kit instructions. Details are given below for the method using Fix and Perm (Caltag, Burlingame, Ca, USA).

Method

Label tubes with the name of the patient, type of specimen, laboratory number and the McAb.

Pipette 100 µl of specimen (whole blood or bone marrow) into a tube.

Add 100 µl of solution A (fixative) and incubate at room temperature for 15 min.

Wash twice in PBS-azide-BSA by centrifuging for 5 min at 2000 rpm.

Add 100 µl of solution B (stabilizing) and the appropriate amount of fluorochrome conjugated McAb.

Incubate at room temperature for 15 min.

Wash twice in PBS-azide-BSA, centrifuging for 5 min at 2000 rpm.

Resuspend in 0.2–0.5 ml of sheath fluid solution (e.g. Isoton).

Read on a flow cytometer.

SIMULTANEOUS DETECTION OF CYTOPLASMIC/ NUCLEAR AND MEMBRANE ANTIGENS (FIG. 14.3)
Method

The first step involves immunostaining for detecting the membrane antigen, followed by cytoplasmic or nuclear antigen detection.

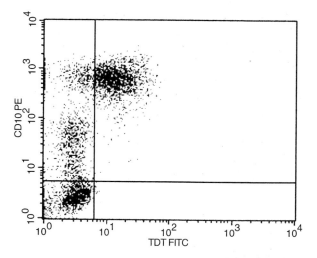

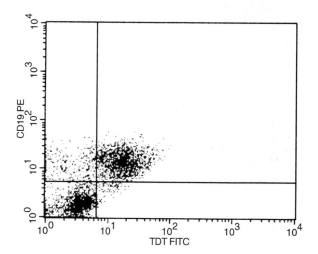

Fig. 14.3 Simultaneous detection of membrane and nuclear antigens.
Upper: Dot plot illustrating the coexpression of CD10 in the cell membrane and nuclear terminal deoxynucleotidyl transferase (TdT) in cells from a case with a common acute lymphoblastic leukaemia.
Lower: Coexpression of membrane CD19 and nuclear TdT in the same case.

Label tubes with the name of the patient, type of specimen, laboratory number and McAb.

Pipette 100 µl of specimen (whole blood or bone marrow) into a tube.

Add the appropriate fluorochrome conjugated McAb, usually PE, to detect the membrane antigen.

Incubate at room temperature for 15 min.

Add 1 ml of lysing solution and incubate for 10 min at room temperature. This solution is commercially available from most manufacturers.

Add 1 ml of PBS-azide-BSA or Hanks solution, centrifuge for 5 min at 2000 rpm and discard the supernatant.

Add 15 µl of solution A (fixative) and incubate at room temperature for 15 min. Then continue with the steps described above.

QUANTIFICATION OF ANTIGENS

Quantification is defined as the measurement of the intensity of staining of cells by flow cytometry to provide an absolute value for the light intensity it measures.[3,4]

Quantification of fluorescence is performed by comparing cell fluorescence with an external standard. By using different commercially available beads, it is now possible to measure the quantity of fluorescence relative to the peak channel obtained by flow cytometry using a standard curve for its calculation. Fluorescence quantification can be expressed in terms of antibody binding capacity (ABC) or molecules equivalent soluble fluorochrome (MESF).

The method involves either *indirect immunofluorescence* or *direct immunofluorescence*. As the latter is simpler, it is the method generally used in routine practice. It comprises four separate steps:

1. choice of quantification kit;
2. staining of cells and beads;
3. acquisition of data;
4. quantification – calculation of the ABC or MESF values.

There are three essential requirements for successful quantification, namely (a) the McAb has to be applied at saturating amounts both for the beads and the cells in the specimen; (b) the same reagent from a specified company and at the same dilution should be used for the test and for any subsequent tests; (c) the instrument fluorescence setting should be maintained unchanged once the beads have been run, and analysis of the unknown sample should be carried out at the same settings.

The type of bead depends on the procedure used for the sample preparation. The beads are commercially available in kits which usually comprise two tubes. One tube contains a mixture of four beads with four different levels of fluorescence uptake: one very dim, one very bright and two intermediate; the other tube contains a blank, e.g. non-fluorescent beads (Fig. 14.4).

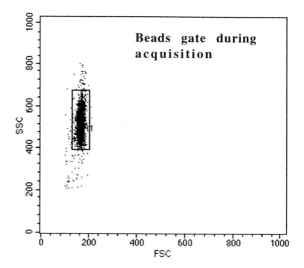

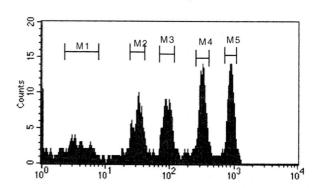

Marker	Left, Right	Events	% Gated	% Total	Peak	Peak Ch
All	1, 9910	1931	100.00	100.00	36	1
M1	2, 8	216	11.19	11.19	6	2
M2	25, 42	292	15.12	15.12	11	31
M3	71, 121	295	15.28	15.28	12	85
M4	262, 414	355	18.38	18.38	18	310
M5	730, 1114	340	17.61	17.61	19	842

Fig. 14.4 Beads for antigen quantification.
Upper: Gate used for the acquisition of the beads to eliminate doublets.
Lower: Beads fluorescence intensity showing five peaks: blank (M1); dim (M2); bright (M5); intermediate (M3 and M4).

1. Choice of quantification kit

Direct immunofluorescence

QSC (Quantum Simply Cellular, Sigma) are beads coated with goat anti-mouse Ig which are used to quantify direct immunofluorescence and to measure the ABC when saturated with the same fluorochrome-conjugated McAb as used in the cell sample. Each level of the standard can bind to a certain amount of mouse Ig. The beads require separate calibration for each McAb.

Indirect immunofluorescence

QIFIKIT (Dako) are beads coated with McAb which mimic McAb-bearing cells. As these receptors bind to the secondary antibody used to stain both the cells and the beads they require only one calibration per experiment.[4]

Direct and indirect immunofluorescence

FCSC (Quantum beads) (Flow Cytometry Standards Corporation, San Juan) are coated with known molecules of fluorochrome and are available conjugated to FITC or PE to measure the MESF. The fluorescence of the cells is compared to that of standard molecules of fluorochrome.

2. Staining of cells and beads

After the quantification beads have been set up, begin the staining of cells by one of the methods described below, depending on the antigen to be quantified. This could be a membrane, nuclear or cytoplasmic antigen or combinations of two of them.

Direct immunofluorescence

Label a 5 ml round bottom tube as the McAb to be quantified with beads.

Add 50 µl of QSC beads and 10 µl of the McAb to the appropriate tubes and incubate for 1 h at 4°C.

Add 2 ml of PBS-azide-BSA to each tube and centrifuge for 5 min at 2000 rpm. Discard the supernatant and resuspend in 250 µl of sheath fluid (e.g. Isoton).

Indirect immunofluorescence

Label a 5 ml round bottom tube as beads.

Add 100 µl of beads and the secondary antibody (anti-mouse) to the tube with the beads and stain for 1 h at 4°C.

Add 2 ml of PBS-azide-BSA to each tube and centrifuge for 5 min at 2000 rpm. Discard the supernatant and resuspend in 250 µl of Isoton.

Direct and indirect immunofluorescence

Label a 5 ml round bottom tube as Quantum beads.

Add 100 µl of beads and stain for 1 h at 4°C.

Then add 2 ml of PBS-azide-BSA to each tube and centrifuge for 5 min at 2000 rpm.

Discard the supernatant and resuspend in 250 µl of sheath fluid (e.g. Isoton).

3. Acquisition of data

The first step involves acquisition of data relating to the beads on a flow cytometer. The data from a single tube with beads are sufficient for quantification with FCSC Quantum beads and QIFIKIT beads. With QSC where a tube is run for each McAb, the tube with the beads for that particular McAb should be run, first followed by all the relevant tubes with beads for each of the different McAbs.

In order to bring the beads into the FSC/SSC dot plot, the SSC voltage must be decreased more than for cells. There may be some doublets if the tube was not shaken vigorously, and these are excluded by placing a tight gate around the beads and acquiring the data only for these gated beads. The instrument should be set up so that the fluorescence signal of the tube with the blank (unlabelled) beads is located in the region between 0 and 101 and four other peaks of fluorescence should be seen along the axis of the relevant fluorochrome. When the fluorescence voltage is established, these settings should be maintained throughout the rest of the analysis of the unknown samples. With QSC, the appropriate settings for each individual McAb must be used.

The data for the samples are then obtained. With the FCSC Quantum Cellular and QIFIKIT, only one set of beads is required as the same fluorescence standard curve can be used for the different McAbs to be quantified (CD5, CD19, CD4, CD8, etc.). With QSC, one set of fluorescence beads is stained for each McAb. The samples for a particular McAb should be run with the fluorescence settings obtained from beads stained with the corresponding McAb, so that one fluorescence standard curve should be obtained for each McAb. Thus, one curve is required with CD5-stained beads for all CD5-stained samples; one curve with CD19-stained beads for CD19-stained samples, etc.

4. Quantification: calculation of ABC or MESF values

Relevant software is provided with the quantification kits. These programs are user friendly and take into account the make of the instrument, voltage used for the sample, the fluorochrome used and the source of the McAb. When the data obtained from the flow cytometer is entered, a standard curve is automatically produced. The standard calibration curve is produced when the values of the peak channels of the blank and the other four peaks obtained from the flow cytometer are entered into the program. The known number of molecules of fluorochrome obtained from the supplier of the beads is also entered into the program. The peak values for the unknown sample and one of the negative control are obtained by running them at the same fluorescence setting as the beads. When the peak value obtained with the sample is entered into the program, the ABC/MESF value of the unknown sample is calculated and the data are saved. For the final estimation of the ABC or MESF, the ABC or MESF value of the control tube is deducted from the ABC or MESF value of the marker.

IMMUNOCYTOCHEMISTRY

The commonest immunocytochemical techniques are the immunoperoxidase (IP) and the alkaline phosphatase anti-alkaline phosphatase (APAAP) methods.[5,6] These detect both membrane and intracellular antigens prior to fixation of the preparation. The APAAP method is suitable for use on blood and bone marrow films and permits good preservation of cell morphology. IP is simpler than APAAP and is useful for the study of mature and immature lymphoid cells, but bone marrow samples containing myeloid cells with endogenous peroxidase may give a false-positive reaction unless steps are taken to inhibit the endogenous peroxidase activity. Unfortunately, these procedures may affect cell morphology and thus defeat one of the purposes of the test.

IMMUNOPEROXIDASE (IP)

The IP method can be carried out with directly labelled antibodies (e.g. anti-human Ig conjugated with peroxidase) or by indirect methods using two or three layers. The first layer is a McAb (mouse Ig); the second layer is an anti-mouse Ig antibody conjugated with horse-radish peroxidase; a third layer is a complex of peroxidase anti-peroxidase which binds to the second layer, and is used to reinforce the reaction. The reaction is completed by testing for peroxidase, using diaminobenzidine (DAB).

Method

Prepare cytocentrifuge slides and allow them to dry for at least 6–8 h at room temperature. If not used immediately, they should be wrapped in foil paper and stored at −20°C. Before testing, frozen material must be thawed at room temperature for 30 min. Make a ring around the chosen area using a diamond pencil.

Fix the slides in pure acetone for 10 min. If they have been kept at room temperature for more than 3 days, fix them for only 5 min.

Dry in the air and then surround the cells with a silicone ring (Dako pen or Sigmacote).

Incubate for 30 min in a moist chamber with 30 μl of McAb diluted in PBS. The dilution of the McAb should be titrated in the individual laboratory for each batch of reagent, using known positive and negative controls.

Wash (flush) carefully with PBS (pH 7.3). Do not let the slides dry and add the second layer antibody immediately after the second wash.

Incubate for 30 min with 30 μl of peroxidase-conjugated rabbit anti-mouse antibody (Dako) diluted 1:20 in PBS (pH 7.3) containing 2% human AB serum.

Wash (flush) carefully with PBS (pH 7.3) twice as above.

Incubate for 30 min in a moist chamber with 30 μl of peroxidase-labelled swine anti-rabbit antibody (Dako) diluted 1:20 in PBS (pH 7.3) containing 2% human AB serum.

Wash (flush) carefully with PBS (pH 7.3) twice as above.

Prepare an IP solution of 30 mg of DAB with 30% hydrogen peroxide in 50 ml of PBS; filter and pour into a coupling jar. Immerse the slides in this solution and incubate for 10 min at room temperature in the dark.

Note that the peroxidase substrate (DAB) is carcinogenic and must be handled with safety precautions, using a fume cupboard and gloves. As an alternative safer procedure, tablets of DAB which are available commercially (Dako) can be diluted in PBS as above.

Rinse in distilled water.

Counterstain with Harris haematoxylin for 10–20 s.

Wash in tap water for 2 min

Wipe off excess water, let the slides dry in the air and mount with DPX.

For assessment of the reactivity with anti-TdT or other rabbit polyclonal antibody, carry out an additional incubation for 30 min with a mouse anti-rabbit antibody diluted 1:20 in PBS (pH 7.3) with 2% human AB serum prior to the incubation with the second layer of peroxidase-conjugated rabbit anti-mouse antibody.

Interpretation

A positive reaction is shown by light microscopy as a dark brown deposit.

IMMUNOALKALINE PHOSPHATASE ANTI-ALKALINE PHOSPHATASE (APAAP)

The APAAP method involves several steps which can be applied to peripheral blood and bone marrow films. The stages include: incubation with the McAb, incubation with a rabbit anti-mouse Ig, and incubation with immune complexes of APAAP. The second and third steps can be repeated to reinforce the reaction.

Method

Make films or cytocentrifuge slides and let them dry for at least 6 or 8 h. If not used immediately, wrap them in foil paper and store at –20°C. If frozen, thaw at room temperature for 30 min before carrying out the test.

Make a ring around the chosen area using a diamond pencil. To test more than one McAb in the same slide, several rings can be marked.

Fix in pure cold acetone for 10 min. If the slides have been kept at room temperature for over 72 hours, fix them for only 5 min.

Allow to dry in the air.

When using peripheral blood or bone marrow films, wash around the encircled areas with a cotton stick wet with PBS to remove the adjacent red blood cells.

Surround the circled areas with a silicone ring (Dako pen or Sigmacote).

Incubate for 30 min with 30 µl of McAb diluted in Tris buffered saline (TBS) 0.05 mol/l, pH 7.6. The appropriate dilution of the McAb must be determined by titrating each batch of reagent, using known positive and negative controls.

For all subsequent procedures, the slides must not be allowed to dry and incubation must be carried out in a moist chamber.

Wash (flush) carefully with TBS 0.05 mol/l and, immediately after the wash, add 20 µl of the second layer consisting of a rabbit anti-mouse Ig (Dako) diluted in TBS 0.05 mol/l with 2% human AB serum.

Incubate for 30 min at room temperature in a moist chamber.

Wash (flush) again with TBS.

Incubate for 45 min with 100 µl of mouse APAAP complexes (Dako) diluted 1:60 in TBS 0.05 mol/l.

Wash (flush) again with TBS.

Cover the circles with the filtered APAAP developing solution for 15–20 min.

Rinse in distilled water.

Counterstain with Harris haematoxylin for 10–20 s.

Wash in tap water for 2 min.

Wipe off excess water and mount with Glycergel (Dako). Do not use DPX to cover preparations.

For estimation of the reactivity with anti-TdT or other polyclonal rabbit antibody, carry out a further incubation step with a mouse anti-rabbit antibody diluted 1:20 in TBS prior to the incubation with the second layer.

Buffers

Tris buffered saline 0.05M, pH 7.6 (to wash and dilute McAb). Make a stock solution with: 60.57 g of tris-hidroxymethyl-methylamine in 500 ml of distilled water. Adjust pH to 7.6 with 385 ml of 1N HCl. Add distilled water to 1 litre and store at 4°C.

To prepare the working solution, dilute the stock solution 1:10 in 9 g/l NaCl.

Tris buffered saline 0.1M, pH:8.2 (to dilute the substrate). Make a stock solution with 1.21 g of

Tris and 80 ml of water. Adjust pH to 8.2 with 4.8 ml of 1N HCl. Add water to 100 ml (this solution can be stored for 1 month at 4°C).

Developing solution (substrate). Mix in the following order 20 mg of naphthol AS-MX phosphate (Sigma), 2 ml of N,N-dimethylformamide (Merck), 98 ml of Tris buffer 0.1 mol/l and 24 mg of levamisole (Sigma).

Store in glass flasks at −20°C in 5 ml aliquots.

Thaw immediately before use; add 5 mg of fast red TR salt (Sigma) per vial and filter.

The developing solution is also available commercially as a kit.

IMMUNOLOGICAL MARKERS IN ACUTE LEUKAEMIA

Panel of McAb for diagnosis and classification

Although there are a large number of McAb-recognizing antigens in haemopoietic cells, for practical reasons a well-defined set of reagents needs to be selected aimed at aiding in the diagnosis of acute leukaemias. The set of markers described below have been largely selected in accordance with the recommendations of the European Group for the Immunological Classification of Leukaemias (EGIL) and the British Committee for Standards in Haematology.[7,8]

An initial McAb panel should aim at distinguishing acute myeloid leukaemia (AML) from acute lymphoblastic leukaemia (ALL) and further classify ALL into B- or T-cell lineage (Table 14.1). This panel is constituted as follows:

1. B-lymphoid markers: CD19, CD10 and cytoplasmic CD22 and CD79a;
2. T-lymphoid markers: CD2, CD7 and cytoplasmic CD3;
3. Myeloid markers: CD13, CD33, CD117 and cytoplasmic myeloperoxidase (anti-myeloperoxidase (MPO));
4. Non-lineage specific markers which are expressed in haemopoietic progenitor cells: CD34, HLA-Dr and TdT.

Two aspects which need to be considered are the degree of lineage specificity of the McAb and whether the antigen is expressed in the membrane or the cytoplasm. Some markers are highly specific and sensitive for a particular lineage, e.g. CD3 for

Table 14.1 Panel of monoclonal antibodies for the diagnosis of acute leukaemias

	ALL		AML
	B-lineage	**T-lineage**	
First line	CD19, CD22 CD79a, CD10*	CD7, CD2 cytCD3	CD13, CD33, CD117, anti-MPO TdT, HLA-Dr, CD34
Second line	cytIgM*, SmIg	CD1a, CD5, CD4, CD8, anti-TCR	CD41, CD42, CD61 anti-glycophorin A

*CD10 and cyt IgM are not essential for a diagnosis of B-lineage ALL but they are important in paediatric cases to identify common-ALL, pro-B-ALL and pre-B-ALL.
Optional markers: CD14, anti-lysozyme, CD36.
ALL, acute lymphoblastic leukaemia; AML, acute myeloid leukaemia; cyt, cytoplasmic; MPO, myeloperoxidase; SmIg, surface immunoglobulin; TCR, T-cell receptor.

T cells, CD79a for B cells and anti-MPO for myeloid cells, while others such as CD10, CD13 or CD7 are less lineage specific. Nevertheless, the latter may support the lymphoid or myeloid commitment in cases which are negative with the most specific markers or when results are equivocal. The second aspect to take into account when performing immunophenotyping is that the most specific markers are either expressed earlier in the cytoplasm than in the membrane during cell differentiation (e.g. CD3) and/or they are only detectable in the cytoplasm (e.g. anti-MPO, CD79a).[9–11] Markers against haemopoietic precursors such as TdT or CD34, although not essential in routine practice, are helpful when problems of differential diagnosis arise between acute leukaemias and large cell lymphomas in leukaemic phase.

A second set of McAb is necessary to classify ALL further into the various subtypes or to identify rare cases of AML derived from cells committed to the megakaryocytic and erythroid lineages. This set comprises cytoplasmic and membrane Ig staining in B-lineage ALL; CD1a, CD4, CD5, CD8 and anti-TCR in T-lineage ALL and, in AML, antibodies which detect membrane glycoproteins present in platelets and megakaryocytes or glycophorin A expressed in erythroid precursors.[7,12]

Identification of cell reactivity with other McAb may include CD14 and anti-lysozyme and CD36. Although CD14 and anti-lysozyme are not specific for acute monoblastic leukaemias, both are more frequently expressed during monocytic differentiation. CD36 is often expressed in poorly differentiated erythroid leukaemias. Although this marker is not specific for erythroid precursors, being expressed also in monoblasts and megakaryocytic cells, when considered together with reactivity with other McAb, e.g. negative HLA-Dr, anti-platelet McAb and CD13/CD33, it is highly indicative of erythroid acute leukaemia.

McAbs against non-haemopoietic cells rarely need to be investigated when performing immunophenotyping for the diagnosis of acute leukaemias. Only rare cases of neuroblastoma or oat-cell carcinoma may mimic acute leukaemia in the bone marrow and in such cases anti-neuroblastoma McAb, and the pan-leucocyte marker CD45 may help in establishing the correct diagnosis.

New markers in acute leukaemias

The following recently reported reagents are potentially useful:

(a) A McAb that recognizes the altered distribution of promyelocytic protein (PML) in cases of AML-M3 with t(15;17). Although the PML is expressed in normal myeloid cells and in blasts from AML other than M3, the pattern of expression, e.g. multiparticulated or cytoplasmic in the cases with t(15;17), is different from that of normal myeloid cells or other myeloblasts. The latter are either negative for anti-PML or have protein expression in the form of large nuclear dots. The reactivity with anti-PML needs to be assessed under fluorescence microscopy or light microscopy if an immunocytochemistry technique is carried out.[13,14]

(b) The McAb 7.1/NG2 and NG1 which is preferentially expressed in a subset of pro-B or early B-cell ALL with 11q23 rearrangement[15] and in a proportion of AML with features of monocytic differentiation (irrespective of the presence of 11q23 rearrangement).[16–18]

Immunological classification of acute leukaemias

There are two major differentiation lineages in the lymphoid system, B and T, and lymphoblastic leukaemias arise from early B- or T-precursor cells. Table 14.2 illustrates that only a few McAbs react positively with the most immature lymphoblasts; with maturation, however, more McAbs become

Table 14.2 Immunological classification of acute leukaemias

Acute lymphoblastic leukaemias (ALL) (TdT+)
B-cell precursor (CD19+ and/or CD79a+ and/or CD22+)
pro-B-ALL (no expression of other B-cell markers)
common-ALL (CD10+, cytoplasmic IgM−)
pre-B-ALL (cytoplasmic IgM+)
mature B-ALL* (surface Ig+)
T-cell precursor (cytoplasmic CD3+, CD7+)
pro-T-ALL (no expression of other T-cell markers)
pre-T-ALL (CD2+ and/or CD5+)
cortical T-ALL (CD1a+)
mature T-ALL (membrane CD3+)
Acute myeloid leukaemias (AML)
AML (M0–M5) (anti-MPO+ and/or CD13+, and/or CD33+ and/or CD117+)
Pure erythroid leukaemia (anti-glycophorin A+, anti-RBC group+, CD36+)
Megakaryoblastic leukaemias (CD41+, CD42+, CD61+).
Miscellaneous
Biphenotypic acute leukaemias (coexpression of myeloid and lymphoid markers)**
Myeloid antigen positive ALL
Lymphoid antigen positive AML

*Mature B-ALL usually is TdT negative.
**Scores for biphenotypic acute leukaemia are described in Table 14.3.

reactive. Thus, to demonstrate all cases of leukaemia of a particular lineage, it is important to always include in the battery of McAbs those which will detect the most immature cells. B-lineage ALL is defined by the expression of at least two B-cell antigens, CD79a, CD19 and/or CD22; T-lineage ALL is defined by the expression of nuclear TdT and CD3. CD7 is also consistently positive in T-ALL. However, the expression of CD7 does not by itself define T-ALL since this McAb is positive in about 20% of cases of AML.

B- and T-ALL can be further subclassified on the basis of cell differentiation or maturation (Table 14.2). Although this subclassification is not essential for diagnosis, it is important because of the correlation between certain B-lineage subtypes and molecular cytogenetics and clinical features.

B-lineage ALL can be classified into four subtypes: pro-B-ALL (previously designated null-ALL), common-ALL (see Fig. 14.3), pre-B-ALL and mature B-ALL (Table 14.2). Mature B-ALL is not considered within ALL in the new WHO classification but is included in the group of high-grade, non-Hodgkin's lymphomas as it corresponds to the leukaemic manifestation (ALL-L3) of Burkitt's lymphoma. There is some correlation between these immunological subtypes and molecular genetics and prognosis. The majority of infant ALL with t(4;11)(q21;q23) and/or rearrangement of the *MLL* gene at 11q23 are pro-B-ALL and often express CD15, while the common-ALL phenotype is associated with hyperdiploidy or t(12;21) involving the *TEL* gene both associated with a good prognosis. The t(1;19)(q23;p13) is more common in the subset of pre-B-ALL.

T-lineage ALL can also be subdivided into several subgroups according to the stage of differentiation of the lymphoblasts. In the most immature form or pro-T-ALL, blasts only express CD7 and cytoplasmic CD3; pre-T-ALL; cortical T-ALL, defined by the expression of CD1a and the rare mature T-ALL in which blasts express membrane as well as cytoplasmic CD3 (Table 14.2). Other T-cell-associated antigens such as CD2, CD5, CD4, CD8 and anti-TCR are expressed with variable frequency in the cortical and mature T-ALL; for instance, coexpression of CD4 and CD8, a phenotype characteristic of normal cortical thymocytes, is frequent in cortical T-ALL. In addition, mature T-ALL can be subclassified in two subgroups on the basis of the membrane expression of the T-cell receptor (TCR) complex molecules, α/β or γ/δ. According to current trials in Germany, these two subgroups of T-ALL seem to have a different outcome.

AML can be defined immunologically by the expression of two or more myeloid markers: CD13, CD33, CD117 and anti-MPO in the absence of lymphoid markers.[7] The most specific marker for the myeloid lineage is anti-MPO followed by CD117; as a rule, both are negative in ALL.[19] According to the French-American-British (FAB) classification there is no marker which allows the distinction between the various subtypes of AML.[20] However, some McAb may be preferentially positive in certain AML subtypes such as CD14 and anti-lysozyme in cases with monocytic differentiation, absence of HLA-Dr expression in M3 AML or expression of CD19 in M2-AML. Furthermore, immunological markers are essential for the diagnosis of poorly different-

iated myeloid leukaemias or M0-AML in which blasts do not show myeloid features by morphology or cytochemistry.[21,22]

In poorly differentiated leukaemias in which the first panel of lymphoid and myeloid markers does not show positive results, McAb against platelet glycoproteins Ib, the complex IIb/IIIa and IIIa, e.g. CD41, CD42 and CD61, should be tested to exclude the diagnosis of acute megakaryoblastic leukaemia,[7,12] and McAb to glycophorin A or to the red blood cell groups such as Gerbich should be used to exclude erythroid leukaemias.

Immunophenotyping enables recognition of an unusual form of acute leukaemia designated acute biphenotypic or mixed lineage acute leukaemia. This leukaemia accounts for 5% of cases and is characterized by the coexpression of a constellation of myeloid and lymphoid antigens in the blast cells (Table 14.3). The lack of agreement among various workers on the definition of biphenotypic leukaemia has made it difficult to establish whether this constitutes a distinct clinicopathological entity. We have described a scoring system[23] that has been adopted by the EGIL group with

Table 14.3 Scoring system for the diagnosis of biphenotypic acute leukaemias

Score	B-lymphoid	T-lymphoid	Myeloid
2	CD79a cytCD22 cytIgM	CD3 anti-TCR $\alpha\beta$ anti-TCR $\gamma\delta$	anti-MPO
1	CD19 CD20 CD10	CD2 CD5 CD8 CD10	CD117 CD13 CD33 CD65
0.5	TdT CD24	TdT CD7	CD14 CD15 CD68

Biphenotypic acute leukaemia is defined when scores for the myeloid and one of the lymphoid lineages are >2 points. Each marker scores the corresponding point. Cases of ALL or AML with expression of myeloid or lymphoid markers respectively but with scores less than 2.5 have been described as Myeloid antigen+ ALL and Lymphoid antigen+ AML. In contrast to biphenotypic acute leukaemias, they do not seem to be cytogenetically or prognostically different from ALL or AML with no aberrant antigen expression.
MPO, myeloperoxidase; TCR, T-cell receptor; TdT, terminal deoxynucleotidyl transferase.

some modifications[7] which aims to distinguish biphenotypic acute leukaemias from cases of ALL or AML with aberrant expression of a marker from another lineage. This scoring is based in the number and lineage specificity of the lymphoid and myeloid markers expressed by the blast cells. The most specific markers score 2, e.g. CD3 for the T-lymphoid lineage, CD79a, Ig and CD22 for the B-lymphoid lineage and anti-MPO for the myeloid lineage.[7,23,24]

IMMUNOLOGICAL MARKERS IN CHRONIC LYMPHOPROLIFERATIVE DISORDERS

Immunophenotyping is essential for the characterization and diagnosis of the chronic lymphoproliferative disorders. Immunological markers enable one to distinguish lymphoblastic leukaemias and lymphomas which are TdT+ from mature or chronic lymphoid diseases which are consistently TdT–. They also demonstrate whether the malignant cells are of B- or T-lymphoid nature and demonstrate clonality in the B-cell cases. Markers may also be useful to confirm or establish the diagnosis of certain entities which show distinct immunological profiles and may provide prognostic information.

Panel of McAb for diagnosis and classification

The diagnosis of a B- or T-cell disorder requires a small battery of McAb. It is convenient to use a two-step procedure with an initial panel applicable to all cases and a second panel based on the results with the first panel and the tentative diagnosis by clinical features and/or cell morphology (Table 14.4).[25]

The first panel of markers is intended to distinguish B-cell from T-cell disorders, to confirm or establish the diagnosis of chronic lymphocytic leukaemia (CLL), to rule out other B-cell conditions and to demonstrate B-cell clonality. It comprises immunostaining with anti-kappa and anti-lambda human Ig, CD2 (anti-T-cell marker), CD5 (T-cell and a subset of B-cell disorders) and four McAbs that detect antigens in subsets of B-cells: CD23, FMC7, CD79b against the β chain of the B-cell receptor and membrane CD22. With the two latter reagents as well as surface Ig, assessment of the fluorescence intensity is important to distinguish between CLL and other B-cell disorders (Fig. 14.5). The results obtained with this

Table 14.4 Panel of monoclonal antibodies for the diagnosis of lymphoid disorders

	B cell	T cell
First line	SmIg (kappa/lambda), CD19, CD23 FMC7, mCD79b, mCD22, CD5*	CD2, CD5*
Second line	CD11c, CD25, CD103, HC2 CD38, CD138, cytIg	CD3, CD4, CD7, CD8

*B subset and T-cell marker.
Optional markers: CD25, CD79a and natural killer associated, e.g. CD16, CD56, CD57 and CD11b.
CytIg, cytoplasmic immunoglobulin; SmIg, surface immunoglobulin.

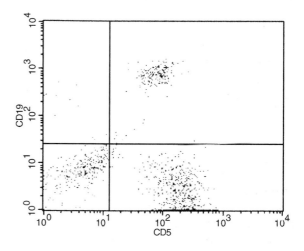

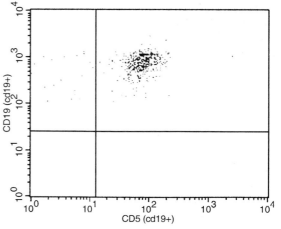

Fig. 14.5 Minimal residual disease detection.
Upper: Dot plot showing a small proportion of lymphocytes coexpressing CD5 and CD19 in a patient with chronic lymphocytic leukaemia following treatment; the majority of lymphocytes are T cells (CD5+, CD19–).
Lower: Dot plot showing enrichment of the CD5+ CD19+ population acquired on a gate for the CD19+ cells in the above case.

set of McAbs can be combined into a scoring system (Table 14.5) to establish the diagnosis of CLL and to distinguish CLL cases with atypical morphology and CLL with increased numbers of prolymphocytes (CLL/PL) from other B-cell diseases such as B-cell prolymphocytic leukaemia (B-PLL) and B-cell lymphomas in leukaemic phase.[26] The characteristic profile of CLL is weak surface immunoglobulin (SmIg), CD5+, CD23+, FMC7− and weak or negative CD79b and CD22.[26-29]

When the marker profile using the first line panel of McAb yields a B-cell phenotype not typical of CLL, a second panel of McAb can be used. This is selected in the light of the review of the cell morphology, clinical information and/or other laboratory features. For example, estimation of the cell reactivity with four McAbs (CD11c, CD25, CD103 and HC2) is useful to distinguish hairy cell leukaemia (HCL) from other disorders with circulating villous cells which may be confused with HCL such as splenic lymphoma with villous lymphocytes (SLVL) or marginal zone lymphoma and the HCL variant. Cells from the majority of HCL cases coexpress the three or four of the markers mentioned above while SLVL and cells from HCL variant are positive with one or at most two of these markers.[30]

When the first line panel of markers suggest a T-cell phenotype (CD2+, CD5+/−), expression of other T-cell markers such as CD3, CD7 and CD4 and CD8 may need to be investigated.

Unusual situations may occur which need to be considered. This is the case in plasma cell leukaemia in which the cells are negative with all T-cell and the majority of B-cell markers including surface Ig expression; cells express Ig only in the cytoplasm (with light chain restriction) and are positive with CD38 and CD138. Normal and malignant plasma cells may also express CD79a, a cytoplasmic epitope of the α chain of the B-cell receptor. CD25 may be used in cases of suspected adult T-cell leukaemia lymphoma.

New monoclonal antibodies
Anti-cyclin D1
McAbs that detect cyclin D1 are preferentially expressed in cells from mantle-cell lymphoma cases and in other cases of lymphoma in which cells carry the t(11;14)(q13;q32).[31,32] These antibodies have been mainly used on tissue sections using immunhistochemistry or on cytospin preparations with immunocytochemistry but it is also possible to estimate the expression of cyclin D1 by flow cytometry with the McAb 5D4 after stabilization and fixation of the cells.[33]

p53 protein
This marker can be detected in cells by immunocytochemistry and flow cytometry with specific antibodies. There is a good correlation between p53 expression and molecular genetics, the latter showing deletion or mutations of the p53 gene. Although not essential for diagnosis, this may be useful as a prognostic indicator because of its correlation with resistance to therapy or disease progression in patients with CLL, B-PLL and other B-cell disorders.[34,35]

Immunological profiles of chronic lymphoproliferative disorders
The most common immunophenotypes of the B- and T-cell disorders are shown in Tables 14.6 and 14.7. CLL has a phenotype that clearly distinguishes this disease from the other B-cell leukaemias. By contrast, there is overlap on the marker expression in the other B-cell malignancies and for this reason, in cases with a B-cell marker profile different from CLL, the immunophenotypic analysis needs to be interpreted in the light of morphology or other laboratory information to establish the precise diagnosis.

There is no specific immunological profile that distinguishes the various T-cell diseases (Table 14.7). However, expression of CD8, with

Table 14.5 Scoring system for the diagnosis of chronic lymphocytic leukaemia (CLL). Scores for CLL range from 3 to 5 while in the other B-cell disorders they range from 0 to 2.

Marker	Points	
	1	0
CD5	Positive	Negative
CD23	Positive	Negative
FMC7	Negative	Positive
SmIg*	Weak	Moderate/strong
CD22/CD79b*	Weak/negative	Moderate/strong

*Membrane expression.

Table 14.6 Membrane markers in mature B-cell disorders (CD2−)

Disease	SmIg	CD5	CD23	FMC7	CD22	CD79b
CLL	Weak	++	++	−/+	Weak/−	Weak/−
B-PLL	Strong	−/+	−	++	+	++
HCL	Strong	−	−	++	++	+
HCL-variant	Strong	−	−	++	++	+
SLVL	Strong	−/+	−/+	++	++	++
FL	Strong	−/+	−/+	++	++	++
Mantle	Strong	++	−	++	++	++
Large-cell	Strong	−/+	−/+	++	++	++
PCL*	Negative	−	−	−	−	−

*Express cytoplasmic Ig (light chain restricted), CD38, CD79a and with a variable frequency other B-cell markers.
B-PLL; B-prolymphocytic leukaemia; CLL, chronic lymphocytic leukaemia; FL, follicular lymphoma; HCL, hairy cell leukaemia; PCL, plasma cell leukaemia; SLVL, splenic lymphoma with villous lymphocytes.
Scoring: (−): negative or positive in less than 10% of cases; (−/+): positive in 10–25% of cases; (+): positive in 25–75% of cases; (++): positive in more than 75% of cases.

Table 14.7 Immunological markers in mature T-cell disorders (CD2+)

Marker	T-PLL	LGL-leukaemia	ATLL	SS	T-NHL
CD3	++	++	++	++	+
CD7	++	+	−/+	+	+
CD4+, CD8−	+	−	++	++	+
CD4+, CD8+	−/+	−	−	−	+
CD4−, CD8+	−/+	++	−	−	+
CD4−, CD8−	−	−/+*	−	−	+

ATLL, adult T-cell leukaemia lymphoma; LGL, large granular lymphocyte; SS, Sézary syndrome; T-NHL, post-thymic T-cell lymphoma; T-PLL, T-prolymphocytic leukaemia.
Scoring: (−): negative or positive in less than 10% of cases; (−/+): positive in 10–25% of cases; (+): positive in 25–75% of cases; (++): positive in more than 75% of cases.
*A proportion of cases are CD3 negative and have a natural killer phenotype: CD56+, CD16+.

or without that of natural killer associated markers such as CD16 or CD56, is characteristic of T-cell large granular lymphocyte (LGL) leukaemia, while such expression is rarely seen in other conditions.[36] By contrast, coexpression of CD4 and CD8 is almost exclusively seen in a subgroup, approximately 25%, of T-cell prolymphocytic leukaemia (T-PLL) (Table 14.7).[37] Other markers may also be differentially expressed in various T-cell malignancies. Thus, for example, there is expression of CD25 in adult T-cell leukaemia lymphoma (ATLL) and very strong reactivity with CD7 in T-PLL.[37,38]

IMMUNOLOGICAL MARKERS FOR THE DETECTION OF MINIMAL RESIDUAL DISEASE

Immunophenotyping can be a useful tool to detect small numbers of residual leukaemic cells in peripheral blood and/or bone marrow specimens which are not detected by standard morphology or histopathology. This can be carried out by double or triple colour immunofluorescent methods with a combination of McAbs aimed to identify 'aberrant' phenotypes not present in normal haemopoietic cells and/or by quantification of antigens which are expressed at a different density in normal and leukaemic cells.[39,40] For example, although normal bone marrows, particularly in infants or when regenerating after therapy, have a minor cell population with a B-cell precursor phenotype, e.g. TdT+, CD10+, CD19+, similar to that of ALL blasts, quantitative studies provide discrimination between the normal precursors (strong TdT and weak CD10 and CD19) and ALL blasts (weak TdT, strong CD10/CD19).[39]

Similarly, there is a small B-cell population in normal blood and bone marrow which coexpresses CD5, a phenotype characteristic of CLL. However, by estimating the proportions of CD5+ cells within the whole B-cell population (CD19+), it is possible to demonstrate whether cells represent residual leukaemia or normal B-lymphocytes (Fig. 14.5).[40]

In bone marrow tissue sections, occasional residual abnormal leukaemic cells can be highlighted and easily recognized using immunohistochemistry with markers known to react with the leukaemic cells, e.g. DBA44 or CD103 in HCL.[41] Detection of minimal residual disease applies to both acute and chronic lymphoid leukaemias and it is likely to have prognostic significance in terms of probability of relapse.

Abbreviations

ABC	antibody binding capacity
ALL	acute lymphoblastic leukaemia
AML	acute myeloid leukaemia
APAAP	alkaline phosphatase anti-alkaline phosphatase
B-PLL	B-cell prolymphocytic leukaemia
BSA	bovine serum albumin
CD	cluster designation
CLL	chronic lymphocytic leukaemia
CLL/PL	chronic lymphocytic leukaemia with increased prolymphocytes
Cyt	cytoplasmic
DAB	diaminobenzidine
EGIL	European Group for the Immunological Classification of Leukaemias
FITC	fluorescein isothiocyanate
FSC/SSC	forward/side scatter
HCL	hairy cell leukaemia
Ig	immunoglobulin
IP	immunoperoxidase
LGL	large granular lymphocyte
McAb	monoclonal antibody
MESF	molecules equivalent soluble fluorochrome
MN	mononuclear
MPO	myeloperoxidase
PBS	phosphate buffered saline
PBS-azide-BSA	PBS containing sodium azide and bovine serum albumin
PE	phycoerythrin
PML	promyelocytic protein
QSC	quantum simply cellular
SLVL	splenic lymphoma with villous lymphocytes
SmIg	Surface immunoglobulin
TBS	Tris buffered saline
TCR	T-cell receptor
TdT	terminal deoxynucleotidyl transferase
T-PLL	T-cell prolymphocytic leukaemia

REFERENCES

1 Groeneveld K, Temarvelde JG, van den Beemd MWM, et al 1996 Flow cytometry detection of intracellular antigens for immunophenotyping of normal and malignant leukocytes. BTS Technical Report. Leukemia 10:1383–1389.

2 Pizzolo G, Vincenzi C, Nadali G, et al 1995 Detection of membrane and intracellular antigens by flow cytometry following ORTHO PermeaFix fixation. Leukemia 9:226–228.

3 Bikoue A, George F, Poncelet LW, et al 1996 Quantitative analysis of leukocyte membrane antigen expression: normal adult values. Cytometry 26:137–147.

4 Poncelet P, George F, Papa S, et al 1996 Quantitation of haemopoietic cell antigens in flow cytometry. European Journal of Histochemistry 40 (Suppl 1):15–32.

5 Erber WN, Mynheer LC, Mason DY 1986 APAAP labelling of blood and bone-marrow samples for phenotyping leukaemia. Lancet i:761–765.

6 Mason DY, Erber WN 1991 Immunocytochemical labeling of leukemia samples with monoclonal antibodies by the APAAP procedure. In: Catovsky D (ed) The leukemic cell. Churchill Livingstone, Edinburgh, ch 7, p. 196.

7 Bene MC, Castoldi G, Knapp W, et al 1995 Proposals for the immunological classification of acute leukemias. Leukemia 9:1783–1786.

8 The British Committee for Standards in Haematology 1994 Immunophenotyping in the diagnosis of acute leukaemias. Journal of Clinical Pathology 47:777–781.

9 Janossy G, Coustan-Smith E, Campana D 1989 The reliability of cytoplasmic CD3 and CD22 antigen expression in the immunodiagnosis of acute leukemia – a study of 500 cases. Leukemia 3:170.

10 Buccheri V, Shetty V, Yoshida N, et al 1992 The role of an anti-myeloperoxidase antibody in the diagnosis and classification of acute leukaemia: a comparison with light and electron microscopy cytochemistry. British Journal of Haematology 80:62–68.

11 Buccheri V, Milhaljevic B, Matutes E, et al 1993 mb-1: a new marker for B-lineage lymphoblastic leukemia. Blood 82:853–857.

12 Tetteroo PAT, Lansdorp PM, Leeksma OC, et al 1983 Monoclonal antibodies against human platelet glycoprotein IIIa. British Journal of Haematology 55:509–522.

13 O'Connor SJ, Forsyth PD, Dalal S, et al 1997 The rapid diagnosis of acute promyelocytic leukaemia using PML (5E10) monoclonal antibody. British Journal of Haematology 99:597–604.

14 Falini B, Flenghi L, Lo Coco F, et al 1997 Immunocytochemical diagnosis of acute promyelocytic leukemia (M3) with the monoclonal antibody PG-M3 (anti-PML). Blood 90:4046–4053.

15 Behm FG, Smith FO, Raimondi SC, et al 1996 Human homologue of the rat chondroitin sulfate proteoglycan, NG2, detected by monoclonal antibody 7.1 identifies childhood acute lymphoblastic leukemias with t(4;11)(q21;q23) or t(11;19)(q23;p13) and MLL rearrangements. Blood 87:1134–1139.

16 Wutchter C, Schnittger S, Schoch C, et al 1998 Detection of acute leukemia cells with 11q23 rearrangements by flow cytometry: sensitivity and specificity of monoclonal antibody 7.1. Blood 92 (Suppl 1):228a.

17 Smith FO, Rauch C, Williams DE, et al 1996 The human homologue of rat NG2, a chondroitin sulfate proteoglycan is not expressed on the cell surface of normal hematopoietic cells but is expressed by acute myeloid leukemia blasts from poor prognosis patients with abnormalities of chromosome band 11q23. Blood 87:1123–1133.

18 Mauvieux L, Delabesse E, Bourquelot P, et al 1999 NG2 expression in MLL rearranged acute myeloid leukaemia is restricted to monoblastic cases. British Journal of Haematology 107:674–676.

19 Bene MC, Bernier M, Casasnovas RO, et al 1998 The reliability and specificity of c-kit for the diagnosis of acute myeloid leukemias and undifferentiated leukemias. Blood 92:596–599.

20 Bennett JM, Catovsky D, Daniel MT, et al 1985 Proposed revised criteria for the classification of acute myeloid leukemia. Annals of Internal Medicine 103:620–625.

21 Matutes E, de Oliveria MP, Foroni L, et al 1988 The role of ultrastructural cytochemistry and monoclonal antibodies in clarifying the nature of undifferentiated cells in acute leukaemia. British Journal of Haematology 69:205–211.

22 Bennett JM, Catovsky D, Daniel MT, et al 1991 Proposals for the recognition of minimally differentiated acute myeloid leukaemia (AML-MO). British Journal of Haematology 78:325–329.

23 Buccheri V, Matutes E, Dyer MJS, et al 1993 Lineage commitment in biphenotypic leukemia. Leukemia 7:919–927.

24 Matutes E, Morilla R, Farahat N, et al 1997 Definition of acute biphenotypic leukemia. Haematologica 82:64–66.

25 The British Committee for Standards in Haematology 1994 Immunophenotyping in the diagnosis of chronic lymphoproliferative disorders. Journal of Clinical Pathology 47:871–875.

26 Matutes E, Owusu-Ankomah K, Morilla R, et al 1994 The immunological profile of B-cell disorders and proposal of a scoring system for the diagnosis of CLL. Leukemia 8:1640–1645.

27 Zomas AP, Matutes E, Morilla R, et al 1996 Expression of the immunoglobulin associated protein b29 in B-cell disorders with the monoclonal antibody SN8 (CD79b). Leukemia 10:1966–1970.

28 Moureau EJ, Matutes E, A'hern RP, et al 1997 Improvement of the chronic lymphocytic leukemia scoring system with the monoclonal antibody SN8 (CD79b). American Journal of Clinical Pathology 108:378–382.

29 Cabezudo E, Morilla R, Carrara P, et al 1999 Quantitative analysis of CD79b, CD5 and CD19 in B-cell lymphoproliferative disorders. Haematologica 84:413–418.

30 Matutes E, Morilla R, Owusu-Ankomah K, et al 1994 The immunophenotype of hairy cell leukemia (HCL). Proposal for a scoring system to distinguish HCL from B-cell disorders with hairy or villous lymphocytes. Leukemia and Lymphoma 14 (Suppl 1):57–61.

31 De Boer CJ, Schuuring E, Dreef E, et al 1995 Cyclin D1 protein analysis in the diagnosis of mantle-cell lymphoma. Blood 86:2715–2723.

32 Delmer A, Ajchenbaum-Cymbalista F, Tang R, et al 1995 Overexpression of cyclin D1 in chronic B-cell malignancies with abnormality of chromosome 11q13. British Journal of Haematology 89:798–804.

33 Elenaei MO, Jadayel DM, Matutes E, et al 2001 Cyclin D1 flow cytometry as a useful tool in the diagnosis of B-cell malignancies. Leukemia Research 25:115–123.

34 Lens D, Dyer MJS, Garcia Marco JA, et al 1997 p53 abnormalities in CLL are associated with excess of prolymphocytes and poor prognosis. British Journal of Haematology 99:848–857.

35 Dohner H, Fischer K, Bentz M, et al 1995 p53 gene deletion predicts for poor survival and non-response to therapy with purine analogs in chronic B-cell leukemias. Blood 85:1580–1589.

36 Matutes E, Catovsky D 1991 T-cell leukemias and leukemia/lymphoma syndromes. Leukemia and Lymphoma 4:81–91.

37 Matutes E, Brito-Babapulle V, Swansbury J, et al 1991 Clinical and laboratory features of 78 cases of T-prolymphocytic leukemia. Blood 78:3269–3274.

38 Ginaldi L, Matutes E, Farahat N, et al 1996 Differential expression of CD3 and CD7 in T-cell malignancies: a quantitative study by flow cytometry. British Journal of Haematology 93:921–927.

39 Farahat N, Lens D, Zomas A, et al 1995 Quantitative flow cytometry can distinguish between normal and B-cell precursors. British Journal of Haematology 91:640–646.

40 Cabezudo E, Matutes E, Ramrattan M, et al 1997 Analysis of residual disease in chronic lymphocytic leukemia by flow cytometry. Leukemia 11:1909–1914.

41 Matutes E, Meeus P, McLennan K, et al 1997 The significance of minimal residual disease in hairy cell leukaemia treated with deoxycoformycin: a long term follow-up study. British Journal of Haematology 98:375–383.

15

Diagnostic radionuclides in haematology

S. Mitchell Lewis

Methods using radionuclides have an important place in haematological diagnosis. Tests which may be undertaken in haematology departments include blood volume, red cell survival studies, vitamin B_{12} absorption (Schilling test) and occasionally ferrokinetic studies. Other investigations are more likely to be referred to a department of medical physics or nuclear medicine. Even when the tests are not carried out directly in the haematology department, it is essential for the haematologist to understand their principles and limitations, and to be able to interpret the results in clinical terms. Anyone handling radionuclides must also be aware of the potential radiation hazard. These aspects will be discussed briefly here. Various text books, e.g. Wagner et al,[1] Bernier et al,[2] Maisey et al,[3] provide more complete accounts of the theory and practice of nuclear medicine techniques, as does a monograph on radionuclides in haematology by Lewis &

Table 15.1 Radionuclides used for diagnostic investigations in haematology

Element	Half-life (T½)	Energies (MeV)*	Pharmaceutical	Application	Activities (MBq)**	Radiation dose (mSv)***
^{57}Co	270 days	0.122 0.136	Vitamin B$_{12}$	Investigation of megaloblastic anaemias	0.04	0.1
^{58}Co	711.3 days	0.811 0.511				0.2
^{51}Cr	27.8 days	0.320	Sodium chromate	Red cell volume	0.8	0.3
				Red cell life-span	2	0.6
				Gastrointestinal bleeding	4	1
				Spleen scan	4	1
				Spleen pool	4	1
^{59}Fe	45 days	1.09 1.29	Ferric chloride or citrate	Oral iron absorption	0.4	4
				Ferrokinetic studies	0.4	4
^{125}I	60 days	0.035	Iodinated human serum albumin	Plasma volume	0.2	0.06†
^{111}In	2.81 days	0.247 0.173	Indium chloride→ oxine/tropolone	Red cell volume	2	1
				Spleen scan	5	2
				Platelet life-span	4	2
^{99m}Tc	6 h	0.141	Pertechnetate	Red cell volume	2	0.02
				Spleen scan	100	1
				Spleen pool	100	1

*eV = electron volt, 10^3eV = 1 keV, 10^3 keV = 1 MeV.
**MBq = megabequeral; 1 MBq = 10^6 Bq = approximately 27 μC.
***Sv = Sievert; 10^3 mSv = 1 Sv.
†Provided that thyroid is blocked and the label is excreted in the urine; if not blocked, about 20% will accumulate in the thyroid, resulting in a radiation dose of c 1 mSv to the thyroid.

Bayly[4] The main properties of the radionuclides useful in diagnostic haematology are summarized in Table 15.1. The units used to express radioactivity and the effects of radiation on the body are given on page 611.

SOURCES OF RADIONUCLIDES

Radionuclides which emit γ-rays are particularly useful as they have the advantage that their emissions penetrate tissues well so that they can be detected at the surface of the body when they have originated within organs. The radionuclide should have as short a half-life ($T_{1/2}$) as is compatible with the duration of the test. A radionuclide with a very short half-life can be administered in much higher amounts than those which are likely to remain active in the body for a considerably longer time.

The longer-lived radionuclides which are used for haematological investigations are generally available from commercial suppliers. The usual way of obtaining certain short-lived radionuclides is by means of a radionuclide generator, in which a moderately long-lived parent radionuclide decays to produce the required short-lived isotope. In this way ^{99m}Tc ($T_{1/2}$ = 6 h) can be derived from ^{99}Mo ($T_{1/2}$ = 66 h).

RADIATION PROTECTION

The quantity of radioactivity used in diagnostic work is usually small and good laboratory practice is all that is necessary for safe working. However, before using radionuclides, workers should familiarize themselves with the regulations concerning radiation protection for themselves, their fellow workers and patients.[5]

The effect of radiation on the body depend on the amount of energy deposited, and is expressed in grays (Gy). The unit which describes the overall effect of radiation on the body, or the 'dose equivalent' is measured in sieverts (Sv) or millisieverts (mSv). The annual whole body dose limit for somebody working with radionuclides is in the order of 20 mSv, whilst 1 mSv is the annual limit for the general public. To put this into perspective, 1 mSv is produced by normal background radiation in 6 months and the radiation dose from a single chest X-ray is 0.02 mSv.[6] No statutory limit of total annual radiation dose has been set for patients, but it is an important requirement that radionuclides should be handled only in approved laboratories under the direction of a trained person who holds a certificate from the appropriate authority which specifies the radionuclides that the individual is authorized to use and the dose limits which must not be exceeded. In the UK, this is the Administration of Radioactive Substances Advisory Committee (ARSAC).[6] Radionuclides should not be given to pregnant women unless the investigation is considered imperative; if an investigation is necessary during lactation, breast-feeding should be discontinued until radioactivity is no longer detectable in the milk. When radionuclide investigations are necessary in children, the dose relative to that for an adult should be based on surface area rather than body weight (Table 15.2).

In general, the radioactive waste from radionuclides used in haematological diagnostic procedures may be poured down a single designated laboratory sink. It should be washed down with a large quantity of running water. If the waste material exceeds the amount allowed for disposal in this way, it should be stored in a suitable place until its radioactivity has decayed sufficiently for it to be disposed of via the refuse system. All working and storage areas and disposal sinks should be clearly labelled with the internationally recognized trefoil symbol.

Decontamination of working surfaces, walls and floors can usually be achieved by washing with a detergent such as Decon 90 (Decon Laboratories Ltd). Glassware can be decontaminated by soaking in Decon 90 and plastic laboratory ware by washing in dilute (e.g. 1%) nitric acid.

Protective gloves must always be worn when handling radionuclides; any activity which does get on to the hands can usually be removed by washing with soap and water, or if that fails, with a detergent solution. For each laboratory in which isotopes are used, a radiological safety officer should be nominated to supervise protection procedures and to ensure that a careful record is kept of all administered radionuclides.

A good account of the general procedures to be followed in handling radioactive materials is given in a monograph published by the International Atomic Energy Agency.[7]

Apparatus for measuring radioactivity in vitro

The radionuclides used for most haematological tests are measured in a scintillation counter with thallium-activated sodium iodide crystals. These are available in various shapes and sizes. A 'well-type' crystal contains a cavity into which is inserted a small container or test-tube holding up to 5 ml of fluid. Since the sample is almost surrounded by the crystal, counting is achieved with high efficiency. As the geometric efficiency of a well-type counter depends on the position of the sample in relation to the crystal, it is important to use the same volume for each sample in a series. Another form of crystal detector is a solid circular cylinder, 2.5–10 cm in diameter. In this form, it is used for in vivo measurements and occasionally for the measurement of bulky samples, e.g. samples of faeces or 24 h urine specimens, thus avoiding the need to concentrate them to a smaller volume.

An alternative method for measuring bulky material is by using two opposed detectors in a single counting system. The sample is placed in a 450 ml waxed cardboard carton with a screw-top

Table 15.2 Radionuclide doses for children as fraction of adult dose

Weight (kg)	Fraction of adult dose
10	0.3
15	0.4
20	0.5
30	0.6
40	0.75
50	0.9
60	0.95
70	1.0

lid, and positioned between two counters placed respectively above and below it, and with a plastic ring over the lower counter to ensure that the specimen in the carton is approximately equidistant from both crystals. The counting system is surrounded by lead and the responses of both crystals are counted together. If a single detector system is used, it is essential to homogenize the samples.

Apparatus for measuring radioactivity in vivo
Surface counting
This depends on shielding the crystals by means of a lead collimator to exclude as far as possible the radiation from outside a well-defined area of the body. It is thus possible to measure the radioactivity in individual organs such as spleen and liver.

Imaging
The most widely used method for imaging is by the scintillation camera. This consists of a lead shielding, a large thin sodium iodide detector, an array of photomultiplier tubes, a collimator with multiple parallel holes and a system for pulse height analysis and for storage and display of the data. By scanning down the body, an image of the distribution of the label is built up and recorded. It can also be used to measure the quantity of the isotope in various organs.

MEASUREMENT OF RADIOACTIVITY WITH A SCINTILLATION COUNTER

Standardization of working conditions
For each radionuclide, it is necessary to plot a spectrum of pulse height distribution and to identify a window corresponding to the energy at which the maximum number of pulses are emitted. Examples of spectra and selected settings are illustrated in Figure 15.1. The setting of the apparatus, once determined, should remain constant for many months.

Counting technique
Measurement of radioactivity
Measurements are usually carried out for a fixed period of time, the results being recorded as counts per s (cps) or counts per min (cpm). Radioactivity is subject to random but statistically predictable variation similar to that in blood cell counts (see

p. 598). The accuracy of the count depends upon the total number of the counts recorded as the variance (σ) of a radioactive count = $\sqrt{}$ total count.

Thus, on a count of 100 the inherent error is 10%; it is 1% on a count of 10 000. Any measured activity represents the difference between the sample count and the background count, in which the errors of both counts are cumulative. In practice, a net count of 2500 over background is adequate for the accuracy required inclinical studies.

Background counts should be measured alongside that of the radioactive material. If the count rate of the sample is not much above background, then the background should be counted for as long a time as the sample. If the sample-count rate is less than the background, accurate measurement requires extremely long counting times.

Correction for physical decay
As physical decay is a continuous process which proceeds at an exponential rate, it is possible to correct mathematically for the loss of radioactivity and to convert any measurement back to the initial reference time. This is necessary when successive observations made at different times after the administration of a radionuclide to a patient are compared.

DOUBLE RADIONUCLIDE MEASUREMENTS

If more than one radionuclide is present in a sample, it is possible to measure the radioactivity of each radionuclide separately by one of the following techniques.

Differential decay
This is of value especially when one of the labels has a very short half-life (e.g. ^{99m}Tc, half-life 6 h). The method is to count the activity in the mixture twice, the second count when the short-lived label has effectively disappeared.

Physical separation
When the two radionuclides produce γ-rays of different energies, they can be identified by their characteristic features and separated using an energy analyzer. Correction for any 'cross talk' is carried out by counting a standard of each radionuclide (A and B) at both channel settings. The proportion of A (P_A) spilling over into

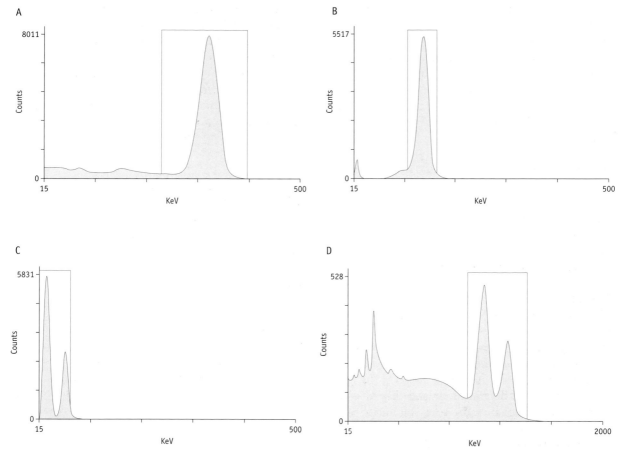

Fig. 15.1 **Spectra of radionuclides obtained on a scintillation spectrometer.** (A) ⁵¹Cr, (B) ⁹⁹ᵐTc, (C) ¹²⁵I, (D) ⁵⁹Fe. The radionuclides should be counted with the window set within the limits indicated by the vertical lines.

channel B = channel B counts/channel A counts from the radionuclide A standard (both corrected for background), and the proportion of B (P_B) spilling over into channel A = channel A counts/channel B counts from the radionuclide B standard. The total counts obtained for labels A and B in their correct channels can then be corrected for the proportion of 'foreign' counts.

BLOOD VOLUME

The haemoglobin content, total red cell count and packed cell volume (PCV) do not invariably reflect the total red cell volume. Whilst in most cases for practical purposes, there is adequate correlation between peripheral blood values and (total) red cell volume,[8] there will be a discrepancy if the plasma volume is reduced or increased disproportionately. Fluctuation in plasma volume may result in haemodilution or conversely in haemoconcen-tration, giving rise to pseudoanaemia or pseudo-polycythaemia, respectively.

An increase in plasma volume occurs in pregnancy, returning to normal soon after delivery. Increased plasma volume may also be found in patients with cirrhosis, nephritis, congestive cardiac failure and when there is marked splenomegaly. Reduced plasma volume occurs in stress, oedema, dehydration, following the administration of diuretic drugs and in smokers. It also occurs during prolonged bed rest.

In contrast to the fluctuations in plasma volume, red cell volume does not fluctuate to any extent if erythropoiesis is in a steady state.

Blood volume should thus be measured whenever the PCV is persistently higher than normal; demonstration of an absolute increase in red cell volume is necessary to diagnose polycythaemia and to assess its severity. The component parts of the blood volume (i.e. red cell and plasma volume) should also be measured separately, in the elucidation of obscure anaemias when the possibility of an increase in plasma volume cannot be excluded.

MEASUREMENT OF BLOOD VOLUME

Principle
The principle is that of dilution analysis. A small volume of a readily identifiable radionuclide is injected intravenously either bound to the red cells or to a plasma component and its dilution is measured after time has been allowed for the injected material to become thoroughly mixed in the circulation, but before significant quantities have left the circulation or become unbound. The most practical method now available is to use a small volume of the patient's red cells labelled with radioactive chromium (^{51}Cr), technetium (pertechnetate) (^{99m}Tc) or indium (^{111}In). The labelled red cells are diluted in the whole blood of the patient and from their dilution the total blood volume can be calculated; the red cell volume, too, can be deduced from knowledge of the PCV. The plasma volume can be measured directly by injecting human albumin labelled with radioactive iodine (I^{125}) which is diluted in the plasma compartment.

In contrast to measurement of red cell volume, plasma volume measurements are only approximations as the labelled albumin undergoes continuous slow interchange between the plasma and extravascular fluids, even during the mixing period. For this reason, it is undesirable to attempt to calculate red cell volume from plasma volume on the basis of the observed PCV. On the other hand, as the red cell volume is generally more stable, calculation of total blood volume from red cell volume is usually more reliable, provided that the difference between whole body and venous PCV is appreciated and allowed for (see

p. 24). Measurement of red cell and plasma volumes separately by direct methods is to be preferred.

DETERMINATION OF RED CELL VOLUME[9]

Radioactive chromium method
Add approximately 10 ml of blood to 1.5 ml of sterile NIH-A acid-citrate-dextrose (ACD) solution (see p. 603), in a sterile bottle with a screw cap. Centrifuge at 1200–1500 g for 5 min. Discard the supernatant plasma and buffy coat and slowly add to the cells, with continuous mixing, 8×10^3 Bq of $Na_2^{51}CrO_4$ per kg of body weight. The sodium chromate should be in a volume of at least 0.2 ml, being diluted in 9 g/l NaCl (saline). Allow the blood to stand for 15 min at 37°C for labelling to take place. Wash the red cells twice in 4 to 5 volumes of sterile saline.* Finally, resuspend the cells in a volume of sterile saline sufficient for an injection of about 5 ml and the preparation of a standard. Take up the appropriate volume into a syringe which is weighed before and after the injection. The volume injected is calculated from the following formula:

Volume injected (ml)
$$= \frac{\text{Weight of suspension injected (g)}}{\text{Density of suspension (g/ml)}}$$
where
Density of suspension =
1.0 + Hb conc. of suspension (g/l) × 0.097/340

(This assumes that packed red cells have a MCHC of 340 g/l and a density of 1.097.)

Inject the suspension intravenously without delay and note the time; at 10, 20 and 30 min later, collect 5–10 ml of the patient's blood and add it to the appropriate amount of a solid anticoagulant (e.g. K_2EDTA). This blood should preferably be withdrawn from a vein other than that used for the injection. However, it is often convenient to insert a self-retaining (e.g. butterfly) needle; in this case, care must be taken to ensure that the isotope is well dispersed into the bloodstream when injected by flushing through with

---

*12 g/l NaCl should be used when red cell osmotic fragility is greatly increased, e.g. in cases of hereditary spherocytosis.

10 ml of sterile saline. When the mixing time is likely to be prolonged as in splenomegaly, cardiac failure or shock, another sample should be taken 60 min after the injection.

Measure the PCV of each sample.* Deliver 1 ml volumes into counting tubes and lyse with saponin; a convenient method is to add 2 drops of 2% saponin. Measure their radioactivity in a scintillation counter. Then dilute an aliquot of the original suspension which was not injected 1 in 500 in water (for use as a standard) and determine the radioactivity of a 1 ml volume. Then:

Red cell volume (RCV) (ml) =

$$\frac{\begin{array}{l}\text{Radioactivity of standard (cpm/ml)}\\ \times \text{Dilution of standard} \times \text{Volume}\\ \text{injected (ml)}\end{array}}{\begin{array}{l}\text{Radioactivity of post-injection}\\ \text{sample (cpm/ml)}\end{array}} \times \begin{array}{l}\text{PCV (on}\\ \text{blood sample)}\end{array}$$

The total blood volume (BV) can be calculated by multiplying the value for RCV by 1/(whole-body PCV) (see p. 322). Plasma volume can be calculated by subtracting RCV from BV.

If a sample has been taken at 60 min in cases where delayed mixing is suspected and there is a significant difference between the measurements at 10–30 min and 60 min, the 60 min measurement should be used for calculating the red cell volume.

TECHNETIUM METHOD

^{99m}Tc is available as sodium pertechnetate. This passes freely through the red cell membrane and will become attached to the cells only if it is present in a reduced form as it enters the cells when it binds firmly to β-chains of haemoglobin. For this to occur, the red cells require to be treated with a stannous (tin) compound by the following in-vivo procedure. Dissolve a vial of Stannous Reagent** in 6 ml of sterile saline and inject intravenously 0.03 ml/kg body weight.

*PCV should be obtained by micro-haematocrit centrifugation for 5 min, or for 10 min if the PCV is more than 0.50 (l/l), and correcting for trapped plasma by deducting 2% from the measurement.

** Stannous fluoride and sodium medronate (Amerscan, Amersham International).

After 15 min, collect 5 ml of blood into a sterile container to which has been added 200 iu of liquid heparin. Add 2 MBq of freshly generated ^{99m}Tc in approximately 0.2 ml of saline or 100 MBq if measurement of splenic red cell pool and scanning are also required. Allow to stand at room temperature for 20 min (or at 37°C for 10 min). Centrifuge; wash twice in cold sterile saline and resuspend in a sufficient volume of cold sterile saline for an injection of 5–10 ml. Take up *c* 5 ml in a syringe which is weighed before and after injection and carry out subsequent procedures as for the chromium method. Because of the short half-life of ^{99m}Tc, radioactivity must be measured on the day of the test. Because 5–10% of the radioactivity is eluted from the red cells within 1 h,[10] the method is less suitable than are the chromium and indium methods when there is splenomegaly or another cause of delayed mixing is suspected.

Indium is available as ^{111}In chloride. The labelling procedure is simpler than with ^{99m}Tc and as there is less elution than with technetium during the first hour,[11] it is particularly suitable for delayed sampling. For labelling blood cells, the indium is complexed with oxine[12] or tropolone.[13] The latter will be described below.

INDIUM METHOD

Preparation of tropolone complex

Prepare a solution of 2.5 mg/ml of tropolone (2-hydroxy-2,4,6-cycloheptatrien-1-one) in HEPES saline buffer pH 7.6 (p. 605). Filter through a 0.22 μm filter. This solution can be used for up-to 3 months if kept at 4°C. Take approximately 5 ml of blood into a sterile container containing 100 iu of liquid heparin, or 10 ml into 1.5 ml of ACD (see p. 603). With heparin as anticoagulant, add *c* 50 μg (20 μl) of the tropolone solution per ml of blood; with ACD add *c* 10 μg (4 μl) per ml of blood. Mix gently for 1 min, then add 2 MBq of freshly generated ^{111}In chloride. Mix on a roller mixer for 5 min, then wash twice in saline. Resuspend in a sufficient volume of saline for an injection of 10 ml and preparation of a standard.

Repeated blood volume measurements

When repeated blood volume measurements are required within a few days, the ^{51}Cr method can be used if the residual radioactivity is measured in the blood immediately before each test. However, the residual radioactivity increases the counting error and it may be necessary to increase the amount of tracer injected. The short-lived radionuclides (^{99m}Tc, ^{111}In) have the advantage that they can be used for repeated tests without this problem and also that the patient will be subjected to lower doses of radioactivity. The radionuclides are slowly eluted in vivo and in vitro. With ^{99m}Tc, elution is slight within the first 10–20 min; it gives results which compare closely with those of ^{51}Cr but because of progressively increasing elution the method is less satisfactory when delayed mixing necessitates sampling at 60 min post-injection.

DETERMINATION OF PLASMA VOLUME

^{125}I-human serum albumin method[9]

Human serum albumin (HSA) labelled with ^{125}I or ^{131}I is available commercially.* The albumin concentration should not be less than 20 g/l. The user must be reassured that only HIV and hepatitis B and C negative donors have been used as the source of albumin. ^{125}I is readily distinguishable from ^{51}Cr, ^{99m}Tc and ^{111}In, and this makes possible the simultaneous direct determination of red cell volume and plasma volume (see p. 323). If further doses of the radionuclide are to be administered for repeat tests, it is advisable to block the thyroid by administering 30 mg of potassium iodide by mouth on the day before the test and daily for 2 to 3 weeks thereafter.

Withdraw c 20 ml of blood into a syringe containing a few drops of sterile heparin solution and transfer to a 30 ml sterile bottle with a screw cap. After centrifuging at 1200–1500 g for 5–10 min, transfer c 7 ml of plasma to a second sterile bottle and add 2.5×10^3 Bq of the radionuclide-labelled HSA per kg body weight (c 0.2 MBq in total). Inject a measured amount (e.g. 5 ml) and retain the residue for preparation of a standard.

After 10, 20 and 30 min, withdraw blood samples from a vein other than that used for the original injection (or after flushing through with 10 ml of sterile 9 g/l NaCl (saline) if a butterfly needle has been used) and deliver into bottles containing EDTA or heparin.

*Available from ISO Pharma, Norway; Mallinckrodt Medical (Nuclear Medicine Division), Northampton.

Measure the PCV (see footnote, p. 321), centrifuge the sample and separate the plasma. Prepare a standard by diluting part of the residue of the uninjected HSA 1 in 100 in saline.

Measure the radioactivity of the plasma samples in a scintillation counter, and by extrapolation on semilogarithmic graph-paper, calculate the radioactivity of the plasma at zero time. If only a single sample is collected 10 min after the injection, the radioactivity at zero time may be obtained approximately by multiplying by 1.015 to allow for early loss of the radionuclide from the circulation. Reliance on a single 10 min sample will lead to error if the mixing of the albumin in the plasma is delayed. After measuring the radioactivity of the standard, the plasma volume (ml) is calculated as follows:

$$\frac{\text{Radioactivity of standard (cpm/ml)} \times \text{Dilution of standard} \times \text{Volume injected (ml)}}{\text{Radioactivity of post-injection sample (cpm/ml, adjusted to zero time)}}$$

DETERMINATION OF TOTAL BLOOD VOLUME

As has already been indicated, the total blood volume is frequently calculated from the red cell volume and PCV. But before this can be done, the observed PCV has to be corrected for the difference between the whole body and venous PCV.

Whole body and venous packed cell volume ratio

PCV measured on venous blood is not identical with the average PCV of all the blood in the body. This is mainly because the red cell:plasma ratio is less in small blood vessels (capillaries, arterioles and venules) than in large vessels. The ratio between the whole body PCV and venous blood PCV is normally about 0.9^9 and it is thus necessary in the calculation of total blood volume from measurements of red cell volume to multiply the observed PCV by 0.9. Thus total blood volume is given by:

$$\text{Red cell volume} \times \frac{1}{\text{PCV} \times 0.9}$$

However, the ratio varies in individuals, especially in splenomegaly, and it is better to estimate red cell volume and plasma volume by separate measurements rather than to attempt to calculate one of these from an estimate of the other.

Simultaneous measurement of red cell volume and plasma volume

Collect blood and label the red cells by one of the methods described above. If ^{99m}Tc is used, it is necessary first to inject stannous reagent (p. 321). Then add ^{125}I HSA (see p. 322) and mix it with the labelled red cell suspension. Inject an accurately measured amount and dilute the remainder 1 in 500 in water for use as a standard. Collect three blood samples at 10, 20 and 30 min, respectively, after the administration of the labelled blood and estimate the radioactivity of a measured volume of each sample and a similar volume of the standard.

When ^{99m}Tc has been used in combination with ^{125}I, count on the same day; then leave for 2 days to allow the ^{99m}Tc to decay and count again for ^{125}I activity. As the radioactivity in the preparation owing to ^{125}I is much smaller than that from ^{99m}Tc, the count from the red cells is not likely to be significantly affected by interference from ^{125}I in the initial count. However, if necessary, a correction can be made by subtracting the ^{125}I counts on day 2 (corrected for decay) from the original counts to obtain a measurement of the counts owing only to the ^{99m}Tc.

When ^{51}Cr has been used in combination with ^{125}I, and a multi-channel counter is available, measure the radioactivity owing to the ^{51}Cr and ^{125}I at the appropriate settings for ^{51}Cr and ^{125}I.

Calculate the radioactivity owing to the red cell label in the blood from the mean of the 10, 20 and 30 min samples, and obtain that owing to ^{125}I from the value extrapolated to zero time. Calculate red cell volume as described on page 321.

Plasma volume is calculated from the formula:

$$\frac{\text{Radioactivity of standard (cpm/ml)} \times \text{Dilution of standard} \times \text{volume injected (ml)}}{\text{Radioactivity of post-injection sample (cpm/ml, corrected to zero time)}} \times 1-PCV$$

Total blood volume = red cell volume + plasma volume

Expression of results of blood volume estimations

Red cell volume, plasma volume and total blood volume are usually expressed in ml/kg of body weight. Because fat is relatively avascular, low values are obtained in obese subjects and the relation between blood volume and body weight varies according to body composition. Blood volume is more closely correlated with lean body mass (LBM).[14,15] Earlier methods for determination of lean body mass were not practical as a routine procedure.[16] Discounting excess fat by using an estimate of so-called 'ideal weight' is arbitrary and tends to overcorrect for the avascularity of fat. Accordingly, various formulae have been devised to predict normal blood volume based on a combination of height, weight and sex. The International Council for Standardization in Haematology[17] analyzed these but concluded that it was not possible to establish which could be recommended as the most reliable. Consequently, ICSH developed two other formulae, based on body surface area, which provide normal reference values in men and women respectively.[17] They are as follows:

Mean normal red cell mass (ml)
Men: $[1486 \times S] - 825$; $\pm 25\%$ includes 98% limits
Women: $[1.06 \times \text{age (yr)}] + [822 \times S]$; $\pm 25\%$ includes 99% limits

Mean normal plasma volume (ml)
Men: $1578 \times S$; $\pm 25\%$ includes 99% limits
Women: $1395 \times S$; $\pm 25\%$ includes 99% limits

$S = [W^{0.425} \times H^{0.725} \times 0.007184]$, where S= surface area (m^2), W = weight (kg), H = height (cm)

However, the problem of establishing the LBM has been overcome to some extent, as there are now available instruments that are simple to use for estimating body composition by the different response of fat and other tissues to electrical impedance.**[15,18]

Thus, RCV can now be obtained by a direct measurement which discounts the effect of fat. The following graph has been designed to normalize the RCV in ml/kg LBM:[15]

On arithmetic graph paper with % Fat on the horizontal (x) axis and RCV in ml/kg total body weight on the vertical (y) axis, plot the intercepts of:

** Body composition analyser', Holtain Ltd, Crosswell, Dyfed, Wales; 'Body fat monitor', Tanita Corporation.

Fat 20% with RCV 29 ml; Fat 50% with RCV 19 ml. Join these two points and extend the line to the right and left.

When the % fat is known in any individual (male or female), draw a line vertically from this reading on the x axis to the slope, and where this intersects the slope draw a horizontal line to the y axis. The reading of this line on the y axis is the normalized RCV for that individual. When the measured RCV is >120% of this figure, it is equivalent to 43 ml/kg LBM and a diagnosis of polycythaemia can be made with confidence in men or women.

Range in health

The total blood volume is 250–350 ml at birth. After infancy, the volume increases gradually until adult life when the red cell volume in men is 30 ± 5 ml (2SD)/kg, and in women 25 ± 5 ml (SD)/kg. Plasma volume (men and women) is 40–50 ml/kg; total blood volume is 60–80 ml/kg.

As a rule, the blood volume remains remarkably constant in an individual and rapid adjustments take place within a few hours after blood transfusion or intravenous infusion.

In pregnancy, both the plasma volume and total blood volume increase. The plasma volume increases especially in the first trimester, the total volume later,[19] and by full term the plasma volume will have increased by c 40% and total blood volume by c 32% or even more. The blood volume returns to normal within a week postpartum.

Bed rest causes a reduction in plasma volume[20] and muscular exercise and changes in posture cause transient fluctuations. In practice, the patient should always be allowed to rest in a recumbent position for 15 min prior to measuring the blood volume.

SPLENIC RED CELL VOLUME

The red cell content of the normal spleen (the red cell 'pool') is less than 5% of the total red cell volume (i.e. <100–120 ml in an adult). In splenomegaly, the pool is increased, e.g. by perhaps as much as 5–10 times in myelofibrosis, polycythaemia, hairy cell leukaemia and lymphoproliferative disorders.[21] Increase in the volume of the splenic red cell pool may itself be a cause of anaemia; measurement of the pool is thus useful in the investigation of anaemia in these conditions. It is also useful in determining the cause of erythrocytosis as the expanded pool in polycythaemia vera contrasts with that in secondary polycythaemia in which it is normal.[22]

An approximate estimate of the splenic red cell volume can be obtained from the difference between the red cell volume calculated from the measurement of the blood sample which has been collected 2–3 min after the injection of labelled cells, and that measured after mixing has been completed, i.e. after a delay of c 20 min.[23] The splenic red cell volume can be estimated more accurately by quantitative scanning, after injecting viable red cells labelled with ^{99m}Tc.[24] The blood volume is measured in the usual way using c 100 MBq of ^{99m}Tc. The splenic area is scanned 20 min after the injection or after 60 min when there is splenomegaly. To delineate the spleen more precisely, it may be necessary to carry out a second scan after an injection of heat-damaged labelled red cells (see p. 333). From the radioactivity in the spleen, relative to that in a standard, and knowledge of the total red cell volume, the proportion of the total red cell volume contained in the spleen can be calculated. This technique has also been used for demonstrating localized accumulation of blood in haemangiomas in the liver,[25] telangiectasia and other vascular abnormalities.[26]

FERROKINETICS

Whilst much can be learnt about the rate and efficiency of erythropoiesis from the red cell count and reticulocyte counts, studies of iron metabolism and measurement of red cell life-span with radioactive isotopes may provide useful additional information.

Radioactive iron (^{59}Fe) has a moderately short half-life, 45 days, and labels haemoglobin after

injection. It also labels the plasma iron pool and this allows the measurement of iron clearance and calculation of plasma iron turnover. Its subsequent appearance in haemoglobin permits the assessment of the rate of haemoglobin synthesis and the completeness of the utilization of iron. Since it is a γ-ray emitter, radioactivity can be measured in vivo, and the sites of distribution of the administered iron and the probable sites of erythropoiesis can thus be determined.

IRON DISTRIBUTION

Principle

Iron is transported to the bone marrow bound to transferrin. At the surface of the erythroblasts, the complex releases its iron which enters the cell to be incorporated into haem, leaving the transferrin free for recycling. Iron not bound to transferrin finds its way to the liver and to other organs rather than to the bone marrow, whilst colloidal particles of iron are rapidly removed by phagocytic cells.

The ferrokinetic studies with ^{59}Fe which provide information on erythropoiesis include the rate of clearance of the radioiron from the plasma, plasma iron turnover and iron incorporation into circulating red cells (iron utilization). These are relatively simple procedures but they do not take account of the recirculation of iron which returns to the plasma from tissues, nor of iron turnover resulting from dyserythropoiesis or haemolysis. To take account of these factors requires much more complex and time-consuming procedures with multiple sampling over an extended period.[27,28] These are essential for the quantitative measurement of effective and ineffective erythropoiesis but the simpler tests provide sufficiently reliable and useful measurements for clinical purposes.

In ferrokinetic studies, it is important to ensure that any iron administered is bound to transferrin. In most cases, plasma has an adequate amount of transferrin. However, the unsaturated iron-binding capacity (UIBC) or transferrin concentration of the patient's plasma should be measured before the test is carried out and, if the UIBC is <1 mg/l (20 µmol/l) or the transferrin concentration is <0.6 g/l, normal donor plasma (HIV and hepatitis B and C negative) should be used instead of that of the patient for the subsequent labelling procedure.

Method

Under sterile conditions, obtain 5–10 ml of plasma from freshly collected heparinized blood. Add 0.4 MBq of ^{59}Fe ferric citrate (specific activity >0.2 MBq/µg). Incubate at room temperature for 15 min. Fill a syringe with all but 1 ml of the mixture. Weigh the syringe to the nearest 10 mg. Inject its content intravenously into the patient, starting a stopwatch at the mid-point of the injection. Reweigh the empty syringe and calculate the volume injected:

$$\text{Volume of plasma (ml)} = \frac{\text{Weight of plasma (g)}}{1.015}$$

Dilute the residual portion of the dose (1 ml) 1 in 100 in water and use as a measure of the total amount of radioactivity and as a standard in subsequent measurements.

PLASMA IRON CLEARANCE

Take a sample at 3 min and four or five further samples over a period of 1–2 h, collecting them into heparin or EDTA. Retain a portion of one sample for measurement of plasma iron. Measure the radioactivity in unit volumes of plasma from the samples and plot the values obtained on loglinear graph paper. A straight line will usually be obtained for the initial slope. The radioactivity at the moment of injection is inferred by extrapolation back to zero time and the time taken for the plasma radioactivity to decrease to half its initial value ($T_{1/2}$-plasma clearance) is read off the graph (Fig. 15.2).

Range of $T_{1/2}$-plasma clearance in health
60–140 min.

The clearance rate is influenced by the intensity of erythropoiesis and also by the activity of the

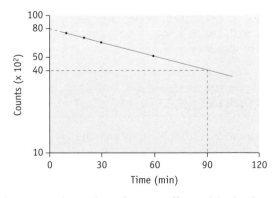

Fig. 15.2 Plasma iron clearance. [59]Fe activity in plasma at 10, 20, 30 and 60 min extrapolated to the vertical axis to obtain activity at zero time. The $T_{1/2}$ was 90 min.

macrophages of the RE system, especially in the liver, spleen and bone marrow, where the iron is retained as storage iron. Also, to a lesser extent, circulating reticulocytes may take up some of the iron. A rapid clearance indicates hyperactivity of one or more of these mechanisms, as for instance in iron-deficiency anaemias, haemorrhagic anaemias, haemolytic anaemias and polycythaemia vera. The clearance rate is decreased in aplastic anaemia. In leukaemia and in myelofibrosis, the results are variable, depending upon the amount of erythropoietic marrow and the extent of extramedullary erythropoiesis; in myelofibrosis, however, rapid clearance is by far the more common finding. In dyserythropoiesis, the clearance may be normal or accelerated.

PLASMA IRON TURNOVER

When the plasma iron clearance is related to the iron content of the plasma, a value can be obtained for plasma iron turnover (PIT) in mg/l or µmol/l of blood per day.

PIT (mg/l/day) is calculated from the formula:

$$\text{Plasma iron (mg/l)}^* \times 0.693^{**} \times \frac{(60 \times 24)}{T_{1/2} \text{(min)}} \times (1 - \text{PCV})$$

which may be simplified to:

$$\frac{\text{Plasma iron (mg/l)} \times 10^3}{T_{1/2} \text{(min)}} \times (1 - \text{PCV}).$$

PIT (µmol/l/day) is calculated from the formula:

$$\frac{\text{Plasma iron (µmol/l)} \times 10^3}{T_{1/2} \text{(min)}} \times (1 - \text{PCV}).$$

The range in normal subjects is 4–8 mg/l/day or 70–140 µmol/l/day.

The PIT is increased in iron-deficiency anaemia, haemolytic anaemias and myelofibrosis. It is increased also in ineffective erythropoiesis, particularly so in thalassaemia. In aplastic anaemia, the PIT is normal or decreased, but when the plasma iron is raised, the PIT may be above normal. The calculation of PIT assumes a constant rate of iron transport and, while it is an indicator of total erythropoiesis, it does not distinguish between effective and ineffective erythropoiesis. For the reasons discussed earlier and because the findings in health and disease overlap, measurement of the PIT has only limited clinical usefulness.

IRON UTILIZATION

Collect blood samples daily or at least on alternate days for a period of about 2 weeks after the administration of the ^{59}Fe. Measure the radioactivity per ml of whole blood and calculate the percentage utilization on each day from the formula:

$$\frac{\text{cpm/ml daily whole blood sample} \times 100 \times f}{\text{cpm/ml whole blood sample at zero time}}$$

where f is a PCV correction factor, i.e. $f = \dfrac{0.9 \text{ PCV}}{1 - 0.9 \text{ PCV}}$

When there is reason to suspect that the body:venous PCV ratio is not 0.9 (see p. 322), measure the red cell volume by a direct method (p. 320)§ and calculate the percentage utilization on each day from the formula:

$$\text{Percentage utilization} = \frac{\text{Red cell volume (ml)} \times \text{cpm/ml red cells} \times 100}{\text{Total radioactivity injected (cpm)}^{‡}}$$

Plot the daily measured percentages against time on arithmetic graph paper. Record the maximum utilization (Fig. 15.3).

The calculation gives a measure of effective erythropoiesis. In normal subjects, red cell radioactivity rises steadily from 24 h, and reaches a maximum of 70–80% utilization on the 10th to 14th day.

A rapid plasma clearance is usually associated with early and relatively complete utilization and the converse also applies. The results are inconsistent in megaloblastic anaemias and in haemoglobinopathies in which there is ineffective

---

*Because of marked diurnal variation, the plasma iron should be measured on a sample of blood collected during the plasma clearance study.

**Natural log of 2.

---

§Calculation of plasma volume from extrapolation of the ^{59}Fe disappearance curve is often unreliable and the figure for plasma volume should not be used as the basis for the calculation of red cell volume.

‡The radioactivity is adjusted for physical decay up to the day of measurement.

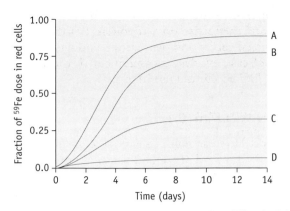

Fig. 15.3 Iron utilization. Red-cell uptake of ^{59}Fe in (A) iron deficiency and polycythaemia, (B) a normal subject, (C) dyserythropoiesis, and (D) severe aplastic anaemia.

erythropoiesis; and also in myelofibrosis, depending on the extent of extramedullary erythropoiesis and whether the red cell life-span is reduced. If there is rapid haemolysis, the utilization curve will be distorted by destruction of some of the labelled red cells; this may be recognized if frequent (daily) samples are measured. In aplastic anaemia, the utilization is usually 10–15%; in ineffective erythropoiesis, it is as a rule 30–50%.

If the iron utilization is known, it is possible to determine the red cell iron turnover expressed as mg/l blood per day (PIT × % maximum utilization). This provides a measure of effective ery-

thropoiesis. In normal subjects, it is about 5 mg/l, but it gives an underestimate if there is increased haemolysis. In normal subjects, the ratio of PIT to red cell iron turnover is 1.2–1.3:1.0.[29]

The ferrokinetic patterns in various diseases are shown in Table 15.3.[9]

BODY IRON DISTRIBUTION

An overall picture of ferrokinetics can be constructed from surface counting with a scintillation probe positioned over the liver, spleen, sacrum (for bone marrow) and heart (for blood pool) after an intravenous injection of ^{59}Fe. By counting over several days, it is possible to identify sites of erythropoiesis from early counts and sites of red cell destruction from later counts. This test is rarely performed nowadays although it has some clinical value for determining the extent of extramedullary erythropoiesis in the spleen before splenectomy.

Where there are facilities for using cyclotron-produced ^{52}Fe and positron emission tomography (PET), high-resolution images of the intra- and extramedullary distribution of erythropoietic tissue can be obtained. This is especially helpful in the myeloproliferative disorders for diagnosing transition of polycythaemia to myelofibrosis and for differentiating essential thrombocythaemia from reactive thrombocytosis.[30] It is also useful in identifying residual skeletal erythropoiesis in aplastic anaemia.

Table 15.3 Ferrokinetic patterns in various diseases

	Plasma clearance $T_{1/2}$	Plasma iron turnover	Red cell utilization*
Normal	60–140 min	70–140 μmol/l/day	80%
Iron deficiency	Shortened	Normal	↑ (90%)
Aplastic anaemia	Prolonged	Normal	↓ (10%)
Chronic infection	Slightly shortened	Normal	Normal
Dyserythropoiesis	Slightly shortened	Increased	↓ (30%)
Myelofibrosis	Shortened	Increased	↓ (50%)
Haemolytic anaemia	Shortened	Increased	↑ (85%)

*↑ = increased; ↓ = decreased. Average figures are shown, but there is a wide range, depending on the stage and severity of the disease.

ESTIMATION OF THE LIFE-SPAN OF RED CELLS IN VIVO

There is an extensive literature on the survival of red cells in haemolytic anaemias using radionuclide labelling of red cells (see review by Bentley & Miller[31]). Although now undertaken less frequently than in the past, measurement of red cell survival can still provide important data in cases of anaemia in which increased haemolysis is suspected but not clearly demonstrated by other tests. In the usual procedure, a population of circulating red cells of all ages is labelled ('random labelling'). By contrast, in 'cohort labelling' a radionuclide is incorporated into haemoglobin during its synthesis by erythroblasts and radioactivity is measured in red cells which appear in the circulation as a cohort of closely similar age. Red cell life-span can be calculated from measurements of red cell iron turnover (p. 326)[32] but the results have to be interpreted with caution because of the re-utilization for haem synthesis of iron derived from red cells at the end of their life-span. Random labelling is a much more practical method than cohort labelling.

RADIOACTIVE CHROMIUM (^{51}Cr) METHOD

^{51}Cr is a γ-ray emitter with a half-life of 27.8 days. As a red cell label, it is used in the form of hexavalent sodium chromate. After passing through the surface membrane of the red cells, it is reduced to the trivalent form which binds to protein, preferentially to the β-polypeptide chains of haemoglobin.[33] In this form, it is not re-utilized nor transferred to other cells in the circulation.

The main disadvantage of ^{51}Cr is that it gradually elutes from red cells as they circulate; there may be, too, an increased loss over the first 1 to 3 days, and uncertainty as to how much has been lost makes it impossible to measure red cell life-span accurately. Chromium, whether radioactive or non-radioactive, is toxic to red cells probably by its oxidizing actions; it inhibits glycolysis in red cells when present at a concentration of 10 μg/ml or more[34] and blocks glutathione reductase activity at a concentration exceeding 5 μg/ml.[35] Blood should thus not be exposed to more than 2 μg of chromium per ml of packed red cells.

$Na_2{}^{51}CrO_4$ is available commercially at a specific activity of c 15–20 GBq/mg Cr. For administration, the stock solution usually requires to be dissolved in 9 g/l NaCl (saline) (see below). ACD must not be used as a diluent as this reduces the chromate to the cationic chromic form.

Care must be taken to avoid lysis when the red cells are washed; and it may be necessary, especially if the blood contains spherocytes, to use a slightly hypertonic solution, e.g. 12 g/l NaCl. This should certainly be used if an osmotic fragility test has demonstrated lysis in 9 g/l NaCl. In patients whose plasma contains high-titre, high-thermal-amplitude cold agglutinins, the blood must be collected in a warmed syringe, delivered into ACD solution previously warmed to 37°C and the labelling and washing in saline carried out in a 'warm room' at 37°C.

Method[36]

The technique of labelling red cells is the same as for blood volume measurement (see p. 320). To ensure as little damage to red cells as possible, with subsequent minimal early loss and later elution, it is important to maintain the blood at an optimal pH. This can be achieved by adding 10 volumes of blood to 1.5 volumes of NIH-A ACD solution (see p. 603).

For a red cell survival study, 0.02 MBq per kg body weight (an average total dose of c 2 MBq) is recommended. If this is to be combined with a spleen scan or pool measurement, a higher dose (4 MBq) should be used, bearing in mind that <2 μg of chromium should be added per ml of packed red cells.

After injection, allow the labelled cells to circulate in the recipient for 10 min (or for 60 min in patients with cardiac failure or splenomegaly in whom mixing may be delayed). Then collect a sample of blood from a vein other than that used for the injection (or after washing the needle through with saline if a butterfly needle is used) and mix with EDTA as anticoagulant. The radioactivity in this sample provides a base line for subsequent observations. Retain part of the labelled cell suspension which was not injected into the patient to serve as a standard. This enables the blood volume to be calculated if required.

Take further 4–5 ml blood samples from the patient 24 h later (day 1) and subsequently at intervals, the frequency of the samples depending on the rate of red cell destruction: in general, three specimens between day 2 and day 7, and then two specimens per week for the duration of the study. Measurements should be continued until at least half the radioactivity has disappeared from the circulation.

Measure the haemoglobin or PCV in a part of each sample; then lyse the samples with saponin, mix well and deliver 1 ml into counting tubes, if possible in duplicate.

Measurement of radioactivity

Estimate the percentage survival (of ^{51}Cr) on any day (t) by comparing the radioactivity of the sample taken on that day with that of the day 0 sample, i.e. the sample withdrawn 10 (or 60) min after the injection of the labelled cells. Thus ^{51}Cr survival on day t (%) is given by:

$$\frac{\text{cpm/ml of blood on Day t}}{\text{cpm/ml of blood on Day 0}} \times 100$$

No adjustment is necessary for the physical decay of the isotope, provided that the standard is counted within a few minutes of the day t sample.

Carry out the measurements in any high-quality scintillation counter, at least 2500 counts being recorded in order to achieve a precision within ±2%.

Processing of radioactivity measurements

Before the data can be analysed and interpreted, factors, other than physical decay, which are involved in the disappearance of radioactivity from the circulation have to be considered. There are two processes: ^{51}Cr-labelled cells are lost from the circulation by lysis, phagocytosis or haemorrhage and, in addition, ^{51}Cr is eluted from intact red cells which still circulate.

Elution

The rate of elution differs to a small extent from one individual to another. It is thought to vary to a greater extent between different diseases, especially when the red cell life-span is considerably reduced. However, in such cases, elution and variation in the rate of elution become unimportant. The rate of elution is also influenced by technique, especially by the anticoagulant solution into which the blood is collected prior to labelling. With the NIH-A ACD solution, the rate of elution is c 1% per day.[36]

Early loss

Sometimes, in addition to the elution that occurs continuously and at a relatively low and constant rate, up to 10% of the ^{51}Cr may be lost within the first 24 h. The cause of this major early loss is obscure and several components may be involved. If this major loss does not continue beyond the first 2 days, it is often looked upon as an artefact, in the sense that it does not denote an increased rate of lysis in vivo, and it can be and usually is ignored by replotting the figures as described on page 331. This procedure is acceptable, at least for clinical studies, but it does not take into account the possibility that a small proportion of red cells are present that lyse rapidly. It is common practice to calculate the T_{50}Cr,* i.e. the time taken for the concentration of ^{51}Cr in the blood to fall to 50% of its initial value, after correcting the data for physical decay but not for elution. The chief objection to the use of T_{50}Cr is that it may be misleading without additional information on the pattern of the survival curve. Moreover, the mean red cell life-span cannot be directly derived from it. With the technique described above, the mean value of T_{50} in normal subjects is c 30 days, range 25 to 33 days (Table 15.4).

Correction for elution

When haemolysis is marked, elution is of minor importance and can be ignored. When haemolysis is not greatly increased, it is essential to correct for elution. This can be done by multiplying the measured survival by the factors given in Table 15.4.

Survival curves

Normal red cell survival (corrected for elution) will be in the range shown in Figure 15.4. When survival is reduced, a survival curve should be drawn, and from this the mean red cell life-span can be derived.

---

*T_{50} is used rather than $T_{1/2}$ as the elimination of the label is not a constant exponential fraction of the original amount.

Table 15.4 Normal range for ^{51}Cr survival curves with correction for elution

Day	%^{51}Cr (corrected for decay; *not* corrected for elution)	Elution correction factors*
1	93–98	1.03
2	89–97	1.05
3	86–95	1.06
4	83–93	1.07
5	80–92	1.08
6	78–90	1.10
7	77–88	1.11
8	76–86	1.12
9	74–84	1.13
10	72–83	1.14
11	70–81	1.16
12	68–79	1.17
13	67–78	1.18
14	65–77	1.19
15	64–75	1.20
16	62–74	1.22
17	59–73	1.23
18	58–71	1.25
19	57–69	1.26
20	56–67	1.27
21	55–66	1.29
22	53–65	1.31
23	52–63	1.32
24	51–60	1.34
25	50–59	1.36
30	44–52	1.47
35	39–47	1.53
40	34–42	1.60

*To correct for elution, multiply the % ^{51}Cr by the elution factor for the particular day.

Plot the % radioactivity figures or count rates per ml of whole blood (corrected for physical decay and for elution) on arithmetic and semilogarithmic graph paper and attempt to fit straight lines passing through the data points.

1. If a straight line *can* be fitted to the arithmetic plot, the mean red cell life-span is given by the point in time at which the line or its extension cuts the abscissa (Fig. 15.5).
2. As a rule, however, a straight line is better fitted to the semilogarithmic plot; the mean red cell life-span can be read as the exponential e^{-1}, i.e. the time when 37% of the cells are still surviving (Fig. 15.6) or calculated by multiplying the half-time of the fitted line by the reciprocal of the natural log of 2 (0.693), i.e. multiplying by 1.44.

A computer programmed curve-fitting procedure is more precise but is not likely to improve overall accuracy of the results for clinical purposes.

Interpretation of survival curves

In the auto-immune haemolytic anaemias, the slope of elimination is usually markedly curvilinear when the data are plotted on arithmetic graph paper. Red cell destruction is typically random and the curve of elimination is thus exponential, and the data give a straight line when plotted on semilogarithmic graph paper.

In some cases of haemolytic anaemia (possibly only when there are intracorpuscular defects), the survival curve appears to consist of two components, an initial steep slope being followed by a

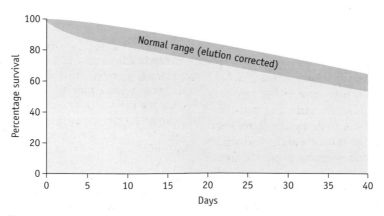

Fig. 15.4 ^{51}Cr red cell survival. The hatched area shows the normal range.

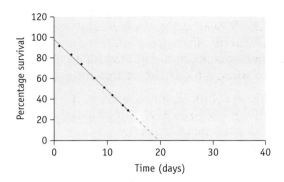

Fig. 15.5 ^{51}Cr red cell survival curve. Patient with hereditary spherocytosis. The results give a straight line when plotted on arithmetic graph paper. The mean cell life-span is indicated by the point at which its extension cuts the abscissa (20 days).

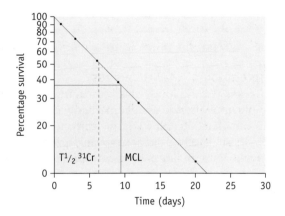

Fig. 15.6 ^{51}Cr red cell survival curve. Patient with auto-immune haemolytic anaemia. The results have been plotted on semilogarithmic graph paper and the mean cell life-span was read as the time when 37% of the cells were still surviving (9 to 10 days). The T_{50}Cr was 6 to 7 days. MCL, mean cell life-span.

much less steeply falling slope. This suggests the presence of cells of widely varying life-span. This type of 'double population' curve is seen in paroxysmal nocturnal haemoglobinuria and in sickle-cell anaemia, and in some cases of hereditary enzyme-deficiency haemolytic anaemia, and when the labelled cells consist of a mixture of transfused normal cells and short-lived patient's cells. The mean cell life-span of the entire cell population can be deduced by plotting the points on semilogarithmic graph paper, as described above. The pro-

portion of cells belonging to the longer-lived population can be estimated by plotting the data on arithmetic graph paper and extrapolating the less steep slope back to the ordinate; the life-span of this population can be estimated by extending the same slope to the abscissa (Fig. 15.7). The life-span of the short-lived cells can be deduced from the formula:

$$MCL_S = \frac{\%S}{\dfrac{100}{MCL_T} - \dfrac{\%L}{MCL_L}}$$

where S = short lived population, L = longer lived population, T = entire cell population, and MCL = mean cell life-span.

Correction for early loss

The simplest method is to ignore the early loss by taking as 100% the radioactivity still present at the end of 24–48 h. Alternatively, the following method can be employed; it has the advantage that the slope of the survival curve is not altered. The data are plotted on arithmetical graph paper, the line of the slope beyond the initial steep part is extrapolated back to the ordinate and the point of

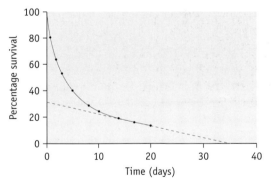

Fig. 15.7 ^{51}Cr red cell survival curve showing a 'double population'. By plotting the data on semilogarithmic graph paper as described in Figure 15.6 and on page 330, the mean cell life-span (MCL) of the entire cell population was deduced as 5 days. When plotted on arithmetic graph paper, by extrapolation of the less steep slope to the ordinate it was deduced that approximately 30% of the red cells belonged to one population, and by extrapolation of the same slope to the abscissa the MCL of this population was deduced as 35 days. The life-span of the remaining 70% of cells was calculated to be 3.6 days (see formula on this page). The T_{50}Cr was 3 to 4 days.

intersection is taken as 100% and the ordinate scale recalibrated accordingly.

Blood volume changes

There is no need to correct the measurements of radioactivity per ml of whole blood for alterations in PCV provided that the total blood volume remains constant throughout the study. However, if it is suspected that the blood volume may be changing, e.g. in patients suffering from haemorrhage or being transfused, serial determinations of blood volume should be carried out and the observed radioactivity should be multiplied by the observed blood volume and divided by the initial blood volume. In practice, if a patient receives a blood transfusion during a survival study, it can, as a general rule, be assumed that the blood volume

will have returned to its pretransfusion level within 24–48 h.

Correction of survival data for blood loss

When there is a relatively constant loss of blood during a red cell survival study, the true mean red cell life-span can be obtained by the following equation:

$$\text{True MCL} = \frac{\text{Ta} \times \text{RCV}}{\text{RCV} - (\text{Ta} \times \text{L})}$$

where Ta = apparent time of MCL (days), RCV = red cell volume (ml), and L = mean rate of loss of red cells (ml/day).

Normal red cell life-span

The mean red cell life-span in health is usually taken as 120 days.

COMPATIBILITY TEST

The behaviour of labelled donor cells in a recipient will provide important information on the compatibility or otherwise of the donor blood:

1. When serological tests suggest that all normal donors are incompatible.
2. When in the presence of an allo-antibody no non-reacting donor can be found.
3. When the recipient has had an unexplained haemolytic transfusion reaction.
4. When the viability of the donor cells may possibly have been affected by suboptimal storage conditions.

Method[36]

Remove 1–2 ml of blood from the donor bag using a sterile technique. Label 0.5 ml of the red cells with 0.8 MBq of ^{51}Cr, 2 MBq of ^{111}In, or 2 MBq of ^{99m}Tc in the standard way (p. 320) and administer to the recipient. Collect 5–10 ml of blood into EDTA or heparin at 3, 10 and 60 min after the injection from a vein other than that used for the injection. Prepare 1 ml samples in counting vials. Centrifuge the remainder of the specimens and pipette 1 ml of the plasma into counting vials. Measure the radioactivity in the usual way. Calculate the activity in the blood and plasma samples as a percentage of the 3 min blood sample.

Interpretation

With compatible blood, the radioactivity in the 60 min sample is, on average, 99% of that of the 3 min sample, but it may vary between 94% and 104%. If the blood radioactivity at 60 min is not less than 70% and the plasma activity is not more than 3%, the donor cells may be transfused with minimal hazard.[36]

Determination of sites of red cell destruction using ^{51}Cr

As ^{51}Cr is a γ-ray emitter, the sites of destruction of red cells, with special reference to the spleen and liver, can be determined by in-vivo surface counting using a shielded scintillation counter placed, respectively, over the heart, spleen and liver. This procedure is now used infrequently. It is laborious, takes 2 to 3 weeks to complete, and even minor fluctuations in positioning of the patient or the counting conditions may result in significant variation in measurements. However, formerly it provided valuable information on the role of the spleen in various types of haemolytic anaemia and helped to define their management, especially by predicting response to splenectomy.[37–39] A standardized method and procedure have been described.[40]

VISUALIZATION OF THE SPLEEN BY SCINTILLATION SCANNING

This procedure was developed as an extension of surface counting described above. It is used:

1. to demonstrate enlargement or abnormal position of the spleen or accessory splenic tissue
2. to identify the nature of a mass in the left hypochondrium
3. to demonstrate the presence of space-occupying lesions within the spleen
4. to demonstrate functional hyposplenism or the presence of splenuncules.

If red blood cells labelled with ^{51}Cr, ^{99m}Tc or ^{111}In are heat damaged, they will be selectively removed by the spleen. ^{99m}Tc-labelled colloid is also removed from circulation by the spleen, but this is not as specific as it is also taken up by reticulo-endothelial cells in the liver and elsewhere. Accumulation of radioactivity within the spleen after administration of heat-damaged labelled cells thus provides a means of demonstrating its size and position, whether it is absent and whether there are any splenuncules. The rate of uptake of the isotope by the spleen is a measure of its function (see below). Imaging by scintillation scanning is usually started about 1 h after the injection of the damaged cells, but it can be performed up to 3–4 h later; satisfactory scans can also be obtained with ^{51}Cr and ^{111}In up to 24 h after the injection.

Methods

With ^{51}Cr as the label[41]

Deliver approximately 10 ml of the patient's blood into 1.5 ml of sterile ACD solution. Centrifuge the sample at 1200–1500 *g* for 5–10 min. Keep the plasma in a sterile container Label the red cells with $Na_2{}^{51}CrO_4$, using *c* 4 MBq. Wash the labelled cells three times in sterile 9 g/l NaCl (saline). Place the packed cells in a sterile 30 ml glass bottle with a screw cap. Heat the bottle in a water-bath at a constant temperature of 49.5–50°C for exactly 20 min with occasional gentle mixing. Resuspend the cells in their own plasma and inject intravenously as soon as possible. Follow a standardized technique meticulously. It is important to use a glass bottle as some plastic containers take considerably longer than glass to reach the required temperature.

With ^{99m}Tc as the label[42]

Carry out pre-tinning in vivo by an injection of a stannous compound as described on page 321. Then collect 5–10 ml of blood into a sterile bottle containing 100 iu of heparin. Wash twice in sterile 9 g/l NaCl (saline), centrifuging at 1200–1500 *g* for 5–10 min. Transfer 2 ml of the packed red cells to a 30 ml glass bottle with a screw cap; heat the bottle in a water-bath at a constant temperature of 49.5–50°C for exactly 20 min with occasional gentle mixing. Wash the cells in saline until the supernatant is free from haemoglobin and discard the final supernatant. Label with 100 MBq of ^{99m}Tc by the method described on page 321. After standing for 5 min, wash twice in saline. Resuspend in about 10 ml of saline and inject as soon as possible.

With ^{111}In as the label

Prepare 2 ml of heat-damaged red cells as for the ^{99m}Tc method. Wash twice in sterile 9 g/l NaCl (saline). Add 5 MBq of ^{111}In, as described on page 321. Then wash twice in saline. Resuspend in about 10 ml of saline and inject as soon as possible.

SPLEEN FUNCTION

Information on splenic activity may be obtained by measuring the rate of clearance of heat-damaged labelled red cells from the circulation. A blood sample is taken exactly 3 min after the mid-point of the injection and further samples are collected at 5 min intervals for 30 min, at 45 min and a final sample at 60 min. The radioactivity in each sample is measured and expressed as a percentage of the radioactivity in the 3 min sample. The results are plotted on semilogarithmic graph paper, the 3 min sample being taken as 100% radioactivity.

For constant results, a carefully standardized technique is necessary to ensure that the red cells are damaged to the same extent.[41]

The disappearance curve is, as a rule, exponential (Fig. 15.8). The initial slope reflects the splenic blood flow; the rate of blood flow is calculated as the reciprocal of the time taken for the radioactivity to fall to half the 3 min value, i.e. $\dfrac{0.693}{T\frac{1}{2}}$, where 0.693 is the natural log of 2.

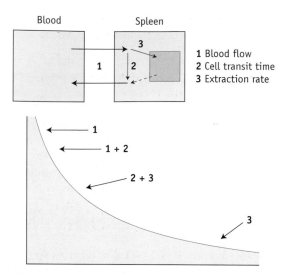

1 Blood flow
2 Cell transit time
3 Extraction rate

Fig. 15.8 Curve of disappearance of heat-damaged red cells from circulation. The curve shows the sequence of blood flow, transient pooling, sequestration and irreversible trapping of cells.

When the spleen is functioning normally the $T_{1/2}$ is 5–15 min and fractional splenic blood flow is 0.05–0.14 ml/min, i.e. 5–14% of the circulating blood per min. The clearance rate is considerably prolonged in thrombocythaemia and in conditions associated with splenic atrophy such as sickle-cell anaemia, coeliac disease and dermatitis herpetiformis.[21] It thus provides some indication of spleen function. However, the disappearance curve is a complex of at least two components. The first (mentioned above) reflects the splenic blood flow, and the second component mainly measures cell trapping, the consequence of both transient sequestration and phagocytosis with irreversible extraction of the cells from circulation.[43,44] Measurement of phagocytosis alone is obtained more reliably with IgG (anti-D) coated red cells.[45]

MEASUREMENT OF BLOOD LOSS FROM THE GASTROINTESTINAL TRACT USING ^{51}Cr

The ^{51}Cr method of red cell labelling can be used to measure quantitatively blood lost into the gastrointestinal tract, as ^{51}Cr is neither excreted nor more than minimally reabsorbed. Accordingly, when the blood contains ^{51}Cr-labelled red cells faecal radioactivity is at a very low level unless bleeding has taken place somewhere within the gastrointestinal tract. Measurement of the faecal radioactivity then gives a reliable indication of the extent of the blood loss.

Method
Label the patient's own blood with approximately 4 MBq of ^{51}Cr, as described on page 320. On each day of the test, collect the faeces in plastic or waxed cardboard cartons. Prepare a standard by adding a measured volume (3–5 ml) of the patient's blood, collected on each day, to approximately 100 ml of water in a similar carton.

Compare the radioactivity of the faecal samples and the corresponding daily standard in a large-volume counting system (see p. 317). Then:

Volume of blood in faeces (in ml) =
$$\frac{\text{cpm/24 h faeces collection}}{\text{cpm/ml standard}}$$

Blood loss from any other source, e.g. surgical operation or menstruation, can be measured in a similar way by counting swabs, dressings, etc., placed in a carton. It is not, however, possible to measure blood or haemoglobin loss in the urine (haematuria or haemoglobinuria) by this method as free ^{51}Cr is normally excreted in the urine.

An imaging procedure has also been described, in which blood is labelled with ^{99m}Tc and a large field scintillation scan is performed after 60–90 min, and if necessary again at intervals for 24 h.[46]

MEASUREMENT OF PLATELET LIFE-SPAN

Principle
The procedure for measuring platelet life-span is broadly similar to that for red cell survival (see p. 328). A method using ^{111}In-labelled platelets was recommended by the International Committee for Standardization in Haematology,[47]

and a modification was described in the eighth edition of this book by means of which it is possible to carry out a survival study on patients with low platelet counts and to combine this with measurement of platelet pooling and identification of sites of platelet destruction.

By this method, normal platelet life-span is 8 to 10 days, but the validity of the analysis is based on the assumption that the blood volume is constant and the pattern of disappearance of platelets from the circulation remains constant during the course of the study.

Platelet survival in disease

In idiopathic thrombocytopenia purpura, platelet life-span is considerably reduced. It is also shortened in consumption coagulopathies, and in thrombotic thrombocytopenic purpura. In thrombocytopenia because of defective production of platelets, the life-span should be normal provided that platelets are not being lost by bleeding during the course of the study. In thrombocytopenia associated with spleno-megaly, the recovery of injected labelled platelets is low, but their survival is usually almost normal. By quantitative scanning with ^{111}In, it is possible to measure the splenic platelet pool and to distinguish the relative importance of pooling and destruction of platelets in the spleen.[30,48,49] The splenic platelet pool is normally about 30% of the total platelet population, and it is thought that each platelet spends one-third of its life-span in the spleen.[49] The size of the pool is increased in splenomegaly, resulting in thrombocytopenia but not necessarily in a reduced mean platelet life-span. In immune thrombocyto-penias, antibody-coated platelets may be destroyed in the liver (whilst a normal pool is present in the spleen) or they may be destroyed in the liver and in the spleen. This complicated pattern means that platelet kinetic studies are often difficult to interpret, and they have only a limited place in diagnosis and routine management of patients with thrombocytopenia.

REFERENCES

1 Wagner HN, Szabo Z, Buchanan JW 1995 Principles of nuclear medicine. Saunders, Philadelphia.

2 Bernier DR, Christian PE, Langan JK 1997 Nuclear medicine technology and techniques. Mosby, St Louis.

3 Maisey MN, Britton KE, Collier BD 1998 Clinical nuclear medicine, 3rd edn. Chapman and Hall, London.

4 Lewis SM, Bayly RJ (eds) 1986 Methods in Hematology14: Radionuclides in haematology. Churchill Livingstone, Edinburgh.

5 National Radiological Protection Board 2000 The ionizing radiation (Medical exposure) regulations 2000. HSE Book, London.

6 ARSAC 1993 Notes for guidance on the administration of radioactive substances to persons for the purposes of diagnosis. United Kingdom Department of Health, London.

7 International Atomic Energy Agency 1973 Safe handling of radionuclides. IAEA Safety Series No. 1. IAEA, Vienna.

8 Bentley SA, Lewis SM 1976 The relationship between total red cell volume, plasma volume and venous haematocrit. British Journal of Haematology 33:301–307.

9 International Committee for Standardization in Haematology 1980 Recommended methods for measurements of red-cell and plasma volume. Journal of Nuclear Medicine 21:793–800.

10 Ferrant A, Lewis SM, Szur L 1974 The elution of ^{99m}Tc from red cells and its effect on red cell volume measurement. Journal of Clinical Pathology 27:983–985.

11 Radia R, Peters AM, Deenemode M, et al 1981 Measurement of red cell volume and splenic red cell pool using [113m]indium. British Journal of Haematology 49:587–591.

12 Goodwin DA 1978 Cell labelling with oxine chelates of radioactive metal ions: techniques and clinical implications. Journal of Nuclear Medicine 19:557–559.

13 Osman S, Danpure HJ 1987 A simple in vitro method of radiolabelling human erythrocytes in whole blood with [113m]In-tropolonate. European Journal of Haematology 39:125–127.

14 Muldowney FP 1957 The relationship of total red cell mass to lean body mass in man. Clinical Science 16:163–169.

15 Berlin NI, Lewis SM 2000 Measurement of total red-cell volume relative to lean body mass for diagnosis of polycythaemia. American Journal of Clinical Pathology. 114:922–926.

16 Lukaski HC 1987 Methods for the assessment of human body composition: Traditional and new. American Journal of Clinical Nutrition 46:537–556.

17 International Council for Standardization in Haematology (Expert panel on radionuclides) 1995 Interpretation of measured red cell mass and plasma volume in adults. British Journal of Haematology 89:747–756.

18 Lukaski HC, Johnson PE, Bolunchuk WW, et al 1985 Assessment of fat-free mass using bioelectrical impedance measurements of the human body. American Journal of Clinical Nutrition 41:810–817.

19 Lund CJ, Sisson TRC 1958 Blood volume and anemia of mother and baby. American Journal of Obstetrics and Gynecology 76:1013–1023.

20 Taylor HL, Erickson L, Henschel A, et al 1945 The effect of bed rest on the blood volume of normal young men. American Journal of Physiology 144:227–232.

21 Pettit JE 1977 Spleen function. Clinics in Haematology 6:639–656.

22 Bateman S, Lewis SM, Nicholas A, et al 1978 Splenic red cell pooling: a diagnostic feature in polycythaemia. British Journal of Haematology 40:389–396.

23 Pryor DS 1967 The mechanism of anaemia in tropical splenomegaly. Quarterly Journal of Medicine 36:337–356.

24 Hegde UM, Williams ED, Lewis SM, et al 1973 Measurement of splenic red cell volume and visualization of the spleen with ^{99m}Tc. Journal of Nuclear Medicine 14:769–771.

25 Miller JH 1987 Technetium-99m-labelled red blood cells in the evaluation of the liver in infants and children. Journal of Nuclear Medicine 28:1412–1418.

26 Front D, Israel O 1981 Tc-99m-labelled red blood cells in the evaluation of vascular abnormalities. Journal of Nuclear Medicine 22:149–151.

27 Cavill I 1986 Plasma clearance studies. Methods in Hematology 14:214–244.

28 Cazzola M, Barosi G, Orlandi E, et al 1980 The plasma ^{59}Fe clearance curve in man; an evaluation of methods of measurement and analysis. Blut 40:325–335.

29 Finch CA, Deubelbeiss K, Cook JD, et al 1970 Ferrokinetics in man. Medicine 49:17–53.

30 Peters AM, Swirsky DM 1998 Blood disorders. In: Maisey MN, Britton KE, Collier BD (eds) Clinical nuclear medicine, 3rd edn. Chapman and Hall, London.

31 Bentley SA, Miller DT 1986 Radionuclide blood cell survival studies. Methods in Hematology 14:245–262.

32 Ricketts C, Cavill I, Napier JAF 1977 The measurement of red cell lifespan using ^{59}Fe. British Journal of Haematology 37:403–408.

33 Pearson HA 1963 The binding of ^{51}Cr to hemoglobin. 1. In vitro studies. Blood 22:218–230.

34 Jandl JH, Greenberg MS, Yonemoto RH, et al 1956 Clinical determination of the sites of red cell sequestration in hemolytic anemias. Journal of Clinical Investigation 35:842–867.

35 Koutras GA, Schneider AS, Hattori M, et al 1965 Studies of chromated erythrocytes. Mechanisms of chromate inhibition of glutathione reductase. British Journal of Haematology 11:360–369.

36 International Committee for Standardization in Haematology 1980 Recommended methods for radioisotope red-cell survival studies. British Journal of Haematology 45:659–666.

37 Lewis SM, Szur L, Dacie JV 1960 The pattern of erythrocyte destruction in haemolytic anaemia, as studied with radioactive chromium. British Journal of Haematology 6:122–139.

38 Ferrant A, Cauwe JL, Michaux C, et al 1982 Assessment of the sites of red-cell destruction using quantitative measurement of splenic and hepatic red-cell destruction. British Journal of Haematology 50:591–598.

39 Ahuja S, Lewis SM, Szur L 1972 Value of surface counting in predicting response to splenectomy in haemolytic anaemia. Journal of Clinical Pathology 25:467–472.

40 International Committee for Standardization in Haematology 1975 Recommended methods for surface counting to determine sites of red-cell destruction. British Journal of Haematology 30:249–254.

41 Marsh GW, Lewis SM. Szur L 1966 The use of ^{51}Cr-labelled heat-damaged red cells to study splenic function. 1. Evaluation of method. British Journal of Haematology 12:161–166.

42 Royal HD, Brown ML, Drum DE, et al 1998 Procedure guideline for hepatic and splenic imaging. Journal of Nuclear Medicine 39:1114–1116.

43 Peters AM, Ryan PFJ, Klonizakis I, et al 1981 Analysis of heat-damaged erythrocyte clearance curves. British Journal of Haematology 49:581–586.

44 Peters AM, Ryan PFJ, Klonizakis I, et al 1982 Kinetics of heat damaged autologous red blood cells. Scandinavian Journal of Haematology 28:5–14.

45 Peters AM, Walport MJ, Elkon KB, et al 1984 The comparative blood clearance kinetics of modified radiolabelled erythrocytes. Clinical Science 66:55–62.

46 Ford PV, Bartold SP, Fink-Bennett DM, et al 1999 Procedure guideline for gastrointestinal bleeding and Meckel's diverticulum scintigraphy. Journal of Nuclear Medicine 40:1226–1232.

47 International Committee for Standardization in Haematology 1988 Recommended methods for ^{111}In platelet survival studies. Journal of Nuclear Medicine 29:564–566.

48 Peters AM, Saverymuttu SH, Bell RN, et al 1985
    The kinetics of short-lived indium-111
    radiolabelled platelets. Scandinavian Journal of
    Haematology 34:137–145.

49 Peters AM, Saverymuttu SH, Wonke B, et al 1984
    The interpretation of platelet kinetic studies for the
    identification of site of abnormal platelet destruction.
    British Journal of Haematology 57:637–649.

16

Investigation of haemostasis

M.A. Laffan & R.A. Manning

COMPONENTS OF NORMAL HAEMOSTASIS

The haemostatic mechanisms have several important functions: (1) to maintain blood in a fluid state whilst it remains circulating within the vascular system; (2) to arrest bleeding at the site of injury or blood loss by formation of a haemostatic plug; (3) to ensure the eventual removal of the plug when healing is complete. Normal physiology thus constitutes a delicate balance between these conflicting tendencies and a deficiency or exaggeration of any one may lead to either thrombosis or haemorrhage. There are at least five different components involved: blood vessels, platelets, plasma coagulation factors, their inhibitors and the fibrinolytic system. In this chapter, a brief review of normal haemostasis is presented followed by a discussion on the general principles of basic tests used to investigate haemostasis and bleeding disorders.

THE BLOOD VESSEL

General structure of the blood vessel

The blood vessel wall has three layers: intima, media and adventitia. The intima consists of endothelium and subendothelial connective tissue and is separated from the media by the elastic lamina interna. Endothelial cells form a continuous monolayer lining all blood vessels. The structure and the function of the endothelial cells vary according to their location in the vascular tree, but in their resting state they all share three important characteristics: they are 'non-thrombogenic', i.e. they promote maintenance of blood in its fluid state; they play an active role in supplying nutrients to the subendothelial structures, and they act as a barrier to macromolecules and particulate matter circulating in the bloodstream. The permeability of the endothelium may vary under different conditions to allow various molecules and cells to pass.

Endothelial cell function[1]

The luminal surface of the endothelial cell is covered by the glycocalyx, a proteoglycan coat. It contains heparan sulphate and other glycosaminoglycans which are capable of activating antithrombin (AT), an important inhibitor of coagulation enzymes. Endothelial cells express a number of coagulation active proteins which play an important regulatory role such as thrombomodulin and the endothelial protein C receptor. Thrombin generated at the site of injury is rapidly bound to a specific product of the endothelial cell, thrombomodulin. When bound to this protein, thrombin can activate the protein C system to degrade and inhibit factors Va and VIIIa and a carboxypeptidase which inhibits fibrinolysis. Thrombin also stimulates the endothelial cell to produce plasminogen activator. The endothelium can also synthesize protein S, the cofactor for protein C. Finally, endothelium produces von Willebrand factor (vWF) essential for platelet adhesion to the subendothelium. This is stored in specific granules called Weibel Palade bodies and is secreted partly into the circulation and partly towards the subendothelium. The expression of these and other important molecules such as adhesion molecules and their receptors are modulated by inflammatory cytokines. The lipid bilayer membrane also contains ADPase, an enzyme which degrades ADP which is a potent platelet agonist (see p. 383). There are also various membrane-lined structures, such as vesicles and 'pits', which participate in transport across the membrane.

The endothelial cell participates in vasoregulation by producing and metabolizing numerous vasoactive substances. On one hand, it metabolizes and inactivates vasoactive peptides such as bradykinin; on the other hand, it can also generate angiotensin II, a local vasoconstrictor, from circulating angiotensin I. Under appropriate stimulation, the endothelial cell can produce vasodilators such as nitric oxide (NO) and prostacyclin or vasoconstrictors such as endothelin and thromboxane. These substances have their principal vasoregulatory effect via the smooth muscle but also have some effect on platelets as well.

The subendothelium consists of connective tissues composed of collagen (principally types I, III and VI), elastic tissues, proteoglycans and non-collagenous glycoproteins, including fibronectin and vWF. After vessel wall damage has occurred, these components are exposed and are then responsible for platelet adherence. This appears to be mediated by vWF binding to collagen, particularly under high shear rate, and also to the microfibrils which have a greater affinity for vWF under some conditions. vWF then undergoes a conformational change and platelets are captured via their surface membrane glycoprotein (Gp) Ib binding to vWF. Platelet activation follows and a conformational change in glycoprotein IIbIIIa allows further binding to vWF via this receptor as well as to fibrinogen.

Vasoconstriction[1,2]

Vessels with muscular coats contract following injury thus helping to arrest blood loss. Although not all coagulation reactions are enhanced by reduced flow, this probably assists in the formation of a stable fibrin plug. Vasoconstriction also occurs in the microcirculation in vessels without smooth muscle cells. Endothelial cells themselves can produce vasoconstrictors such as angiotensin II. In addition, activated platelets produce thromboxane A_2 (TXA_2) which is a potent vasoconstrictor.

PLATELETS[3,4]

Platelets are small fragments of cytoplasm derived from megakaryocytes. On average they are

1.5–3.5 μm in diameter but may be larger in some disease states. They do not contain a nucleus and are bounded by a typical lipid bilayer membrane. Beneath the outer membrane lies the marginal band of microtubules which maintain the shape of the platelet and depolymerize when aggregation begins. The central cytoplasm is dominated by the three types of platelet granules: the δ granules, α granules and lysosomal granules. The contents of these various granules are detailed in Table 16.1. Finally, there exists the dense tubular system and the canalicular membrane system; the latter communicates with the exterior. It is not clear how all these elements act together to perform such functions as contraction and secretion, which are characteristic of platelet activation.

The platelet membrane is the site of interaction with the plasma environment and with damaged vessel wall. It consists of phospholipids, cholesterol, glycolipids and at least nine glycoproteins, named GpI–GpIX. The membrane phospholipids are asymmetrically distributed, with sphingomyelin and phosphatidylcholine predominating in the outer leaflet, and phosphatidyl-ethanolamine, -inositol and -serine in the inner leaflet. The membrane also expresses specific receptors for several coagulation proteins such as factor XI and factor VIII. The contractile system of the platelet consists of the dense microtubular system and the circumferential microfilaments which maintain the disc shape. Actin is the main constituent of the contractile system, but myosin and a regulatory calcium binding protein, calmodulin, are also present.

Platelet function in the haemostatic process[5]

The main steps in platelet functions are adhesion, activation with shape change, and aggregation. When the vessel wall is damaged, the subendothelial structures, including basement membrane, collagen and microfibrils, are exposed. Surface-bound vWF binds to GpIb on circulating platelets resulting in an initial monolayer of adhering platelets. Binding via GpIb initiates activation of the platelet via a G-protein mechanism. Once activated, platelets immediately change shape from a disc to a tiny sphere with numerous projecting pseudopods. After adhesion of a single layer of platelets to the exposed subendothelium, platelets stick to one another to form aggregates. Fibrinogen, fibronectin and the glycoprotein Ib-IX and IIbIIIa complexes are essential at this stage to increase the cell to cell contact and facilitate aggregation. Certain substances (agonists) react with specific platelet membrane receptors to promote platelet aggregation and further activation. The agonists include: exposed collagen fibres, ADP, thrombin,

Table 16.1 Some contents of platelet granules

Dense (δ) granules	α Granules	Lysosomal vesicles
ATP	PF4	Galactosidases
ADP	β-Thromboglobulin	Fucosidases
Calcium	Fibrinogen	Hexosaminidase
Serotonin	Factor V	Glucuronidase
Pyrophosphate	Thrombospondin	Cathepsin
P selectin (CD62)	Fibronectin	Glycohydrolases
Transforming growth factor-beta (1)	PDGF	+ others
Catecholamines (noradrenaline/adrenaline)	PAI-1	
GDP/GTP	Histidine-rich glycoprotein α_2 Macroglobulin Plasmin inhibitor P selectin (CD62)	

ADP, adenosine 5′-diphosphate; ATP, adenosine 5′-triphosphate; GDP, guanosine 5′-diphosphate; GTP, guanosine 5′- triphosphate; PAI-1, plasminogen activator inhibitor-1; PDGF, platelet-derived growth factor.

adrenaline, serotonin and certain arachidonic acid metabolites including TXA_2. In areas of non-linear blood flow such as may occur at the site of an injury, locally damaged red cells release ADP which further activates platelets.

Platelet aggregation

Platelet aggregation may occur by at least two independent but closely linked pathways. The first pathway involves arachidonic acid metabolism. Activation of phospholipase enzymes (PLA_2) releases free arachidonic acid from membrane phospholipids (phosphatidylcholine). About 50% of free arachidonic acid is converted by a lipo-oxygenase enzyme to a series of products including leucotrienes which are important chemoattractants of white cells. The remaining 50% of arachidonic acid is converted by the enzyme cyclo-oxygenase into labile cyclic endoperoxides, most of which are in turn converted by thromboxane synthetase into TXA_2. TXA_2 has profound biological effects, causing secondary platelet granule release and local vasoconstriction, as well as further local platelet aggregation via the second pathway below. It exerts these effects by raising intracellular cytoplasmic free calcium concentration and binding to specific granule receptors. TXA_2 is very labile with a half-life of less than 1 min before it is degraded into the inactive thromboxane B_2 (TXB_2) and malonyldialdehyde.

The second pathway of activation and aggregation can proceed completely independently from the first one: various platelet agonists, including thrombin, TXA_2 and collagen, bind to receptors and via a G protein mechanism activate phospholipase C. This generates diacylglycerol and inositol triphosphate which in turn activate protein kinase C and elevate intracellular calcium respectively. Calcium is released from the dense tubular system to form complexes with calmodulin; this complex and the free calcium act as co-enzymes for the release reaction, for the activation of different regulatory proteins, as well as of actin and myosin and the contractile system, and also for the liberation of arachidonic acid from membrane phospholipids and the generation of TXA_2.

The aggregating platelets align together into loose reversible aggregates, but after the release reaction of the platelet granules, a larger, firmer aggregate forms. Changes in the platelet membrane configuration now occur: 'flip-flop' rearrangement of the surface brings the negatively charged phosphatidylserine and inositol on to the outer leaflet, thus generating platelet factor 3 (procoagulant) activity. At the same time, specific receptors for various coagulation factors are exposed on the platelet surface and help coordinate the assembly of the enzymatic complexes of the coagulation system. Local generation of thrombin will then further activate platelets.

Platelets are not activated if in contact with healthy endothelial cells. The 'non-thrombogenicity' of the endothelium is due to a combination of control mechanisms exerted by the endothelial cell: synthesis of prostacyclin, capacity to bind thrombin and activate the protein C system, and ability to inactivate vasoactive substances, etc. (see p. 345). Prostacyclin released locally binds to specific platelet membrane receptors and then activates the membrane-bound adenylate cyclase (producing c-AMP). c-AMP inhibits platelet aggregation by inhibiting arachidonic acid metabolism and the release of free cytoplasmic calcium ions.

BLOOD COAGULATION[6]

The central event in the coagulation pathways is the production of thrombin which acts upon fibrinogen to produce fibrin and thus the fibrin clot. This clot is further strengthened by the crosslinking action of factor XIII which itself is activated by thrombin. The two commonly used coagulation tests, the activated partial thromboplastin time (APTT) and the prothrombin time (PT), have been used historically to define two pathways of coagulation activation; the intrinsic and extrinsic paths, respectively. However, this bears only a limited relationship to the way coagulation is activated in vivo. For example, deficiencies of the contact factors or of factor VIII both produce marked prolongation of the APTT but only deficiency of the latter is associated with a haemorrhagic tendency. Moreover, there is considerable evidence that activation of factor IX (intrinsic pathway) by factor VIIa (extrinsic pathway) is crucial to establishing coagulation after an initial stimulus has been provided by factor VIIa-tissue factor (TF) activation of factor X (see Fig. 16.1).

Investigation of the coagulation system centres on the coagulation factors but the activity of these

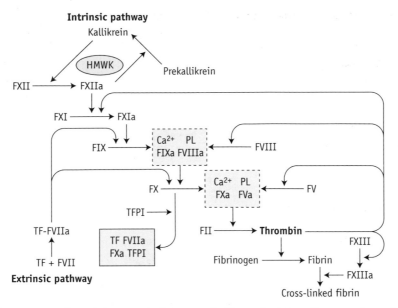

Fig. 16.1 Schematic representation of the coagulation network. The major interactions are shown by the bold arrows. Inhibitory factors and clot-limiting mechanisms are not shown. PL, phospholipid; HMWK, high molecular weight kininogen; TFPI, tissue factor pathway inhibitor.

proteins is also greatly dependent on specific surface receptors and phospholipids largely presented on the surface of platelets but also by activated endothelium. The necessity for calcium in many of these reactions is frequently utilized to control their activity in vitro. The various factors are described below, as far as possible in their functional groups, and their properties are detailed in Table 16.2.

The contact activation system[7]

This system comprises factor XII (Hageman factor), high molecular weight kininogen (HMWK) (Fitzgerald factor) and prekallikrein/kallikrein (Fletcher factor). As mentioned above, these factors do not appear to be essential for haemostasis in vivo. There is evidence that their ability to activate the fibrinolytic system may be functionally more important as may their ability to generate vasoactive peptides: in particular, bradykinin is released from HMWK by prekallikrein or FXIIa cleavage. Kallikrein and factor XIIa also function as chemo-attractants for neutrophils. When bound to a negatively charged surface in vitro, factor XII and prekallikrein are able to reciprocally activate one another by limited proteolysis but the initiating event is not clear. Possibly a conformational change

in factor XII on binding results in limited auto-activation which triggers the process. HMWK acts as a (zinc dependent) co-factor by facilitating the attachment of prekallikrein and factor XI, with which it circulates in a complex, to the negatively charged surface. It has been shown in in-vitro studies that platelets or endothelial cells can provide the necessary negatively charged surface for this mechanism and also possess specific receptors for factor XI. The contact system can activate fibrinolysis by a number of mechanisms: plasminogen cleavage, uPA activation and tissue plasminogen activator (t-PA) release. Most importantly from the laboratory point of view, the contact activation system results in the generation of factor XIIa which is able to activate factor XI, thus initiating the coagulation cascade of the intrinsic pathway.

Tissue factor

Tissue factor (TF) is the co-factor for the extrinsic pathway and the physiological initiator of coagulation. It is a lipoprotein which is membrane bound and constitutively present in many tissues outside the vasculature and on the surface of stimulated inflammatory cells such as monocytes. TF combines with factor VIIa in the presence of calcium ions and this complex is then capable of activating factor X to

Table 16.2 The coagulation factors

No.	Factor	RMM (Daltons)	Half-life	Concentration in plasma	
				µg/ml	nmol/l
I	Fibrinogen	340 000	90 h	1.5–4 × 10	–
II	Prothrombin	70 000	60 h	100–150	1400
V	–	330 000	12–36 h	5–10	20
VII	–	48 000	6 h	0.5	10
VIII	–	200 000	12 h	0.2	0.7
vWF	–	800 000–140 000 000	24 h	10	–
IX	–	57 000	24 h	4	90
X	–	58 000	40 h	10	170
XI	–	158 000	60 h	6	30
XII	–	80 000	48–52 h	30	375
Pre-kallikrein	–	85 000	48 h	40	450
HMWK	–	120 000	6.5 days	80	700
XIII	–	32 000	3–5 days	30 (A+B)	900 (tetramer)

RMM, Relative molecular mass (molecular weight); h, hours; HMWK, high molecular weight kininogen; vWF, von Willebrand factor.

factor Xa. Small amounts of factor VIIa are present in the circulation but have virtually no enzymic activity unless bound to TF. The factor VIIa-TF complex can activate both factor X and factor IX and therefore two routes to thrombin production are stimulated. Factor Xa subsequently binds to tissue factor pathway inhibitor (TFPI) and then to factor VIIa to form a quaternary (Xa-TF-VIIa-TFPI) complex. This mechanism therefore functions to shut off the extrinsic pathway after an initial stimulus to coagulation has been provided.

The vitamin K-dependent factors

This group comprises coagulation factors II, VII, IX and X. However, it is important to remember that the anticoagulant proteins S, C and Z are also vitamin K dependent. Each of these proteins contains a number of glutamic acid residues at its amino terminus that are γ-carboxylated by a vitamin K-dependent mechanism. This results in a novel amino acid, γ-carboxyglutamic acid, which appears to be important in promoting a conformational change in the protein which promotes binding of the factor to phospholipid. Because this binding is crucial for coordinating the interaction of the various factors, the proteins produced in the absence of vitamin K (PIVKAs) which are not γ-carboxylated are essentially functionless. The vitamin K-dependent factors are pro-enzymes or zymogens which require cleavage sometimes with release of a small peptide (activation peptide) in order to become functional. Measurement of these activation peptides has become a useful test for measuring coagulation activation.

Labile factors

Factors VIII and V are the two most labile of the coagulation factors and they are rapidly lost from stored blood or heated plasma. They share considerable structural homology and are co-factors for the serine proteases factor IX and factor X respectively, and both require proteolytic activation by factor IIa or Xa in order to function. Factor VIII circulates in combination with vWF which is present in the form of large multimers of a basic 200 kD monomer. vWF serves to stabilize factor VIII and protect it from degradation. In the absence of vWF, the survival of factor VIII in the circulation is extremely short, i.e. 2 h instead of the normal 8–12 h. vWF may also serve to deliver factor VIII to platelets adherent to a site of vascular injury. Once factor VIII has been cleaved and activated by thrombin, it no longer binds to vWF.

Fibrinogen[8,9]

Fibrinogen is a large dimeric protein, each half consisting of three polypeptides named Aα, Bβ and γ held together by 12 disulphide bonds. The two monomers are joined together by a further three disulphide bonds. Fibrin is formed from fibrinogen by thrombin cleavage of the A and B peptides from fibrinogen. This results in fibrin monomers that associate to form a polymer that is the visible clot. The central E domain exposed by thrombin cleavage binds with a complementary region on the outer or D domain of another monomer. The monomers thus assemble into a staggered overlapping two-stranded fibril. More complex interactions subsequently lead to branched and thickened fibre formation. Fibrinogen in plasma is heterogeneous owing to removal of a 35 kD fragment from the carboxyterminus of some Aα chains.

Factor XIII

The initial fibrin clot is held together by non-covalent interactions and can be deformed and resolubilized. Factor XIII which is also activated by thrombin is able to covalently cross-link these fibrin monomers. Factor XIII is a transglutaminase which joins a glutamine residue on one chain to a lysine on an adjacent chain. This loss of resolubility is the basis of the screening test for factor XIII deficiency.

INHIBITORS OF COAGULATION[10,11]

A number of mechanisms exist to ensure that the production of the fibrin clot is limited to the site of injury and is not allowed to propagate indefinitely. First, there are a number of proteins which bind to and inactivate the enzymes of the coagulation cascade. Probably the first of these to become active is TFPI which rapidly quenches the factor VIIa-TF complex that initiates coagulation. It does this in combination with factor Xa so that coagulation is thereafter dependent on the small amount of thrombin that has been generated.

The principal physiological inactivator of thrombin is AT which belongs to the serpin group of proteins. This binds to factor IIa forming an inactive thrombin–antithrombin complex (TAT) which is subsequently cleared from the circulation by the liver. This process is greatly enhanced by the presence of heparin. AT is responsible for approximately 60% of thrombin inactivating capacity in the plasma, the remainder is provided by heparin co-factor II and less specific inhibitors such as α2 macroglobulin. AT is also capable of inactivating factors X, IX, XI and XII but to lesser degrees than thrombin.

As thrombin spreads away from the area of damage, it is also bound by thrombomodulin on the surface of endothelial cells. In doing so it is changed from a primarily procoagulant protein to an anticoagulant one. Whilst remaining available for binding to AT, thrombin bound to thrombomodulin no longer cleaves fibrinogen. It now has a greatly enhanced preference for protein C as a substrate. Protein C activated by thrombin cleavage acts to limit and arrest coagulation by inactivating factors Va and VIIIa. This action is further enhanced by its co-factor protein S which does not require prior activation. In larger vessels, where the effective concentration of thrombomodulin is low, the binding of protein C is enhanced by the endothelial protein C receptor (EPCR). Protein C is subsequently inactivated by its own specific inhibitor.

THE FIBRINOLYTIC SYSTEM[12]

The deposition of fibrin and its removal are regulated by the fibrinolytic system. Although this is a complex multicomponent system with many activators and inhibitors, it centres around the fibrinogen- and fibrin-cleaving enzyme plasmin. Plasmin circulates in its inactive precursor form, plasminogen, which is activated by proteolytic cleavage. The principal plasminogen activator (PA) in man is t-PA which is another serine protease. t-PA and plasminogen are both able to bind to fibrin via the amino acid lysine. When they are both bound, the rate of plasminogen activation is markedly increased and thus plasmin is generated preferentially at its site of action and not free in plasma. The second important physiological PA in humans is called urokinase (u-PA). This single chain molecule (scu-PA) is activated by plasmin or kallikrein to a two-chain derivative (tcu-PA) which is not fibrin-specific in its action. However, the extent to which this is important in vivo is not clear and the identification of cell surface receptors for u-PA suggests that its primary role may be extravascular. The contact activation system also appears to generate some plasminogen activation via factor XIIa, and bradykinin stimulates release of t-PA. The degradation products released by the action of plasmin on fibrin are of diagnostic use and are discussed below. The activation of plasmin on fibrin is restricted by the action of a carboxypeptidase which removes the amino terminal lysine binding sites for plasminogen and t-PA. This carboxypeptidase is activated by thrombomodulin-bound thrombin and is referred to as thrombin-activated fibrinolysis inhibitor (TAFI).

PAI-1 (plasminogen activator inhibitor-1) is a potent inhibitor of t-PA, produced by endothelial cells, hepatocytes, platelets and placenta. Levels in plasma are highly variable. It is a member of the serpin family and is active against t-PA and tcu-PA but not scu-PA. A second inhibitor PAI-2 has also been identified, originally from human placenta, but its role and importance are not yet established.

The main physiological inhibitor of plasmin in plasma is plasmin inhibitor (α2-antiplasmin) which inhibits plasmin function by forming a 1:1 complex (plasmin–antiplasmin complex; PAP). This reaction in free solution is extremely rapid but depends on the availability of free lysine-binding sites on the plasmin. Thus, fibrin-bound plasmin in the clot is not accessible to the inhibitor. Deficiencies of the fibrinolytic system are rare but have sometimes been associated with a tendency to thrombosis or haemorrhage.

GENERAL APPROACH TO INVESTIGATION OF HAEMOSTASIS

This section begins with some general points regarding the clinical and laboratory approach to investigation of haemostasis. Following this, the basic or first-line screening tests of haemostasis are described. These tests are generally used as the first step in investigation of an acutely bleeding patient, a person with a suspected bleeding tendency or as a precaution before an invasive procedure is carried out. They have the virtue that they are easily performed and the patterns of abnormalities obtained point clearly to the appropriate next set of investigations. It should be remembered, however, that these tests may be normal in the presence of a mild but significant bleeding diathesis such as von Willebrand disease (vWD) or disorders of platelets or vessels. Hence a normal 'clotting screen' should not be taken to mean that haemostasis is normal.

CLINICAL APPROACH

The investigation of a suspected bleeding tendency may begin from three different points:

1. *Investigating a clinically suspected bleeding tendency.* The investigation properly begins with the bleeding history which may suggest an acquired or congenital disorder of primary or secondary haemostasis. If the bleeding history or family history is significant, appropriate specific tests and assays should be performed, notwithstanding the results of screening tests such as the PT, APTT, etc.

2. *Following up an abnormal first-line test.* The abnormalities already detected will determine the appropriate further investigations (see below).

3. *Investigation of acute haemostatic failure.* This is often required in the context of an acutely ill or postoperative patient. Investigations are therefore directed towards detecting disseminated intravascular coagulation (DIC) or a previously undetected coagulation defect. The availability of a normal pre-morbid coagulation screen and further questioning to determine a bleeding history can be extremely useful in this respect.

In all cases, comprehensive clinical evaluation, including the patient's history, the family history and the family tree, as well as the details of the site, frequency and the character of haemorrhagic manifestations (purpura, bruising, large haematomata, haemarthroses, etc.), is required to establish a definitive diagnosis. If considered in conjunction with laboratory results, they will help avoid misinterpretation. It is also desirable to undertake a series of screening tests before proceeding to more specific tests. The results of the screening investigations, taken in conjunction with clinical information, usually point to the appropriate additional procedure.

Despite their simplicity, it is clearly important that the results obtained from the first-line tests are reproducible and accurate. This requires attention to blood sample collection and processing, selection, preparation and storage of reagents and the use of appropriate controls and standards. Laboratories should participate in local or national quality assessment schemes.

PRINCIPLES OF LABORATORY ANALYSIS

It is worth remembering that the tests of coagulation performed in the laboratory are attempts to mimic in vitro processes that normally occur in vivo. Not surprisingly, this may give rise to misleading results. One of the most striking is the gross prolongation of the APTT in complete factor XII deficiency in the absence of any bleeding tendency. Similarly, the amount of factor VII required to produce a normal PT is greatly in excess of the amount required for normal haemostasis. Conversely, normal screening tests do not necessarily imply that the patient has entirely normal haemostasis. The only in-vivo test of coagulation that is commonly performed is the bleeding time and even with this test there are notable discrepancies between the results and the clinical bleeding propensity.

The more detailed investigations of coagulation proteins also require caution in their interpretation depending on the type of assay performed. These can be divided into three principal categories.

1. Immunological

These include immuno-diffusion, immuno-electrophoresis, radioimmunometric assays, latex agglutination tests and tests using enzyme-linked antibodies (ELISA). Fundamentally, all these tests rely on the recognition of the protein in question by polyclonal or monoclonal antibodies. They are often easy to perform, particularly convenient for large batches, and can be bought as kits with standardized controls. The obvious drawback of these assays is that they may tell you nothing about the functional capacity of the antigen detected. If possible they should always be carried out in parallel with a functional assay.

2. Assays using chromogenic peptide substrates (amidolytic assays)[13]

The serine proteases of the coagulation cascade have narrow substrate specificities. It is possible to synthesize a short peptide specific for each enzyme that has a dye (p-nitroaniline; p-NA) attached to the terminal amino acid. When the synthetic peptide reacts with the specific enzyme, the dye is released and the rate of its release or the total amount released can be measured photometrically. This gives a measure of the enzyme activity present. Chromogenic substrate assays can be classified into direct and indirect assays. Direct assays can be further sub-classified into primary assays in which a substrate specific for the enzyme to be measured is used and secondary assays in which the enzyme or pro-enzyme measured is used to activate a second protease for which a specific substrate is available. Specific substrates are available for many coagulation enzymes. However, the substrate specificity is not absolute and most kits include inhibitors of other enzymes capable of cleaving the substrate in order to improve specificity. Indirect assays are used to measure naturally occurring inhibitors and some platelet factors.

It should be remembered that the measurement of amidolytic activity is not the same as the measurement of biological activity in a coagulation assay and in some cases may not accurately reflect this. This is particularly important when dealing with the molecular variants of various coagulation factors. Nevertheless, the continuing development of more specific substrates with good solubility and high affinity for individual enzymes, together with rapid advances in automation, make chromogenic substrate assays increasingly popular. The assays can be carried out in a microtitre plate or in a tube when a spectrophotometer is used to measure the intensity of the colour development.

3. Coagulation assays

These assays are functional bioassays and rely on comparison with a control or standard preparation with a known level of activity. The assay can be performed using either a one-stage or two-stage system. In the one-stage system, optimal amounts of all the clotting factors are present except the one to be determined, which should be as near to nil as possible. The best one-stage system is provided by a substrate plasma either obtained from a patient with severe congenital deficiency or artificially depleted by immuno-adsorption. In the two-stage assay, the coagulation enzyme is generated in a two-step system and there is no requirement for a factor-deficient substrate plasma. The principles of bioassay, its standardization and limitations are considered in detail on page 362.

Coagulation techniques are also used in mixing tests to identify a missing factor in an emergency, or to identify and estimate quantitatively an inhibitor or anticoagulant. The advantage of this type of assay is that it most closely approximates to the activity in vivo of the factor in question. However, they can be technically more difficult to perform than the other types described above.

Other assays

These include measurement of coagulation factors using snake venoms, assay of ristocetin co-factor and the clot solubility test for factor XIII.

NOTES ON EQUIPMENT

Water-baths

A 37°C water-bath is required for manual coagulation tests, incubation steps and the rapid thawing of frozen specimens. Water-baths set at 37°C should vary by no more than ± 0.5°C because slight variation in temperature will markedly affect the speed of clotting reactions. A water-bath with plastic or glass sides is preferable and some type of cross-illumination helps to determine the exact time and appearance of fibrin clot formation. Check that the temperature is 37°C before and during use. Distilled or deionized water should be used to fill and maintain the water level.

Refrigerators and freezers

Check that the temperature has not been out of the acceptable range of 4° ± 2°C for refrigerators and −20° ± 2°C for freezers, re-checking during the day. Records must be kept.

Centrifuges

Check to ensure each machine is clean before and after use, plus a visual inspection of rotors, buckets and liners for corrosion and cracks. Thorough maintenance records should be kept.

Reagents and buffers

Attention must be paid to the age and condition of solutions. This is particularly important with the calcium chloride solution. Whenever a solution is prepared, it should be correctly labelled and dated. Buffers should be inspected before use for bacterial growth. Contamination with microorganisms can cause errors and assay failures owing to the release of enzymes and other active biological substances into solution. Azide may be added as a preservative to some buffers, but should not be used in reagents for platelet studies or ELISA substrates. Chromogenic substrates should be reconstituted with sterile distilled water, contamination with bacterial enzymes may cause para nitroaniline (pNA) release and yellow discolouration of the reagent. Records of batch numbers and expiry dates should be kept.

Plastic and glass tubes

For clotting tests, 75×10 mm glass rimless test tubes should be used. Plastic tubes should be used for sample dilutions, storage and reagent preparation.

Pipettes

A range of graduated glass (certified Class A) and automatic pipettes must be obtained. The latter should be accurate and durable. Fluids should not be drawn into the pipette barrels and acids should not be pipetted with instruments containing metal piston assemblies, which may become pitted or corroded. Attention to technique is vital, as contamination of reagents with used pipette tips may occur; there may be errors of volume because of fluid on the exterior of the pipette tip, or the manner of addition of a reagent may alter the results obtained. The amount of fluid drawn into the tip should be inspected visually with each pipetting procedure. Records of pipette accuracy and precision should be kept.

Stopwatches and clocks

Stopclocks are useful for timing incubation periods of several minutes or more, but stopwatches which may be held in the hand, and controlled rapidly, should be used for measuring clotting times and for short incubations. At least four stopwatches are needed unless an automatic coagulometer is used.

Automated coagulation analysers

A wide variety of automated and semi-automated coagulation analysers are available. The choice of analyser depends on predicted workload, repertoire and cost implications. A thorough evaluation of the current range of analysers is recommended. This is aided by reports of instrument evaluation, and reports available, e.g. from the NHS Medical Devices Agency.*

If coagulation analysers are used, it is important to ensure that their temperature control and the mechanism for detecting the end-point are functioning properly. Although such instruments reduce observer error when a large number of samples are tested, it is important to apply stringent quality control at all times to ensure accuracy and precision.

Safety

Each laboratory should have its own safety recommendations, taking into account the use of specialized equipment and reagents, and have procedures to follow in case of accident or contamination. Attention should be paid to fire, chemical, mechanical and microbiological safety aspects, and the handling of automated equipment.

PRE-ANALYTICAL VARIABLES INCLUDING SAMPLE COLLECTION

It is evident that many misleading results in blood coagulation arise not from errors in testing but from carelessness in the pre-analytical phase. Ideally the results of blood tests should accurately reflect the values in vivo.

When blood is withdrawn from a vessel, changes begin to take place in the components of blood coagulation. Some occur almost immediately, such as platelet activation and the initiation of the clotting mechanism dependent on surface contact.

It is essential to take precautions at this early stage to prevent, or at least minimize, in-vitro changes by conforming to recommended criteria during collection and storage. These criteria, as described below, have been laid down by the National Committee for Clinical Laboratory Standards (NCCLS).

Collection of venous blood

Venous blood samples should be obtained whenever possible, even from the neonate. Capillary blood tests require modification of techniques, experienced operators and locally established normal ranges; they are not an easy alternative to tests on venous blood. All blood samples must

be collected by personnel who are trained and experienced in the technique. Patients requiring venepuncture should be relaxed and in warm surroundings. Excessive stress and vigorous exercise cause changes in blood clotting and fibrinolysis. Stress and exercise will increase factor VIII, vWF antigen and fibrinolysis.

Whenever possible, venous samples should be collected without a pressure cuff, allowing the blood to enter the syringe by continuous free flow or by the negative pressure from an evacuated tube. Venous occlusion causes haemoconcentration, increase of fibrinolytic activity, platelet release and activation of some clotting factors. In the majority of patients, however, light pressure using a tourniquet is required; this should be applied for the shortest possible time, i.e. less than 1 min. The venepuncture must be 'clean'; blood from indwelling catheters should not be used for tests of haemostasis, as they are prone to dilution or heparin contamination.

The most accessible site for venepuncture in an adult is the antecubital fossa of the arm. A clean puncture should be made through the vein wall. A sufficiently wide bore needle (21 G or larger) should be used to avoid unnecessary frothing or shear stress.

To minimize the effects of contact activation, good quality plastic or polypropylene syringes

---

* The NHS Medical Devices Agency, Hannibal House, London SEI 6 TQ. See also www.medical-devices.gov.uk

should be used. If glass blood containers are used they should be evenly and adequately coated with silicon.

The blood is thoroughly mixed with the anticoagulant by inverting the container several times. The samples should be brought to the laboratory as soon as possible. If urgent fibrinolysis tests are contemplated, the blood samples should be kept on crushed ice until delivered to the laboratory. Assays of t-PA and of PAI-1 antigen are preferably performed on samples taken into CTAD to prevent continued t-PA–PAI-1 binding (see p. 407).

If an evacuated tube system is used, the coagulation sample should be the second or third tube obtained.

Patient identification is of utmost importance. Care must be taken in labelling the patient sample both at the bed-side and within the laboratory.

Blood sample anticoagulation

The most commonly used anticoagulant for coagulation samples is 32 g/l (0.109 M) trisodium citrate (see p. 604). Other anticoagulants, including oxalate, heparin and EDTA, are unacceptable. The labile factors (factors V and VIII) are unstable in oxalate, while heparin and EDTA directly inhibit the coagulation process and interfere with end-point determinations.

For routine blood coagulation testing, nine volumes of blood are added to one volume of anticoagulant. When the haematocrit is grossly abnormal in polycythaemia or severe anaemia this ratio should be adjusted to ensure the correct plasma citrate concentration (see p. 390).[56]

Time of sample collection

The time of day when the sample is collected can be an important factor in the interpretation of results. Fibrinolytic activity follows a definite circadian pattern with a trough at around 6 am. The timing of the collection of the blood sample in relation to drug administration should also be taken into consideration, e.g. the APTT for monitoring heparin therapy.

The timing following administration of factor concentrate samples is very important. The following times are recommended.

Factor VIII	at 15 min
Factor IX	at 30 min
DDAVP	at 45 min.

Transportation to the laboratory

An efficient and regular collection service is necessary. It is important that samples are delivered as quickly as possible to prevent deterioration of the labile clotting factors such as factors V and VIII. For certain investigations, it is necessary for the samples to be placed on ice once taken and delivered immediately to the laboratory.

Centrifugation, preparation of platelet-poor plasma

Most routine coagulation investigations are performed on platelet-poor plasma (PPP) which is prepared by centrifugation at 2000 g for 15 min at 4°C (approximately 4000 rpm in a standard bench cooling centrifuge). The sample should be kept at room temperature if it is to be used for prothrombin time tests, or factor VII assays, and at 4°C for other assays; the testing should preferably be completed within 2 h of collection. Care must be taken not to disturb the buffy coat layer when removing the PPP.

Samples for platelet function testing, lupus anticoagulant and the activated protein C resistance (APCR) test should not be centrifuged at 4°C. These samples should be prepared by centrifugation at room temperature to prevent activation of platelets and release of platelet contents such as phospholipid and factor V. For lupus anticoagulant testing and APCR it is very important that the number of platelets and platelet debris in the samples are minimized. The platelet count should be below $10^4/\mu l$. This is best achieved by double centrifugation, or filtration of the plasma through a 0.2 μm filter.

Storage of plasma and sample thawing

Some tests such as the PT and APTT are carried out on fresh samples. Certain coagulation assays, unless urgently required, can be performed in batches at a later date on deep frozen plasma. Storage of small aliquots of samples in liquid nitrogen (−196°C) is the optimum although samples may be frozen at −40°C or −80°C for several weeks without significant loss of most haemostatic activities. Gentle but thorough mixing of samples is essential after thawing and before testing. Once thawed, the sample should never be refrozen.

Some common 'technical' errors

An artifactual abnormality of the clotting time occurs in the following situations:

1. Faulty collection of the sample, resulting in it undergoing partial clotting, can lead to a shortening of the clotting times.
2. Under- or over-filling of bottle or high or low haematocrit so that the volume of citrate in relation to the plasma volume is incorrect.
3. An unsuitable anticoagulant, such as EDTA, used in collecting the sample.
4. Collection of blood through a line that has at some stage been in contact with heparin. This leads to a marked prolongation of the APTT and thrombin time (TT).
5. Contamination of the kaolin/platelet substitute reagent with a trace of thromboplastin. This can shorten the APTT.
6. Undue delay in sample analysis.
7. Use of inaccurate pipettes. (Documented pipette calibration is essential.)
8. Machine malfunction.
9. Incorrect water-bath temperature.
10. Calcium chloride that is not the correct concentration or is not freshly prepared.

CALIBRATION AND QUALITY CONTROL

Reference standard

International (WHO) and national standards are available for a number of coagulation factors (see p. 608). For diagnostic tests, it is necessary to have a calibrated normal reference preparation tested alongside the patients' plasmas.

The concentration of some coagulation factors may vary as much as fourfold in different normal plasma samples and it is therefore inadvisable to use plasma from any one person as representing 100% clotting activity. The larger the number of donors in the pool, the more likely the pool clotting activity will be 100% or 1.0 u/ml. A suggested minimum for the normal pool is 20 donors.

Calibration of standard pools and suggested calibration procedure

Whenever possible, the normal pool should be calibrated as described below against a freeze-dried reference material already calibrated against the international standard. The reference material may be a national standard (e.g. NIBSC) or a commercial standard. In the absence of reference materials, the laboratory should obtain as large a normal pool as possible and assign it a value of 100 u/dl (1.0 u/ml).

The most important principle of calibration is repetition to minimize possible errors at each stage of calibration. It is necessary to carry out at least four independent assays, and preferably six. An independent assay is an assay for which a new ampoule of standard is opened, or if a freeze-dried standard is not available, for which a new set of dilutions are prepared from frozen previous reference plasma. Each plasma must be tested in duplicate; two replicate assays should be carried out each day, and the procedure repeated on at least 4 days (four independent assays). Whenever possible more than one operator should be involved.

Comparison should always be made with the previous normal pool. The potency of the new normal pool is calculated for each assay on each day and an overall mean value calculated. This calibration also enables an assessment of the precision of the method used.

Control plasma

Controls are included alongside patient samples in a batch of tests. Inclusion of both normal and abnormal controls will enable detection of non-linearity in the standard curve. Whilst a reference standard (calibrator) is used for accuracy, controls are used for precision. Precision control, the recording of the day to day variation in control values, is an important procedure in laboratory coagulation. Participation in an external assessment scheme (e.g. NEQAS) is also important to ensure interlaboratory harmonization. The use of lyophilized reference standard and control plasmas has become widespread whilst locally calibrated standard pools are used especially in under-resourced countries.

A control must be stable and homogeneous; the exact potency is not important although the approximate value should be known in order to select a preparation at the upper or lower limit of the normal reference range.

Fresh control blood is required for procedures such as platelet aggregation and should be obtained from 'normal' healthy subjects. Fresh controls should be prepared in exactly the same way as the patient sample. Normal and abnormal controls are usually obtained from commercial companies.

Variability of coagulation assays

Within a laboratory, variability is most commonly due to a dilution error, differences in the composition of reagents, failure to take the time-trend into account, and because of differences in experience and technique between operators. A coefficient of variation of 15–20% is not uncommon for factor VIII:C assay. Furthermore, the variability increases if like is not compared with like, e.g. if concentrate preparations are assayed against plasma.

Variability between laboratories is much higher. Apart from the factors described for the within-laboratory variability, there is the major effect of differences in methods and in the composition of reagents. Comparability between laboratories improves if standardized reagents are used.

The unavoidable variability associated with coagulation assays makes the use of reliable reference materials imperative.

Commonly used reagents

Some reagents are common to the majority of first-line tests. They are described here, whereas the reagents specific for one test or assay only are described with the details of the relevant test.

$CaCl_2$

The working solution is best prepared from a commercial molar solution. Small volumes of 0.025 mol/l concentration should be frequently prepared and stored for short periods of time to avoid proliferation of microorganisms. Prewarmed $CaCl_2$ should always be discarded at the end of the working day.

Barbitone buffered saline

Barbitone buffered saline pH 7.3–7.4 is recommended for most clotting tests. See page 605 for preparation of barbitone buffered saline, pH 7.4.

Glyoxaline buffer

Dissolve 2.72 g of glyoxaline (imidazole) and 4.68 g of NaCl in 650 ml of water. Add 148.8 ml of 0.1 mol/l HCl and adjust the pH to 7.4. Adjust the volume to 1 litre with water.

Owren's veronal buffer

Sodium acetate	3.89 g
Barbitone sodium	5.89 g
Sodium chloride	6.8 g

Dissolve the salts in 800 ml of water. Add 21.5 ml of 1 mol/l HCl, then make up to 1 litre with water; mix and check that the pH is 7.4.

Factor-deficient plasmas

Plasmas deficient in specific factors are required for many bioassays. They may be obtained from individuals with congenital deficiency of the factor but frequently these patients will have been treated with plasma concentrates and there is a danger of infection. This practice also raises some ethical questions. Many laboratories now use commercial plasmas rendered deficient in the factor by immunodepletion and then lyophilized. Once reconstituted, lyophilized plasmas should be gently mixed and left to stand for 20 min before use. If an automated coagulation analyzer is used, the factor-deficient plasma should be placed in position 10 min prior to testing.

PERFORMANCE OF COAGULATION TESTS

Handling of samples and reagents

All plasma samples should be kept in plastic or siliconized glass tubes and placed on melting ice or at 4°C until used, except when cold activation of factor VII and platelets is to be avoided, in which case the plasma is kept at room temperature. All pipetting should be performed using disposable plastic pipettes or automatic pipette tips. The actual clotting tests are performed at 37°C in new round-bottom glass tubes of standard size (10 or 12 mm external diameter). Ideally, all glassware should be disposable. If the tubes have to be re-used, scrupulous cleaning using chromic acid and a detergent such as 2% Decon 90 is essential.

Eliminating a time trend

The potential instability of biological reagents used in tests of haemostasis makes it desirable to arrange results so as to reduce time-related errors. Thus, if there is a significant length of time between the results with the patient's plasma and the results with the control sample, the difference may be due to the deterioration of one or more of the reagents or of the plasma itself rather than to a true defect or deficiency. In the simplest case, if there are two samples A and B, the readings should be carried out in the order A_1, B_1, B_2, A_2. Additional specimens are allowed for by inserting further letters into the design.

The end-point

Detecting clot formation as the end-point depends to some extent on the rate of its formation: the shorter the clotting time the more opaque is the clot and the easier it is to detect. A slowly forming clot may appear as mere fibrin wisps. In manual work, the observer must try to adopt a uniform convention in selecting the moment in clot formation which will be accepted as the end-point. It is also important to ensure that the tube can be watched with its lower part under the water or while quickly dipped in and out so as to avoid cooling and a slowing down of the clot formation. Bubbles also make the determination of the end-point difficult. In instrumental work the coagulometer must be shown to detect long clotting times reliably and reproducibly. The various coagulometers available have different means of detecting the end-point which may make comparison of results difficult.

THE 'CLOTTING SCREEN'

Basic tests of coagulation are often performed with no specific diagnosis in mind and in the absence of any clinical indication of a haemostatic disorder. There may be numerous reasons for this and the tests performed may give clues to diagnosis or may detect an unsuspected hazard which increases the risk of postoperative bleeding. The choice and extent of tests performed in this screening process will vary between hospitals. Our current practice is to perform a PT, APTT, TT and a fibrinogen assay. Many hospitals omit one or more of these tests but few will do more for this purpose.

PROTHROMBIN TIME

Principle

The test measures the clotting time of plasma in the presence of an optimal concentration of tissue extract (thromboplastin) and indicates the overall efficiency of the extrinsic clotting system. Although originally thought to measure prothrombin, the test is now known to depend also on reactions with factors V, VII and X, and on the fibrinogen concentration of the plasma.[14]

Reagents
Patient and control plasma samples

Platelet poor plasma (PPP) from the patient and control are obtained as described on page 350. Note that plasma stored at 4°C may have a shortened PT as a result of factor VII activation in the cold.[15]

Thromboplastin

Thromboplastins were originally tissue extracts obtained from different species and different organs containing tissue factor and phospholipid. Because of the potential hazard of viral and other infections from handling human brain, as well as for ethical reasons, its use as a source of thromboplastin is not recommended. The majority of animal thromboplastins now in use are extracts of rabbit brain or lung. A laboratory method for a rabbit brain preparation is described on p. 606.

Recently the introduction of recombinant thromboplastins has resulted in a move away from rabbit brain thromboplastin. They are manufactured using recombinant human tissue factor produced in *E. coli* and synthetic phospholipids which do not contain any other clotting factors such as prothrombin, factor VII and factor X. Therefore they are highly sensitive to factor deficiencies and oral anticoagulant-treated patient plasma samples and have an international sensitivity index (ISI) close to 1.

Each preparation has a different sensitivity to clotting factor deficiencies and defects, in particular the defect induced by oral anticoagulants (see p. 416). For control of oral anticoagulation, a preparation calibrated against the international reference thromboplastin should be used; a calibrated commercially available thromboplastin will have its ISI determined and clearly labelled. It is important to remember that some thromboplastins are not sensitive to an isolated factor VII deficiency and that use of animal thromboplastin for analysis of human samples may produce abnormalities owing solely to species differences. If the manufacturer does not state in the accompanying literature that the reagent is sensitive to factor VII, it is advisable to check whether it is capable of detecting this deficiency by performing a PT on a known factor VII deficient plasma.

CaCl₂. 0.025 mol/l.

Method
Deliver 0.1 ml of plasma into a glass tube placed in a water-bath and add 0.1 ml of thromboplastin. Wait 1–3 min to allow the mixture to warm. Then add 0.1 ml of warmed $CaCl_2$ and mix the contents of the tube. Start the stopwatch and record the end-point. Carry out the test in duplicate on the patient's and the control plasma. When a number of samples are to be tested as a batch, the samples and controls must be suitably staggered to eliminate the time bias. Some thromboplastins contain calcium chloride in which case 0.2 ml of thromboplastin is added to 0.1 ml plasma and timing begun immediately.

Expression of results
The results are expressed as the mean of the duplicate readings in seconds or as the ratio of the mean patient's time to the mean normal control time. The control plasma is obtained from 20 normal men and women (non-pregnant and not on oral contraceptives) and the logarithmic mean normal PT (LMNPT) calculated. For further details and a discussion of the importance of the one-stage PT test in oral anticoagulant control, when results may be reported as an international normalized ratio (INR), see Chapter 18.

Normal values
Normal values depend on the thromboplastin used, the exact technique and whether visual or instrumental end-point reading is used. With most rabbit thromboplastins, the normal range of the prothrombin time is between 11 and 16 s; for recombinant human thromboplastin, it is somewhat shorter (10–12 s). Each laboratory should establish its own normal range.

Interpretation
The common causes of prolonged one-stage PTs are:

1. Administration of oral anticoagulant drugs (vitamin K antagonists).
2. Liver disease, particularly obstructive.
3. Vitamin K deficiency.
4. DIC.
5. Rarely, a previously undiagnosed factor VII, X, V or prothrombin deficiency or defect (see pp. 364 and 366). *Note*: With prothrombin, factor X or factor V deficiency the APTT will also be prolonged.

ACTIVATED PARTIAL THROMBOPLASTIN TIME

This test is also known as the partial thromboplastin time with kaolin (PTTK) and the kaolin cephalin clotting time (KCCT) reflecting the methods used to perform the test.

Principle
The test measures the clotting time of plasma after the activation of contact factors but without added tissue thromboplastin, and so indicates the overall efficiency of the intrinsic pathway. To standardize the activation of contact factors, the plasma is first pre-incubated for a set period of time with a contact activator such as kaolin or elagic acid. During this phase of the test, factor XIIa is produced which cleaves factor XI to factor XIa but coagulation does not proceed beyond this in the absence of calcium. After recalcification, factor XIa activates factor IX and coagulation follows. A standardized phospholipid is provided to allow the test to be performed on PPP. The test depends not only on the contact factors and on factors VIII and IX, but also on the reactions with factors X, V, prothrombin and fibrinogen. It is also sensitive to the presence of circulating anticoagulants (inhibitors) and heparin.

Reagents

Platelet-poor plasma. From the patient and a control, stored as described previously.

Kaolin. 5 g/l (laboratory grade) in barbitone buffered saline, pH 7.4 (p. 605). Add a few glass beads to aid resuspension. The suspension is stable at room temperature. Other insoluble surface active substances such as silica, celite or elagic acid can also be used.

Phospholipid. Many reagents are available; these contain different phospholipids.

When choosing a reagent for the APTT, it is important to establish that the activator–phospholipid combination is sensitive to deficiencies of factors VIII:C, IX and XI at concentrations of 0.35 to 0.4 iu/ml. Reagents which fail to detect reductions of this degree are too insensitive for routine use. The system should also be responsive to heparin over the therapeutic range of approximately 0.3–0.7 u/ml. In addition, some laboratories will wish the system to be sensitive to the presence of lupus-like anticoagulants.

A laboratory preparation of the reagent is described on p. 607.

CaCl₂. 0.025 mol/l.

Method

Mix equal volumes of the phospholipid reagent and the kaolin suspension and leave in a glass tube in the water-bath at 37°C. Place 0.1 ml of plasma into a new glass tube. Add 0.2 ml of the kaolin–phospholipid solution, mix the contents and start the stopwatch simultaneously. Leave at 37°C for 10 min with occasional shaking. At exactly 10 min, add 0.1 ml of pre-warmed $CaCl_2$ and start a second stopwatch. Record the time taken for the mixture to clot. Repeat the test at least once on both the patient's and the control plasma. It is possible to do four tests at 2-min intervals if sufficient stopwatches are available.

Expression of results

Express the results as the mean of the paired clotting times.

Normal range

30–40 s. The actual times depend on the reagents used and the duration of the pre-incubation period which varies in manufacturer's recommendations for different reagents. These variables also greatly alter the sensitivity of the test to minor or moderate deficiencies of the contact activation system. Laboratories can choose appropriate conditions to achieve the sensitivity they require. Each laboratory should calculate its own normal range.

Interpretation

The common causes of a prolonged APTT are:

1. DIC.
2. Liver disease.
3. Massive transfusion with stored blood.
4. Administration of heparin or contamination with heparin.
5. A circulating anticoagulant.
6. Deficiency of a coagulation factor other than factor VII.

The APTT is also moderately prolonged in patients on oral anticoagulant drugs and in the presence of vitamin K deficiency. Occasionally, a patient with previously undiagnosed haemophilia or another congenital coagulation disorder presents with an isolated prolonged APTT. If the patient's APTT is abnormally long, the equal mixture test must be set up (see below).

Deficiency or circulating anticoagulant?

In cases with a long APTT, a 50:50 mixture of normal and test plasma should be tested to distinguish between factor deficiency and the effect of an inhibitor (see p. 367).

THROMBIN TIME

Principle

Thrombin is added to plasma and the clotting time measured. The TT is affected by the concentration and reaction of fibrinogen, and by the presence of inhibitory substances, including fibrinogen/fibrin degradation products (FDP) and heparin. The clotting time and the appearance of the clot are both informative.

Reagents

Platelet-poor plasma. From the patient and a control.

Thrombin solution. A commercial bovine thrombin is used. It is stored frozen as a 50 NIH unit solution, and freshly diluted in barbitone buffered saline in a plastic tube so as to give a clotting time of normal plasma of 17 s (usually 7–8 NIH thrombin units per ml). Shorter times with normal plasma may fail to detect mild abnormalities.

Method

Add 100 µl thrombin solution to 200 µl of control plasma in a glass tube at 37°C and start the stopwatch. Measure the clotting time and observe the nature of the clot, e.g. whether transparent or opaque, firm or wispy, etc. Repeat the procedure with two tubes containing patient's plasma in duplicate, and then with a second sample of control plasma.

Expression of results
The results are expressed as the mean of the duplicate clotting times in seconds for the control and the test plasma.

Normal range
A patient's TT should be within 2 s of the control (i.e. 15–19 s). Times of 20 s and over are definitely abnormal.

Interpretation of results
The common causes of prolonged TT are:

1. Hypofibrinogenaemia as found in DIC and, more rarely, in a congenital defect or deficiency.
2. Raised concentrations of FDP, as encountered in DIC or liver disease.
3. Extreme prolongation of the TT is nearly always due to the presence of heparin which interferes with the thrombin–fibrinogen reaction. If the presence of heparin is suspected, a Reptilase time test should be carried out (see p. 362). Low molecular weight heparin (LMWH) produces only a slight prolongation at therapeutic levels.
4. Dysfibrinogenaemia, found either inherital or acquired (in liver disease), or physiologically in neonates.
5. Hypoalbuminaemia

Shortening of the TT occurs in conditions of coagulation activation.

A transparent bulky clot is found if fibrin polymerization is abnormal, as is the case in liver disease and some congenital dysfibrinogenaemias.

A gross elevation of the plasma fibrinogen concentration may also prolong the TT. Correction can be obtained by diluting the patient's plasma with saline (see p. 361).

MEASUREMENT OF FIBRINOGEN

Numerous methods of determining fibrinogen concentration have been devised including clotting, immunological, physical and nephelometric techniques and all tend to give slightly different results,

presumably owing in part to the heterogeneous nature of plasma fibrinogen.[16] Many automated analysers will now provide a measure of fibrinogen concentration estimated from the coagulation changes during the PT (PT-derived fibrinogen). This is simple, cheap and widely used. However, it tends to give higher estimates of fibrinogen than the Clauss assay and is inaccurate in some disease states and in anticoagulated patients.[17,18]

FIBRINOGEN ASSAY (CLAUSS TECHNIQUE)[19]

Principle
Diluted plasma is clotted with a strong thrombin solution; the plasma must be diluted to give a low level of any inhibitors, e.g. FDPs and heparin. A strong thrombin solution must be used so that the clotting time over a wide range is independent of the thrombin concentration.

Reagents
Calibration plasma. With a known level of fibrinogen calibrated against an international reference standard.

Citrated platelet-poor plasma. From the patient and a control.

Thrombin solution. Freshly reconstituted to 100 NIHu per ml in 9 g/l NaCl.

Owren's veronal buffer. pH 7.4. See p. 352.

Method
A calibration curve is prepared each time the batch of thrombin reagent is changed or there is a drift in control results and this is used to calculated the results of unknown plasma samples. Make dilutions of the calibration plasma in veronal buffer to give a range of fibrinogen concentrations, i.e. 1 in 5, 1 in 10, 1 in 20 and 1 in 40. 0.2 ml of each dilution is warmed to 37°C, 0.1 ml of thrombin solution is added and the clotting time is measured. Each test should be performed in duplicate. Plot the clotting time in seconds against the fibrinogen concentration in g/l on log/log graph paper. The 1 in 10 concentration is considered to be 100% and there should be a straight line correlation between clotting times of 5–50 s. Make a 1 in 10 dilution of each patient's sample and clot 0.2 ml of the dilution with 0.1 ml of thrombin.

The fibrinogen level can be read directly off the graph if the clotting time is between 5 and 50 s. However, outside this time range, a different assay dilution and mathematical correction of the result will be required, i.e. if the fibrinogen level is low and a 1 in 5 dilution is required, divide answer by 2 and for a 1 in 20 dilution multiply answer by 2.

The clot formed in this method may be 'wispy' because of the plasma being diluted, and end-point detection may be easier with automated equipment.

Normal range
2–4 g/l.

Interpretation
The Clauss fibrinogen is usually low in inherited dysfibrinogenaemia but is insensitive to heparin unless the level is very high (>0.8 u/ml). High levels of FDPs >190 µg/ml may also interfere with the assay.[20] As the chronometric Clauss assay is a functional assay, it will generally give a relevant indication of fibrinogen function in plasma. When an inherited disorder of fibrinogen is suspected, a physico-chemical estimation should be obtained, e.g. clot weight estimate of fibrinogen or total clottable fibrinogen (see p. 370). If a dysfibrinogenaemia is present, it will reveal a discrepancy between the (functional) Clauss assay and the physical amount of fibrinogen present.

PLATELET COUNT

Before considering further investigation of a suspected bleeding disorder, always check the platelet count (see Ch. 3) and morphology (Ch. 5).

INTERPRETATION OF FIRST-LINE TESTS

The pattern of abnormalities obtained using the first-line tests described above often gives a reasonably clear indication of the underlying defect and determines the appropriate further tests required to define it. The patterns are outlined in Table 16.3. The further tests which include specific factor assays and tests for DIC are described below.

SECOND-LINE INVESTIGATIONS

Relevant second-line investigations are described with each of the patterns of abnormalities detected by the first-line tests.

1.

PT	Normal
APTT	Normal
TT	Normal
Fibrinogen	Normal
Platelet count	Normal

If all the first-line investigations are normal in a patient who continues to bleed from the site of an injury or after surgery (or has a history of such bleeding), there are seven possible diagnoses:

1. A disorder of platelet function, either congenital or acquired.
2. vWD in which the factor VIII is not sufficiently low to cause prolongation of the APTT. This is quite common in mild cases.
3. A mild coagulation disorder that is below the sensitivity of the routine tests to detect or which has been masked by the administration of blood products. This will include mild factor VIII deficiency (e.g. 30% of normal).
4. Factor XIII deficiency.
5. A vascular disorder of haemostasis.
6. Bleeding from a severely damaged vessel or vessels with normal haemostasis.
7. A disorder of fibrinolysis such as anti-plasmin or PAI-1 deficiency.

Second-line investigations required in this situation are specific factor assays for the suspected deficiencies or appropriate screening tests such as the bleeding time or clot solubility test.

2.

PT	Long
APTT	Normal
TT	Normal

Table 16.3   First-line tests used in investigating acute haemostatic failure

	Test					
	PT	**APTT**	**TT**	**Fibrinogen**	**Platelet count**	**Condition**
1.	N	N	N	N	N	Normal haemostasis. Disorder of platelet function. Factor XIII deficiency. Disorder of vascular haemostasis. Mild/masked coagulation factor deficiency. Mild von Willebrand disease. Disorder of fibrinolysis.
2.	Long	N	N	N	N	Factor VII deficiency. Early oral anticoagulation. Lupus anticoagulant (with some reagents). Mild II, V, or X deficiency.
3.	N	Long	N	N	N	Factor VIII, IX, XI, XII, prekallikrein, HMWK deficiency. Von Willebrand's disease. Circulating anticoagulant, e.g. lupus. Mild II, V or X deficiency.
4.	Long	Long	N	N	N	Vitamin K deficiency. Oral anticoagulants. Factor V, X or II deficiency. Multiple factor deficiency, e.g. liver failure. Combined V + VIII deficiency.
5.	Long	Long	Long	N or Abnormal	N	Heparin (large amount). Liver disease. Fibrinogen deficiency/disorder. Inhibition of fibrin polymerization. Hyperfibrinolysis.
6.	N	N	N	N	Low	Thrombocytopenia.
7.	Long	Long	N	N or Abnormal	Low	Massive transfusion. Liver disease.
8.	Long	Long	Long	Low	Low	Disseminated intravascular coagulation Acute liver disease.

HMWK, high molecular weight kininogen; N, normal.

Fibrinogen   Normal
Platelet count   Normal
This combination of results is found in:

1. Factor VII deficiency – congenital or secondary to liver disease or vitamin K deficiency.
2. At the start of oral anticoagulant therapy.
3. Lupus anticoagulants. Some thromboplastins are sensitive to lupus-like anticoagulants and some APTT reagents insensitive, giving rise to this pattern of results.

4. Depending on reagents used, mild deficiencies of II, V or X may cause prolongation of PT whilst the APTT remains in the normal range.

A mixing test should be performed. Factor VII assay is described below. It is usually possible to establish from the history whether the patient has received oral anticoagulant drugs. Specific tests for lupus and specific factor assays should be performed, as indicated by the mixing test results. Biochemical measures of liver function should be obtained.

3.

PT	Normal
APTT	Long
TT	Normal
Fibrinogen	Normal
Platelet count	Normal

An isolated prolonged APTT is found in:

1. Congenital deficiencies or defects of the intrinsic pathway, i.e. factor VIII, factor IX, factor XI and factor XII deficiency, as well as in prekallikrein and HMWK deficiencies.
2. Depending on reagents used, mild deficiencies of II, V or X may cause prolongation of APTT whilst the PT remains in the normal range.
3. vWD owing to low levels of factor VIII and when it may be associated with a prolonged bleeding time.
4. In the presence of circulating anticoagulants (inhibitors).
5. A common cause of a prolonged APTT is heparin, either because the patient is on treatment or because of sample contamination. However, the TT is extremely sensitive to heparin and will also be prolonged. A Reptilase time will confirm this if necessary.

The next diagnostic step is to establish whether the patient has a deficiency or an inhibitor by performing the 50:50 mixture test described on page 367. Mixing tests should be done immediately, followed by the specific assay or tests.

4.

PT	Long
APTT	Long
TT	Normal
Fibrinogen	Normal
Platelet count	Normal

The main causes of a prolonged PT and APTT are:

1. Lack of vitamin K. In this case the PT is usually relatively more prolonged than is the APTT.
2. The administration of oral anticoagulant drugs. The PT is usually more prolonged than is the APTT.
3. Liver disease giving rise to multiple factor deficiencies. (In some cases the fibrinogen may also be abnormal.)

4. Rare congenital or acquired defects of factors V, X, prothrombin, and combined V and VIII deficiency.

Mixing experiments using the PT may be useful if there is no history of anticoagulant therapy and no obvious reason for failure of vitamin K absorption, e.g. parenteral feeding, long-term antibiotic treatment. If correction is obtained, specific factor assays should be performed.

5.

PT	Long
APTT	Long
TT	Long
Fibrinogen	Normal/abnormal
Platelet count	Normal

Abnormalities in all three screening coagulation tests are found:

1. In the presence of heparin (TT usually disproportionately long).
2. In hypo-, a- and dys-fibrinogenaemias.
3. In some cases of liver disease.
4. In systemic hyperfibrinolysis.

To distinguish between these conditions, perform a Reptilase or ancrod time, measure the fibrinogen concentration and measure the level of FDPs or D-dimers in plasma.

6.

PT	Normal
APTT	Normal
TT	Normal
Fibrinogen	Normal
Platelet count	Low

If the only abnormality is a low platelet count, possible causes must be investigated. The usual approach is to perform a bone marrow aspirate to exclude marrow failure and establish whether megakaryocytes are present. If the number and morphology of megakaryocytes in the marrow are normal, further investigations are undertaken to establish the cause of the presumed peripheral destruction of platelets. Heparin and other drugs are common causes in hospital practice.

7.

PT	Long
APTT	Long

TT	Normal
Fibrinogen	Normal/abnormal
Platelet count	Low

This pattern of abnormalities of the screening test is found:

1. After massive transfusion with stored/plasma reduced blood which is deficient in coagulation factors.
2. In some cases of chronic liver disease, especially cirrhosis.

In both instances, the clotting tests should correct by mixing with normal plasma and fibrinogen assay will be normal. Specific factor assays may be useful if the situation persists. Consider the possibility that the low platelet count has a separate aetiology and that the situation is in fact the same as in **4**.

8.

PT	Long
APTT	Long
TT	Long
Fibrinogen	Low
Platelet count	Low

All the first-line tests are abnormal in:

1. Acute DIC.
2. Some cases of acute liver necrosis with DIC.

It may sometimes be necessary to confirm the diagnosis of DIC with additional tests, e.g. by estimating FDP concentration or by carrying out a screening test for the presence of fibrin monomers. Consider the possibility that more than one pathology is present.

CORRECTION TESTS USING THE PT OR APTT

Principle
Unexplained prolongation of the PT or APTT can be investigated with simple correction tests, by mixing the patient's plasma with normal plasma. Correction indicates a possible factor deficiency, whereas failure to correct suggests the presence of an inhibitor, but interpretation should initially be cautious (see below).

Reagents
Plasmas for correction
Normal plasma contains all the coagulation factors and therefore mixing tests with normal plasma will

only identify the presence of an inhibitor or a factor deficiency. The factor which is deficient in the patient's sample can be identified by correction tests using the following plasmas (containing these factors):

1. Specific factor-deficient plasma	(all except the specific factor)
2. Aged normal human serum	(VII, IX, X, XI, XII)
3. Adsorbed normal human plasma	(I, V, VIII, XI, XII)

Notes
Aged normal human serum. In many cases, untreated serum is over-activated. This can be minimized by using aged human serum, i.e. serum that has been stored at 4°C for several weeks before use.

Adsorbed normal human plasma. Treatment of normal human plasma with inorganic chemicals such as aluminium hydroxide or barium sulphate results in the adsorption of coagulation factors II, VII, IX and X. A stock suspension of aluminium hydroxide is prepared by thoroughly mixing 1 g moist gel (BDH) in 4 ml distilled water. One-tenth volume of the suspension is mixed with plasma at 37°C for 3 min, and then deposited by centrifugation.

However, these correction reagents may give misleading results if not used with great care. It is better to proceed directly to specific factor assays if appropriate factor-deficient plasmas are available.

Platelet-poor plasma. From the patient and a control.

Other reagents. As described under APTT (p. 354).

Method
Perform a PT and/or APTT on control, patient's and a known deficient plasma, followed by a PT and/or APTT on 50:50 (0.05 ml of each) mixtures of (a) the control and a known deficient plasma and (b) patient's and a known deficient plasma. Perform all the tests in duplicate using a balanced order to avoid time bias; or perform PT and/or APTT on mixtures of control, test, aged and absorbed plasma. Note that mixing experiments to detect factor VIII inhibitors may require incubation for 2 h (see p. 368).

Interpretation
If the prolongation is due to deficiency of a clotting factor, the PT or APTT of the mixture should

return to within a few seconds of normal and at least to less than 50% of the difference between the two individual clotting times. It is then necessary to identify the specific factor(s) that are deficient. Further mixing experiments may be performed using factor-deficient plasmas. Correction of the clotting time by mixing with another plasma indicates that any factor(s) missing in the patient is (are) present in the second (deficient) plasma (see Tables 16.4 and 16.5). In many instances, only a partial correction is possible because the congenitally deficient plasma samples may have been stored for long periods of time or are freeze-dried commercially-obtained preparations. It is therefore essential always to include a control normal plasma and mixtures with a control normal plasma in every experiment. If possible, it is preferable to proceed directly to factor assays if correction is obtained with normal plasma.

If the APTT is prolonged, and normal plasma fails to correct the APTT, an inhibitor should be suspected. An inhibitor screen and tests for a lupus anticoagulant should be performed. However mixing tests may be misleading in two particular circumstances: (1) Some inhibitors (typically anti-factor VIII antibodies) are time dependent in their action and testing immediately after mixing may show correction whereas testing after 2 h incubation reveals an inhibitory effect. (2) Some lupus-like anticoagulants are relatively weak and may only be apparent if 25:75 mixes of normal and test plasma are used. For details of testing for inhibitors, see page 367.

Comment

Correction tests are sometimes not as clear cut as the literature and theory would suggest. A marginal correction can be difficult to interpret. If the correction tests fall into the 'grey' area, specific factor levels should be measured, and tests for the presence of a lupus anticoagulant performed, checking for time-dependent effects and non-linearity.

CORRECTION TESTS USING THE THROMBIN TIME

Principle

The tests utilize certain physicochemical properties of reagents to bind to inhibitors or abnormal molecules and normalize the prolonged TT. Protamine sulphate has a net electropositive charge and interacts with heparin, as well as binding to FDP, neutralizing the inhibitory effects of both. Toluidine blue is also a charged reagent which will neutralize heparin but has no effect on FDP. Interestingly, toluidine blue normalizes the TT in some dysfibrinogenaemias, probably by interacting with the excess of sialic acid attached to the fibrinogen molecules.

Reagents

Patient's and control plasma.

Protamine sulphate. 1% and 10% in 9 g/l NaCl.

Toluidine blue. 0.05 g in 100 ml of 9 g/l NaCl.

Bovine thrombin. As described under TT (p. 351).

Method

Perform the test as described for TT, adding 0.1 ml of saline to the controls and replacing in the test

Table 16.4 Interpretation of mixing experiments with the APTT activated partial thromboplastin time (prothrombin time normal)

APTT of test plasma corrected with		
Aged plasma	Al (OH)₃ plasma	Interpretation
No	Yes	Factor VIII deficiency
Yes	No	Factor IX deficiency
Yes	Yes	Factor XI or XII deficiency

Table 16.5 Interpretation of mixing experiments using the prothrombin time (PT) (activated partial thromboplastin time also prolonged)

PT of test plasma corrected with		
Aged plasma	Al (OH)₃ plasma	Interpretation
No	Yes	Factor V deficiency
Yes	No	Factor X deficiency
Yes	Partial	Prothrombin deficiency

with protamine sulphate or toluidine blue solution. Also perform a TT on a 50:50 mixture of control and test plasma.

Interpretation

See Table 16.6.

Comment

The end-point may be difficult to see in samples with a low fibrinogen content in the presence of toluidine blue owing to the dark colour of the reagent. Grossly elevated fibrinogen concentrations or the presence of a paraprotein can cause a prolonged time not corrected by either protamine or toluidine blue. Diluting the test plasma in saline will shorten the TT.

REPTILASE OR ANCROD TIME[21]

Reptilase, a purified enzyme from the snake *Bothrops atrox*, and ancrod (Arvin), a similar enzyme from the snake *Agkistrodon rhodostoma*, may be used to replace thrombin in the TT test.

The venoms are reconstituted as directed by the manufacturers, and the test is performed exactly as described for the TT. The snake venoms are not inhibited by heparin and will give normal times for the clotting of normal plasma in the presence of heparin. The clotting times will, however, remain prolonged in the presence of raised FDP or abnormal or reduced fibrinogen or hypoalbuminaemia.

Table 16.6 Interpretation of correction tests using the thrombin time (TT)

| Saline | TT of test plasma corrected with | | | Interpretation |
	Normal plasma	Protamine sulphate	Toluidine blue	
No	Yes	No	No	Deficiency
No	Var	No	Yes	Dysfibrinogenaemia of liver disease
No	Var	Yes	No	High concentration of FDP

FDP, fibrin degradation products; var, variable.
It is essential to exclude the possibility of heparin contamination.

INVESTIGATION OF A BLEEDING DISORDER OWING TO A COAGULATION FACTOR DEFICIENCY OR DEFECT

When the screening tests indicate that an individual has a coagulation defect, the plasma concentration of the coagulation factors should be assayed. Such assays not only establish the diagnosis of the deficiency or defect, but they also assess its severity, and can be used to monitor replacement therapy and to detect the carrier state in families in which one or more members are affected by a congenital bleeding disorder.

An individual may have a congenital deficiency of a coagulation factor because of impaired synthesis or because a variant of the molecule is synthesized which is deficient in clotting activity. In both instances the results of assays based on coagulation tests will be subnormal, but when a variant molecule is being produced, the result of

an immunological assay may be normal or near normal.

GENERAL PRINCIPLES OF PARALLEL LINE BIOASSAYS OF COAGULATION FACTORS

If two materials containing the same coagulation factor are assayed in a specific assay system in a range of dilutions, and the clotting times are plotted against the plasma concentration on linear graph paper, curved dose response lines are obtained. If the plot is redrawn on double-log paper, a sigmoid curve with a straight middle section is obtained (Fig. 16.2). If the dilutions of the test and standard materials are chosen carefully, it should be possible to draw two straight

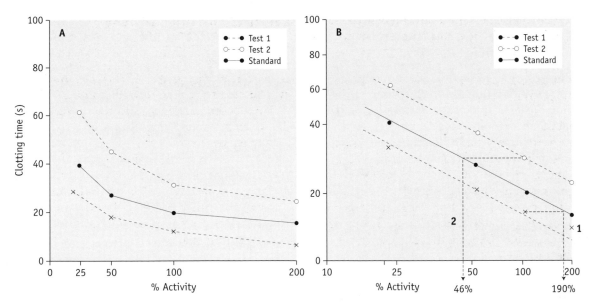

Fig. 16.2 Parallel line bioassay of factor VII. (A) Clotting times with 1 in 5, 1 in 10, 1 in 20 and 1 in 40 dilutions of test and standard plasma plotted on linear graph paper. (B) The same data plotted on double log paper. Three parallel straight lines are obtained. The horizontal shift of the test line represents the difference in potency. In this case, test 1 has a potency of 190% and test 2 a potency of 46%. The 1 in 10 dilution of the standard plasma is assigned a potency of 100%.

parallel lines. The horizontal distance between the two lines represents the difference in potency ('strength' or concentration) of the factor assayed. If the test line is to the right of the standard, it contains less of the factor than the standard; if to the left, it contains more.

When setting up and performing a parallel line assay, a number of measures must be taken to ensure that the assay is valid and reliable:

1. *Dilution range.* This should be chosen so that the coagulation times lie on the linear portion of the sigmoid curve. For example, when assaying factor VIII:C by one-stage assay, dilutions giving times between 60 and 100 s are chosen if the blank clotting time is over 120 s. (The blank consists of a mixture of buffer and substrate or deficient plasma which provides all factors except the one to be measured.)
2. *Number of dilutions.* At least three dilutions of the standard and the test are assayed to give the best graphical or mathematical solution.
3. *Responses.* Dilutions of the test sample should be chosen so that the clotting times fall within the range obtained for the standard. If it transpires that the test result falls outside this range, the standard curve should not be extra-

polated but the dilutions of the test and/or the standard must be adjusted.
4. *Duplicates and replicates.* Duplicates are obtained from the same dilution of the sample and sometimes by sub-sampling from the same incubation mixture. Replicates are true repeats involving a fresh dilution and fresh reagents. Normally, coagulation times are measured on duplicates. Replicates are sometimes used for particularly difficult assays.
5. *Temporal drift.* This has already been discussed. Duplicates in a coagulation assay should always be tested in a balanced order, e.g. ABCCBA.

Note on single point factor assays

Factor assay results are dependent on obtaining parallel lines for the test and reference plasmas. Many automated coagulation analysers will give an assay result obtained from a single dilution assuming that this condition is met. However, this is not always true and if an inhibitor is suspected results from more than one dilution should be obtained for comparison and to determine parallelism. Similarly, if the result is above the linear part of the standard curve further dilutions should be tested.

ASSAYS BASED ON THE PROTHROMBIN TIME, E.G. SUSPECTED FACTOR VII DEFICIENCY OR DEFECT

The investigation of an isolated prolonged one-stage PT in an individual with a life-long history of bleeding includes a one-stage factor VII assay. If a reduced concentration of factor VII is found, further tests may include immunoassays of factor VII and, when possible, a family study.

ONE-STAGE ASSAY OF FACTOR VII
Principle

The assay of factor VII is based on the PT. The assay compares the ability of dilutions of the patient's plasma and of a standard plasma to correct the PT of a substrate plasma. It is easily adapted to assay prothrombin, FV or FX.

Reagents

Platelet-poor plasma from the patient.

Standard/reference plasma.   See page 351.

Factor VII deficient plasma.   Commercial or from a patient with known severe deficiency.

Barbitone buffered saline.   See page 605.

Thromboplastin.   It is recommended that a recombinant human thromboplastin is used for the assay of human FVII. Rabbit brain thromboplastin known to be sensitive to factor VII deficiency has been used but there is a danger of the interspecies differences giving misleading results. The thromboplastin should be reconstituted according to the manufacturer's instructions and may contain sufficient Ca for the assay. Warm sufficient thromboplastin for the assay to 37°C.

$CaCl_2$.   0.025 mol/l (if not present in the thromboplastin preparation).

Method

Prepare 1 in 5, 1 in 10, 1 in 20 and 1 in 40 dilutions of the standard and test plasma in buffered saline. Transfer 0.1 ml of each dilution to a glass tube and add to it 0.1 ml of deficient (substrate) plasma. Mix and allow to warm to 37°C. Add 0.1 ml of dilute thromboplastin and start the stopwatch. Record the clotting time. If the thromboplastin does not contain calcium, start the stopwatch after adding 0.1 ml of $CaCl_2$. A blank must be included with every assay and all tests carried out in duplicate, and in balanced order.

Calculation of results

Plot the clotting times of the test and standard against the concentration of factor VII on log-log graph paper. Read the concentration as shown in Figure 16.2.

Normal range

0.5–2.0 u/ml (for discussion of units see p. 369).

Interpretation

Patients with a congenital deficiency have factor VII levels of 0.30 u/ml and less. The concentration measured may vary according to the thromboplastin used in the assay so recombinant human thromboplastin is preferable. A small proportion of patients have normal factor VII antigen despite abnormal functional activity.

ASSAYS BASED ON THE ACTIVATED PARTIAL THROMBOPLASTIN TIME, e.g. FACTOR VIII

An APTT-based assay may be indicated after obtaining correction of a prolonged APTT by mixing with normal plasma. An assay for factor VIII is described but this is easily adapted to FIX, FXI or contact factor assay by substituting the relevant factor-deficient plasma.

ONE-STAGE ASSAY OF FACTOR VIII[22,23]
Principle

The one-stage assay for factor VIII:C is based on the APTT according to the bioassay principle described above.

Reagents

Platelet-poor plasma.   From the patient.

Standard/reference plasma.   See page 351.

Factor VIII deficient plasma (substrate plasma). If using a commercial plasma, the reagent should be reconstituted according to the manufacturer's instructions. If a haemophiliac donor is used, the factor VIII concentration should be less than 1% and the plasma should be free of inhibitors. The plasma should be stored in suitable volumes, e.g. 2 ml, at −20°C or lower until used. All samples obtained from patients must be considered potentially infective. Patient samples should be tested for antibodies to HIV and hepatitis C virus and for HBs antigen after obtaining the patient's informed consent.

Barbitone buffered saline. See page 605.

Reagents for APTT

Plastic tubes. To avoid contact activation while preparing samples.

Ice-bath.

Method

Place the APTT reagent and $CaCl_2$ at 37°C, and the patient's, standard and substrate plasma in the ice-bath until used.

Make 1 in 10 dilutions of the test and standard plasma in buffered saline in plastic tubes in the ice-bath. Using 0.2 ml volumes, make doubling dilutions in buffered saline to obtain 1 in 20 and 1 in 40 dilutions. Place 0.1 ml of the three dilutions (1 in 10, 1 in 20 and 1 in 40) in glass tubes. If the test plasma is suspected of having a very low factor VIII content, make 1 in 5, 1 in 10 and 1 in 20 dilutions of the test instead.

Add to each dilution 0.1 ml of freshly reconstituted or thawed substrate plasma and warm up at 37°C. Perform APTTs according to the laboratory protocol following a balanced order of duplicates.

The dilutions should be tested at 2-min intervals on the master stopwatch. The assay must end with a blank consisting of 0.1 ml of buffered saline and 0.1 ml of substrate plasma.

Calculation of results

Plot the clotting times of the test and standard against the concentration of factor VIII on semi-log paper. Read the concentration as shown in Figure 16.2. It is important to obtain straight and parallel lines if the result is to be accurate. The reasons for non-parallelism and curvature are:

1. Technical error. Repeat the assay with fresh dilutions.
2. Activation of the plasma by poor collection. A new sample should be collected.
3. A low concentration of factor VIII in the test plasma gives rise to non-parallel lines. Stronger

concentration of plasma should be prepared and tested.
4. The presence of an inhibitor. The tests described on page 367 should be carried out.

Some automated coagulometers produce computed values using mathematical formulae. If the standard plasma is calibrated in terms of international units, the result can be expressed in iu. For example, if the standard plasma has a factor VIII concentration of 0.65 iu/ml and the test is shown to have 20% of the activity of the standard, the test plasma will have a factor VIII concentration of 0.13 iu/ml (20% of 65 iu/ml).

Normal range

45–158 iu/dl (0.45–1.58 iu/ml). Each laboratory should determine its own normal range.

Interpretation

Some clinically normal people have factor VIII concentrations of 35–50 iu/dl. Values below 30 iu/dl are unequivocally abnormal; values below 50 iu/dl are significant in carriers.

A reduced factor VIII concentration is found in:

1. Haemophilia A.
2. Some carriers of haemophilia A (heterozygotes).
3. vWD, types I and III, and some cases of type II.
4. Rare congenital combined deficiency of factors VIII and V.
5. DIC.
6. Acquired haemophilia (anti-factor VIII antibodies).

An elevated level of factor VIII has now been shown to have an association with thrombosis.[24]

Further tests in haemophilia A

Reduction in factor VIII secondary to vWD should be excluded. vWF:Ag and ristocetin co-factor (RiCoF) (described below) should be measured and the patient's family investigated. A low factor VIII with normal vWF:Ag and RiCoF may also result from the Normandy type vWD (Type 2N) which should be suspected from a recessive type family history and can be confirmed by a vWF-FVIII binding assay.

Two-stage and chromogenic assays for factor VIII

The one-stage factor VIII assay is sensitive to pre-activation of coagulation factors in the patient sample. The two-stage and chromogenic assays circumvent this problem by preactivating all the available factor VIII to generate Xa and then assaying this in a separate system. In general, these have proved too cumbersome or expensive for widespread use and preactivation is rarely a significant problem. However, a clinically significant discrepancy between the two types of assay has been reported in some cases of mild haemophilia. In these cases, mutations destabilizing the interaction between the A1 and A2 domains result in a one-stage assay result which is higher than that obtained by two stage. Most significantly, the patient's clinical problem is more in keeping with the two-stage assay result.[26,27]

TESTS REQUIRED FOR MONITORING REPLACEMENT THERAPY IN COAGULATION FACTOR DEFECTS AND DEFICIENCIES

Replacement therapy requires the following:

1. Calculation of the dose of the material to be administered and its frequency.
2. Assessment of the response to the dose.
3. Monitoring of any untoward effects.

The *dose* to be administered is calculated from the patient's body weight and the rise in the plasma concentration of the defective coagulation factor that is desired. Thus, the patient's plasma concentration of the factor and the potency or strength of the therapeutic material must be known. For the vast majority of patients where the defect is known and its plasma concentration has been measured, and for whom a commercial freeze-dried factor concentrate is used, this means a calculation based on the following formulae:

- For factor VIII, the dose in iu per kg body weight = rise required in iu per dl divided by 2.
- For factor IX, the dose in iu per kg body weight = rise required in iu per dl.

The rise required depends on the type of bleeding, the half-life and stability of the clotting factor used, and on the concentration of the defective factor in the patient's plasma prior to treatment.

Assessment of the response to the therapy requires regular measurements of the plasma concentration of the coagulation factor infused, by means of a functional assay. The response can be assessed from the formula:

Rise in iu per dl divided by dose in iu per kg body weight = K, which is approximately 2 for haemophilia A, and approximately 1 for haemophilia B (if plasma concentrates are used).

The response is usually measured immediately after the administration of the therapeutic material. If the response is inadequate, this may have been due to an error in calculating the dose, or because the potency of the therapeutic material is less than expected, or because the patient is developing an inhibitor. Problems of determining potency of concentrates and comparisons with plasma standards are discussed on page 351.

The main *untoward effects* are transmission of infection and the development of inhibitors. If the presence of an inhibitor is suspected, it must be confirmed using the tests described on page 367 and later assessed quantitatively. Monitoring replacement and other types of therapy in patients with inhibitors are described by White & Roberts.[28]

Estimations of factor VIII in patients with haemophilia treated with factor VIII concentrates often yield discrepant results. This is primarily because the factor VIII concentrate (diluted in haemophilic plasma) is compared with a plasma standard. In general, two-stage or chromogenic assays reveal greater potency than one-stage assays in this situation. This has been particularly noted in patients who have been treated with B domain-less factor VIII. In these cases, an alternative product-specific reference preparation may be available from the company. In most other cases, the clinical experience of using results from one-stage assays remains valid. Assays of factor VIII concentrates are fraught with difficulty and beyond the scope of this chapter.[29]

INVESTIGATION OF A PATIENT WHOSE APTT AND PT ARE PROLONGED

A prolonged APTT and PT but a normal TT in a patient with a bleeding disorder may be due to a defect or deficiency of one of the factors of the common pathway: factor X, factor V or prothrombin. In addition, the patient could be suffering from the much rarer combined deficiency of factors V and VIII:C. Liver disease and vitamin K deficiency should always be excluded, even in the presence of a family history of bleeding. Mixing tests illustrated on page 368 may help to pinpoint the defect; the missing factor or factors should be estimated quantitatively. Factor X, factor V and prothrombin can all be assayed satisfactorily using a prothrombin-based assay as described for factor VII. The Taipan venom assay for prothrombin and the Russell's viper venom assay for factor X are described in the 8th edition.

INVESTIGATION OF A PATIENT WITH A CIRCULATING ANTICOAGULANT (INHIBITOR)[30]

Circulating anticoagulants or acquired inhibitors of coagulation factors are immunoglobulins arising either in congenitally deficient individuals as a result of the administration of the missing factor or in previously haemostatically normal subjects as a part of an auto-immune process. Typically, an inhibitor is suspected when a prolonged clotting test does not correct after mixing 50:50 with normal plasma or if an apparent factor deficiency does not fit with a patient's clinical history.

The commonest anticoagulant in haemostatically normal people is the lupus anticoagulant, but despite the prolongation of clotting tests in vitro, this anticoagulant predisposes to thrombosis and its diagnosis and investigation are therefore considered on page 392. Of the anticoagulants which cause a bleeding tendency, antibodies to factor VIII:C are most common. They are present in 15% or more of haemophiliacs but also arise as auto-antibodies in previously normal individuals. They fall into two general categories: those with simple kinetics, and those with complex kinetics. Patients with haemophilia usually develop antibodies with simple kinetics; this inhibitor reacts with factor VIII:C in a linear fashion and the antigen/antibody complex has no factor VIII:C activity. Antibodies in non-haemophilic individuals or patients with mild/moderate haemophilia usually develop antibodies with complex kinetics: inactivation of factor VIII:C is at first rapid, but it then slows as the antigen/antibody complex either dissociates or displays some factor VIII:C activity. Addition of further factor VIII results in the same residual (equilibrium) factor VIII activity.

Inhibitors directed against other coagulation factors are very rare but an acquired form of vWD commonly associated with a paraprotein has been increasingly recognized in recent years. Only the factor VIII inhibitor assays are described in detail in this section.

Confusion may arise in the presence of inhibitor if different clotting factors are assayed. For instance, if a patient's plasma contains an inhibitor directed against factor VIII and the factor IX level in that plasma is assayed using factor IX deficient plasma, the clotting times in the factor IX assay will be prolonged. This may lead to the mistaken conclusion that the patient has factor IX deficiency, particularly if a single dilution of test plasma is used. Clotting factors should always be assayed at multiple dilutions. If the inhibitor is specifically directed against one clotting factor, that factor will appear to be equally deficient at all dilutions of patient's plasma. The assayed level of other clotting factors will increase with increasing dilution as the inhibitor is diluted out.

CIRCULATING INHIBITOR (ANTICOAGULANT) SCREEN BASED ON THE APTT[30]

Principle

Circulating anticoagulants or inhibitors affecting the APTT may act immediately or be time dependent. Normal plasma mixed with a plasma containing an immediately acting inhibitor will have little or no effect on the prolonged clotting time. In contrast, if normal plasma is added to a plasma containing a time-dependent inhibitor, the clotting time of the latter will be substantially shortened. However, after 1–2 h, correction will be abolished, and the clotting time will become long again. In order to detect both types of inhibition, normal plasma and test plasma samples are tested immediately after mixing and also after incubation together at 37°C for 120 min.

Reagents

Normal plasma. Commercial lyophilized normal plasma or a plasma pool from 20 donors as described on page 351.

Platelet-poor plasma. From the patient.

Reagents for the APTT (see p. 354).

Method

Prepare three plastic tubes as follows: place 0.5 ml of normal plasma in a first tube, 0.5 ml of the patient's plasma in a second tube, and a mixture of 0.25 ml of normal and 0.25 ml of patient's plasma in a third tube. Incubate the tubes for 120 min at 37°C and then place all three tubes in an ice-bath or on crushed ice. Next make a 50:50 mixture of the contents of tubes 1 and 2 into a 4th tube: which serves to check for the presence of an immediate inhibitor. Perform APTTs in duplicate on all four tubes.

Results and interpretation

See Table 16.7. Note that the incubation period results in a prolongation of the normal plasma APTT.

QUANTITATIVE MEASUREMENT OF FACTOR VIII INHIBITORS[30]

Principle

Factor VIII inhibitors are usually time dependent. Thus if factor VIII is added to plasma containing an inhibitor and the mixture is incubated, factor VIII will be progressively neutralized. If the amount of factor VIII added and the duration of incubation are standardized, the strength of the inhibitor may be measured in units according to how much of the added factor VIII is destroyed.

In the Bethesda method, the unit is defined as the amount of inhibitor which will neutralize 50% of 1 unit of factor VIII:C in normal plasma after 2 h incubation at 37°C.

Dilutions of test plasma are incubated with an equal volume of the normal plasma pool at 37°C. The normal plasma pool is taken to represent 1 unit of factor VIII. Dilutions of a control normal plasma containing no inhibitor are treated in the same way. An equal volume of normal plasma mixed with buffer is taken to represent the 100% value.

At the end of the incubation period, the residual factor VIII is assayed and the inhibitor strength calculated from a standard graph of residual factor VIII activity versus inhibitor units.

Reagents

Glyoxaline buffer. See page 352.

Kaolin. 5 mg/ml and *Platelet substitute.* Phospholipid or preferred APTT reagent.

Factor VIII:C deficient plasma.

Standard plasma. Normal plasma pool.

Method

Pipette into each of a series of plastic tubes 0.2 ml of normal pool plasma. Add 0.2 ml of glyoxaline buffer to the first tube (this tube serves as the 100% value); add 0.2 ml of test plasma dilutions in glyoxaline buffer to each of the other tubes. If the patient's inhibitor has been assayed previously, this can be used as a guide to the dilutions that should be used. If the patient has not been tested before, a range of dilutions should be set up ranging from undiluted plasma to a 1 to 50 dilution.

Cap, mix and incubate all the tubes for 2 h at 37°C. Then immerse all the tubes in an ice-bath.

Table 16.7 Interpretation of the inhibitor screen based on the activated partial thromboplastin time

Tube	Content	Clotting time		
1	Normal plasma	Normal	Normal	Normal
2	Patient's plasma	Long	Long	Long
3	50:50 mixture, patient:normal; incubated 2 h	Normal	Long	Long
4	50:50 mixture, patient:normal; no incubation	Normal	Long	Normal
Interpretation		Deficiency	Immediately acting inhibitor	Time-dependent inhibitor

Perform factor VIII assays on all the incubation mixtures.

Calculation of results

Record the residual factor VIII percentage for each mixture assuming the assay value of the control to be 100%. The dilution of test plasma that gives the residual factor VIII percentage nearest to 50% (between 30% and 60%) is chosen for calculating the strength of inhibitor. Results are calculated as shown in Table 16.8 for three different patients with a mild inhibitor only detected in undiluted plasma, a stronger inhibitor with simple kinetics and an inhibitor with complex kinetics, respectively.

Interpretation

If the residual factor VIII activity is between 80% and 100%, the plasma sample does not contain an inhibitor. If the residual activity is less than 60%, the plasma unequivocally contains an inhibitor. Values between 60% and 80% are borderline and repeated testing on additional samples is needed before the diagnosis can be established.

Inhibitor assay modifications

The Bethesda assay and Nijmegen modification[31] give similar results at high levels of factor VIII inhibition. However, at low levels (below 1.0), the Bethesda method can give false-positive levels of inhibition whereas the Nijmegen method would give zero levels of inhibition. Reports have shown

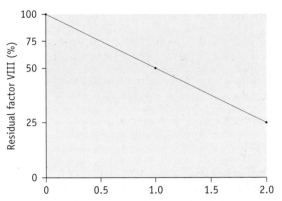

Fig. 16.3 Measurement of factor VIII:C inhibitors. Relationship between the residual factor VIII:C activity in normal plasma and the inhibitor activity of the test plasma can be read off this plot. At 50% inhibition, the test plasma contains, by definition, 1 Bethesda inhibitor unit per ml. Note that the y axis is a logarithmic scale. See also Table 16.9.

that shifts in pH and protein concentrations will lead to changes in factor VIII stability and inactivation. Factor VIII inactivation increases with pH and reduced protein concentration leads to further inactivation of factor VIII activity. The Nijmegen modification prevents these discrepancies by buffering normal plasma with 0.1 mol/l imidazole buffer at pH 7.4 and using immunodepleted factor VIII deficient plasma in the control mixture.[31] The assay can also be modified to use factor VIII concentrate (Oxford method) or by increasing the incubation time to 4 h (New Oxford method).

Table 16.8 Example of the calculation of Bethesda units (u) in three plasma samples

Patient	Plasma dilution	% residual VIII:C	Calculation u × dilution	Inhibitor in Bethesda u
A	Undiluted	61	0.70 × 1	= 0.07
B	1 in 5	33	1.60 × 5	= 8.0
	1 in 10	55	0.85 × 10	= 8.5
	1 in 15	68	0.55 × 15	= 8.3
C	1 in 5	40	1.30 × 5	= 6.5
	1 in 10	55	0.85 × 10	= 8.5
	1 in 15	61	0.70 × 15	= 10.5
	1 in 20	65	0.60 × 20	= 12

Patient A has a mild inhibitor, patient B an inhibitor with simple kinetics and patient C an inhibitor with complex kinetics. All values are chosen for the percent residual factor VIII:C activity close to 50%. The units for the calculation are read from Figure 16.3 using the % residual VIII:C. (Modified from Kasper C.K, Ewing NP. 1982 The haemophilias: measurement of inhibitor to factor VIII C (and IX C). Methods in Haematology 5:39).

Note that in patients B and C the results should be reported as 8.5 Bethesda units; in C, the calculated level of inhibitor may continue to rise with increasing dilution.

Tests for other inhibitors

Factor IX inhibitors can be measured in a system identical to that described above. Because factor IX inhibitors act immediately, there is no need for prolonged incubation: the mixtures can be assayed after 5 min at 37°C. The activity of the inhibitor against porcine factor VIII can be measured by substituting Hyate C (porcine factor VIII, concentrate, appropriately diluted in factor VIII deficient plasma) for normal plasma.

INVESTIGATION OF A PATIENT SUSPECTED OF AFIBRINOGENAEMIA, HYPOFIBRINOGENAEMIA OR DYSFIBRINOGENAEMIA

The patient usually has a prolonged PT, APTT and TT. The prolongation of the PT is usually less marked than that of the APTT and TT. There may be either a history of bleeding or of recurrent thrombotic events but many patients (~50%) are asymptomatic. It is important that a physical estimation of fibrinogen (such as the clot weight) is obtained as well as a function-based assay (e.g. Clauss) (see p. 356).

FIBRINOGEN ESTIMATION (DRY CLOT WEIGHT)

Principle

Fibrinogen in plasma is converted into fibrin by clotting with thrombin and calcium. The resulting clot is weighed. The resulting clot may include other proteins including some FDPs. It is, however, simpler than the total clottable protein method used for the international standard[32] and provides a useful comparison for the Clauss.

Reagents

Citrated platelet-poor plasma.

CaCl$_2$. 0.025 mol/l.

Bovine thrombin. 50 NIH u/ml.

Method

Pipette 1 ml of plasma into a 12 × 75 mm glass tube and warm to 37°C. Place a wooden applicator or swab stick in the tube, add 0.1 ml of CaCl$_2$ and 0.9 ml of thrombin and mix. Incubate for 15 min at 37°C.

Gently wind the fibrin clot onto the stick, squeezing out the serum. Wash the clot in a tube containing at first 9 g/l NaCl, then water. Blot the clot carefully with filter paper, remove the fibrin from the stick and put into acetone for 5–10 min. Dry the clot in a hot air oven or over a hot lamp for 30 min. Allow it to cool and then weigh.

Results

The fibrinogen level is expressed as g/l, i.e. the weight of fibrin obtained from 1 ml of plasma × 1000.

Normal range

1.5–4.0 g/l.

Further investigations

Whenever a congenital fibrinogen abnormality is suspected, DIC and hyperfibrinolysis must be excluded: FDPs should not be in excess and there should be no evidence of the consumption of other coagulation factors and platelets (see p. 386). Immunological or chemical determination of fibrinogen is the next step in investigation. In dysfibrinogenaemias there is often a normal or even raised plasma fibrinogen concentration using these methods although the functional assays indicate a deficiency. Other tests which may be helpful are the Reptilase time, fibrinopeptide release, factor XIII cross-linking, tests of polymerization, binding to thrombin and lysis by plasmin. In some cases, genomic DNA analysis can be performed.[33] Testing the parents or other family members is sometimes a useful means for establishing whether a hereditary fibrinogen abnormality is present.

DEFECTS OF PRIMARY HAEMOSTASIS

INVESTIGATION OF THE VASCULAR DISORDERS OF HAEMOSTASIS

Vascular disorders of haemostasis are those which arise owing to defect or deficiency of the vessel wall. This may be due to one of the inherited disorders of collagen or to an acquired disorder such as amyloid or scurvy.

In general, the tests of coagulation available in the laboratory will be of little help in elucidating such defects. The only test of any use is the bleeding time. Tests of capillary resistance are of little value. A careful clinical history and physical examination are most likely to provide the basis for diagnosis. Particular attention should be paid to previous scars, associated signs of the inherited syndromes and evidence of systemic disease. In some cases, a tissue biopsy may be useful but confirmation of the diagnosis requires analysis of collagen from cultured fibroblasts or DNA analysis of the relevant candidate genes.[34]

BLEEDING TIME

Principle

A standard incision is made on the volar surface of the forearm and the time the incision bleeds is measured. Cessation of bleeding indicates the formation of haemostatic plugs which are in turn dependent on an adequate number of platelets and on the ability of the platelets to adhere to the subendothelium and to form aggregates.[35]

STANDARDIZED TEMPLATE METHOD[36]

Materials

Sphygmomanometer.

Cleansing swabs.

Template bleeding time device.   Such as 'Simplate ®R' with a single retractable blade (Organon Teknika).

Filter paper.   1 mm thick.

Stopwatch.

Method

Place a sphygmomanometer cuff around the patient's arm above the elbow, inflate to 40 mmHg and keep it at this pressure throughout the test. Clean the area with 70% ethanol or isopropylalcohol swabs and allow to dry. Choose an area of skin on the volar surface of the forearm which is devoid of visible superficial veins. Use a commercial template device to make one or two standard longitudinal incisions. If not available, then press a sterile metal template with a linear slit 7–8 mm long firmly against the skin aligned along the long axis of the arm and use a scalpel blade with a guard so arranged that the tip of the blade protrudes 1 mm through the template slit. In this way, make an incision 6 mm long and 1 mm deep. Modifications of the template and blade making two simultaneous cuts with a spring mechanism are commercially available.

With the edge of a filter paper at 15 s intervals, blot off the blood exuding from the cut. Avoid contact with the wound during this procedure because this may disturb the formation of the platelet plug. When bleeding has ceased, carefully bring together the edges of the incision and apply an adhesive strip to lessen the risk of keloid formation and an unsightly scar.

Normal range

2.5–9.5 min. Ideally, every laboratory should determine its own normal range and if possible ensure that the test is performed by the same operator.

IVY'S METHOD[37]

The test is similar to the template method, but instead of a standardized incision two separate punctures, 5–10 cm apart, are made in quick succession using a disposable lancet. Any microlance with a cutting depth of 2.5 mm and width of just over 1 mm is suitable; it can be inserted to its maximum depth without fear of penetrating too deeply. A source of inaccuracy with Ivy's method is the tendency for the puncture wound to close before bleeding has ceased.

Normal range

2–7 min. But a lower range of 0–4 min has been found in a study of a large number of healthy subjects who had not taken aspirin.[55] Ideally, every laboratory should determine its own normal range and if possible ensure that the test is performed by the same operator.

Interpretation of results

A prolonged bleeding time may be due to:

1. *Thrombocytopenia*. It is advisable to check the platelet count before carrying out the bleeding time test. Patients with a platelet count below $50 \times 10^9/l$ may have a very long bleeding time and the bleeding may be difficult to arrest.
2. *Disorders of platelet function*. They may be congenital, such as thrombasthenia, storage pool defect, etc. (see below), or acquired, owing to drugs or the presence of a paraprotein, or in myelodysplastic/myeloproliferative syndromes.
3. vWD, owing to defective platelet adherence to the subendothelium in the absence of a normal amount of or of normally functioning vWF (see below).
4. Vascular abnormalities, as found in Ehlers–Danlos's syndrome, or in pseudoxanthoma elasticum.
5. Occasionally, severe deficiency of factor V or XI, or afibrinogenaemia.
6. The bleeding time is subject to a large number of variables and confounding factors. It is important to standardize the sphygmomanometer pressure, longitudinal orientation of the incision, volar aspect of arm and the blotting technique. Attempting to repeat the test within a short period will usually give a shorter bleeding time. A normal bleeding time does not imply normal haemostasis and the result of the test has been shown not to correlate with bleeding at other sites.

LABORATORY TESTS OF PLATELET–vWF FUNCTION

PFA-100 system

The most widely used screening test for platelet disorders, the bleeding time, suffers from inherent variability and does not correlate well with the incidence of clinically significant bleeding.

An in-vitro system for measuring platelet–vWF function – PFA-100 (Dade Behring) – is now available. The instrument aspirates a blood sample under constant vacuum from the sample reservoir through a capillary and a microscopic aperture cut into a membrane. The membrane is coated with collagen and either adrenaline or adenosine 5′-diphosphate. It therefore attempts to reproduce under high shear rates vWF binding, platelet attachment, activation and aggregation, which slowly builds a stable platelet plug at the aperture. The time required to obtain full occlusion of the aperture is reported as the 'closure time'. Collagen/adrenaline is the primary screening cartridge and the collagen/ADP is used to identify possible aspirin use.

Studies have shown this system to be sensitive to platelet adherence and aggregation abnormalities and to be dependent on normal vWF, glycoprotein Ib and glycoprotein IIbIIIa levels but not on plasma fibrinogen or fibrin generation.

The PFA-100 system may reflect vWF platelet function better than the bleeding time but it is not sensitive to vascular–collagen disorders.[38,39]

INVESTIGATION OF SUSPECTED VON WILLEBRAND DISEASE[40,41]

A diagnosis of vWD should be considered in individuals with a relevant history or family history of bleeding, particularly of the mucosal type. Although a prolonged bleeding time and APTT in screening tests are suggestive, these are normal in many patients with vWD and specific assays must be performed. Preliminary screening with a test such as the PFA-100 may be useful in excluding borderline cases. All factor VIII activities, i.e. VIII:C concentration, vWF:Ag concentration and activity RiCoF, should be measured.

If an abnormality is detected, the multimer analysis of the plasma should be performed. In normal plasma, each multimer of vWF (a large molecule consisting of 4 to over 20 subunits of vWF) is seen to be composed of a 'triplet', a dark central band sandwiched between two lighter bands; high molecular weight multimers predominate. In vWD, the multimer analysis may be superficially normal, there may be either no vWF:Ag detectable, or the high molecular weight forms necessary for normal platelet adhesion may be lacking, or the triplet pattern may be abnormal. On the basis of these results, vWD can be classified as shown in Table 16.9.[40]

ENZYME-LINKED IMMUNOSORBENT ASSAY FOR VON WILLEBRAND FACTOR ANTIGEN[42]
Principle

Enzyme-linked immunosorbent assay (ELISA) involves coating a special microtitre plate with a

Table 16.9 Classification of von Willebrand disease

Type	Inheritance	VIII:C	vWF:Ag	RiCoF	Multimer analysis	Comments
1	Autos. dominant	L/N	L	L	Normal pattern	—
2A	Autos. dominant	L/N	L/N	L	Absent large and intermediate size multimers, some forms have abnormal triplets	—
2B	Autos. dominant	L/N	L	L/N	Large multimers absent normal triplets	Aggregation with low dose Ristocetin in platelet-rich plasma Thrombocytopenia
2M	Autos. dominant	N	N	L	Normal pattern	—
2N	Autos. recessive	L	N	N	Normal pattern	Abnormal FVIII binding
3	Autos. recessive	L	L	L	Virtually absent	—

Autos., autosomal; L, low; N, normal; RiCoF, ristocetin cofactor; vWF, von Willebrand factor.

primary antibody to vWF:Ag. A suitable dilution of the test plasma is added to the wells allowing the vWF:Ag to bind to the primary antibody. After removal of excess antigen by washing the plate, a second antibody, conjugated to an enzyme, usually peroxidase, and called the 'tag' antibody, is added and this binds to the vWF:Ag already bound to the plate. On addition of a specific substrate, a colour change occurs. After the reaction has been stopped with acid, the optical density (OD) of each well can be measured using an electronic plate reader; the OD is directly proportional to the amount of vWF:Ag present in the test plasma.

The primary antibody can be substituted by a monoclonal antibody specifically raised against the glycoprotein Ib binding site on the vWF (available from Porton, Cambridge). This modification was found to correlate with the functional activity of the vWF measured as RiCoF activity. However, as a number of exceptions to this relationship have been identified the RiCoF assay remains the gold standard for estimation of vWF functional activity.

Reagents

0.05 M Carbonate buffer. 1.59 g Na_2CO_3, 2.93 g $NaHCO_3$, 0.2 g NaN_3 in 1 litre of water (pH 9.6).

0.01 M Phosphate buffered saline. 0.39 g $NaH_2PO_4.2H_2O$, 2.68 g $Na_2HPO_4.12H_2O$, 8.47 g NaCl in 1 litre water (pH 7.2).

0.1 M Citrate phosphate buffer. 8.8 g citric acid, 24.0 g $Na_2HPO_4.12H_2O$ in 1 litre water (pH 5.0).

Anti-vWF:Ag antiserum.

Anti-vWF:Ag conjugated with peroxidase.

Platelet-poor (100%) calibration plasma.

Platelet-poor plasma (tests and control).

1,2-o-Phenylenediamine dihydrochloride (OPD).

1M Sulphuric acid.

Hydrogen peroxide 20 vol.

Tween 20.

Method

Dilute the anti-human vWF:Ag 1:500 in 0.05 mol/l carbonate buffer (e.g. 40 μl antibody in 20 ml buffer) and add 100 μl to each well of the microtitre plate. Incubate for 1 h at room temperature in a moist chamber. Discard antibody and wash three times by immersion in a trough of phosphate buffered saline with 0.5 ml/l Tween for 2 min, followed by inversion onto absorbent paper.

Prepare dilutions of the 100% standard 1:10, 1:20, 1:40 and 1:60 in phosphate buffered saline with 1 ml/l Tween. Dilute patients' and control plasmas 1:10, 1:20 and 1:40 in the same way and add 100 μl of each dilution in duplicate to the wells of the microtitre plate. Incubate for 1 h as before and repeat washing.

Dilute the anti-human vWF:Ag-peroxidase conjugate 1:500 in 1 ml/l phosphate buffered saline-Tween (i.e. 40 μl antibody in 20 ml buffer) and add 100 μl to each well. Incubate for 1 h. Wash twice in 0.5 ml/l phosphate buffered saline-Tween and once in 0.1 mol/l citrate phosphate buffer.

Dissolve 40 mg of substrate (OPD) in 15 ml citrate phosphate buffer. Add 10 μl of 20 volume hydrogen peroxide to the substrate solution immediately before use, and then add 100 μl to each well.

When the yellow colour has reached an intensity where a mid-yellow ring is clearly visible in the bottom of the wells, stop the reaction by the addition of 150 μl of 1 mol/l sulphuric acid. Read the optical density across the plate at 492 nm using a microtitre plate reader. Plot the standard curve on log-linear graph paper. vWF:Ag levels are obtained by reading from the reference curve.

Normal range
0.5–2.0 iu/ml.

Interpretation
The results must be interpreted in conjunction with the results of factor VIII:C assay and the RiCoF assay (Table 16.9). vWF:Ag can also be measured by an immunoelectrophoretic assay. The Laurell rocket method for this is described in the 7th edition of this book.

RISTOCETIN CO-FACTOR ASSAY[43]
Principle
Washed platelets do not 'agglutinate' in the presence of ristocetin unless normal plasma is added as a source of vWF. 'Agglutination' follows a dose-response curve dependent upon the amount of plasma/vWF added. Fresh washed platelets or formalin-fixed platelets can be used in the assay. Fixed platelets take longer to prepare, but are not susceptible to aggregation (as distinct from 'agglutination') with ristocetin, and they can be stored so that they are available for emergency use. Fresh washed platelets are quicker to prepare, and retain a functional platelet membrane, but they cannot be retained for later use.

Commercial lyophilized fixed washed platelet preparations are available. Once reconstituted, these preparations are stable for several weeks and should enhance assay standardization.

ASSAY USING FRESH PLATELETS
Reagents

K₂ EDTA. 0.134 mol/l.

Citrate-saline. One volume of 31.1 g/l trisodium citrate + 9 volumes of 9 g/l NaCl.

EDTA-citrate-saline. One volume of 0.134 mol/l K₂EDTA + 9 volumes of citrate-saline.

Method
Collect 40–60 ml of normal blood into a one-tenth volume of EDTA-saline in flat-bottom plastic, universal containers. Do not use conical-bottom containers. Centrifuge at 150–200 *g* at room temperature (*c* 20°C) for 15 min.

Pipette, using a plastic pipette, the platelet-rich plasma into a plastic container. Mark the level of plasma on the tube. Centrifuge at 1500–2000 *g* to obtain a platelet button.

Discard the PPP. Resuspend the platelet button in a 2 ml volume of EDTA-citrate-saline by gently squeezing the liquid up and down a pipette until a smooth suspension is formed. Add EDTA-citrate-saline to the 20 ml mark.

Centrifuge at 1500–2000 *g* for 15 min. Discard the supernatant. Resuspend in EDTA-citrate-saline and leave at room temperature for 20 min to elute the RiCoF off the platelets.

Centrifuge again, discard the supernatant, resuspend in EDTA-citrate-saline two more times to a total of four washes.

Centrifuge at 1500–2000 *g* for 15 min. Discard the supernatant and resuspend in citrate-saline using a volume slightly under the original plasma volume (marked on the container). Centrifuge at 800 *g* for 5 min to remove platelet clumps, white cells and red cells.

Remove the platelet-rich supernatant carefully. Perform a platelet count and dilute the platelet-rich suspension with citrate-saline until the platelet count is about 200×10^9/l.

Leave the platelets at room temperature for 30–45 min to allow the platelets to recover from the trauma of washing and centrifugation.

Reagents for assay
Citrate-saline.

Ristocetin. 100 mg/ml. Stored frozen in 1 ml volumes.

Plasma standard.

Platelet-poor plasma. From the patient(s).

Assay method

Confirm that the washed platelets do not 'agglutinate' with ristocetin in the absence of added plasma. Deliver 0.5 ml of citrate-saline into an aggregometer cuvette and 0.4 ml of the platelet suspension + 0.1 ml of citrate-saline into another cuvette. Place in the warming block and leave for 3 min to warm. Add 5 µl of ristocetin and record at 1 cm/min for 2 min. The absorbance owing to citrate-saline alone is taken to represent 100% agglutination, and that owing to platelets alone represents zero (%) agglutination (blank). The absorbance owing to the platelet suspension must not exceed five divisions on the chart paper. If it is greater, the platelets must be washed again and the procedure repeated. The reading of this blank must be repeated every hour.

All plasma samples and ristocetin should be kept in an ice-bath.

Standard curve

A standard curve is obtained by making doubling dilutions, 1 in 2 to 1 in 32 in citrate-saline, of the standard plasma (donor pool, commercial reference plasma or other reference materials). The absorbance owing to a mixture of 0.4 ml of citrate-saline and 0.1 ml of plasma dilution is taken to represent 100% agglutination and that owing to the mixture of 0.4 ml of platelet suspension and 0.1 ml of plasma dilution zero (0%) agglutination.

Add 5 µl of ristocetin to the cuvette containing the mixture giving zero agglutination and record the agglutination for 2 min. Test each dilution of the standard plasma in a similar way.

The patient's plasma is tested at two dilutions, depending on the expected concentration of vWF in the plasma. Both dilutions should give agglutination within the range of that of the standard curve.

Reset 100% and zero aggregation for each patient.

A reading of the platelet blank should be repeated at hourly intervals. If the reading differs from the original, the difference must be subtracted from the results of subsequent tests.

Results

Measure 'agglutination' at 1 or 2 min depending on the strength of 'agglutination'. All responses must be compared on the same time scale and not read at maximum 'agglutination'.

Plot the standard curve on semi-log paper with 'agglutination' on the linear scale and the concentration of vWF in u/dl on the log scale (Fig. 16.4). For assay purposes, assign the 1 in 2 dilution of standard plasma a value of 0.50 iu/ml. (Each batch of standard is precalibrated and may not necessarily be 1.0 iu/ml.)

Read the patient's vWF concentration directly off the standard curve, correct for the dilution factor and average the two results from the different dilutions.

Normal range

0.5–2.0 iu/ml.

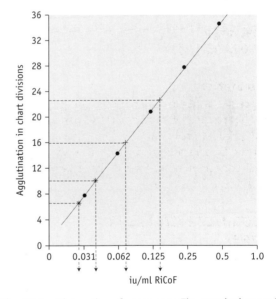

Fig. 16.4 Ristocetin cofactor assay. The standard curve is plotted on semi-log paper. Each test plasma is assayed in two dilutions. Plasma 1 (+) produced the following readings: 1 in 4 dilution: 16 divisions of the chart paper = 7 u (× 4 (dilution factor) = 0.28 iu/ml); 1 in 2 dilutions: 22 divisions = (0.013 iu/ml (× 2 dilution factor) = 0.026 iu/ml. The mean of the two readings is 0.27 iu/ml. Plasma 2 (*) gave the following results. 1 in 2 dilution: 7 divisions = 0.025 iu/ml (× 2 dilution factor) = 0.05 iu/ml). 1 in 4 dilutions: 5 divisions (not shown). This result was similar to the blank and the plasma was next tested undiluted, giving a reading of 10 divisions = 0.04 iu/ml. The mean is 0.045 iu/ml (very low).

Interpretation

The vWF concentration measured by RiCoF assay can only be interpreted in conjunction with other factor VIII:C and vWF:Ag assays, as shown in Table 16.9.

ASSAY USING FORMALIN-FIXED PLATELETS
Reagents

Sodium citrate solution.   32 g/l trisodium sodium citrate ($Na_3C_6H_5O.2H_2O$).

K_2EDTA.   0.134 mol/l.

2% formalin (40% formaldehyde).   In 9 g/l NaCl.

0.05% sodium azide.   In 9 g/l NaCl.

Method

Suitable preparations can be obtained from citrated blood in a blood donation bag, from a normal individual or from a therapeutic venesection carried out on a patient with a normal platelet count. ACD or CPD solution from the donor bag is ejected through the taking needle and replaced by the equivalent volume of sodium citrate. Collect *c* 500 ml of blood.

Centrifuge the blood at 300 *g* for 15 min at room temperature. Separate the platelet-rich plasma (PRP) and add 9 volumes of PRP to 1 volume of EDTA solution. Incubate for 1 h at 37°C to reverse the effect of ADP released during the preparation. Add an equal volume of 2% formalin and leave at 4°C for 1 h. Centrifuge at 200 *g* for 10 min at 4°C. Decant the supernatant and recentrifuge it at 250 *g* for 20 min at 4°C. Discard the supernatant and resuspend the platelet sediment in chilled (4°C) 9 g/l NaCl. Wash the platelets twice more. After the final wash, resuspend the platelets in the sodium azide solution. Adjust the platelet count to $300–500 \times 10^9$/l. The suspension is stable for 1 month at 4°C.

Commercial fixed platelets are also available.

Reagents for assay

Buffer for plasma dilutions.   Barbitone buffer, pH 7.4, containing 40 mg/ml of bovine serum albumin (p. 605).

Ristocetin, plasma standard and patient's platelet-poor plasma.   As described in the previous assay.

Assay method

Follow the method described for washed fresh platelets. Prepare all plasma dilutions in the albumin-containing buffer.

Results, interpretation and normal range

As described for the washed platelet assay.

MULTIMERIC ANALYSIS OF VON WILLEBRAND FACTOR ANTIGEN IN PLASMA SAMPLES[44]
Principle

Plasma samples are diluted in a buffer containing 8 mol/l urea and sodium dodecylsulphate (SDS) to ensure mobility of protein is related to size and not molecular charge. Samples are electrophoresed through an agarose stacking gel at pH 6.8, and then through a running gel of higher agarose concentration at pH 8.8. After running overnight on a cooling platen, the protein is fixed in the gel, washed, and incubated with radiolabelled antibody to vWF followed by extensive washing. An X-ray film is exposed to the dried gel and an autoradiograph produced.

The technique described here uses an agarose gel in a discontinuous buffer system. The method appears less prone to technical problems than an acrylamide/agarose system, and yet can distinguish clearly the known patterns of vWD subtypes.

Reagents

Rabbit anti-human vWF:Ag.   DAKO Limited.

[125]Iodine.   Amersham International.

Chloramine T.

Sodium metabisulphite.

PD-10 Sephadex G-25 M Columns.   Pharmacia.

Bovine serum albumin or Infant powdered milk feed.

Bio-Rad DNA grade ultrapure agarose.

Sodium dodecyl sulphate (SDS).

Glycine.

Sodium EDTA.

Hydrochloric acid.

Propan-2-ol.

Acetic acid.

Trizma base. Sigma.

Bromophenol blue.

Bovine IgG fraction.

Rabbit plasma.

Deionized water.

Sodium phosphate.

Preparation of ^{125}I labelled antibody

Mix 50 μl of antiserum with c 2 mCi (20 μl) ^{125}I. Add 10 μl of freshly prepared chloramine T (50 mg in 10 ml 0.5 mol/l sodium phosphate buffer) and mix for exactly 30 s. Add 100 μl sodium metabisulphite (12 mg in 10 ml sodium phosphate buffer). Pass the mixture down a Sephadex column. The column is equilibrated in phosphate buffered saline and the eluant is phosphate buffered saline containing 1% bovine serum albumin. Collect a total of ten 1 ml fractions; the radioactive-labelled antibody will appear in the third and fourth fraction, the remaining fractions contain free iodine and are discarded. Pool the fractions containing the radioactive-labelled antibody. Dispose of the column containing free iodine. Aliquot the labelled antibody and store in working aliquots (approximately 10 aliquots of 0.2 ml) at –40°C for up to a maximum of 3 months. Usual precautions should be observed for working with radioactive material.

Each gel will require 100 ml of 1.2×10^6 cpm/ml activity.

Stock solutions

2 mol/l Tris.

3 mol/l HCl.

0.01 mol/l Na$_2$ EDTA.

The above three reagents may be stored at 4°C for up to 3 months.

Preparation of buffers and reagents

Stacking buffer

12.5 ml–2 mol/l Tris.

7.9 ml–3 mol/l HCl.

Make up to 50 ml with water; check pH is 6.8.

May be stored at 4°C for up to 2 weeks.

Running buffer

37.5 ml 2 mol/l Tris.

4.45 ml 3 mol/l HCl.

Make up to 50 ml with water; check pH is 8.8.

May be stored at 4°C for up to 2 weeks.

Sample buffer stock

0.5 ml 2 mol/l Tris.

10 ml stock EDTA.

Make up to 100 ml with water.

May be stored at 4°C for up to 4 weeks.

For use

9.61 g urea.

0.4 g SDS.

Dissolve in sample buffer and make up to 20 ml. May need warming to dissolve. Carefully adjust the pH to 8.0 with 1 mol/l HCl – use within 1 day of preparation.

10% SDS. 1 g SDS dissolved in deionized water to a final volume of 10 ml. Store at 4°C to prevent bacterial growth; warm to room temperature just before use. Discard after 4 weeks of storage.

Electrophoresis buffer

57.6 g glycine.

12.0 g Tris base.

2.0 g SDS.

Dissolve and make up to 2 litres with water; make up fresh on day of use.

Fixative

100 ml propan-2-ol.

40 ml acetic acid

Make up to 400 ml with water.

Washing solutions

Prepare 9 g/l and 30 g/l NaCl solutions from a stock solution of 180 g/l NaCl.

Preparation of gels

Running gel (1.6% agarose, 0.1% SDS)

0.8 g agarose.

12.5 ml running buffer.

37.0 ml water.

0.5 ml 10% SDS.

Dissolve the agarose by boiling; it is essential that the agarose is completely dissolved. Add the SDS to the molten agarose last to prevent frothing. Loss of water must be kept to a minimum to maintain the correct agarose concentration. The hydrophilic side of standard gel bond is stuck to a clean glass slide (110 × 205 mm) by a few drops of water. The gel is cast between the hydrophobic side and a clean glass plate separated by a 1-mm spacer. Bulldog clips are used to clamp the mould together. The mould is warmed at 37°C prior to the addition of molten agarose. The running gel is carefully poured and then allowed to set at 4°C.

Stacking gel (0.8% agarose, 0.1% SDS)
0.16 g agarose
5.0 ml stacking buffer.
14.8 ml water.
0.2 ml 10% SDS.

Carefully disassemble the running gel mould and remove the top 1.5 cm of gel using a clean scalpel. After re-assembly, pour the stacking gel to fill the mould. Allow the gel to set at 4°C for several hours.

Preparation of samples
Plasma samples are diluted in the sample buffer:
50 µl sample.
700 µl sample buffer.
15 µl 1% bromophenol blue dye.

Electrophoresis
Set the cooling system at 8°C to achieve a gel temperature of 13°C. Wicks are prepared from J-cloths and Whatman No. 1 24-cm filter papers, cut to the length of the agarose gel. 500 ml of electrophoresis buffer is placed in each reservoir of the electrophoresis tank. The mould is carefully disassembled and the gel-bond removed, leaving the gel on the glass plate. Using a template, 8 or 10 wells (10 × 2 mm) are cut into the stacking gel 8 mm from the running/stacking gel interface. The gel is placed on the cooling platen. Two filter paper wicks are soaked in electrophoresis buffer and positioned over the gel by 5 mm at either end. Two J-cloth* wicks are soaked in electrophoresis buffer; one is placed completely over the paper wick at the running gel end; the other is placed over the paper wick at the stacking gel end leaving a small portion of the paper wick visible.

   0.02 ml (20 µl) of diluted sample are pipetted into each well taking care not to touch the wick. The gel is electrophoresed at a constant current of 5 mA (approx. 65 V). When the blue dye has migrated 1 cm from each well, the electrophoresis is stopped. Residual liquid is carefully removed from

* Johnson and Johnson.

each well, and each well refilled with molten stacking gel. Electrophoresis is restarted at the same current. After a total of 18–20 h, the dye will have run off the gel into the wick and electrophoresis is complete. The gel is gently removed from the glass plate and fixed for 1 h in a suitable container. Once fixed, the gel is washed for 3 h in several changes of distilled water. The gel is transferred to a small plastic tray and washed successively with 100 ml 1% bovine IgG (in phosphate buffered saline), phosphate buffered saline and 10% rabbit plasma (in phosphate buffered saline), each wash being for about 20 min. Alternatively, wash successively in 1% and 10% solutions of baby milk powder in phosphate buffered saline. The gel is then washed in phosphate buffered saline for 3 hours. An aliquot of iodinated anti-vWF antibody is thawed and added to 100 ml phosphate buffered saline (100 ml of 1.2×10^6 cpm/ml activity). This is then added to the gel in the tray and mixed overnight behind a lead shield. The labelled antibody solution is carefully removed and poured to waste down a designated radioactive sink. The gel is then washed for 24 hours in 3% saline changing the solution 5–10 times. The next day, the gel is washed three times for 1 h in 9 g/l NaCl followed by distilled water for 4 h. The gel is mounted on the hydrophilic side of the gel bond and dried rapidly in a hot air oven. Alternatively, the gel can be dried in a 37°C oven overnight. The dried gel is placed against a Kodak X Omat X-ray film in between intensifying screens in a cassette. The cassette is kept at –70°C overnight, warmed for 30 min, and then developed.

Interpretation[41]
See Figure 16.5.

INVESTIGATION OF A SUSPECTED DISORDER OF PLATELET FUNCTION, INHERITED OR ACQUIRED

(For assays of vWD, see p. 372; for diagnosis of thrombocytopenia, see p. 39 and 596.)

   Abnormalities of platelet function all lead to signs and symptoms characteristic of defects of primary haemostasis: bleeding into the mucous membranes, epistaxes, menorrhagia and small skin ecchymoses. The patient may also suffer from abnormal intra- or postoperative bleeding and oozing from small cuts or wounds.

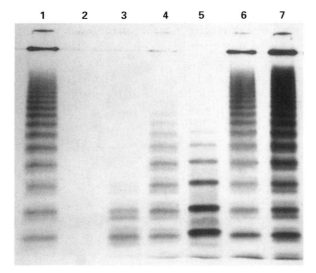

Fig. 16.5 Autoradiograph of the electrophoretic analysis of vWF multimer patterns. The largest multimers appear at the top of the gel. The normal pattern with numerous large multimers and a triplet pattern visible in the smaller multimers are shown in lane 7. Lanes 1 and 6 are compatible with Type 1 vWD in which there is a generalized decrease in multimer numbers but retaining the normal triplet pattern. In lane 2, there is virtually no vWF detected indicating Type 3 vWD. Lanes 3 and 5 show both abnormality of vWF amount and multimer pattern, indicating Type 2A. In lane 4, there is a selective loss of the large multimers typical of type 2B vWD.

LABORATORY INVESTIGATION OF PLATELETS AND PLATELET FUNCTION[45]

The peripheral blood platelet count and the skin bleeding time or PFA-100 are the first-line tests of platelet function. If the results of these tests are within the normal limits, it is unlikely that a clinically important platelet defect is responsible for the bleeding tendency. Additional information may be obtained by inspecting a fresh blood film which may show abnormalities of platelet size or morphology which may be of diagnostic importance.

If the screening procedures suggest a disorder of primary haemostasis and vWF function is normal, further tests should be organized. Drugs and certain foods (Table 16.10) may affect platelet function tests, and the patient must be asked to refrain from taking such substances for at least 7 days before the test.

The usual sequence of investigation is shown in Figure 16.6. Platelet function tests can be divided

Table 16.10 Substances which commonly affect platelet function

Agents which affect prostanoid synthesis
Aspirin
Non-steroidal anti-inflammatory drugs
Corticosteroids
Agents which bind to platelet receptors and membranes
α-antagonists
β-blockers
Antihistamines
Tricyclic antidepressants
Local anaesthetics
Ticlopidine
Clopidogrel
IIb, IIIa blocking agents
Antibiotics
Penicillin
Cephalosporins
Agents which increase cyclic adenosine monophosphate (c-AMP) levels
Dipyridamole
Aminophylline
Prostanoids
Others
Heparin
Dextran
Ethanol
Clofibrate
Phenothiazine
Garlic

into six main groups (Table 16.11): adhesion tests, aggregation tests, assessment of the granular content and the release reaction, investigation of the prostaglandin pathways and tests of platelet coagulant activity and flow cytometry.

The *granular content* of the platelets can be assessed by electron microscopy or by measuring the substances released (Table 16.11). Adenine nucleotide and serotonin release from the dense granules are probably best measured by a specialist laboratory. The release of β-thromboglobulin and platelet factor 4 can be measured using commercial radio-immunoassay kits, but there are problems with reproducibility and interpretation of the results. The release from the α granules is mostly investigated as a marker of in-vivo platelet activation and thrombotic tendency. Platelet vWF is measured to diagnose some variants of vWD.

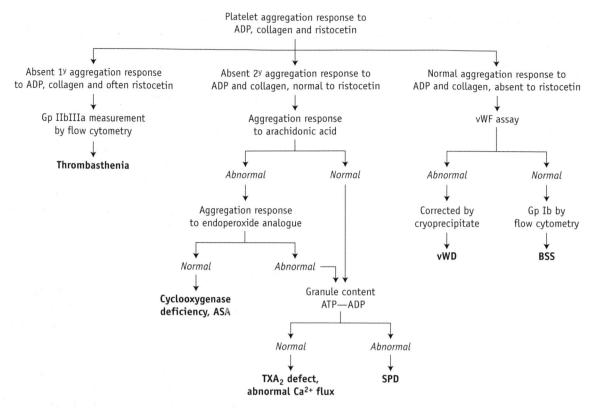

Fig. 16.6 Flowchart for investigation of suspected platelet dysfunction. Gp, glycoprotein; SPD, storage pool defect; vWD, von Willebrand's disease; BSS, Bernard–Soulier syndrome; ASA, effect of aspirin ingestion.

If the initial aggregation studies suggest a defect in the prostaglandin pathways, TXB_2 can be estimated quantitatively by radio-immune assay. Highly specific assays of various steps in arachidonic acid metabolism are also available but are outside the scope of a routine laboratory.

Platelet coagulant activity – the completion of the membrane 'flip-flop' – can be indirectly measured using the prothrombin consumption index. This test is rarely performed now, but is abnormal in Scott syndrome, a rare bleeding disorder; it was described in the 7th edition of this book.

PLATELET AGGREGATION

Principle

The light absorbance of platelet-rich plasma falls as platelets aggregate. The amount and the rate of fall are dependent on platelet reactivity to the added agonist provided that other variables, such as temperature, platelet count and mixing speed, are controlled. The absorbance changes are monitored on a chart recorder.

Reagents

Test and control platelet-rich plasma. The patient and control subject should be off all drugs, beverages and foods which may affect aggregation for at least 10 days (see Table 16.10) and preferably should have fasted overnight as the presence of chylomicra may also disturb the aggregation patterns. 20 ml of venous blood are collected with minimal venous occlusion and added to a one-tenth volume of trisodium citrate (see p. 604) contained in a plastic or siliconized container. The blood should not be chilled because cold activates the platelets. PRP is obtained by centrifuging at room temperature (*c* 20°C) for 10–15 min at 150–200 *g*. The PRP is carefully removed, avoiding contamination with red cells or buffy coat, and placed in a stoppered plastic tube. PRP should be stored at room temperature until tested and is stable for about 3 h. It is impor-

Table 16.11 Platelet function tests

Adhesion tests
Retention in a glass-bead column
Baumgartner's technique
PFA-100

Aggregation tests
Turbidometric technique using
   ADP
   Collagen
   Ristocetin
   Adrenaline
   Thrombin
   Arachidonic acid
   Endoperoxide analogues
   Calcium ionophore

Investigation of granular content and release
Dense bodies
   Electron microscopy
   ADP and ATP content (bioluminescence)
   Serotonin release
Granules
   β-Thromboglobulin
   Platelet factor 4
   vWF
   Fluorescence by flow cytometry

Prostaglandin pathways
TXB$_2$ radio-immunoassay

Platelet coagulant activity
Prothrombin consumption index

Flow cytometry
Glycoprotein surface expression
Activation
   P-selectin (CD62) surface expression
   Fibrinogen binding
   Annexin binding (to phosphatidyl serine)
   Conformational changes in IIbIIIa
Platelet granule fluorescence

ADP, adenosine 5'-phosphatase; ATP, adenosine 5'-triphosphatase; vWF, non Willebrand factor.

tant to test all samples after a similar interval of time (say 1 h) and to store them at the same temperature in order to minimize variation.

Test and control platelet-poor plasma. The remaining blood is centrifuged at $2000\,g$ for 20 min to obtain PPP.

Standardization of platelet-rich plasma. A platelet count is performed on the PRP. The number of platelets will influence aggregation response if the count falls outside $200-400 \times 10^9/l$. For very high PRP counts, the count should be adjusted by diluting the PRP in the patient's PPP. Platelet counts below $200 \times 10^9/l$ give rise to diminished aggregation responses. Further centrifugation of PRP is not recommended because it induces platelet activation. The control PRP should be diluted to the same count and tested as a comparison.

PRP should always be stored in tightly stoppered tubes which are filled nearly to the top, to avoid changes in pH which also affect platelet aggregation and tests of nucleotide release.

Aggregating agents
The five aggregating agents listed below should be sufficient for the diagnosis of most functional disorders. For research purposes and when investigating unusual kindreds, other agonists listed in Table 16.11 may also be used.

Adenosine 5'-diphosphate. The anhydrous sodium salt of adenosine 5'-diphosphate (ADP) is used. A stock solution is prepared by dissolving 4.93 mg of the trisodium salt or 4.71 mg of the disodium salt in 10 ml of 9 g/l NaCl, pH 6.8. This makes a 1 mmol/l solution. It is stored in 0.5-ml volumes at –40°C until use and remains stable for up to 3 months at this temperature. Once thawed, the solution must be used within 3 h and then discarded. For aggregation testing, prepare 100, 50, 25, 10 and 5 μmol/l solutions.

Collagen 1 mg/ml (Mascia Brunelli, Sigma, Helena). This is a 1 mg/ml stock solution. For use, it is diluted in the buffer supplied with the collagen or in 5% dextrose to obtain concentrations of 10 and 40 μg/l. When diluted 1:10 in PRP (see below), the final concentrations will be 1 and 4 μg/ml.

Ristocetin sulphate (American Biochemical & Pharmaceutical Corporation, ABP). Each vial contains 100 mg of ristocetin and should be stored at 4°C until dissolved; 8 ml of 9 g/l NaCl are added to each vial so as to obtain a 12.5 mg/ml solution. This is stored at –40°C in 0.5-ml volumes until used. Ristocetin may be refrozen after use. It should never be used in concentrations greater than 1.4 mg/ml as protein precipitation may occur in plasma and give rise to false results.

Arachidonic acid. Na-salt, 99% pure. The contents of a 10-mg vial are dissolved in 1.5 ml of sterile water by gentle mixing to give a 20 mmol/l stock solution. This may be frozen in 0.5-ml volumes at –20°C for later use. A working solution is prepared by making doubling dilutions of the stock in saline to give 5- and 10-mmol/l solutions.

Adrenaline. 1-Epinephrine bitartarate. 3.33 mg are dissolved in 10 ml of water to prepare a 1 mmol/l stock solution. It is stored in 0.5-ml volumes at –40°C. 20- and 200-μmol/l solutions are prepared for use in barbitone buffered saline, pH 7.4.

Note. All aggregation reagents should be kept on ice until used.

Method

Centrifugation may cause cellular release of ADP and platelet refractoriness to aggregation, and the actual aggregation test should not be started before 30 min after preparing the PRP. However, the tests should be completed within 3 h and whenever possible within 2 h of preparing the PRP. Platelets left standing at room temperature (*c* 20°C) become increasingly reactive to adrenaline and in some cases to collagen; the rate of change increases after 3 h.

Switch the aggregometer on about 30 min before the tests are to be performed to allow the heating block to warm up to 37°C. Set the stirring speed to 900 rpm. Pipette the appropriate volume of PRP (this varies depending on the make of the aggregometer used) into a plastic tube or cuvette. Place the tube in the heating block. After 1 min, insert the stirrer into the plasma. Set the transmission to 0 on the chart recorder. Replace with a cuvette containing PPP and set the transmission to 100%. Repeat this procedure until no further adjustments are needed and the pen traverses most of the width of the chart paper in response to the difference in absorbance between the PRP and PPP.

Allow the PRP to warm up to 37°C for 2 min and then add 1:10 vol of the agonist. Record the change in absorbance until the response reaches a plateau or for 3 min (whichever is sooner). Repeat this procedure for each agonist. The starting amount for each agonist is the lowest concentration prepared as described above (see Fig. 16.7). If no release is obtained, increase the concentration until a satisfactory response is obtained.

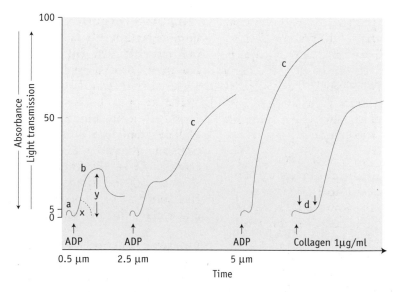

Fig. 16.7 Traces obtained during the aggregation of platelet-rich plasma. (a) Shape change. (b) Primary wave aggregation. (c) Secondary wave aggregation. x°, angle of the initial aggregation slope; y, height of the aggregation trace; d, lag phase; μm = μmol/l.
(Reproduced with the permission of the authors and the publisher from Yardumian DA, Mackie IJ, Machin SJ. 1986 Laboratory investigation of platelet functions: a review of methodology. Journal of Clinical Pathology 39:701.)

Interpretation

Normal platelet aggregation curves are shown in Figure 16.7.

ADP. Low concentrations of ADP (<0.5 to 2.5 µmol/l) cause primary or reversible aggregation. First, ADP binds to a membrane receptor and releases Ca^{2+} ions. A reversible complex with extracellular fibrinogen forms and the platelets undergo a shape change reflected by a slight increase in absorbance. After this, the bound fibrinogen adds to the cell-to-cell contact and reversible aggregation occurs. At very low concentrations of ADP, platelets may disaggregate after the first phase. In the presence of higher concentrations of ADP, an irreversible secondary wave aggregation is associated with the release of dense and α-granules owing to activation of the arachidonic acid pathway. If only high doses of ADP are used, defects in the primary wave (measuring the second pathway as described on p. 342) will be missed.

Collagen. The aggregation response to collagen is preceded by a short 'lag' phase lasting between 10 and 60 s. The duration of the lag phase is inversely proportional to the concentration of collagen used and to the responsiveness of the platelets tested. This phase is succeeded by a single wave of aggregation owing to the activation of the arachidonic acid pathway and the release of the granules. Higher doses of collagen (>2 µg/ml) cause a sudden increase in intraplatelet calcium concentration and this may bring about the release reaction without activating the prostaglandin pathway. Collagen responses should therefore always be measured using 1 and 4 µg/ml concentrations.

Ristocetin. Ristocetin reacts with vWF and the membrane receptors to induce platelets to clump together ('agglutination'). It does not activate any of the three aggregation pathways and does not initially cause granule release. The response is assessed on the basis of the angle of the initial slope. The platelet response to 1.2 mg/ml is initially studied. Concentrations above 1.4 mg/ml may cause nonspecific platelet 'agglutination' owing to an interaction between ristocetin and fibrinogen and protein precipitation.

Arachidonic acid. Arachidonic acid induces TXA_2 generation and granule release even if there is a defect of agonist binding to the surface membrane or of the phospholipase-induced release of endogenous arachidonate. If steps further along the pathway are impaired, such as absence or inhibition of cyclo-oxygenase (e.g. aspirin effect), arachidonic acid will not produce normal aggregation.

Adrenaline. No shape change precedes aggregation, but the response thereafter resembles the ADP response. Such a response is usually obtained with concentrations of 2–10 µmol/ml. Some clinically normal people have severely reduced responses to adrenaline.

Calculation of results[45,46]

Results can be expressed in one of three ways:

1. As a percentage fall in absorbance measured at 3 min after the addition of an agonist (see Fig. 16.7; y). This does not provide any information on the shape of the curve.
2. By the initial slope of the aggregation tracing (see Fig. 16.7; x°). This indicates the rate of aggregation but does not show whether or not secondary aggregation has occurred.
3. By the minimum amount of agonist required to induce a secondary response.

Normal range

The platelets of normal subjects usually produce a single reversible primary wave with 1 µmol/l ADP or less, biphasic aggregation with ADP at 2.5 µmol/l, and a single irreversible wave at 5 or 10 µmol/l. A single phase response is observed after a lag phase lasting not more than 1 min with 1 and 4 µg/ml of collagen. A single phase or biphasic response is seen with 1.2 mg/ml of ristocetin and after 50 and 100 µmol/l of arachidonic acid. Biphasic aggregation is observed with 2–10 µmol/l of adrenaline. A response to a low concentration of ristocetin (0.5 mg/ml) is abnormal and is a feature of type 2 B vWD (see above).

Interpretation and technical artifacts

The volumes of PRP used will depend on the aggregometer and cuvettes used. The smaller the cuvette, the more responses can be tested with a given volume of PRP, but the poorer the optical quality (because of a shorter lightpath), and the more likely the influence of factors such as debris or air bubbles.

Care should be taken to exclude red cells and granulocytes from PRP as these will interfere with the light transmittance and cause reduced response heights which can be mistaken for abnormal aggregation. In diseases such as thalassaemia, where there may be red cell fragments and membranes, these may be removed by further centrifugation of PRP at 150 **g** for 2 min, or after settling has occurred.

If cryoglobulins are present, they may cause changes in transmittance like spontaneous aggregation. Warming the PRP to 37°C for 5 min allows aggregation to be performed in the normal way.

Lipaemic plasma may cause problems in adjusting the aggregometer and the responses may be compressed owing to the small difference in transmitted light between PRP and PPP. Care should be taken in the interpretation of results from such samples.

The pattern of responses in various disorders of platelet function is shown in Table 16.12. For a discussion of hyperaggregability, see page 408.

Some common technical problems associated with platelet aggregation are described in Table 16.13.

FURTHER INVESTIGATION OF PLATELET FUNCTION

If an abnormal aggregation pattern is observed, it is advisable to check the assessment on at least one further occasion. If the aggregation tests are persistently abnormal, and the patient is not taking any drugs or substances known to interfere with platelet function, the following tests should be done (see also Fig. 16.6 and Table 16.12):

1. If thrombasthenia or the Bernard–Soulier syndrome is suspected, an analysis of membrane glycoproteins is necessary, most conveniently by flow cytometry.
2. If a release abnormality is suspected, additional agonists including synthetic endoperoxide analogues and calcium ionophores should be used in testing for aggregation. In addition, the total adenine nucleotide content of the platelets and the amount released after maximal stimulation should be measured using a firefly bioluminescence technique.[45,47]
3. Whenever possible, electron microscopic studies of platelet ultrastructure should be carried out.

Table 16.12 Differential diagnosis of disorders of platelet function

Condition	Platelet		Aggregation with:					Comment/further tests
	Count	Size	ADP	Col	Ri	AA	A23187	
Thrombasthenia	N	N	0	0	1	0	0	IIbIIIa expression
Bernard–Soulier syndrome	Low	Large	N	N	0	N	N	GpIb expression
Storage pool defect (δ)	N	N	1	R	1	1/0	R	ATP:ADP pools
Cyclo-oxygenase deficiency	N	N	1/N	R	N	R	R	Responds to endoperoxide
Thromboxane synthetase deficiency	N	N	1/N	R	N	R/0	N	
Aspirin ingestion	N	N	1	R	N	R/0	N/R	Stop aspirin/ NSAID and retest
Ehlers–Danlos syndrome	N	N	N	N	N	N	N	
von Willebrand disease	N	N	N	N	0/R	N	N	Assay vWF:Ag and RiCoF

N, normal; 0, absent; 1, primary wave only; R, reduced; Col, collagen; Ri, ristocetin; AA, arachidonic acid; A23187, calcium ionophore; ATP, adenosine 5′-triphosphatase; ADP, adenosine 5′-diphosphatase; NSAID, non-steroidal anti-inflammatory drug; RiCoF, ristocetin co-factor; vWF, von Willebrand factor.
Note that many other defects, such as found in oculocutaneous albinism, Chediak–Higashi syndrome and grey platelet syndrome, have also been described.

Table 16.13 Technical factors which may influence platelet aggregation tests

Centrifugation. At room temperature, *not* at 4°C. Should be sufficient to remove red cells and white cells but not the largest platelets. Residual red cells in the PRP may cause apparently incomplete aggregation.
Time. For 30 min after the preparation of PRP, platelets are refractory to the effect of agonists. Progressive increase in reactiveness occurs thereafter; more marked from 2 h onward.
Platelet count. Slow and weak aggregation observed with platelet counts below 150 or over 400 × 10⁹/l.
pH. <7.7 inhibits aggregation; pH >8.0 enhances aggregation.
Mixing speed. <800 rpm or >1200 rpm slows aggregation.
Haematocrit. >0.55 is associated with less aggregation, especially in the secondary phase owing to the increased concentration of citrate in PRP. It may also be difficult to obtain enough PPP. Centrifuging twice may help.
Temperature. <35°C causes decreased aggregation except to low dose ADP which may be enhanced.
Dirty cuvette. May cause spontaneous platelet aggregation or interfere with the optics of the system.
Air bubbles in the cuvette. Cause large irregular oscillations even before the addition of agonists.
No stir bar. No response to any agonist obtained.

PPP, platelet-poor plasma; PRP, platelet-rich plasma.

4. Factor VIII:C, vWF:Ag and RiCoF assays should be carried out on all patients investigated for an abnormality of platelet function who show abnormal ristocetin 'agglutination', or in whom all platelet function tests are normal.

5. Plasma assays of β-thromboglobulin and platelet factor 4 are described in Chapter 18 (p. 408) as tests of hypercoagulability. They are also used to detect α-granule deficiency states, such as the grey platelet syndrome.

CLOT SOLUBILITY TEST FOR FACTOR XIII

Principle
Fibrin clots formed in the presence of factor XIII and thrombin are stable (owing to cross-linking) for at least 1 h in 5 mol/l urea, whereas clots formed in the absence of factor XIII dissolve rapidly. Quality assurance surveys in the UK have shown that the solubility test for factor XIII is more sensitive when the sample is clotted with thrombin rather than calcium.

Reagents

Platelet-poor plasma. From the patient and a control subject.

Thrombin 10 NIH unit solution.

Urea. 5 mol/l in 9 g/l NaCl.

Method
In duplicate, 0.2 ml patient plasma is mixed with 0.2 ml 10 NIH thrombin solution in a glass test-tube and incubated at 37°C for 20 min. Set up a normal plasma control in the same way; EDTA plasma can be included as a negative control. Each tube is filled with approximately 3 ml of urea solution, carefully dislodging the clot, and left undisturbed at 37°C for 24 h. Inspect each tube for the presence of a clot at regular intervals.

Interpretation
The control clot, if normal, shows no sign of dissolving after 24 h. However, in the absence of factor XIII, the clot will have dissolved. The test is reported as normal if the clot is present and abnormal if the clot is absent. The clot solubility test has

poor sensitivity and may only detect levels below approximately 0.01 u/ml. However, since the level of activity required for adequate haemostasis is low, the technique is suitable in most cases. In suspected cases, the factor XIII subunits can be determined by immunoelectrophoresis with commercial antisera. Kits are now available for direct assays of factor XIII antigen.

DISSEMINATED INTRAVASCULAR COAGULATION

The term DIC encompasses a wide range of clinical phenomena of varying degrees of severity. It is also sometimes referred to as consumptive coagulopathy because its characteristic feature is excessive and widespread activation of the coagulation mechanism with consequent consumption of clotting factors and inhibitors with loss of the normal regulatory mechanisms. In acutely ill patients, this typically results in defibrination and a haemorrhagic diathesis. In some situations, however, the activation may be less marked and partially compensated resulting in a tendency to thrombosis. This latter phenomenon is typical of the coagulation activation seen in association with malignancy and may be associated with slightly shortened clotting times.

The diagnosis of acute DIC can generally be made from the basic first-line screening tests described above. Characteristically, the PT, APTT and TT are all prolonged and the fibrinogen level is markedly reduced. In association with the consumption of clotting factors responsible for these abnormalities, there is also a fall in platelet count also owing to consumption.

Concomitantly, there is activation of the fibrinolytic system and an increase in circulating fibrin(ogen) degradation products. These abnormalities form the basis for the diagnosis of DIC. More elaborate tests are not usually performed but can demonstrate reductions in individual clotting factors, ATIII and antiplasmin and increased levels of thrombin–antithrombin and plasmin–antiplasmin complexes and of activation peptides such as prothrombin F1+2. some analyaers provide a profile of fibrin formation that can detect early stages of DIC.

DETECTION OF FIBRINOGEN/FIBRIN DEGRADATION PRODUCTS USING A LATEX AGGLUTINATION METHOD[48]

Principle
A suspension of latex particles is sensitized with specific antibodies to the purified FDP fragments D and E. The suspension is mixed on a glass slide with a dilution of the serum to be tested. Aggregation indicates the presence of FDP in the sample. By testing different dilutions of the unknown sample, a semi-quantitative assay can be performed.

Reagents

Venous blood. Collected into a special tube (provided with the kit) containing the anti-fibrinolytic agent and thrombin.

Thrombo-Wellcotest kit (Abbott Laboratories Ltd).

Positive and negative controls. Provided by the manufacturer.

Glycine buffer. Part of the kit.

Method
Allow the tube with blood to stand at 37°C until clot retraction commences. Then centrifuge the tube and withdraw the serum for testing. It is important that the fibrinogen in the sample is completely clotted or this will be detected by the test. This may be a problem in the presence of heparin or a dysfibrinogenaemia or high levels of FDPs. Addition of a few drops of 100 u (NIH)/ml thrombin will enhance clotting in these cases.

Make 1 in 5 and 1 in 20 dilutions of serum in glycine buffer. Mix one drop of each serum dilution with one drop of latex suspension on a glass slide. Rock the slide gently for 2 min while looking for macroscopic agglutination. If a positive reaction is observed in the higher dilution, make doubling dilutions from the 1 in 20 dilution until macroscopic agglutination can no longer be seen.

Interpretation
Agglutination with a 1 in 5 dilution of serum indicates a concentration of FDP in excess of 10 µg/ml; agglutination in a 1 in 20 dilution indicates FDP in excess of 40 µg/ml.

Normal range

Healthy subjects have an FDP concentration less than 10 µg/ml. Concentrations between 10 and 40 µg/ml are found in a variety of conditions including acute venous thromboembolism, acute myocardial infarction, severe pneumonia and after major surgery. High levels are seen in systemic fibrinolysis associated with DIC and thrombolytic therapy with streptokinase.

SCREENING TESTS FOR FIBRIN MONOMERS[49-51]

Principle

When thrombin acts on fibrinogen some of the monomers do not polymerize but give rise to soluble complexes with plasma fibrinogen and FDP. These complexes can be associated in vitro by ethanol or protamine sulphate.

Reagents

Platelet-poor plasma. From the patient and a control.

Positive control. This is prepared by adding 0.1 ml of thrombin (0.2 NIH units/ml) to 0.9 ml of control plasma and incubating at 37°C for 30 min. Fibrin threads formed during the incubation are removed by centrifugation.

Protamine sulphate. 1% (10 g/l).

Ethanol. 50% (v/v) in water.

Method

1. *Protamine sulphate test.* Add 0.05 ml of protamine sulphate to 0.5 ml of patient's plasma and to 0.5 ml of positive control plasma. Incubate undisturbed at 37°C for 30 min. A positive result is indicated by the formation of a fine fibrin network or fibrin strands. The presence of amorphous material only is a negative result.

2. *Ethanol gelation test.* Add 0.15 ml of ethanol to 0.5 ml of patient's plasma and to 0.5 ml of the positive control plasma at room temperature (c 20°C). After gentle agitation, inspect the tubes at 1-min intervals. A positive result is the formation of a definite gel within 3 min.

Interpretation

Positive gelation tests are found in:

1. The early stages of acute DIC.
2. After major surgery.
3. Severe inflammatory illness, in particular lobar pneumonia.
4. Liver disease.

DETECTION OF CROSS-LINKED FIBRIN D-DIMERS USING A LATEX AGGLUTINATION METHOD

Principle

This is identical to the test previously described for fibrinogen/fibrin degradation products, but in this case the latex beads are coated with a monoclonal antibody directed specifically against fibrin D-dimer in human plasma or serum. As there is no reaction with fibrinogen, the need for serum is eliminated and measurements can be performed on plasma samples.

Reagents

Several manufacturers market kits for the measurement of D-dimers. These usually contain the latex suspension, dilution buffer and positive and negative controls.

Method

The manufacturer's protocol should be followed. Undiluted plasma is mixed with one drop of latex suspension on a glass slide and the slide is gently rocked for the length of time recommended in the kit. If macroscopic agglutination is observed, dilutions of the plasma are made until agglutination can no longer be seen.

Interpretation

Agglutination with the undiluted plasma indicates a concentration of D-dimers in excess of 200 mg/l. The D-dimer level can be quantified by multiplying the reciprocal of the highest dilution showing a positive result by 200 to give a value in mg/l.

Normal range

Plasma levels in normal subjects are <200 mg/l. There has been much study of D-dimer assays as a useful way of excluding thrombosis but there is naturally a compromise between sensitivity and specificity, especially when a rapid turnaround time is required. The lack of an international standard and the poor correlation between kits means that the use of kits for this purpose should be validated individually. A number of kits using ELISA methods for the detection of D-dimers are now available which have greater sensitivity but are more cumbersome to perform. Latex test using automated analysers may provide an acceptable compromise.[52]

INVESTIGATION OF CARRIERS OF A CONGENITAL COAGULATION DEFICIENCY OR DEFECT[53,54]

Carrier detection is important in genetic counselling, and antenatal diagnosis may enable heterozygotes to consider abortion of a severely affected fetus as well as optimizing management of the pregnancy and delivery. The information of value in carrier detection is derived from family studies, phenotype investigations and the determination of genotype.

FAMILY STUDIES

Haemophilia A and B (factor VIII and factor IX deficiency) are inherited by X-linked genes. This means that all the sons of a haemophiliac will be normal and all his daughters carriers. The children of a carrier have 0.5 chance of being affected if they are sons, and 0.5 chance of being carriers if they are daughters. The other coagulation factor defects are inherited as autosomal traits. Heterozygotes possess approximately half the normal concentration of the coagulation factor and are generally not affected clinically; only homozygotes have a significant bleeding tendency. Factor XI is an exception to this where heterozygotes sometimes bleed excessively after trauma or surgery. The most common form of vWD (type 1) is inherited as an autosomal dominant.

A detailed family study is important in all coagulation factor defects in order to establish the true nature of the defect and its severity. Patients often describe any familial bleeding tendency as haemophilia, and it is therefore essential to prove the exact defect in every new patient and family. In inbred kindreds, the likelihood of homozygotes emerging is increased.

Phenotype investigation

Theoretically one might expect the concentration of the affected coagulation factor in the heterozygote or carrier to be roughly half that of normal. However, in the case of factor VIII and factor IX, this is complicated by the phenomenon of X chromosome inactivation (XCI). Women possess two X chromosomes but in each cell only one of these two is utilized and the other is largely inactivated. The choice of which X is active is essentially random and varies over a normal distribution. Thus, in carriers of haemophilia A or B, the level of factor VIII or IX also varies over roughly a normal distribution depending on the proportions of the normal and haemophiliac-containing Xs that are utilized. As a result, some carriers may have an entirely normal level of factor VIII or factor IX and others may be significantly deficient. This chromosome inactivation is sometimes referred to as Lyonization after Mary Lyon by whom it was first described.

In the case of factor VIII, the level of vWF has sometimes been found to be useful. The ratio of VIII:C to vWF:Ag is reduced in most carriers and can be used in conjunction with the family history to determine a probability that the subject is a carrier. These estimations are further complicated by the fact that factor VIII levels behave as an acute phase reactant and may be elevated by a number of intercurrent factors including pregnancy, stress and exercise.

When a detailed family study has been carried out, it may be possible to establish the statistical chance of inheriting a coagulation defect. For a review, see Graham et al.[53]

Genotype assignment

The advent of molecular biology and the cloning of many of the genes for coagulation factors, especially factor VIII and factor IX, have revolutionized the approach to carrier determination. The discovery of genetic polymorphisms, some of which are multi-allelic, within the coagulation factor genes has meant that in most families the affected gene can be tracked and the carrier state determined with a high degree of probability. Increasingly, and particularly for factor IX, the genetic defect itself can be identified resulting in unequivocal genotypic assignment in every member of a family. The techniques for these analyses are described in Chapter 21. Carrier determination and antenatal diagnosis has been dealt with in a comprehensive review.[54]

REFERENCES

1 Cines DB, Pollak ES, Buck CA, et al 1998 Endothelial cells in physiology and in the pathophysiology of vascular disorders. Blood 91:3527–3561.

2 May AE, Neumann FJ, Preissner KT 1999 The relevance of blood cell–vessel wall adhesive interactions for vascular thrombotic disease. Thrombosis and Haemostasis 82:962–970.

3 Ruggeri ZM 1997 Mechanisms initiating platelet thrombus formation Thrombosis and Haemostasis 78:611–616. [published erratum appears in Thrombosis and Haemostasis (1997) 78:1304].

4 Nurden AT 1999 Inherited abnormalities of platelets. Thrombosis and Haemostasis 82:468–480.

5 George J 2000 Platelets. Lancet 355:1531–1539.

6 Mann KG 1999 Biochemistry and physiology of blood coagulation. Thrombosis and Haemostasis 82:165–174.

7 Colman R, Schmaier A 1997 Contact system: a vascular biology modulator with anticoagulant, profibrinolytic, antiadhesive and proinflammatory attributes. Blood 90:3819–3843.

8 Mosesson MW 1998 Fibrinogen structure and fibrin clot assembly. Seminars in Thrombosis and Hemostasis 24:169–174.

9 Matsuda M, Sugo T, Yoshida N, et al 1999 Structure and function of fibrinogen: insights from dysfibrinogens. Thrombosis and Haemostasis 82:283–290.

10 van Boven HH, Lane DA 1997 Antithrombin and its inherited deficiency states. Seminars in Hematology 34:188–204.

11 Dahlback B 1997 Factor V and protein S as cofactors to activated protein C. Haematologica 82:91–95.

12 Collen D 1999 The plasminogen (fibrinolytic) system. Thrombosis and Haemostosis 82:259–270.

13 Hutton RA 1987 Chromogenic substrates in haemostasis. Blood Reviews 1:201–206.

14 Quick AJ 1973 Quick on Quick's test. New England Journal of Medicine 288:1079.

15 Miller GJ, Seghatchian MJ, Walter SJ, et al 1986 An association between the factor VII coagulant activity and thrombin activity induced by surfaced/cold exposure of normal human plasma. British Journal of Haematology 62:379–384.

16 Palareti G, Maccaferri M, Manotti C, et al 1991 Fibrinogen assays: a collaborative study of six different methods. C.I.S.M.E.L. Comitato Italiano per la Standardizzazione dei Metodi in Ematologia e Laboratorio. Clinical Chemistry 37:714–719.

17 Lawrie AS, McDonald SJ, Purdy G, et al. 1998 Prothrombin time derived fibrinogen determination on Sysmex CA-6000. Journal of Clinical Pathology 51:462–466.

18 De Cristofaro R, Landolfi R 1998 Measurement of plasma fibrinogen concentration by the prothrombin-time-derived method: applicability and limitations. Blood Coagulation and Fibrinolysis 9:251–259.

19 Clauss A 1957 Rapid physiological coagulation method in determination of fibrinogen. Acta Haematologica 17:237.

20 Jespersen J, Sidelmann J 1982 A study of the conditions and accuracy of the thrombin time assay of plasma fibrinogen. Acta Haematologica 67:2–7.

21 Funk C, Gmur J, Herold R, et al 1971 Reptilase-R – a new reagent in blood coagulation. British Journal of Haematology 21:43–52.

22 Williams KN, Davidson JM, Ingram GI 1975 A computer program for the analysis of parallel-line bioassays of clotting factors. British Journal of Haematology 31:13–23.

23 Kirkwood TB, Snape TJ 1980 Biometric principles in clotting and clot lysis assays. Clinical and Laboratory Haematology 2:155–167.

24 Koster T, Blann A, Briet E, et al. 1995 Role of clotting factor VIII in effect of von Willebrand factor on occurrence of deep vein thrombosis. Lancet 345:152–155.

25 Jorieux S, Tuley EA, Gaucher C, et al 1992 The mutation Arg (53) → Trp causes von Willebrand disease Normandy by abolishing binding to factor VIII. Studies with recombinant von Willebrand factor. Blood 79:563–567.

26 Pipe SW, Eickhorst AN, McKinley SH, et al 1999 Mild hemophilia A caused by increased rate of factor VIII A2 subunit dissociation: evidence for nonproteolytic inactivation of factor VIIIa in vivo. Blood 93:176–183.

27 Keeling DM, Sukhu K, Kemball Cook G, et al 1999 Diagnostic importance of the two-stage factor VIII:C assay demonstrated by a case of mild haemophilia associated with His 1954→ Leu substitution in the factor VIII A3 domain. British Jounal of Haematology 105:1123–1126.

28 White GC, Roberts HR 1996 The treatment of factor VIII inhibitors – a general overview. Vox Sanguinis 70 Suppl 1:19–23.

29 Barrowcliffe TW, Raut S, Hubbard AR 1998 Discrepancies in potency assessment of recombinant FVIII concentrates. Haemophilia 4:634–640.

30 Kasper CK 1984 Measurement of factor VIII inhibitors. Progress in Clinical and Biological Research 150:87–98.

31 Verbruggen B, Novakova I, Wessels H, et al 1995 The Nijmegen modification of the Bethesda assay for factor VIII:C inhibitors: improved specificity and reliability. Thrombosis and Haemostasis 73:247–251.

32 Gaffney PJ, Wong MY 1992 Collaborative study of a proposed international standard for plasma fibrinogen measurement. Thrombosis and Haemostasis 68:428–432.

33 Haverkate F, Samama M 1995 Familial dysfibrinogenemia and thrombophilia. Report on a study of the SSC Subcommittee on Fibrinogen. Thrombosis and Haemostasis 73:151–161.

34 Pepin M, Schwarze U, Superti Furga A, et al. 2000 Clinical and genetic features of Ehlers–Danlos syndrome type IV, the vascular type. New England Journal of Medicine 342:673–680.

35 Rodgers RP, Levin J 1990 A critical reappraisal of the bleeding time. Seminars in Thrombosis and Hemostasis 16:1–20.

36 Mielke CH, Jr., Kaneshiro MM, Maher IA, et al. 1969 The standardized normal Ivy bleeding time and its prolongation by aspirin. Blood 34:204–215.

37 Ivy A, Nelson D, Bucher G 1940 The standardization of certain factors in the cutaneous 'venostasis' bleeding time technique. Journal of Laboratory and Clinical Medicine 26: 1812.

38 Fressinaud E, Veyradier A, Truchaud F, et al 1998 Screening for von Willebrand disease with a new analyzer using high shear stress: a study of 60 cases. Blood 91:1325–1331.

39 Cattaneo M, Federici AB, Lecchi A, et al 1999 Evaluation of the PFA-100 system in the diagnosis and therapeutic monitoring of patients with von Willebrand disease. Thrombosis and Haemostasis 82:35–39.

40 Sadler JE, Matsushita T, Dong Z, et al 1995 Molecular mechanism and classification of von Willebrand disease. Thrombosis and Haemostasis 74:161–166.

41 Sadler JE 1994 A revised classification of von Willebrand disease. For the Subcommittee on von Willebrand Factor of the Scientific and Standardization Committee of the International Society on Thrombosis and Haemostasis. Thrombosis and Haemostasis 71:520–525.

42 Bartlett A, Dormandy KM, Hawkey CM et al 1976 Factor-VIII-related antigen: measurement by enzyme immunoassay. British Medical Journal 1:994–996.

43 Macfarlane DE, Stibbe J, Kirby EP, et al 1975 Letter: A method for assaying von Willebrand factor (ristocetin cofactor). Thrombosis et Diathesis Haemorrhagica 34: 306–308.

44 Enayat MS, Hill FG 1983 Analysis of the complexity of the multimeric structure of factor VIII related antigen/von Willebrand protein using a modified electrophoretic technique. Journal of Clinical Pathology 36:915–919.

45 British Society for Haematology 1988 Guidelines on platelet function testing. BCSH Haemostasis and Thrombosis Task Force. Journal of Clinical Pathology 41:1322–30.

46 Yardumian DA, Mackie IJ, Machin SJ 1986 Laboratory investigation of platelet function: a review of methodology. Journal of Clinical Pathology 39:701–712.

47 David JL, Herion F 1972 Assay of platelet ATP and ADP by the luciferase method: some theoretical and practical aspects. Advances in Experimental Medicine and Biology 34:341–354.

48 Garvey MB, Black JM 1972 The detection of fibrinogen–fibrin degradation products by means of a new antibody-coated latex particle. Journal of Clinical Pathology 25:680–682.

49 Lipinski B, Worowski K 1968 Detection of soluble fibrin monomer complexes in blood by means of protamine sulphate test. Thrombosis et Diathesis Haemorragica 20:44–49.

50 Breen FA, Jr., Tullis JL 1968 Ethanol gelation: a rapid screening test for intravascular coagulation. Annals of Internal Medicine 69:1197–1206.

51 Breen FA, Jr., Tullis JL 1969 Ethanol gelation test improved. Annals of Internal Medicine 71:433–434.

52 Keeling DM, Wright M, Baker P, et al. 1999 D-dimer for the exclusion of venous thromboembolism: comparison of a new automated latex particle immunoassay (MDA D-dimer) with an established enzyme-linked fluorescent assay (VIDAS D-dimer). Clinical and Laboratory Haematology 21:359–362.

53 Graham J, Elston R, Barrow E, et al 1982 The hemophilias: statistical methods for carrier detection in hemophilias. Methods in Hematology 5:156.

54 Peake IR, Lillicrap DP, Boulyjenkov V, et al 1993 Report of a joint WHO/WFH meeting on the control of haemophilia: carrier detection and prenatal diagnosis Blood Congulation and Fibrinolysis 4: 313–344. [published erratum appears in Blood Coagulation and Fibrinolysis (1994): 148].

55 Bain BJ, Forster T, Baner A 1983 An assessment of the sensitivity of three bleeding time techniques. Scandinavian Journal of Haematology 30:311–316.

56 Ingram GI, Hills M 1976 The Prothrombin time test: effect of varying citrate concentration. Thrombosis and Haemostasis 36:230–236.

17

Investigation of a thrombotic tendency

M.A. Laffan & R.A. Manning

INTRODUCTION

Investigations to exclude an acquired or inherited thrombotic tendency are carried out in neonates, children and young adults who develop venous thrombosis, those who have a strong family history of such events or have thrombosis at an unusual site, and in individuals of all ages with recurrent episodes of thrombo-embolism. These investigations are most commonly instituted in venous thrombosis, but some unexplained arterial events, especially in young people, are also studied. In general, the contribution of the inherited factors described here is less evident for arterial than venous thrombosis because their effect is then usually obscured by atherosclerosis. It should be remembered that many thromboses are almost entirely the result of circumstantial factors. These include trauma, fractures, operations, acute phase inflammatory responses and pregnancy. Further investigation of coagulation is often unnecessary in these circumstances

In this chapter, the investigations to diagnose or exclude an acquired thrombotic tendency are presented first, followed by a simplified battery of tests needed to establish the diagnosis of the more common inherited 'thrombophilias'. Although the number of coagulation factors known to contribute to a thrombotic tendency has increased greatly in the last few years, it remains clear that not all factors have been identified. Hence the failure to detect one of the traits described does not imply that the individual risk of thrombosis is not increased. An acquired thrombotic tendency is common and occurs in many conditions. The large number of traits identified, often with a small associated relative risk, makes their individual utility equally small. Until the interactions of these

numerous factors is more completely understood the clinical history remains a dominant factor in clinical management. The British Committee for Standards in Haematology has published guidelines on the investigation and management of thrombophilia.[1] An outline of appropriate investigations in different circumstances is described below and also shown in Figure 17.1.

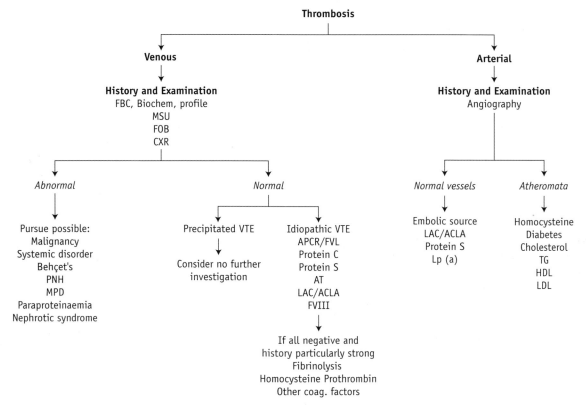

Fig. 17.1 Investigations used to diagnose thrombosis. ACLA, anticardiolipin antibody; APCR, activated protein C resistance; AT, antithrombin; CXR, chest X-ray; FBC, full blood count; FOB, faecal occult blood; FVL, factor V Leiden; HDL, high-density lipoprotein; LAC, lupus anticoagulant; LDL, low-density lipoprotein; Lp(a), lipoprotein (a); MPD, myeloproliferative disorder; MSU, midstream specimen of urine; PNH, paroxysmal nocturnal haemoglobinuria; TG, triglyceride; VTE, venous thromboembolism.

INVESTIGATIONS FOR THE PRESENCE OF A LUPUS ANTICOAGULANT

The lupus anticoagulant (LAC) is an acquired autoantibody found in a variety of auto-immune disorders and sometimes in otherwise healthy individuals.[2] LACs are immunoglobulins which bind to complexes of various proteins with phospholipids active in coagulation and thus prolong the clotting times of phospholipid-dependent tests

such as the PT or APTT. The name 'anticoagulant' is misleading since patients do not have a bleeding tendency. Instead, there is a clear association with recurrent venous thromboembolism, cerebrovascular accidents and other arterial events and, in women, with recurrent abortions and fetal loss. Therefore tests for the presence of the LAC should be carried out in all young individuals with unexplained venous or arterial thrombosis, and also in women with recurrent early or late pregnancy loss. The detection of an LAC should not preclude further investigation for other prothrombotic defects, such as co-existent antithrombin (AT), protein C (PC) and protein S (PS) deficiency and factor V Leiden (FVL).

The presence of an LAC may be detected by the clotting screen, depending on the reagents and methods used as well as on the potency and avidity of the antibody. However, the sensitivity of both APTT and PT to LAC varies considerably so that these tests may well be normal and, if clinically suspected, specific tests should always be performed.[3] The test for activated protein C (APC) resistance (see below) is also sensitive to the presence of an LAC.

Patients with the LAC may show other abnormalities, including thrombocytopenia, a positive direct antiglobulin test and a positive antinuclear factor test. In some rare cases, specific antibodies against coagulation factors are also found. Such patients may have a bleeding tendency. The specific tests most commonly used are: (1) kaolin clotting time (KCT), (2) dilute Russell's viper venom time (DRVVT) in conjunction with the platelet neutralization test and (3) tissue thromboplastin inhibition time. It is essential that all the samples of plasma tested for the LAC should be as free of platelets as possible. This is achieved by further centrifugation of plasma at 2000 *g* or by passing the test plasma through a 0.2 μm microfilter under pressure using a syringe. A platelet count of less than 10×10^9/l should be achieved. The plasma is centrifuged at room temperature to avoid platelet activation because platelet microvesicles may also invalidate the test. Guidelines for the investigation of antiphospholipid syndrome and detection of LACs have been published.[4]

KAOLIN CLOTTING TIME[5]

Principle
When the APTT is modified by omitting platelet substitute reagent, it is particularly sensitive to the LAC. If the test is performed on a range of mixtures of normal and patient's plasma, different patterns of response are obtained indicating the presence of LAC, deficiency of one or more of the coagulation factors or the 'lupus co-factor' effect.

Reagents
Kaolin. 20 mg/ml in Tris buffer, pH 7.4 (see p. 354). This may need to be reduced to 5 mg/ml in some automated analysers.

Normal platelet-poor plasma. Depleted of platelets by second centrifugation or microfiltration.

Patient's plasma. Also platelet-depleted.

CaCl₂. 0.025 mol/l.

Method
Mix normal and patient's plasma in plastic tubes in the following ratios of normal to patient's plasma: 10:0, 9:1, 8:2, 5:5, 2:8, 1:9 and 0:10. Pipette 0.2 ml of each mixture into a glass tube at 37°C. Add 0.1 ml of kaolin and incubate for 3 min, then add 0.2 ml of $CaCl_2$ and record the clotting time.

Results
Plot the clotting times against the proportion of normal: patient's plasma on graph paper as shown in Figure 17.2.

Interpretation
The pattern obtained for each patient must be critically assessed. A convex pattern (pattern 1) indicates a positive result, whilst a concave pattern (pattern 4) indicates a negative result. Pattern 2 indicates a coagulation factor deficiency as well as LAC. Pattern 3 is found in plasma containing the anticoagulant and also deficient in a co-factor necessary for the full inhibitory effect. The initial rate of slope is very important as a steep slope indicates a positive result. This allows the test to be simplified so that only the tests of 100% normal and 80% normal/20% test plasmas are performed. The slope can be calculated using the ratio of KCT at 20% test plasma and KCT at 100% normal control plasma (N). For a positive result, the ratio at this point should be 1.2 or greater, i.e.

$$\frac{KCT\ (80\%N{:}20\%Test)}{KCT\ (100\%\ N)} \geq 1.2$$

A control KCT of <60s may indicate contamination of the control plasma with phospholipid.

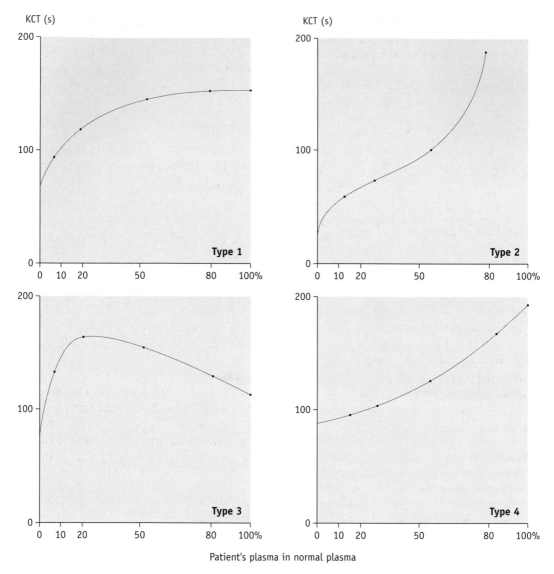

Fig. 17.2 Curves obtained using the kaolin clotting time (KCT) to test for the presence of the lupus anticoagulant. For explanation, see text.

DILUTE RUSSELL'S VIPER VENOM TIME[6]

Principle

Russell's viper venom (RVV) activates factor X leading to a fibrin clot in the presence of factor V, prothrombin, phospholipid and calcium ions. LAC prolongs the clotting time by binding to the phospholipid and preventing the action of RVV. In the test described below, dilution of the venom and phospholipid makes it particularly sensitive for detecting the LAC. Since RVV activates factor X directly, defects of the contact system and factor VIII, IX or XI deficiencies will not influence the test. The DRVVT is usually combined with a platelet/phospholipid neutralization procedure to add specificity and this is incorporated into several commercial kits.

Reagents

Platelet-poor plasma. From the patient and a control.

Pooled normal plasma.

Glyoxaline buffer. 0.05 mol/l, pH 7.4 (p. 352).

Russell's viper venom. Stock solution: 1 mg/ml in saline. For working solution dilute approximately 1 in 200 in buffer. The working solution is stable at 4°C for several hours.

Phospholipid. Platelet substitute (p. 607); also available commercially.

CaCl$_2$. 0.025 mol/l.

Reagent preparation

The RVV concentration is adjusted to give a clotting time of 30–35 s when 0.1 ml of RVV is added to the mixture of 0.1 ml of normal plasma and 0.1 ml of undiluted phospholipid. The test is then repeated using doubling dilutions of phospholipid reagent. The last dilution of phospholipid before the clotting time is prolonged by 2 s or more is selected for the test (thus giving a clotting time of 35–37 s).

Method

Place 0.1 ml of pooled normal plasma and 0.1 ml of dilute phospholipid reagent in a glass tube at 37°C. Add 0.1 ml of dilute RVV and, after warming for 30 s, add 0.1 ml of CaCl$_2$. Record the clotting time. Repeat the sequence using the test plasma. Calculate the ratio of the clotting times of the test and control (normal pool) plasma.

Interpretation

The normal ratio should be determined in each laboratory: it is usually between 0.9 and 1.05. Ratios greater than 1.05 suggest the presence of the LAC, but could also arise from an abnormality of factors II, V, X or fibrinogen or the presence of some other inhibitor. The presence of an inhibitor can be confirmed by testing a mixture of equal volumes of patient's and control plasma, and phospholipid dependence by using the platelet neutralization test described below. The addition of normal plasma will correct an abnormal dilute RVV test result owing to factor deficiency or defect, but will not do so in the presence of the LAC. The platelet neutralization procedure will shorten the clotting time in the dilute RVV test of plasma containing the LAC (see next test).

PLATELET NEUTRALIZATION TEST

Principle

When platelets are used instead of phospholipid reagents in clotting tests, the tests become insensitive to the LAC. This appears to be due to the ability of the platelets to adsorb the LAC. To utilize this property of platelets, they must be washed to remove contaminating plasma proteins, and activated or 'fractured' to expose their coagulation factor binding sites.

Reagents

Commercial platelet extract reagent or washed normal platelets.

ACD anticoagulant solution (see p. 603) pH 5.4 (for washed platelets). For use, 6 parts of blood are added to one part of this anticoagulant.

Na$_2$ EDTA. 0.1 mol/l in saline.

Calcium-free Tyrode's buffer. Dissolve 8 g NaCl, 0.2 g KCl, 0.625 g Na$_2$HPO$_4$, 0.415 g MgCl$_2$ and 1.0 g NaHCO$_2$ in 1 litre of water. Adjust pH if necessary to 6.5 with 1 mol/l HCl.

Method

Collect normal blood into ACD and centrifuge at 270 *g* for 10 min. Pipette the supernatant platelet-rich plasma (PRP) into a plastic container, and centrifuge again to obtain more PRP, which is added to the first lot. Dilute the PRP with an equal volume of the calcium-free buffer, and add 1/10th volume of EDTA to give a final concentration of 0.01 mol/l. Centrifuge the mixture in a conical or round-bottom tube at 2000 *g* for 10 min, and discard the supernatant. Gently resuspend the platelet pellet in buffer and 0.01 mol/EDTA. Centrifuge again, discard the supernatant, and resuspend the pellet in buffer alone. Then centrifuge the platelets a third time, and resuspend the pellet in buffer without EDTA to give a platelet count of at least 400×10^9/l. The washed platelets may be stored below –20°C in volumes of 1–2 ml. Before use, they must be activated by repeatedly thawing and refreezing 3–4 times.

Use the washed platelets or the commercial reagent in the dilute RVV test or in the APTT in place of the usual phospholipid reagent. First, determine a suitable dilution by testing a range of doubling dilutions in the test system with control plasma. A suitable dilution will give a similar clotting time to that obtained using control plasma and the phospholipid reagent.

Interpretation

The addition of platelets or a commercial 'confirm' phospholipid reagent to the DRVVT system will shorten the clotting time when the LAC is present. It will not shorten the time when the prolongation is due to a factor deficiency or an inhibitor directed against a specific coagulation factor. However, the ability of different batches of platelets to perform this correction is variable and may vary further with storage. Accordingly, each time the test is performed a plasma sample known to contain an LAC should be tested in parallel to establish the efficacy of the platelets.

Many commercial kits are now available for performing the tests described above. As with all such tests, there is an inevitable trade-off between sensitivity and specificity. This varies with different techniques, kits and coagulometer. A recent survey of reagents found that the best discriminator of positivity was by using a normalized correction ratio (CR) of DRVVT clotting times as follows:

$$CR = \frac{\left(\dfrac{P_D}{N_D}\right) - \left(\dfrac{P_C}{N_C}\right)}{\left(\dfrac{P_D}{N_D}\right)}$$

Where P is patient and N is normal plasma, D represents the detection procedure and C represents the confirmation (platelet/phospholipid neutralization) procedure.[7] A correction of >10% is regarded as positive but care should be taken to establish a local normal range and other calculations may also be used.[4]

False-positive results may be obtained in patients on intravenous heparin, and the interpretation is unreliable in patients receiving oral anticoagulants. The latter can sometimes be overcome by performing the test on a 50:50 mix with normal plasma.

DILUTE THROMBOPLASTIN INHIBITION TEST[8]

Principle

The principle is similar to other tests. When the thromboplastin used for the PT is diluted, the PT becomes prolonged. At a certain point (usually 1:50–1:500 dilution), the concentration of phospholipid is low enough for the test to become sensitive to phospholipid binding antibodies and when an LAC is present the ratio of the test plasma to normal plasma clotting time increases. This test is now considered more useful as some thromboplastin reagents (e.g. Innovin) are more sensitive to LAC. However, it should be noted that diluting thromboplastin makes the system sensitive to low levels of factor VIII as are encountered in mild haemophilia and acquired haemophilia and low levels of factor VII or factor V. Care should be taken that these disorders are not confused. In one study, the test was determined to be positive when the dilute prothrombin time ratio (test/mean normal) using Innovin at 1:200 dilution was greater than 1.15.[8]

TEXTARIN/ECARIN RATIO

Principle

The Textarin/Ecarin ratio is a sensitive and relatively specific test for the LAC based on fractions of two snake venoms. Textarin is a protein fraction of *Pseudonaja textilis* venom (Australian Eastern brown snake), that activates prothrombin in the presence of phospholipid, factor V and calcium ions.[9] Ecarin is a protein fraction of *Echis carinatus* venom that activates prothrombin in the absence of any co-factors. The activation of prothrombin by Textarin yields thrombin while Ecarin yields meizothrombin (an intermediate of prothrombin activation). In the presence of an LAC, the Textarin time is prolonged whilst the Ecarin time remains unaffected.

Results

The test results are reported as a ratio of Textarin/Ecarin times. A positive result is indicated by a ratio greater than 1.3.

Polybrene is incorporated with Textarin when testing heparinized samples for the LAC. False-positive results may be obtained in the presence of factor V deficiency and specific inhibitors of factor V.

Interpretation of tests for LAC

No single test will detect all lupus-like anticoagulants and if suspected clinically, then two or, if possible, three tests should be performed before concluding that one is not present.[3,10,11] Conversely, a single positive test should be repeated 6 to 8 weeks later because a transient positive may be the result of intercurrent illness or medication.

It is crucial to distinguish LAC from specific anti-factor VIII antibodies which are more typically time dependent but may have some immediate effect as well: specific factor assays may be of use. Similarly, some weak LAC are neutralized by 50:50 mixing with normal plasma and sometimes exhibit a time-dependent effect.

ANTI-CARDIOLIPIN ASSAY[12]

The LAC effect is produced by members of the antiphospholipid group of antibodies. These antibodies do not bind to phospholipid itself but to a number of different proteins to which binding is facilitated by the presence of phospholipid. The proteins that are bound in this way include β2-glycoprotein I, prothrombin, annexin V and cardiolipin. The most frequent of these are anti-cardiolipin antibodies. These antibodies are detected using the relevant protein in immuno-assay on microtitre plates or in coated polystyrene tubes. It is possible that the test for anticardiolipin which is currently most prevalent will be superseded by tests for anti-β2-glycoprotein 1 antibodies as these may have a closer relationship with thrombosis. However, this is not exclusively so and no standardization is yet available. Commercial kits for these assays are available.

Care must be taken in the selection of control sera and in setting the cut-off point for normal values. It is also important to remember that anti-cardiolipin antibodies may be found after viral infections, including glandular fever, and after myocardial infarction.

OTHER ACQUIRED PROTHROMBOTIC STATES[13]

There are numerous other disorders which are associated with an increased risk of thrombosis but which are not usually diagnosed using coagulation-based tests. Their position in the investigation of thrombosis is illustrated in Figure 17.1 and appropriate tests for some of these such as myelo-proliferative disorders and paroxysmal nocturnal haemoglobinuria will be found elsewhere in this book. One of the most important factors precipitating thrombosis is malignancy. However, studies have shown that a history and examination combined with a few simple tests as indicated in Figure 17.1 will detect virtually all cases of malignancy as well as other systemic disorders.

INVESTIGATION OF SUSPECTED INHERITED THROMBOTIC SYNDROMES

Testing for thrombotic syndromes is becoming increasingly frequent.[14,15] Patients with disorders of pregnancy as well as those with thrombotic disorders are often referred for investigation. Screening must start by excluding the common causes of an acquired thrombotic tendency as described above. A careful family history must be taken next; however, a negative history does not exclude an inherited thrombotic tendency because the defects have variable penetration or a new mutation may have been responsible. As with a bleeding tendency, laboratory investigation is a step-wise procedure, starting with the simpler, first-line tests (as shown in Fig. 17.1) The relevant tests are described below.

INVESTIGATION OF ANTITHROMBIN DEFICIENCY[16,17]

AT (previously known as antithrombin III) is the major physiological inhibitor of thrombin, and also inhibits factors Xa, IXa and XIa. AT deficiency is found in approximately 2% of cases of thrombosis and may be acquired or congenital. A variety of methods are available for measuring either functional activity or antigenic quantity of AT. The functional methods are based on the reaction with thrombin or factor Xa and can be coagulation or chromogenic assays. A chromogenic assay is described below.

ANTITHROMBIN MEASUREMENT USING A CHROMOGENIC ASSAY
Principle
In the presence of heparin, AT reacts rapidly to inactivate thrombin by forming a 1:1 complex. The chromogenic AT assay is a two-step procedure. In the first step, the plasma sample is incubated with a fixed quantity of thrombin and heparin. In the second step, the residual thrombin is measured spectrometrically by its action on a

synthetic chromogenic substrate which results in the release of para-nitroaniline dye (pNA). The use of bovine thrombin avoids interference in the assay by heparin co-factor II; this can also be achieved by measuring the Xa neutralizing capacity of the AT and an appropriate chromogenic substrate. The assay thus measures heparin co-factor activity rather than progressive AT activity and may therefore also detect AT variants with altered heparin binding.

Method

Carry out the procedure on dilutions of a standard plasma so as to construct a standard graph. Then test dilutions of the test plasma in an identical manner and read the results directly from the standard graph.

The reagents provided and details of the method vary from manufacturer to manufacturer and should be closely followed. There may also be variation between different batches of the same reagent.

Normal range

Generally between 0.75 and 1.25 iu/ml. Some manufacturers suggest a slightly narrower range (i.e. 0.8–1.20 iu/ml), but it is preferable for each laboratory to establish its own normal range. Repeated freezing and thawing of samples, as well as storage at or above –20°C result in a reduction in AT concentration.

Interpretation

In an inherited deficiency, the AT concentration is usually <0.7 iu/ml. Most cases are heterozygotes for null mutations and have levels of approximately 50% of normal. Be aware that a large number of variants have been described, some of which give assay results that are close to normal. Further tests such as AT antigen or crossed immunoelectrophoresis may be required. A low level of AT may be acquired during active thrombosis, liver disease, heparin therapy, nephrotic syndrome or asparaginase therapy: very low values are sometimes encountered in fulminant disseminated intravascular coagulation (DIC) or liver failure. Normal newborns have a lower AT concentration (0.60–0.80 iu/ml) than adults. In congenitally deficient neonates, very low values (0.30 iu/ml and lower) may be found. Very high values are encountered after myocardial infarction and in some forms of vascular disease. It is also important to remember that oral anticoagulant therapy may raise the AT concentration by c 0.1 iu/ml in cases of congenital deficiency.

ANTITHROMBIN ANTIGEN DETERMINATION

AT antigen can be assessed using various methods such as ELISA, immuno-electrophoresis assays and latex agglutination (nephelometry).

Principle

Latex agglutination assays are based on the agglutination of a suspension of antibody-coated, micro-latex particles in the presence of plasma containing AT antigen (the antibody is attached by covalent bonding). The wavelength is such that light can pass through the latex suspension unabsorbed. However, in the presence of AT antigen, when the antibody-coated latex particles agglutinate to form aggregates of diameter greater than the wavelength of the light; the latter is absorbed. There is a direct relationship between the observed absorbance value and the concentration of the antigen being measured. The convenience of this form of test is that it can be performed on automated analysers.

INVESTIGATION OF PROTEIN C DEFICIENCY[18]

Protein C (PC) is a vitamin-K-dependent protein. After activation by thrombin, which is accelerated in the presence of thrombomodulin on the vascular endothelium, PC complexes with phospholipids and protein S (PS) to degrade factors Va and VIIIa. Inherited heterozygous PC deficiency is found in 2–4% of first-episode thromboses and 5–7% of all recurrent thrombo-embolic episodes in young adults.[14,15] The importance of the PC–PS system is evidenced by the catastrophic syndrome of purpura fulminans in neonates with homozygous PC or PS deficiency.[19] Acquired PC deficiency is found in all conditions associated with vitamin-K deficiency or defect, including oral anticoagulant therapy. A low plasma concentration is also found in DIC, liver disease and in the early postoperative period.

PC can be measured using a chromogenic assay, a coagulation assay or an antigenic method.

MEASUREMENT OF FUNCTIONAL PROTEIN C BY THE PROTAC METHOD
Principle
In the presence of a specific snake venom activator, PC is converted into its active form (APC). This allows the activation to be carried out in whole plasma without separation of PC. APC is measured by its action on one of the specific synthetic substrates (such as S-2366, CBS 65.25). The reaction is stopped by the addition of 50% acetic acid and the p-nitroalanine produced measured at 405 nm in a spectrometer.

Reagents

Platelet-poor plasma. Standard and test samples are centrifuged at 1500–2000 g for 15 min. After centrifugation, plasma can be stored indefinitely at –40°C or below.

Protac. This is an activator derived from the venom of *Agkistrodon contortrix contortrix*. It is obtained commercially; each vial contains lyophilized powder which is reconstituted and stored according to the manufacturer's instructions.

Specific chromogenic substrate. Reconstituted and stored according to the manufacturer's instructions.

Barbitone buffered saline. See page 605.

Acetic acid. 50%.

Method
Construct the standard curve according to the instructions. Some manufacturers recommend the use of commercial calibrators or control plasma in preference to the normal pool.

The assay is carried out by a two-step method. In the first step, plasma and activator are incubated for an exact period of time. In the second step, the specific chromogenic substrate is added and the reaction is stopped with acetic acid again at a precise point in time. Read the amount of the dye produced against a blank as follows: acetic acid, activator and chromogenic substrate are first mixed; then standard or patient's plasma is added to the mixture and the absorbance measured at 405 nm. The manufacturer's instructions must be closely followed. Plot the PC activity against the corresponding absorbance reading on linear graph paper.

Normal range
0.70–1.40 iu/ml. Each laboratory should preferably establish its own normal range.

Further investigation
If inherited PC deficiency is suspected, an immunological assay should also be carried out with an ELISA-based kit. The amidolytic assay described here will not detect the rare type II PC deficiency owing to mutations in the Gla domain although they will be detected by a coagulation-based assay. A problem with the coagulation-based assay is its susceptibility to interference from FVL. Although the chromogenic substrate is said to be specific, this is not true. Specificity is conferred by the inclusion of substances which will inhibit other enzymes capable of cleaving the substrate. In some circumstances, this can fail and spuriously high PC activities can be obtained which may obscure a PC deficiency.[20] PC activity and antigen are reduced in patients taking oral vitamin K antagonists: although it is sometimes possible to make a provisional diagnosis of PC deficiency by using a PC:VIIc ratio.[21] It is also important to exclude vitamin-K deficiency by assaying other vitamin-K-dependent factors which should be normal. Family studies should be carried out whenever possible.

CLOTTING-BASED PROTEIN C ASSAY
Principle
PC-clotting assays use an APTT reagent incorporating a PC activator derived from the Southern copperhead snake venom (*Agkistrodon contortrix contortrix*), PC-deficient plasma and calcium chloride. The APTT reagent activates both PC and the factors of the intrinsic pathway. The clotting time of normal plasma is long (>100 s), while that of PC-deficient plasma is normal (30 s). The degree of prolongation of the clotting time when patient plasma is mixed with PC-deficient plasma is proportional to the concentration of PC in the patient plasma.

Unlike chromogenic PC assays, PC-clotting assays are sensitive to functional PC defects such as PS binding and calcium binding. However, they are also sensitive to activated PC resistance (FVL), LACs and raised factor VIII levels.

PROTEIN C ANTIGEN
PC antigen can be measured using a conventional ELISA. Commercial kits are available.

INVESTIGATION OF PROTEIN S DEFICIENCY

PS is also a vitamin-K-dependent protein which acts as a co-factor for APC. It is similar to the serine proteases of the coagulation system in having a Gla domain and four epidermal growth factor domains; however, instead of a protease domain, it has a large terminal domain closely homologous to sex hormone binding globulin (SHBG). In plasma, 60% of PS is bound to C4b-binding protein (C4bBP) via the SHBG domain[22] and does not possess any APC co-factor activity; the remaining 40% is free and available to interact with APC. The functional assays of PS are based on the capacity of PS to augment the prolongation of a clotting test time by APC. However, PS has some APC independent anticoagulant activity which can also be measured in coagulation assays.[23] Measurement of the total and free PS antigen is possible using enzyme-linked immunoassays. Interpretation of PS assay results is frequently difficult and the three measurements are considered together below.

ENZYME-LINKED IMMUNOSORBENT ASSAY OF FREE AND TOTAL PROTEIN S[24]
Principle
The total PS in plasma is detected by a standard ELISA using polyclonal antibodies. The analysis is then repeated using plasma in which C4bBP-bound PS has been removed by polyethylene glycol (PEG) precipitation. This gives a measure of free PS.

Reagents

Polyethylene glycol precipitation solution. Dissolve 100 g of PEG 8000 in 200 ml of sterile water. Prepare approximately 50 ml of working PEG by diluting the stock solution to exactly 18.75% with sterile water. Store in 2 ml aliquots at −20°C.

Coating buffer (phosphate buffered saline, pH 7.2). 0.39 g $NaH_2PO_4.2H_2O$, 2.68 g $Na_2HPO_4.12H_2O$, 8.474 g NaCl. Make up to 1 litre and adjust to pH 7.2, store at 4°C.

Wash buffer. This is the same as the coating buffer, but contains 0.5 M NaCl and 0.2% v/v Tween 20. Add 10.37 g of NaCl to 1 litre of coating buffer and 0.2% Tween 20 (mix well). Store at 4°C.

Dilution buffer. This is the washing buffer with 30 g/l PEG 8000. Store at 4°C.

Substrate buffer (citrate phosphate buffer, pH 5.0). 7.3 g citric acid, 23.87 g. $Na_2HPO_4.12H_2O$. Make up to 1 litre with water. Adjust pH to 5.0.

o-phenylenediamine.

Anti-Protein S and peroxidase conjugated anti-Protein S. (Dako Ltd)

Sulphuric acid 1 M.

Microtitre plates. (Greiner Labortechnick Ltd)

Standards and controls.

Hydrogen peroxide. '30 vols'.

Methods
Dilute the anti-human PS immunoglobulin 1:1000 in coating buffer, i.e. 20 μl in 20 ml of buffer. Add 0.1 ml to each well of a microtitre plate, cover with parafilm and leave overnight in a moist chamber at 4°C. On the day the assay is to be performed, warm an aliquot of working PEG solution to 30°C. Accurately pipette 200 μl of standard, patient's and control plasma samples into conical Eppendorf tubes, warm for 5 min at 37°C. Add exactly 50 μl of warmed PEG; immediately cap and vortex mix twice for exactly 5 s each. Place in water/crushed ice mixture. In turn, treat all the samples identically. Leave for 30 min on the melted ice. Centrifuge for 30 s in the Eppendorf centrifuge. Then return to ice and remove 100 μl in a labelled tube (taking care not to remove any precipitate).

Prepare dilutions of control and patient's samples in PEG dilution buffer as follows. For total PS, dilute 0.05 ml of reference plasma in 8 ml of diluent. Use the PEG-precipitated reference plasma for measuring free PS; add 0.1 ml to 4 ml of dilution buffer.

Prepare a range of standards from these stock solutions using the same dilution schedule for free and total PS.

A. Stock solution = 1.25 u/ml.
B. 0.8 ml stock + 0.2 ml buffer = 1.0 u/ml.
C. 0.6 ml stock + 0.4 ml buffer = 0.75 u/ml.
D. 0.4 ml stock + 0.6 ml buffer = 0.5 u/ml.
E. 0.2 ml stock + 0.8 ml buffer = 0.25 u/ml.
F. 0.1 ml stock + 0.9 ml buffer = 0.125 u/ml.
G. 0.05 ml stock + 0.95 ml buffer = 0.0625 u/ml.

Control and patient's samples are tested at two dilutions – total PS plasma: 1:200 and 1:400; free PS PEG supernatants: 1:50 and 1:100. Shake out the contents of the previously prepared plate, blot on tissue. Wash the plate three times in wash buffer by filling all the wells, leaving for 2 min, shaking out the contents, blotting and repeating. Add 100 µl of each dilution of standard, control or patient's plasma in duplicate across the plate. Cover and incubate for 3 h in a wet box at room temperature. Wash the plate as described earlier. Dilute 2 µl of peroxidase-labelled antibody in 24 ml of dilution buffer. Add 100 µl of diluted tag (peroxidase-conjugated) antibody to each well and leave in a wet box for 2–3 h at room temperature. Wash the plate as described earlier. Make up the substrate solution by adding 8 mg of *o*-phenylene-diamine to 12 ml of citrate phosphate buffer. Immediately before use, add 10 µl of hydrogen peroxide. Add 100 µl of substrate solution to each well. When the weakest standard has a visible yellow colour, add 150 µl of 1 M sulphuric acid to each well. Read the optical densities on a plate reader at 492 nm. Plot the optical densities against plasma dilutions on double-log graph paper and read the patient's values from the corresponding calibration curve, i.e. total against total and free against free.

The polyclonal antibody should have similar affinities for free and bound PS: high-plasma dilutions and long incubation times help to avoid differential affinity leading to error. Alternatively, two monoclonal antibodies (capture and tag) with the same affinity for free and bound PS can be used (Asserchrom).

A new test using two separate antibodies to measure free and total PS in now available.[25]

PROTEIN S FUNCTIONAL ASSAY
Principle
Functional PS can be assessed using coagulation-based assays activated by different means. In one commercial assay (American Diagnostica), dilutions of normal and test plasmas are mixed with PS-deficient plasma. Activation of these mixtures is achieved by a reagent containing factor Xa, activated PC and phospholipid. After a 5-min activation time, clot formation is initiated by the addition of calcium chloride. Under these conditions, the prolongation of the clotting time is

directly proportional to the concentration of PS in the patient plasma. The use of factor Xa as the activator minimizes the potential interference by high levels of factor VIII.

A PS function assay may also be based on the PT in which case the effect of factor VIII is again bypassed. The PT-based PS assay uses PS-depleted plasma activated by Protac, thus providing APC. The PT is increased by the APC–PS mediated destruction of factor Va, which occurs in the presence of PS from the test and control plasmas. The PT is measured using bovine thromboplastin and prolongation is proportional to PS activity.

The details of the tests are performed according to the manufacturer's instructions and many tests can be automated.

Because the assays are subject to interference by other plasma factors, it is recommended that the test plasma is assayed at two different dilutions to ensure parallelism with the standard curve.

PS functional assays are designed to measure the PC co-factor activity of PS, but as discussed above, this is not its only anticoagulant activity. PS that is bound to C4bBP, or is inadequately γ-carboxylated or which has been cleaved by thrombin will have an indeterminate effect on these assays but will not contribute via PC co-factor activity.

Interpretation of PS functional and antigenic assays
PS deficiency has been classified into three sub-types according to the pattern of results obtained in functional and antigenic assays:

Category	Total PS	Free PS	Functional PS
Type I	Low	Low	Low
Type II	Normal	Normal	Low
Type III	Normal	Low	Low

Recent studies have suggested that the Type I and Type III patterns are both the result of the same genetic defect and that the difference may be the result of an age-related rise in C4bBP.[26,27] Many examples of what were thought to be Type II PS deficiency have subsequently been shown to be due to the presence of FVL which causes a spuriously low result in the functional PS assay.

Note that whilst bound PS does not have any APC co-factor activity it does have some other anticoagulant activities. Because the functional assay is usually performed on whole plasma, not just on free PS in a PEG supernatant, one should expect discrepancies between the two results and this is frequently seen. The use of whole patient plasma also renders the assay sensitive to other plasma factors: most notably FVL (see below) but also LACs which may elevate or reduce the apparent functional PS.[28] High levels of factor VIIa have been reported to cause underestimation of PS function by shortening of the clotting time. An assay on free PS removed from plasma using a monoclonal antibody has been described and avoids these problems but is not in general use.[29]

Low levels of PS may be an acquired phenomenon during pregnancy, oral anticoagulation, nephrotic syndrome, use of oral contraceptives, with systemic lupus erythematosus and liver disease. Catastrophically low levels have been reported in children after varicella infection.[30] It is important to note that the normal range for pre-menopausal women is significantly lower than in other groups and local normal ranges should be determined to avoid misinterpretation paying attention to the additional effects of hormonal therapy and artefactual reduction in PS as described above.[31,32] Although C4bBP is elevated during an acute phase reaction, the PS binding β chain does not rise and as a result free PS does not fall.[33]

ACTIVATED PROTEIN C RESISTANCE

In 1993, Dahlback and colleagues described an inherited tendency to thrombosis characterized by a defective plasma response to APC.[34] This became known as activated protein C resistance (APCR) and was subsequently shown to be due in >90% of cases to result from a mutation Arg506Glu in factor V (FVL). This mutation destroys a cleavage site for APC which greatly slows APC inactivation of Va. It also blocks the conversion by APC of factor V into factor VI which acts as a co-factor for APC degradation of factor VIIIa. APCR is found in approximately 20% of patients with a first episode of venous thrombosis.

Principle[35]
When APC is added to plasma and an APTT performed, there is normally a prolongation of the clotting time as a result of factor V and factor VIII degradation. The original detection of this phenomenon was by means of a modified APTT but it can also be detected using modifications of the PT, RVVT, and Xa clotting time. These tests all vary somewhat in their sensitivity and specificity for the FVL mutation which is generally improved by mixing the test plasma with factor V-deficient plasma. This reduces the effect of other factors such as factor VIII which can alter estimation of APCR[36] and restores the sensitivity of the test in patients who are taking oral anticoagulants. However, the test remains sensitive to interference by LACs. A number of commercial kits are available for these tests.

Expression of results
APCR was originally reported as a simple ratio of clotting times with and without APC. The result can be normalized by expressing this as a ratio of the same result obtained with normal plasma, i.e.

$$\text{Normalized APCR} = \frac{T+APC}{T-APC} \div \frac{N+APC}{N-APC}$$

The use of a normalized ratio improves day-to-day precision and may also improve accuracy. However, it is extremely important that the pooled normal plasma contains no FVL as very small amounts (2.5%) will markedly affect the response to APC. A normal range should be established locally, and its relationship to the presence of FVL investigated.

Interpretation
The Leiden thrombophilia survey estimated the relative risk of thrombosis for APCR to be approximately 7.[37] Studies using DNA analysis alone have generally found lower relative risks.[38] Most testing strategies have been directed towards producing tests which have a high sensitivity and specificity for FVL but this may not be appropriate. It seems likely that 'acquired APCR' or APCR owing to other causes represents a prothrombotic state even in the absence of FVL. This conjecture is supported by a recent report from the Leiden thrombophilia survey[39] and also by the presence of acquired APCR in prothrombotic states such as pregnancy. These will not (except LACs) be detected after mixing with factor V-deficient plasma. Many laboratories use a combination of plasma and DNA testing to assess patients' status.

ELEVATED PROTHROMBIN, FACTOR VIII AND OTHER FACTORS

A later finding from the Leiden thrombophilia survey was that elevated levels of prothrombin were significantly associated with thrombosis.[40] The majority of elevated levels were themselves associated with a mutation in the 3' untranslated region of the gene (G20210A). The mutation is detected by a simple PCR-based test (see Ch. 21). Subsequently, other factors including factor VIII, factor XI and factor IX have been shown to have an association with thrombosis when elevated.[41–43]

INVESTIGATION OF HEPARIN CO-FACTOR II DEFICIENCY

A deficiency of heparin co-factor II (HCII) is found in some individuals with recurrent thrombo-embolism. However, there is no clear evidence that HCII deficiency is more prevalent in this group than in the normal population. Its concentration may be measured in the presence of a strong family history if the assays of other physiological inhibitors give normal results.

HEPARIN CO-FACTOR II ASSAY

Principle

HCII present in test and standard plasma is activated by dermatan sulphate and incubated with human thrombin. The residual, uninhibited thrombin is then measured by cleavage of a chromogenic substrate.

Reagents

Reagents are commercially available in a kit form. *Buffer*, pH 8.2. 0.05 mol/l Tris, 0.15 mol/l NaCl, 6.8 mmol/l Na_2EDTA, 2 mg/l Polybrene,

10 g/l bovine serum albumin, pH adjusted with HCl.

Dermatan sulphate (free of heparin).

Human thrombin.

Chromogenic substrate for thrombin.

50% Acetic acid.

Pooled normal plasma as standard.

Test plasma.

Method

It is important to follow the manufacturer's instructions which come with the kit. Prepare a range of dilutions of pooled normal plasma in order to construct a calibration curve. Prepare also a single dilution of each test plasma. Incubate the dilutions with dermatan sulphate at 37°C in a plastic tube or a microtitre plate. Then add thrombin, followed, after a further incubation, by the chromogenic substrate. After a suitable reaction time, in accordance with the manufacturer's instructions, add acetic acid to stop the reaction, and measure the absorbance at 405 nm in a spectrometer or a microtitre plate reader, as appropriate.

Calculation

Read the absorbance of the test plasma from the calibration curve and express as percentage normal.

Normal range

Generally 0.55–1.45 u/ml.

Interpretation

The plasma concentration may be increased in healthy women on oral contraceptive pills. HCII is reduced in congenital deficiency, liver disease and DIC.

INVESTIGATION OF A SUSPECTED DYSFIBRINOGENAEMIA

Congenital dysfibrinogenaemia associated with thrombosis should be suspected in individuals with a prolonged thrombin time and a slightly or moderately reduced fibrinogen concentration in

plasma. The presence of a dysfibrinogen is proved when a significant (usually twofold) discrepancy is found between the Clauss and clot weight assays. For details of investigation, see page 370.

INVESTIGATION OF THE FIBRINOLYTIC SYSTEM

GENERAL CONSIDERATIONS

The investigation of fibrinolysis has an uncertain place in haemostasis. It seems well established that uncontrolled fibrinolytic capacity owing to anti-plasmin or plasminogen activator inhibitor (PAI)-1 deficiency can lead to a haemorrhagic tendency, although these are rare.[44,45] In contrast, there is no good evidence that an impaired fibrinolytic capacity results in a tendency to venous thrombosis. This may be attributed in part to the poor repro-ducibility of the global tests of euglobulin clot lysis or fibrin plate lysis, but the uncertainty has not been removed by use of either specific assays or genetic polymorphic markers.[46] Whilst reduced fibrinolysis is a common finding in patients who have had a venous thrombosis it appears to have no prospective value. Similarly, high (sic) levels of t-PA were shown to be predictive of myocardial infarction in the ECAT study but it seems likely that in both cases the association can be best interpreted as demonstrating an abnormality of endothelial function rather than a problem with fibrinolysis per se.[47–50]

Fibrinolysis shows considerable diurnal vari-ation as well as interference from plasma lipids and stress. It is therefore generally preferred to perform these tests in the morning after an overnight fast, no smoking and after the subject has lain resting for ≥ 15 min (the plasma half-life of t-PA is approximately 5 min). Great care is required in obtaining and handling samples for the assays described below.[51] Tests for fibrin and fibrinogen degradation products are described in Chapter 16.

INVESTIGATION OF A SUSPECTED PLASMINOGEN DEFECT OR DEFICIENCY

Inherited plasminogen deficiency or defect may be found in 2–3% of unexplained thromboses in young people.[52,53] However, the relationship between the deficiency and thrombosis is not clear. The laboratory screening should be carried out using a functional assay based on full transform-ation of plasminogen into plasmin by activators. Such assays can be caseinolytic, fibrin substrate or chromogenic.

CHROMOGENIC ASSAY FOR PLASMINOGEN
Principle
In this two-step amidolytic assay, plasminogen is first complexed with excess streptokinase. In the second step, the plasmin-like activity of the streptokinase–plasminogen complex is measured by its effect on a plasmin-specific peptide. The amount of the dye released is proportional to the amount of plasmin-ogen available in the sample for complexing with streptokinase. The plasminogen–streptokinase complex is not significantly inhibited by the plasma plasmin inhibitors.

Reagents and method
Details can be found in the manufacturer's instruc-tions. They vary with manufacturer and even from batch to batch of the same kit.

Normal range
0.75–1.60 u/ml.

Interpretation
Plasminogen concentration is reduced in the newborn, in patients with cirrhosis, with DIC and during and after thrombolytic therapy, but the assay is less reliable in these circumstances when FDPs (or high levels of fibrinogen) may augment plasmin activity. Plasminogen is an acute phase reactant and an increased concentration is found in infection, trauma, myocardial infarction and malignant disease. The diagnosis of inherited plas-minogen deficiency must be confirmed by func-tional tests using other activators, immunological assays and family studies.

INVESTIGATION OF 'FIBRINOLYTIC POTENTIAL'

The 'fibrinolytic potential' is measured as the combined effect of plasminogen activators and inhibitors. The concentration of activators may be increased by venous occlusion or by the adminis-tration of DDAVP. The tests used are, first, the assays of plasminogen activators, using a fibrin sub-strate (euglobulin lysis time, fibrin plate lysis and many others) or a chromogenic substrate or ELISA techniques; and second, assays of inhibitors. The commonly used tests for inhibitors are the chromogenic assays of PAI and of α_2 antiplasmin (AP).[54,55] The finding of an increased or reduced fibrinolytic potential should be followed by assays of specific firbrinolytic factors.

EUGLOBULIN LYSIS TIME

Principle
When plasma is diluted and acidified, the precipitate (euglobulin) which forms contains plasminogen activator (mostly t-PA), plasminogen and fibrinogen. Most of the plasmin inhibitors are left in the solution. The precipitate is redissolved, the fibrinogen clotted with thrombin and the time for clot lysis measured.

Reagents

Acetic acid. 0.01%

Bovine thrombin. 10 NIH u/ml.

Fresh platelet-poor plasma from the patient and control. As t-PA is very labile, blood must be collected into cooled sample tubes, placed on ice and processed immediately.

Glyoxaline buffer, pH 7.4. See page 352.

Method
Place venous blood in a plastic tube containing citrate; after mixing, keep the tube in an ice-bath. Centrifuge the sample as soon as possible (never later than 30 min after collection) at 4°C at 1200–1500 g. Pipette 1.0 ml of plasma into 9 ml of acetic acid. Mix well and keep on ice for 15 min. Centrifuge at 4°C for 15 min at 1500 g, to deposit the white euglobulin precipitate. Discard the supernatant, invert the tubes, then wipe the walls with cotton wool on an applicator stick until completely dry inside. Add 0.5 ml of glyoxaline buffer and dissolve the precipitate. Place duplicate 0.3 ml volumes of patient's and control plasma-dissolved euglobulin fraction in glass tubes and clot with 0.1 ml of thrombin. Leave undisturbed at 37°C and inspect for clot lysis at 15-min intervals.

Normal range
90–240 min.

Interpretation
A technical problem leading to a long lysis time is the failure to maintain a low temperature through-

out all the stages of the test. Furthermore, the fact that a variable amount of PAI-1 precipitates in the euglobulin fraction makes it essential to analyse a normal control on each occasion the test is performed. Exercise and prolonged venous stasis shorten the lysis times. There is also a significant diurnal variation: lysis time is longer in the morning than at noon or in the afternoon. Prolonged fibrinolysis (as found during fibrinolytic therapy) may result in plasminogen depletion and give rise to a falsely long time. In DIC, a low fibrinogen concentration in the patient's plasma gives a wispy clot which dissolves rapidly and results in a falsely short lysis time. Conversely, high levels of fibrinogen will result in a prolonged lysis time.

Long lysis times are found in the last trimester of pregnancy, in the postoperative period, after myocardial infarction, in obese individuals and in many cases of recurrent venous thrombosis. Very short lysis times are seen in some haematological or disseminated malignancies, and in cirrhosis. A short lysis time is also seen in factor XIII deficiency.

LYSIS OF FIBRIN PLATES[56]

Principle
Most commercially available fibrinogen preparations are contaminated with plasminogen. If a standard fibrinogen solution is poured into a Petri dish and clotted with $CaCl_2$ and thrombin, a solid fibrin plate is obtained. If the euglobulin fraction under test is placed on the plate, the plasminogen in the plate will be converted into plasmin and a zone of lysis will appear around the sample. The area of lysis will be proportionate to the concentration of plasminogen activator in the euglobulin fraction.

Reagents

Bovine fibrinogen.

Bovine thrombin. 50 NIH u/ml.

Calcium. 0.025 mol/l.

Barbitone buffered saline. (See p. 605).

Platelet-poor plasma. From the patient and a control collected as described for euglobulin lysis time.

Equipment

Plastic Petri dishes.

Method

To prepare the fibrin plate, dilute the fibrinogen in buffered saline to obtain a final concentration of 1.5 g/l. Pipette 10 ml of diluted fibrinogen into a Petri dish. Place it on a level tray. Add 0.5 ml of $CaCl_2$ and 0.2 ml of thrombin solution. Mix the contents by swirling quickly. The plate clots within 10 to 20 s; it must clot evenly to be suitable for the test. Leave the plate undisturbed for 20 min. The prepared plates can then be kept for 3 to 4 days at 4°C.

Carefully apply 30 µl of the euglobulin fraction, prepared as described in the previous test, to the surface of the plate. There is no need to cut a well. Place in an incubator at 37°C for 24 h. This preparation time can be shortened by the addition of exogenous plasminogen.[56]

Perform all tests (patient and control) in duplicate.

Results

Calculate the zone of lysis by measuring two diameters in mm at right angles to each other. Multiply the two values to obtain the approximate area of lysis in mm^2.

Normal range

Variable, but usually between 40 and 60 mm^2.

Interpretation

The area of lysis may be difficult to define because of incomplete lysis. Only areas of complete, clear lysis should be measured. In other respects the interpretation is as for the euglobulin lysis time except that the levels of plasminogen and fibrinogen in the test plasma do not affect the result. The same problems in preparing the euglobulin fraction apply as does the necessity for a normal control.

VENOUS OCCLUSION TEST[57]

Principle

Localized venous occlusion of an arm for a standardized period of time is used as a stimulus for release of t-PA from the vessel wall. The original intention was that this would be a better measure of functional defects in fibrinolysis than a resting sample. Pre- and post-occlusion lysis times, using the above-described euglobulin lysis or the fibrin plate lysis tests, are measured. In normal subjects, fibrinolysis is greatly enhanced by occlusion. However, given the problems associated with global assays of fibrinolysis it seems preferable to perform specific measurements of t-PA pre- and post-occlusion.

Method

Withdraw blood from the arm to be tested without stasis, place it in a citrate-containing tube and keep in an ice-bath. Inflate the sphygmomanometer cuff to a pressure midway between the systolic and diastolic pressure. Leave the inflated cuff on for 10 min. Take a sample of venous blood from below the cuff immediately before deflation and place on ice. Measure the lysis in both samples, as described previously. This test is uncomfortable and some patients may not be able to tolerate as much as 10 min occlusion. Petechiae are commonly seen after the test is completed.

Results

The post-occlusion lysis times should be shorter than the pre-occlusion times. Shortening by at least 30 min is found in most normal subjects.

Interpretation

Failure to enhance lysis is found in some cases of recurrent venous thrombosis, in obese people and after surgery, trauma or severe illness and in Behçet's syndrome.[55,57] It may also be due to a failure to release the activator because insufficient pressure was applied or the occlusion time was too short. Normal people vary in the degree of response: 'good' responders increase the concentration of t-PA by three- to four-fold, whereas 'poor' responders may consistently show only a very slight enhancement of fibrinolysis even with longer occlusion times. When comparing plasma levels of proteins pre- and post-occlusion, an adjustment for changes in haematocrit may be required.[58] The effect of the venous occlusion test and the levels of t-PA are very variable over time.[59,60]

TISSUE PLASMINOGEN ACTIVATOR AMIDOLYTIC ASSAY[61,62]

Principle

Different amidolytic assays for t-PA have been described. One relies on the activation of purified plasminogen to plasmin in the presence of fibrinogen fragments which stimulate the t-PA activity in the test plasma. The plasmin is measured using a specific chromogenic substrate. In the second method, t-PA is captured on specific antibodies bound to a solid phase matrix such as a microtitre plate; the various plasma inhibitors of t-PA and plasmin are washed away, plasminogen is added together with a stimulator of t-PA activity, and the plasmin produced measured with chromogenic substrates. Alternatively, chromogenic substrates specific for t-PA may be used, but there are specificity problems, especially in the plasma assays.

Interpretation

t-PA is secreted into plasma in its active form but rapidly complexes with its principal inhibitor PAI-1. The amount of active t-PA in the plasma is a result of this equilibrium and represents only a small fraction of the total (antigenic) t-PA. This process continues after blood sampling unless taken into appropriate acidic anticoagulant pH 6, e.g. Stabilyte tubes (Biopool) and processed rapidly. t-PA can also be measured by ELISA using monoclonal antibodies on microtitre plates, Although this closely parallels the PAI-1 concentration and says little about the proportion of free, active t-PA, it has been found to have a predictive effect in patients with angina.[49] The t-PA levels have a very large number of disease associations.[63]

PLASMINOGEN ACTIVATOR INHIBITOR ASSAY

Principle

A fixed amount of t-PA is added in excess to undiluted plasma. Part of it rapidly complexes with the t-PA inhibitor (PAI). Plasminogen in plasma is then activated into plasmin by the residual, uncomplexed t-PA. The amount of plasmin formed is directly proportional to the residual t-PA activity and inversely proportional to the PAI activity of the sample. The amount of plasmin generated is measured using a plasmin-specific substrate.

Reagents are available in kit form and the manufacturer's instructions must be closely followed. The normal range is as yet poorly defined, and each laboratory should establish its own range until reliable normal values become available.

The time of sampling must be standardized. Early morning (7 a.m.) samples have much greater levels of activity then those later in the day. Sample processing is extremely important as PAI leaks from platelets in sampled blood and PAI-1 in plasma rapidly converts to a latent (inactive) form. An ELISA assay is also available to measure the total PAI-1 which is present.

PLASMINOGEN ACTIVATOR INHIBITOR ANTIGEN ASSAY

Principle

Microplate wells coated with an anti-PAI-1 monoclonal antibody are incubated with samples and standards. PAI-1 present in the samples and standards is bound to the solid phase during this incubation. Unbound substances are then removed by washing. An enzyme-labelled anti-PAI-1 monoclonal antibody (conjugate) is added. The conjugate will bind to the antibody–antigen complexes formed in the previous incubation. Unbound conjugate is then removed by washing. Finally enzyme substrate is added. The action of the bound enzyme on the substrate produces a blue colour which turns yellow after stopping the reaction with acid. The absorbances are read in a microplate reader at 450 nm. The amount of colour is proportional to the concentration of PAI-1. The assay is specific for total PAI-1, including both free and complexed forms.

Specimen collection

Blood should be collected into CTAD tubes (CTAD is a buffered tri-sodium citrate solution with theophylline, adenosine and dipyridamole), Vacutainer coagulation tubes with CTAD (Becton-Dickinson) or Diatube H (Stago) to stabilize and immediately platelets cooled on ice. Samples can be stored on ice for up to 7 h in the collection tubes. If the sample is not tested immediately, it should be separated and frozen as soon as possible.

Reagents and method

Available in kit form based on an ELISA (Chromogenix).

Normal range

Usually 11–69 ng/mL. However, each laboratory should establish its own normal range.

PLASMIN INHIBITOR (ANTIPLASMIN) AMIDOLYTIC ASSAY

Principle

Plasma dilutions are incubated with excess plasmin, a proportion of which will be inhibited by antiplasmins. The residual, uninhibited plasmin is measured using a specific chromogenic substrate. α_2-antiplasmin is the major circulating inhibitor of plasmin and forms complexes much faster than other inhibitors: if the reaction times are short, the assay effectively measures α_2-antiplasmin only.

Different commercial kits are available containing all the necessary reagents. The manufacturer's instructions should be carefully followed. Specificity is achieved by keeping the reaction times short. Care is required when aliquoting the plasmin solution which has a high viscosity owing to its glycerol content. Note that plasmin bound to α_2-macroglobulin may escape inhibition, thus underestimating inhibitor activity.

The usual normal range is between 0.80 and 1.20 u/ml. Congenital α_2-antiplasmin deficiency is associated with a severe bleeding tendency. A reduced concentration is also found in liver disease, DIC and during thrombolytic therapy. α_2-antiplasmin increases with age and is higher in Caucasians than in Africans.

INVESTIGATION OF PLATELET 'HYPERREACTIVITY' AND ACTIVATION

Platelets may be more reactive than normal as a consequence of in-vivo activation by thrombin or non-endothelial surfaces, such as prosthetic valves or Dacron grafts. This can sometimes be detected by a lowered threshold (increased sensitivity) for aggregating agents. Because there is considerable variation in response to aggregating agents in normal people, attempts to show platelet hyper-aggregability are rarely successful and the results are frequently inconsistent. Spontaneous aggregation of platelets in the blood can also be demonstrated.[64]

Platelets which have formed a part of a platelet thrombus and have been released into the circulation may show a measurable decrease in aggregability owing to a loss of some of the granular content. The released contents can be measured in plasma: the α-granule proteins, β-thromboglobulin (β-TG) and platelet factor 4 (PF4) are the constituents most commonly measured. Shortened platelet survival using [111]Indium-labelled platelets can also be used as a marker of platelet activation by a thrombotic process (see p. 334).

β-THROMBOGLOBULIN AND PLATELET FACTOR 4 ASSAYS

Principle

ELISA and RIA methods are available for the measurement of these proteins using specific antisera. In the former, a double antibody sandwich technique is used, in which the surface of a tube or microplate is coated with antibody against β-TG or PF4, and plasma is added. Protein is then bound to the antibody, and may be detected by the binding of a second antibody carrying an enzyme tag. In the RIA methods, there is competition between β-TG or PF4 from the test sample and radiolabelled (usually ^{125}I) tracer protein for binding to a specific antibody. A high plasma concentration of the protein released from the platelets displaces the tracer from the immune complex.

Sample collection

Blood has to be collected and handled carefully to avoid artefactual release of β-TG and PF4 from the platelets. Samples are collected from free-flowing blood, drawn without venous stasis, and the first 2–3 ml discarded. The blood is immediately added to a tube chilled in a beaker filled with melting ice, which contains a special mixture of inhibitors of platelet activation, as well as calcium chelators. Plasma must be separated strictly at 4°C.

Reagents and method

Sample collection tubes and reagents are provided with the commercial kits used for the two tests. It is important to follow the manufacturer's instructions carefully. The calculation of results depends on whether an ELISA or a RIA method is used.

Interpretation

The normal concentration of β-TG is less than 50 ng/ml and that of PF4 less than 10 ng/ml.

Falsely high results may be encountered in RIA methods if diagnostic isotope techniques (such as leg scanning for thrombosis using ^{125}I fibrinogen) have been used on the patient. The tests cannot be performed for a week or so after the scanning or until ^{125}I is cleared from the patient's plasma.

PF4 is rapidly cleared from plasma by the vascular endothelium; it may be displaced from the endothelial binding by heparin. Thus a high PF4 concentration may be found in patients receiving heparin. β-TG is cleared from plasma by the kidney, and its concentration is commonly high in renal failure. In patients without these clinical problems, both proteins should be measured in order to distinguish in-vivo release from an in-vitro artefact. With in-vivo activation of platelets, the plasma concentration of both proteins rises, but the concentration of β-TG remains much higher owing to the rapid endothelial clearance of PF4. The ratio of β-TG to PF4 is usually greater than 5:1. If venepuncture has been difficult or sample handling inadequate, in-vitro platelet release occurs and the concentration of both proteins is high (ratio less than 2:1). Overall the problems with these tests make them of doubtful utility.[48]

PLATELET ACTIVATION: FLOW CYTOMETRY

The problems associated with previous tests of platelet activation have been circumvented to some extent by the application of flow cytometric analysis of platelets in whole blood samples.

Principle

The activation of platelets is associated with the appearance of new antigenic determinants on the platelet surface. Some of these are molecules present in platelet granules brought to the surface during degranulation (e.g. CD62) and others are new conformations of existing molecules (e.g. GpIIbIIIa). These can by detected using fluorescein-conjugated antibodies and the degree of expression quantified by flow cytometry. This gives a measure of platelet activation with a much greater degree of sensitivity than PF4 or β-TG estimation. A number of alternative surface molecules are available (Table 17.1). These tests have not yet entered routine laboratory practice but are proving increasingly useful in research.[65,66]

An alternative approach is offered by the new PFA-100 (see p. 428) in which short closure times may be indicative of platelet hyperractivity and/or hyperreactive vWF species.

Table 17.1 Indicators of platelet activation detectable by flow cytometry

Name	CD designation	Comment
GpIb, IX, V	CD42	Decreases
GpIIbIIIa	CD41	Increases
Phosphatidyl serine	–	Increases Detected by Annexin V binding
Lysosomal Integral membrane protein (gp53, granulophysin)	CD63	Indicates lysosomal degranulation
P-selectin	CD62	Indicates α granule release
Fibrinogen	–	Surface bound fibrinogen increases
IIbIIIa activation	–	Conformation change in IIbIIIa produced by activation, detected by PAC-1 antibody

HOMOCYSTEINE[67]

Following the observation that patients with homocystinuria have venous and arterial thromboses with accelerated vascular damage, there has been considerable interest in patients with less marked elevation of plasma homocysteine (hyper-homocystinaemia). This has been shown to have an association with arterial and venous thrombosis. Until recently, homocysteine has been measured by high-performance liquid chromatography or mass spectroscopy but an ELISA-based assay is now available which allows it to fit more easily into coagulation laboratory practice. In order to standardize study results, homocysteine is either measured while fasting or after a methionine load. Rapid processing of samples is required as homocysteine quickly leaches out of red blood cells.

MARKERS OF COAGULATION ACTIVATION

A number of commercial kits are now available for measuring molecules produced by coagulation activation.

Principle

The activation of many proteins active in coagulation is mediated by proteolytic cleavage with the release of small peptides: activation peptides. The most frequently measured of these is prothrombin fragment 1 + 2 which is released when prothrombin is converted to thrombin. It has an appreciable half-life of approximately 45 min which allows a measurable concentration to accumulate in plasma and provides an indication of the rate at which thrombin is being generated.

An alternative is to measure the concentration of thrombin–antithrombin (TAT) complexes which provides similar information. Plasmin–antiplasmin complexes provide corresponding information about fibrinolysis. These can all be measured using commercially available ELISA kits but are not used routinely and are not required for normal diagnostic work.[68] Other tests such as fibrinopeptide A require exceptional care and the use of special anticoagulants to prevent in-vitro activation of the sample.

ACTIVATED FACTOR VIIa

As discussed in Chapter 16, factor VIIa is thought to be the physiological initiator of coagulation in vivo and is therefore a potentially important thrombogenic factor. The majority of factor VII circulates in its inactive, zymogen form but approximately 1% is activated (factor VIIa). Factor VIIa has an unusually long half-life in plasma of approximately 2.5 h which helps explain this level and makes its measurement possible.

Principle[69]

The assay is based on the availability of recombinant soluble tissue factor which functions as a co-factor for factor VIIa but does not support conversion of factor VII to factor VIIa. The clotting time after addition of soluble tissue factor is thus dependent on the amount of factor VIIa in the test sample. The test is performed on a dilution of the test plasma in factor VII deficient plasma to improve specificity. A standard curve is produced using purified factor VIIa.

Interpretation

The clinical utility of factor VIIa assays is not established; however, elevated levels have been found in some thrombotic disorders such as diabetes mellitus and have been implicated as a predictor of ischaemic heart events. Reduced levels are found in patients with factor IX but not factor VIII deficiency.

REFERENCES

1 British Committee for Standards in Haematology 1990 Guidelines on the investigation and management of thrombophilia. Journal of Clinical Pathology 43:703–709.

2 Greaves M 1999 Antiphospholipid antibodies and thrombosis. Lancet 353:1348–1353.

3 Brandt JT, Barna LK, Triplett DA 1995 Laboratory identification of lupus anticoagulants: results of the Second International Workshop for Identification of Lupus Anticoagulants. Thrombosis and Haemostasis 74:1597–1603.

4 British Committee for Standards in Haematology 2000 Guidelines on the investigation and management of the antiphospholipid syndrome. British Journal of Haematology 109:704–715.

5 Exner T, Rickard KA, Kronenberg H 1978 A sensitive test demonstrating lupus anticoagulant and its behavioural patterns. British Journal of Haematology 40:143–151.

6 Thiagarajan P, Pengo V, Shapiro SS 1986 The use of the dilute Russell viper venom time for the diagnosis of lupus anticoagulants. Blood 68:869–874.

7 Lawrie AS, Mackie IJ, Purdy G, et al 1999 The sensitivity and specificity of commercial reagents for the detection of lupus anticoagulant show marked differences in performance between photo-optical and mechanical coagulometers. Thrombosis and Haemostasis 81:758–762.

8 Arnout J, Vanrusselt M, Huybrechts E, et al 1994 Optimization of the dilute prothrombin time for the detection of the lupus anticoagulant by use of a recombinant tissue thromboplastin. British Journal of Haematology 87:94–99.

9 Hoagland LE, Triplett DA, Peng F, et al 1996 APC-resistance as measured by a Textarin time assay: comparison to the APTT-based method. Thrombosis Research 83:363–373.

10 Jennings I, Kitchen S, Woods TA, et al 1997 Potentially clinically important inaccuracies in testing for the lupus anticoagulant: an analysis of results from three surveys of the UK National External Quality Assessment Scheme (NEQAS) for Blood Coagulation. Thrombosis and Haemostasis 77:934–937.

11 Triplett DA 1996 Antiphospholipid-protein antibodies: clinical use of laboratory test results (identification, predictive value, treatment). Haemostasis 26(Suppl 4):358–367.

12 Kandiah DA, Krilis SA 1996 Laboratory detection of antiphospholipid antibodies. Lupus 5:160–162.

13 Wright SD, Tuddenham EG 1994 Thrombophilia. Myeloproliferative and metabolic causes. Baillière's Clinical Haematology 7:591–635.

14 Lane DA, Mannucci P, Bauer K, et al 1996 Inherited thrombophilia: part 1. Thrombosis and Haemostasis 76:651–662.

15 Lane DA, Mannucci P, Bauer K, et al 1996 Inhertied thrombophilia: part 2. Thrombosis and Haemostasis 76:824–834.

16 Tollefsen DM 1990 Laboratory diagnosis of antithrombin and heparin cofactor II deficiency. Seminars in Thrombosis and Haemostasis 16:162–168.

17 van Boven HH, Lane DA 1997 Antithrombin and its inherited deficiency states. Seminars in Hematology 34:188–204.

18 Bertina RM 1990 Specificity of protein C and protein S assays. Ricerca in Clinica E in Laboratorio 20:127–138.

19 Marlar RA, Neumann A 1990 Neonatal purpura fulminans due to homozygous protein C or protein S deficiencies. Seminars in Thrombosis and Haemostasis 16:299–309.

20 Mackie IJ, Gallimore M, Machin SJ 1992 Contact factor proteases and the complexes formed with alpha 2-macroglobulin can interfere in protein C assays by cleaving amidolytic substrates. Blood Coagulation and Fibrinolysis 3:589–595.

21 Jones DW, Mackie IJ, Winter M, et al 1991 Detection of protein C deficiency during oral anticoagulant therapy – use of the protein C:factor VII ratio. Blood Coagulation and Fibrinolysis 2:407–411.

22 Van Wijnen M, Stam JG, Chang GT, et al. 1998 Characterization of mini-protein S, a recombinant variant of protein S that lacks the sex hormone binding globulin-like domain. Biochemical Journal 330:389–396.

23 van Wijnen M, van't Veer C, Meijers JC, et al 1998 A plasma coagulation assay for an activated protein C-independent anticoagulant activity of protein S. Thrombosis and Haemostasis 80:930–935.

24 Comp PC, Doray D, Patton D, et al 1986 An abnormal plasma distribution of protein S occurs in functional protein S deficiency. Blood 67:504–508.

25 Aillaud MF, Pouymayou K, Brunet D, et al 1996 New direct assay of free protein S antigen applied to diagnosis of protein S deficiency. Thrombosis and Haemostasis 75:283–285.

26 Simmonds RE, Zoller B, Ireland H et al 1997 Genetic and phenotypic analysis of a large (122 member) protein S deficient kindred provides an explanation for the co-existence of type I and type III plasma phenotypes. Blood 89:4364–4370.

27 Zoller B, Garcia dFP, Dahlback B 1995 Evaluation of the relationship between protein S and C4b-binding protein isoforms in hereditary protein S deficiency demonstrating type I and type III deficiencies to be phenotypic variants of the same genetic disease. Blood 85:3524–3531.

28 Lawrie AS, Lloyd ME, Mohamed F, et al 1995 Assay of protein S in systemic lupus erythematosus. Blood Coagulation and Fibrinolysis 6:322–324.

29 D'Angelo A, Vigano D'Angelo S, Esmon CT, et al 1988 Acquired deficiencies of protein S. Protein S activity during oral anticoagulation, in liver disease,

and in disseminated intravascular coagulation. Journal of Clinical Investigation 81:1445–1454.

30 Levin M, Eley BS, Louis J, et al 1995 Postinfectious purpura fulminans caused by an autoantibody directed against protein S. Journal of Pediatrics 127:355–363.

31 Gari M, Falkon L, Urrutia T, et al 1994 The influence of low protein S plasma levels in young women, on the definition of normal range. Thrombosis Research 73:149–152.

32 Faioni EM, Valsecchi C, Palla A, et al 1997 Free protein S deficiency is a risk factor for venous thrombosis. Thrombosis and Haemostasis 78:1343–1346.

33 Garcia de Frutos P, Alim RI, Hardig Y, et al 1994 Differential regulation of alpha and beta chains of C4b-binding protein during acute-phase response resulting in stable plasma levels of free anticoagulant protein S. Blood 84:815–822.

34 Dahlback B, Carlsson M, Svensson PJ 1993 Familial thrombophilia due to a previously unrecognized mechanism characterized by poor anticoagulant response to activated protein C: prediction of a cofactor to activated protein C [see comments]. Proceedings of the National Academy of Sciences of the USA 90:1004–1008.

35 Bertina RM 1997 Laboratory diagnosis of resistance to activated protein C (APC-resistance). Thrombosis and Haemostasis 78:478–482.

36 Laffan MA, Manning R 1996 The influence of factor VIII on measurement of activated protein C resistance. Blood Coagulation and Fibrinolysis 7:761–765.

37 Koster T, Rosendaal FR, de Ronde H, et al 1993 Venous thrombosis due to poor anticoagulant response to activated protein C: Leiden Thrombophilia Study. Lancet 342:1503–1506.

38 Ridker PM, Glynn RJ, Miletich JP, et al 1997 Age-specific incidence rates of venous thromboembolism among heterozygous carriers of factor V Leiden mutation. Annals of Internal Medicine 126:528–531.

39 de Visser MCH, Rosendaal FR, Bertina RM 1999 A reduced sensitivity for activated protein C in the absence of factor V Leiden increases the risk of venous thrombosis. Blood 93:1271–1276.

40 Poort S, Rosendaal F, Reitsma P, et al 1996 A common genetic variation in the 3′ untranslated region of the prothrombin gene is associated with elevated plasma prothrombin levels and an increase in venous thrombosis. Blood 88:3698–3703.

41 Koster T, Blann A, Briet E, et al 1995 Role of clotting factor VIII in effect of von Willebrand factor on occurrence of deep vein thrombosis. Lancet 345:152–155.

42 Meijers JC, Tekelenburg WL, Bouma BN, et al 2000 High levels of coagulation factor XI as a risk factor for venous thrombosis. New England Journal of Medicine 342:696–701.

43 O'Donnell J, Tuddenham EG, Manning R, et al 1997 High prevalence of elevated factor VIII levels in patients referred for thrombophilia screening: role of increased synthesis and relationship to the acute phase reaction. Thrombosis and Haemostasis 77:825–882.

44 Lind B, Thorsen S 1999 A novel missense mutation in the human plasmin inhibitor (alpha2-antiplasmin) gene associated with a bleeding tendency. British Journal of Haematology 107:317–322.

45 Fay WP, Parker AC, Condrey LR, et al 1997 Human plasminogen activator inhibitor-1 (PAI-1) deficiency: characterization of a large kindred with a null mutation in the PAI-1 gene. Blood 90:204–208.

46 Lane D, Grant P 2000 Role of hemostatic gene polymorphisms in venous and arterial thrombotic disease. Blood 95:1517–1532.

47 Thompson SG, Kienast J, Pyke SD, et al 1995 Hemostatic factors and the risk of myocardial infarction or sudden death in patients with angina pectoris. European Concerted Action on Thrombosis and Disabilities Angina Pectoris Study Group. New England Journal of Medicine 332:635–641.

48 Pyke SD, Thompson SG, Buchwalsky R, et al 1993 Variability over time of haemostatic and other cardiovascular risk factors in patients suffering from angina pectoris. ECAT Angina Pectoris Study Group. Thrombosis and Haemostasis 70:743–746.

49 Juhan VI, Pyke SD, Alessi MC, et al 1996 Fibrinolytic factors and the risk of myocardial infarction or sudden death in patients with angina pectoris. ECAT Study Group. European Concerted Action on Thrombosis and Disabilities. Circulation 94:2057–2063.

50 Ridker PM, Vaughan DE, Stampfer MJ, et al 1993 Endogenous tissue-type plasminogen activator and risk of myocardial infarction. Lancet 341:1165–1168.

51 Kluft C, Meijer P 1996 Update 1996: Blood collection and handling procedures for assessment of plasminogen activators and inhibitors (Leiden fibrinolysis workshop). Fibrinolysis 10 (supplement 2):171–179.

52 Dolan G, Greaves M, Cooper P, et al 1988 Thrombovascular disease and familial plasminogen deficiency: a report of three kindreds. British Journal of Haematology 70:417–421.

53 Heijboer H, Brandjes DP, Buller HR, et al 1990 Deficiencies of coagulation-inhibiting and fibrinolytic proteins in outpatients with deep-vein thrombosis [see comments]. New England Journal of Medicine 323:1512–1516.

54 Wiman B, Chmielewska J 1985 A novel fast inhibitor to tissue plasminogen activator in plasma, which may be of great pathophysiological significance. Scandinavian Journal of Clinical and Laboratory Investigation Supplement 177:43–47.

55 Nilsson IM, Ljungner H, Tengborn L 1985 Two different mechanisms in patients with venous thrombosis and defective fibrinolysis: low concentration of plasminogen activator or increased concentration of plasminogen activator inhibitor. British Medical Journal 290:1453–1456.

56 Marsh NA, Gaffney PJ 1977 The rapid fibrin plate – a method for plasminogen activator assay. Thrombosis and Haemostasis 38:545–551.

57 Juhan VI, Valadier J, Alessi MC, et al 1987 Deficient t-PA release and elevated PA inhibitor levels in patients with spontaneous or recurrent deep venous thrombosis. Thrombosis and Haemostasis 57:67–72.

58 Wieczorek I, Ludlam CA, MacGregor I 1993 Venous occlusion does not release von Willebrand factor, factor VIII or PAI-1 from endothelial cells – the importance of consensus on the use of correction factors for haemoconcentration. Thrombosis and Haemostasis 69:91–93.

59 Marckmann P, Sandstrom B, Jespersen J 1992 The variability of and associations between measures of blood coagulation, fibrinolysis and blood lipids. Atherosclerosis 96:235–244.

60 Stegnar M, Mavri A 1995 Reproducibility of fibrinolytic response to venous occlusion in healthy subjects. Thrombosis and Haemostasis 73:453–457.

61 Mahmoud M, Gaffney PJ 1985 Bioimmunoassay (BIA) of tissue plasminogen activator (t-PA) and its specific inhibitor (t-PA/INH). Thrombosis and Haemostasis 53:356–359.

62 Holvoet P, Cleemput H, Collen D 1985 Assay of human tissue-type plasminogen activator (t-PA) with an enzyme-linked immunosorbent assay (ELISA) based on three murine monoclonal antibodies to t-PA. Thrombosis and Haemostasis 54:684–687.

63 Collen D 1999 The plasminogen (fibrinolytic) system. Thrombosis and Haemostasis 82:259–270.

64 Wu KK, Hoak JC 1976 Spontaneous platelet aggregation in arterial insufficiency: mechanisms and implications. Thrombosis and Haemostasis 35:702–711.

65 Abrams CS, Ellison N, Budzynski AZ, et al 1990 Direct detection of activated platelets and platelet-derived microparticles in humans. Blood 75:128–138.

66 Michelson AD 1996 Flow cytometry: a clinical test of platelet function. Blood 87:4925–4936.

67 D'Angelo A, Selhub J 1997 Homocysteine and thrombotic disease. Blood 90:1–11.

68 Bauer KA, Rosenberg RD 1994 Thrombophilia: Activation markers of coagulation. Baillière's Clinical Haematology 7:523–540.

69 Morrissey JH, Macik BG, Neuenschwander PF, et al 1993 Quantitation of activated factor VII levels in plasma using a tissue factor mutant selectively deficient in promoting factor VII activation. Blood 81:734–744.

18

Laboratory control of anticoagulant, thrombolytic and anti-platelet therapy

M.A. Laffan & R.A. Manning

Anticoagulant and antithrombotic therapy is given in various doses to prevent formation or propagation of thrombus. Apart from those that act via fibrinolysis, anticoagulant drugs have little if any effect on an already formed thrombus. There are five main classes of drugs that require consideration:

1. Oral anticoagulants; coumarins and indanediones, which act by interfering with the γ-carboxylation step in the synthesis of the vitamin-K-dependent factors (see p. 346).
2. Heparin and heparinoids (low molecular weight and synthetic compounds) which have a complex action on haemostasis, the main effect being the potentiation and acceleration of the effect of antithrombin on thrombin and factor Xa.
3. Defibrinating agents such as ancrod (Arvin) and Reptilase which induce hypocoagulability by the removal of fibrinogen from the blood.
4. Hirudin (natural or recombinant) which is a highly specific inhibitor of thrombin and thus a potent anticoagulant. New orally active thrombin inhibitors are now under development.
5. Antiplatelet drugs such as aspirin, non-steroidal anti-inflammatory drugs, dipyridamole and clopidogrel.

ORAL ANTICOAGULANT TREATMENT[1]

It is not possible to produce a therapeutic derangement of haemostasis without increasing the risk of haemorrhage. The purpose of laboratory control is to maintain a level of hypocoagulability which effectively minimizes the combined risks of haemorrhage and thrombosis: the therapeutic range. Individual responses to oral anticoagulant treatment are extremely variable and so must be regularly and frequently controlled by laboratory tests to ensure that the anticoagulant effect remains within the therapeutic range.

Selection of patients

Haemostasis is not usually investigated before starting oral anticoagulant treatment but it is advisable to perform the first-line coagulation screen (PT, APTT, TT and platelet count) before commencing treatment. An abnormality of these tests must be investigated, as a contra-indication to the use of oral anticoagulants may be revealed. History and examination should be used to ensure that no local or general haemorrhagic diathesis exists.

Methods used for the laboratory control of oral anticoagulant treatment

The one-stage prothrombin time of Quick is the most commonly used test. Originally, lack of standardization of the thromboplastin preparations and methods of expressing the PT results led to great discrepancies in the reported results and hence also in anticoagulant dosage. The use of the International Sensitivity Index (ISI) to assess the sensitivity of any given thromboplastin, and the use of the International Normalized Ratio (INR) to report the results have minimized these difficulties and greatly improved uniformity of anticoagulation and interpretation throughout the world.

Chromogenic substrates have been used for the control of anticoagulant treatment in factor X, VII or II assays. Although it is possible to use such a single factor measurement, it must be remembered that the one-stage PT measures the effect of three vitamin-K-dependent factors (factors VII, X and II) and is also affected by the presence of PIVKAs* or the acarboxy forms of vitamin-K-dependent factors. It thus gives a better assessment of the situation in vivo.

Chromogenic substrate assays may be of use where the presence of an inhibitor invalidates the PT and coagulation-based assays.

The Thrombotest of Owren and **the prothrombin and proconvertin (P & P) method** of **Owren and Aas** have been described in previous editions of this book. They are not now recommended for oral anticoagulant control.

STANDARDIZATION OF ORAL ANTICOAGULANT TREATMENT

Standardization of oral anticoagulant therapy comprises the following steps:

1. A thromboplastin is chosen and its ISI determined by comparison with a reference thromboplastin.

2. The log mean normal PT is determined for that thromboplastin.

3. PTs are performed on patient samples and the results converted to an INR.

Reference thromboplastins (rabbit and bovine) are available as WHO Reference Preparations or certified reference materials from the European Union Bureau of Reference (BCR) (see p. 608). All the reference preparations have been calibrated in terms of a primary WHO human brain thromboplastin established in 1967 which is no longer in existence.

The following terms are employed in the calibration procedure which is described below:

International Sensitivity Index[2] This is the slope of the calibration line obtained when the prothrombin times obtained with the reference preparation are plotted on the vertical axis of log-log paper and the prothrombin times obtained by the test thromboplastin are plotted on the horizontal axis. The same normal and anticoagulated patient's plasma samples are used for both sets of results.

International Normalized Ratio. This is the PT ratio which, by calculation, would have been obtained had the original primary, human reference thromboplastin been used to perform the PT.

CALIBRATION OF THROMBOPLASTINS[2]

Principle
The test thromboplastin must be calibrated against a reference thromboplastin of the same species (rabbit *v* rabbit, bovine *v* bovine). All reference preparations are calibrated in terms of the primary material of human origin and have an ISI which is assigned after a collaborative trial involving many laboratories from different countries.

Reagents
Normal citrated plasma. From 20 healthy donors.
Anticoagulated plasma. From 60 patients stabilized on oral anticoagulant treatment for at least 6 weeks.

The tests need not all be done at the same time but may be carried out on freshly collected samples on successive days.

---

*Proteins induced by vitamin K absence or antagonism.

Reference and test thromboplastins.

CaCl₂. 0.025 mol/l.

Method

Carry out PT tests as described on page 353. Allow the plasma and thromboplastin to warm up to 37°C for at least 2 min before mixing or adding CaCl₂. Test each plasma in duplicate with each of the two thromboplastins in the following order with minimum delay between tests:

	Reference thromboplastin	Test thromboplastin
Plasma 1	Test 1	Test 2
	Test 4	Test 3
Plasma 2	Test 5	Test 6
	Test 8	Test 7 etc.

Record the mean time for each plasma. If there is a discrepancy of more than 10% in the clotting times between duplicates, repeat the test on that plasma.

Calibration

Plot the PTs on log-log graph paper, with results using the reference preparation (y) on the vertical axis and results with the test thromboplastin (x) on the horizontal axis (Fig. 18.1). On arithmetic graph paper it is necessary to plot the logarithms of the PTs (Fig. 18.2). The relationship between the two thromboplastins is determined by the slope of the line (b). A rough estimate of the slope can be obtained as shown in Figure 18.1 and 18.2; this can then be used to obtain an approximation of the ISI of the test thromboplastin.

Whenever possible, however, to obtain a reliable measurement, the following more complicated calculation should be used instead.

Calculation of ISI

The natural logarithms of the PTs obtained using the reference thromboplastin and the test thromboplastin are called y_i and x_i respectively where $i = 1,2,3 \dots N$ for N pairs of results. The following designations are then made:

x_0 and y_0 are the arithmetic means of the N values of x_i and y_i respectively.
Q_1 and Q_2 are the sums of the squares of $(x_i - x_0)$ and $(y_i - y_0)$ respectively.

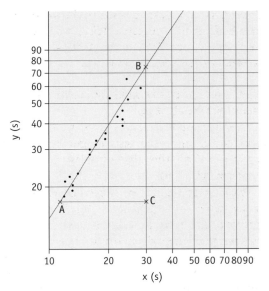

Fig. 18.1 Calibration of thromboplastin. The PTs (in seconds) with the test thromboplastin are plotted on the horizontal axis (x) and with the reference thromboplastin on the vertical axis (y) on double log graph paper. The best-fit line is drawn by eye, and the slope is obtained as follows: Points (a) and (b) are marked on the line just below the lowest recorded PT and just above the longest recorded PT, respectively, (c) is a point where a horizontal line through (a) and a vertical through (b) meet. The distance between (b) and (c) is measured accurately in mm. The slope

$$b = \frac{[B \text{ to } C]}{[A \text{ to } C]}.$$ In this example B to C = 55 mm,

A to C = 35 mm, $b = 55/35 = 1.57$. The ISI of the reference thromboplastin was 1.11. Therefore, the ISI of the test thromboplastin = $1.11 \times 1.57 = 1.74$.

P is the sum of their products $\Sigma(x_i - x_0)(y_i - y_0)$

$$E = (Q_2 - Q_1)^2 + 4P^2$$

$$\text{and } b = \frac{Q_2 - Q_1 + E^{1/2}}{2P}$$

where b is the slope of the graph. The ISI of the preparation under test (ISI_t) is then given by:

$$ISI_t = ISI_{IRP} \times b$$

(IRP = International Reference Preparation)

LOCAL CALIBRATION

Although the ISI system has been very effective in standardizing anticoagulant control and improving

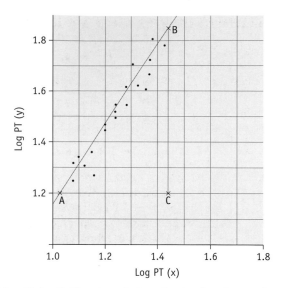

Fig. 18.2 Calibration of thromboplastin. The PTs (in seconds) are converted to their logarithms which are plotted on arithmetic graph paper. The slope is calculated as in Figure 18.1. In this example, A to C = 42 mm, B to C = 65 mm, *b* = 65/42 = 1.54. Therefore, ISI = 1.11 × 1.54 = 1.71.

INR = PT ratio obtained using the test thromboplastin to the power of the ISI of the test reagent.

The PT ratio is calculated using the patient's test result and the log mean normal prothrombin time (LMNPT) from 20 normal donors,

i.e. INR = (PT patient/LMNPT)^{ISI}

For example, a ratio of 2.5 using a thromboplastin with ISI of 1.4 can be calculated from the formula to be: $2.5^{1.4} = 3.61$
which is either read from a logarithmic table or calculated on an electronic calculator.

The LMNPT is the logarithmic mean normal prothrombin time. (i.e. $e^{(\Sigma \ln PT)/N}$). In this way, the level of anticoagulation in all plasma samples can be compared and a meaningful therapeutic range established regardless of the thromboplastin used.

agreement between laboratories, it is not perfect. One problem is that the ISI of a thromboplastin may vary according to the coagulometer used and even with different models of the same instrument. To circumvent this, a system of local calibration has been suggested. In this system, a set of plasmas with an assigned INR are tested with the local thromboplastin-machine combination. These results are used to generate a standard curve from which the INRs of further test plasmas can be read by interpolation. In effect, the ISI of the system is determined in a reverse fashion.[3,4]

DETERMINATION OF THE INR

It is essential to use a thromboplastin whose ISI has been determined either by the commercial supplier or (preferably) according to a local, regional or national procedure. The PT result can then be expressed as an INR. Using the INR/ISI system, the patient's INR should be the same in any laboratory in the world. To ensure safety and uniformity of anticoagulation, the results should be reported as an INR, either alone or in parallel with the locally accepted method of reporting.

CAPILLARY REAGENT

Principle
Reagents are commercially available for monitoring the INR using samples of capillary blood. These are usually a mixture of thromboplastin, calcium and absorbed plasma so that when whole blood is added the reagent measures the overall clotting activity; it is sensitive to deficiency of factors II, VII and X. The reagents have an ISI assigned to them in the same way as individual thromboplastins and the INR is calculated from the PT ratio. These reagents are frequently used in anticoagulant clinics when a large number of INRs need to be performed rapidly and in point-of-care testing (p. 554).

THERAPEUTIC RANGE AND CHOICE OF THROMBOPLASTIN[1,5]

Several different authorities have now published recommended therapeutic ranges denoting the appropriate degree of anticoagulation in different clinical circumstances.[5] These are partly based on controlled clinical trials but to some extent also represent a consensus on practice that has emerged over many years.

The choice of thromboplastin greatly determines the accuracy with which anticoagulant control can be maintained. If the ISI of the thromboplastin is high, then a small change in PT represents a large change in the degree of anticoagulation. This affects the precision of the analysis and the coefficient of variation for the test increases with the ISI.

Moreover, the prothrombin ratio range becomes very small for any given range of INR. This is illustrated in Figure 18.3 and Table 18.1. For these reasons, it is strongly recommended that a thromboplastin with a low ISI (i.e. close to 1) is used.

MANAGEMENT OF OVER-ANTICOAGULATION

The approach to management of a patient whose INR exceeds the therapeutic range with or without bleeding is shown in Table 18.2.[5]

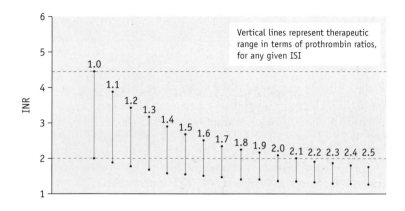

Fig. 18.3 The ratios obtained with thromboplastins with given ISI values equivalent to INR therapeutic range of 2.0–4.5. (Slightly modified, from Poller L 1987 Oral anticoagulant therapy. In: Bloom AL, Thomas DP (eds) Haemostasis and thrombosis, 2nd edn. Churchill Livingstone, Edinburgh with the permission of the editors and the publisher.)

Table 18.1 Therapeutic ranges equivalent to an INR of 2.0–4.0 using different commercial thromboplastins. (Modified from Poller L 1987 Oral anticoagulant therapy. In: Bloom AL, Thomas DP (eds) Haemostasis and thrombosis, 2nd edn. Churchill Livingstone, Edinburgh, p 870.)

Thromboplastin	ISI	Ratios equivalent to INR 2.0–4.0
Thrombotest	1.03	2.0–3.8
Thromborel	1.23	1.7–3.1
Dade FS	1.35	1.65–2.8
Simplastin	2.0	1.3–2.0
Boehringer	2.1	1.35–1.9
Ortho	2.3	1.3–1.8

ISI, International Sensitivity Index; INR, International Normalized Ratio.

Table 18.2 Recommendations for management of bleeding and excessive anticoagulation

3.0< INR <6.0 (target INR 2.5)	1. Reduce warfarin dose or stop
4.0< INR <6.0 (target INR 3.5)	2. Restart warfarin when INR <5.0
6.0< INR <8.0 No bleeding or minor bleeding	1. Stop warfarin 2. Restart when INR <5.0
INR >8.0 No bleeding or minor bleeding	1. Stop warfarin 2. Restart warfarin when INR <5.0 3. If other risk factors for bleeding give 0.5–2.5 mg of vitamin K (oral or IV)
Major bleeding	1. Stop warfarin 2. Give prothrombin complex concentrate 50 units/kg or FFP 15 ml/kg 3. Give 5 mg of vitamin K (oral or IV)

FFP, fresh-frozen plasma; INR, International Normalized Ratio.

HEPARIN TREATMENT

The anticoagulant action of heparin is primarily due to its ability to bind to antithrombin (AT), thereby accelerating and enhancing the latter's rate of inhibition of the major coagulation enzymes, i.e. factors IIa and Xa and to lesser extents IXa, XIa and XIIa. The two main effects of heparin, the AT and the anti-Xa effects, are differentially dependent on the size of the heparin molecule. The basic minimum sequence needed to obtain anticoagulant activity has been identified as a pentasaccharide unit. Of the molecules containing this pentasaccharide, those comprising less than 18 saccharide units and of molecular weight less than 5000 can only augment inhibitory activity of AT against Xa. In contrast, longer chains can augment AT activity as well by formation of a tertiary complex bridging both AT and thrombin molecules.

Hence, low molecular weight heparins (LMWH) which have an average molecular mass of 5000 Da have a ratio of anti-Xa to AT effect of 2–5 compared to that of unfractionated heparin (UFH) which is defined as 1. However, all heparin preparations are heterogeneous mixtures of molecules with different molecular weights and many do not contain the crucial pentasaccharide sequence. Heparin also produces some anticoagulant effect by promoting the release of tissue factor pathway inhibitor (TFPI) from the surface endothelium (see p. 345).

Selection of patients

It is advisable to perform the first-line tests of haemostasis as described in Chapter 16 before starting treatment. In the presence of a reduced platelet count or deranged coagulation, heparin may be contra-indicated or, if used, the dose must be reduced.

LABORATORY CONTROL OF HEPARIN TREATMENT[6]

The pharmacokinetics of heparins are extremely complicated, partly because of the variation in molecule size. Large molecules are cleared by a rapid saturable cellular mechanism and bind to numerous acute phase proteins such as vWF and fibronectin. Smaller molecules are cleared by a non-saturable renal route and bind less to plasma proteins. As a result therapeutic doses of UFH result in a variable degree of anticoagulation and require close monitoring (Table 18.3). The dose–response relationship is much more predictable for the LMWHs and most trials have not monitored therapy with these agents which are simply given on a units per kg basis.

Low-dose prophylactic therapy with either UFH or LMWH is given by subcutaneous injection and is usually not monitored. However,

Table 18.3 Tests used in the laboratory control of heparin treatment

Test	Advantages	Disadvantages
Whole blood clotting time	Simple, inexpensive, no equipment needed	Time-consuming, can only be carried out at the bedside, one at a time, insensitive to <0.4 iu, and to LMW heparins
APTT	Simple, many tests can be carried out in parallel	Not all reagents sensitive to heparin, insensitive to <0.2 iu and to LMW heparins, affected by variables other than heparin
TT	Simple, many tests can be carried out in parallel	Insensitive to <0.2 iu and to LMW heparins
Protamine neutralization	Sensitive to all concentrations	Time-consuming and insensitive to LMW heparins
Anti-Xa assays	Sensitive to all concentrations and to LMWT heparins	Expensive if commercial kits used; time-consuming if home-made reagents used

APTT, activated partial thromboplastin time; LMW, low molecular weight; TT, thrombin time.

prophylactic treatment and therapeutic LMWH may be monitored in some circumstances when it is expected that pharmacokinetics may be altered such as during pregnancy and in renal failure. A blood sample is taken 2–4 h after subcutaneous injection to detect the peak heparin level. Some authors have also measured trough levels prior to injection.

Therapeutic treatment with UFH is given by continuous intravenous infusion and is usually monitored using the APTT which is repeated 6 h after every dose change. Rarely, therapeutic UFH is given twice daily by subcutaneous injection, in which case samples for testing should be taken at the midpoint between injections. Low-dose prophylactic heparin therapy and LMWH produce relatively little effect on the APTT and if monitoring is required, a specific heparin assay must be used. The result will then be reported as heparin activity in iu/ml. In general, unless stated otherwise, this is measured as anti-Xa activity. An international standard for LMWH is now available.[7] The dose–response curve of the thrombin time is too steep to make it useful for monitoring heparin therapy. However, it is very sensitive to the presence of UFH and is a useful laboratory indicator of its presence.

ACTIVATED PARTIAL THROMBOPLASTIN TIME FOR HEPARIN MONITORING

Principle
The APTT is currently the most widely used test for monitoring UFH therapy.[6] It is very sensitive to heparin but has a number of shortcomings which must be kept in mind: first, different APTT reagents have different sensitivities to heparin. It is important to establish that the reagent in use has a linear relationship between clotting times and heparin concentration in the therapeutic range (0.3–0.7 iu/ml). An example of different responses is shown in Figure 18.4. The result is expressed as a ratio of the time obtained with that for the normal pool containing no heparin (often called 'the heparin ratio').

The second shortcoming of the APTT in the control of heparin treatment is that the APTT is affected by a number of variables not related to heparin. The most important of these are fibrinogen and factor VIII:C concentration and the presence of FDP. When these factors are abnormal

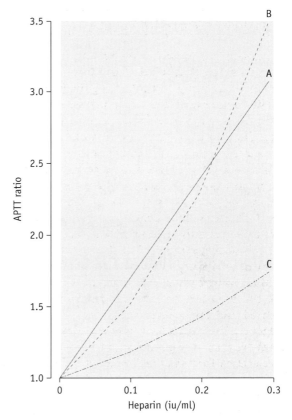

Fig. 18.4 APTT response to heparin added to plasma in vitro. APTT response expressed as ratio (APTT of heparinized plasma/APTT of plasma without heparin). Three different reagents and methods shown. (Slightly modified, from Thomson JM (ed) 1985 Blood coagulation and haemostasis. A practical guide. Churchill Livingstone, Edinburgh, p 370, with the permission of the editor and the publisher.)

there may be dissociation of the APTT and heparin level causing 'apparent heparin resistance'. In these circumstances, a heparin assay must be performed. Lastly, the use of the APTT may be rendered invalid by the presence of inhibitors, factor deficiency (including liver disease) or other coagulation-active drugs.

Reagents and method
The reagents and method are described on p. 354.

Therapeutic range
The therapeutic range for heparin is 0.3–0.7 iu/ml by anti-Xa assay and 0.2–0.4 units by protamine titration. The prolongation of the APTT achieved

with these concentrations varies between reagents according to the reagents and coagulometer used. The results may be expressed as clotting time in seconds or as a ratio. For the majority of sensitive reagents, ratios of 1.5–3.0 cover the therapeutic range but this must be determined for each reagent and, ideally, each batch of reagent. It is important that samples from patients treated with heparin are used for calibration as these give significantly different results from those obtained when normal plasma is 'spiked' with heparin. Regression analysis is used to determine the normal range and a better fit may be obtained using logarithmically transformed APTT values.

HEPARIN MONITORING AT THE BEDSIDE[8]

The whole blood activated clotting time (ACT) is routinely used to assess heparin effects during cardiac surgery. However, the ACT is not a specific assay for heparin and may be influenced by several other factors such as hypothermia, haemodilution and platelet dysfunction. For these reasons, the ACT may be misleading with regard to the proper administration of heparin and protamine.

Principle

The ACT is determined by using one of several different clotting cascade activators, such as kaolin or celite (diatomaceous earth activator), and a method of end-point detection such as optical or electromagnetic. No additional phospholipid is added.

ACT monitors include the Hemochron ACT monitors (International Technidyne, Inc., Edison, NJ), and the HemoTec Automated Coagulation Timer (HemoTec, Inc., Englewood, CO). The Hemochron ACT monitor uses 2.0 ml of whole blood in glass tubes with celite. The HemoTec ACT monitor uses 0.8 ml of whole blood in dual-chamber, high-range kaolin cartridges. The ACT is thus primarily a system with little laboratory involvement.

ANTI-Xa ASSAY FOR HEPARIN

Principle

Plasma anti-Xa activity owing to AT is enhanced by the addition of heparin, and either a coagulation or amidolytic (chromogenic) assay of anti-Xa activity can be adapted to measure this effect. A standard curve is constructed by adding varying amounts of heparin to a normal plasma pool which provides the source of the AT. A known amount of Xa is added and after incubation, the amount of Xa remaining is assayed by chromogenic or coagulation-based assay. A number of commercial kits such as Heptest and Hepaclot, as well as various kits based on chromogenic substrates, are in use and give linear and reproducible responses. A standard curve should be constructed that is appropriate for the level of heparin expected.

Chromogenic

The assay is performed as instructed with the kit. The concentration of heparin is read off a standard curve constructed according to the manufacturer's instructions.

CLOTTING
Principle

The anti-Xa activity of AT is enhanced by the addition of heparin. The inhibition of factor Xa by heparin is measured in a modified factor-X assay.

Reagents

Pooled normal plasma. From 20 normal donors.

Patient's plasma. Citrated platelet-poor plasma (PPP) should be collected between 2 and 4 h after the injection of heparin; it should be tested as soon as possible after the collection and kept at 4°C or on crushed ice until tested.

Buffer. Trisodium citrate 30 volumes, glyoxaline buffer (p. 352) 150 volumes, and 20% bovine albumin 1 volume.

Commercially prepared artificial factor-X-deficient plasma. Reconstitute according to instructions.

Platelet substitute. Mix equal volumes of factor-X-deficient plasma and platelet substitute. This is the working reagent and is kept at 37°C.

Factor Xa. Reconstitute as instructed by the manufacturer. Dilute further in the buffer to give a 1 in 100 dilution. Keep on crushed ice until used.

Heparin. 1000 iu/ml. Dilute in 9 g/l NaCl to 10 iu/ml. Ideally, the same batch of heparin as the patient is receiving should be used.

CaCl₂. 0.025 mol/l.

Table 18.4 Preparation of a standard curve for an anti-Xa assay

Reagent	Tube					
	1	2	3	4	5	6
Heparin (10 iu/ml)	0.05	0.10	0.15	0.20	0.25	0.30
Saline (ml)	0.95	0.90	0.85	0.80	0.75	0.70
Concentration of heparin (iu/ml)	0.5	1.0	1.5	2.0	2.5	3.0
Final conc. of heparin after addition to normal plasma pool	0.05	0.10	0.15	0.20	0.25	0.30

Method

A standard curve is constructed as shown in Table 18.4. Add 0.05 ml of each dilution to 0.45 ml of the normal plasma pool. This will give final concentrations of heparin from 0.05 to 0.30 iu/ml in 0.05 iu steps.

Pipette 0.3 ml of diluted factor Xa into a large glass tube at 37°C.

Add 0.1 ml of the first standard dilution. Start the stopwatch. At 1 min and 30 s exactly, transfer duplicate 0.1 ml volumes of the mixture into two tubes each containing 0.1 ml of pre-warmed CaCl$_2$.

At 2 min after sub-sampling, add 0.2 ml of the mixture of factor-X-deficient plasma and platelet substitute, start the stopwatch, mix and record the clotting time.

Repeat for each dilution of standard. The patient's sample is tested undiluted in pooled normal plasma if the clotting time is longer than the times used to construct the standard curve.

Calculation

Plot the clotting times against the heparin concentration on log-linear graph paper, with the clotting times on the linear axis. The concentration of heparin in the patient's sample can be read directly from the standard curve. It is multiplied by the dilution factor if necessary.

PROTAMINE NEUTRALIZATION ASSAY

Principle

This test is an extension of the TT, various amounts of protamine sulphate being added to the plasma before the addition of thrombin. When all the heparin present in plasma has been neutralized, the clotting time should become normal. The concentration of heparin in the plasma can be calculated from the amount of protamine sulphate required to produce this effect. The protamine neutralization test is used mainly to calculate the dose of protamine sulphate needed to neutralize circulating heparin after cardiopulmonary surgery and haemodialysis, but it is also used to control treatment or to calculate the dose of protamine to be administered if the patient needs rapid reversal of heparinization.

Reagents

Protamine sulphate. Prepare dilutions (0–50 mg/ml) in barbitone buffer, pH 7.4. Dilute 5 ml of protamine sulphate (10 g/l) 1 in 20 with buffer to give 1 dl of a stock solution containing 500 µg/ml. Then make working solutions to cover the range of 0–500 µg/ml in 50 µg steps from the stock solution by dilution with buffer. The solutions keep indefinitely at 4°C.

Thrombin. Dilute thrombin in barbitone buffer to a concentration of about 20 NIH units/ml. Adjust the concentration so that 0.1 ml of thrombin clots 0.2 ml of normal plasma at 37°C in 10 ± 1 s.

Keep the thrombin in a plastic tube in melting ice during the assay.

Plasma. Citrated PPP from the patient.

Method

Place 0.2 ml of test plasma and 20 µl of barbitone buffer in a glass tube kept in a water-bath at 37°C. Allow the mixture to warm and then add 0.1 ml of thrombin. Record the clotting time. If this is *c* 10 s, there is no demonstrable heparin in the plasma. If the thrombin time is prolonged, repeat the test using 20 µl of the 500 µg/ml protamine solution instead of buffer. Repeat the test if necessary, until a concentration of protamine is found which gives a clotting time of *c* 10 s.

Calculation

If 20 µl of 150 µg/ml protamine sulphate produce a normal TT (whereas the clotting time is prolonged with 100 µg/ml protamine), then the concentration of 15 µg of protamine is sufficient to neutralize the heparin in 1 ml of plasma. Assuming weight-for-weight neutralization, the patient's plasma contains 15 µg of heparin per ml or 1.5 iu, assuming that 1 mg of heparin is equivalent to 100 iu. This figure can be further converted to concentration of heparin per ml of whole blood by multiplying by 1–PCV.

In the above example, for in-vivo neutralization of heparin by protamine sulphate, assuming a total blood volume of 75 ml per kg body weight, the required dose of protamine would be:

$$\frac{15 \times 75 \times \text{body weight} \times (1-\text{PCV})}{1000} \text{ mg.}$$

HEPARIN-INDUCED THROMBOCYTOPENIA

Most patients receiving UFH experience a small and immediate drop in their platelet count. This is referred to as type I heparin-induced thrombocytopenia (HIT) and is completely harmless. It is thought to arise as result of heparin binding to platelets. A second more serious thrombocytopenia (type II HIT) is seen in approximately 5% of patients receiving UFH and is due to development of antibodies against heparin-PF4 complexes. These bind to and activate platelets via the FCRγII resulting in accelerated clearance. Type II HIT develops 5 to 12 days after starting heparin therapy and causes a profound fall in platelets to <50% of pre-heparin value and usually $<50 \times 10^9$/l. The process of activation sometimes results in arterial and venous platelet thrombus formation particularly in ill or septic patients, and skin necrosis has also been reported. This syndrome of heparin-induced thrombocytopenia and thrombosis (HITT) has a high mortality. Heparin must be stopped immediately and alternative immediate-acting anticoagulation instituted.

The diagnosis of HIT is primarily clinical and there is no test that can be performed with sufficient speed, sensitivity and specificity to be of use in making the primary decision to stop heparin. However, confirmatory information is useful and a number of tests can be performed to substantiate the diagnosis. The 'gold standard' test is thought to be the serotonin release assay[9] but this is too cumbersome and inconvenient for routine use. The simplest for routine use is a modified platelet aggregation test as described below. However, other tests exist including an ELISA for heparin-PF4 antibodies and flow cytometry-based tests.[10,11]

DETECTION BY PLATELET AGGREGATION

Addition of heparin to the patient's PPP results in PF4–heparin complexes which are bound by the pathological antibody. The antibody–PF4–heparin complexes then bind to and activate the platelets. Platelet activation is detected as aggregation.

Principle
Blood is centrifuged gently to obtain platelet-rich plasma (PRP), which is stirred in a cuvette at 37°C, between a light source and a photocell.

Reagents
Normal control platelet-rich plasma. Preferably blood group O or the same group as the patient. The control should be off all drugs, beverages and foods which may affect aggregation for at least 10 days. 20 ml of venous blood are collected with minimal venous occlusion and added to a one-tenth volume of trisodium citrate contained in a plastic or siliconized container. The blood should not be chilled because cold activates the platelets. PRP is obtained by centrifuging at room temperature (c 20°C) for 10–15 min at 150–200 *g*. The PRP is carefully removed, avoiding contamination with red cells or buffy coat, and placed in a stoppered plastic tube. PRP should be stored at room temperature until tested and is stable for about 3 h. It is important to test all samples after a similar interval of time (say 1 h) and to store them at the same temperature in order to minimize variation. A platelet count is performed on the PRP. The number of platelets will influence aggregation response if the count falls outside $200–400 \times 10^9$/l. If necessary the PRP is adjusted to give a platelet count of 300×10^9/l by diluting with control PPP.

Patient and normal control PPP is obtained by centrifuging at 2000 *g* for 20 min. Check that the platelet count is zero.

Heparin. A sample of the type (batch identical) of heparin previously given to the patient is required. The heparin is diluted to give working concentrations of 10 and 20 iu/ml (final concentration of 1.0 and 2.0 iu/ml).

Method
Following the scheme shown in Table 18.5, four aggregation cuvettes are set up. 300 µl of normal PRP is added to each cuvette. 200 µl of the appro-

Table 18.5 The combinations of platelets, plasma and heparin required to test for heparin-induced thrombocytopenia

	Cuvette	Cuvette	Cuvette	Cuvette
Normal control PRP	300 μl	300 μl	300 μl	300 μl
Patient PPP	None	200 μl	None	200 μl
Normal control PPP	200 μl	None	200 μl	None
Heparin (10 or 20 iu/ml)	None	None	50 μl	50 μl
Saline (0.85%)	50 μl	50 μl	None	None

PPP, platelet-poor plasma; PRP, platelet-rich plasma.

priate patient or control PPP are added, along with a magnetic stir bar. The 100% baselines are set with the normal control PPP and the 0% baselines with PRP and PPP. The stir rate is set at 1200 rpm. The baselines are observed for 1 min. Aggregation is initiated by the addition of 50 μl of either heparin or saline. Aggregation is observed for a minimum of 15 min.

Interpretation

If aggregation is observed in cuvette 4 with a final heparin concentration of 1.0 and 2.0 iu/ml, the test is repeated using normal platelets, patient plasma and a final heparin concentration of 0.2 iu/ml.

Aggregation observed in cuvette 4 only, with subsequent demonstration of heparin induced aggregation at a final concentration of 0.2 iu/ml, is considered positive for heparin-induced platelet aggregation.

Alternatively aggregation testing can be repeated with a much higher final concentration of heparin (10 iu/ml). Inhibition of aggregation by a higher concentration of heparin is suggestive of heparin-induced platelet aggregation.

Aggregation observed in cuvette 4 with or 2 iu/ml but without demonstration of aggregation with the lower concentration of heparin is considered questionable.

Aggregation observed in cuvettes 1, 2 or 3 indicates that the reaction may be due to something other than heparin-induced platelet aggregation and the test is repeated using different normal donor platelets and control PPP.

With experience, subjective assessment of aggregation responses is usually sufficient for clinical interpretation. The total amount of aggregation seen may be reported.

Technical problems
See platelet aggregation, page 380.

The literature suggests that test sensitivity can be improved by the use of the patient's own platelets, platelets from selected donors known to be reactive in the assay, or washed platelets. Test specificity may be enhanced by the use of two point assays that include neutralization of the reaction by a high dose of heparin.

HIRUDIN

Recombinant manufactured hirudin is now available and licensed for both prophylactic and therapeutic use in some indications. It is a direct thrombin inhibitor and is given intravenously or subcutaneously. It is most easily monitored using the APTT with the same target range as for heparin. The TT may be prolonged but the Reptilase time is normal.

THROMBOLYTIC THERAPY

The thrombolytic agents currently in use are urokinase, streptokinase, staphylokinase and the tissue type plasminogen activator (t-PA) obtained by recombinant technology or from tissue culture. A number of plasminogen activator molecules with binding properties modified via recombinant techniques are also being developed and studied.

Urokinase. This is a trypsin-like protease found in urine. It binds directly to plasminogen but the presence of urokinase receptors on several cell types suggest that it may have an important extravascular role. Urokinase directly converts plasminogen into plasmin by cleaving a single Arg-Val bond. The active enzyme is isolated in either a two-chain or a one-chain form. Genes for both forms have been cloned and their products can be used therapeutically and are administered intravenously.

Streptokinase. This is a purified fraction of the filtrate from cultures of *Streptococcus haemolyticus*. Streptokinase interacts with plasminogen or plasmin to form a plasminogen activator in plasma. The activator complex in turn cleaves a bond in the plasminogen molecule to give rise to free plasmin. Streptokinase therefore results in systemic fibrinogenolysis as well as lysis of fibrin clot. Streptokinase is a foreign protein and induces antibody production in man, limiting a course of treatment to 3 to 5 days. It is recommended that 2 years should elapse before repeated administrations of streptokinase. It also cross-reacts with anti-streptococcal antibodies which may cause resistance to therapy, although this is usually overcome with large doses. Its half-life in plasma is approximately 25 min.

Tissue-type plasminogen activator (t-PA). This is a single or double chain polypeptide obtained by recombinant techniques or from tissue cultures. It is a potent activator of plasminogen when the two molecules are bound to fibrin for which it has a strong affinity. It thus causes less systemic fibrinogenolysis than any of the previously mentioned agents although some fall in circulating fibrinogen does occur, particularly with prolonged administration. It induces a thrombolytic state of longer duration then either streptokinase or urokinase infusion. It half-life in plasma is approximately 5 min.

Staphylokinase. Staphylokinase acts in a similar way to streptokinase by forming a complex with plasminogen which activates other plasminogen molecules. However, this occurs poorly with free plasminogen and much more efficiently with plasminogen bound to fibrin. Moreover, the plasmin generated within the clot is protected from neutralization by circulating plasmin inhibitor. Intravenous administration of staphylokinase is associated with very little change in plasma fibrinogen, plasminogen or plasmin inhibitor confirming that it is highly clot specific. It is also rapidly cleared from plasma in a biphasic pattern with α and β half-lives of 6.3 and 37 min respectively.[12]

Selection of patients

Thrombolytic treatment carries a serious risk of bleeding and thrombolytic agents should not be given to individuals suffering from a variety of illnesses where there is a high risk of bleeding. In addition, each patient should have haemostatic function and platelet count measured before treatment is started.

LABORATORY CONTROL OF THROMBOLYTIC THERAPY[13]

Many laboratory tests are abnormal during thrombolytic therapy, but a perfect and specific procedure for monitoring is not available. In practice, thrombolytic therapy is given rapidly according to protocol with no time or need for adjustment of dosage. During thrombolytic therapy, all screening tests of coagulation are prolonged, reflecting the hyperplasminaemic state with the reduction in the fibrinogen concentration and the presence of FDP. The prolongation is most marked with streptokinase and streptokinase–plasminogen complex; it is less marked with urokinase and least with t-PA and staphylokinase. The fibrinogen-concentration commonly falls to below 0.05 g/l and the FDP concentration may rise to over 1000 ng/l.

Monitoring of therapy is only recommended for treatment lasting longer than 24 h. If possible, a sample should be obtained prior to treatment. Samples taken after fibrinolysis has begun should be taken into citrate plus an inhibitor of fibrinolysis such as aprotinin (250 u/ml) or ε-aminocaproic acid (EACA: 0.07 mol/l). The fibrinolytic state will affect several tests.

APTT. With effective fibrinolysis, the APTT is likely to be prolonged >1.5 times control. This is a result of fibrinogen, FV and FVIII depletion as well as interference from FDPs. There are however no data to correlate APTT with therapeutic effect.

TT. The TT can be used to monitor therapy. A few hours after the start of the infusion, the TT is prolonged to 40 s or more (control 15 ± 1 s); it then settles to approximately 20–30 s. Very long thrombin times carry a high risk of bleeding and are indicative of severe hyperplasminaemia.

Plasma fibrinogen. Depending on duration of therapy and the specific PA used, there is a variable fall in fibrinogen. The fibrinogen should be measured by a method dependent on clottable fibrinogen (e.g Clauss technique, p. 356). The PT-derived fibrinogen is likely to be unreliable. Fibrin(ogen) degradation products will be elevated but this is unlikely to be helpful.

Follow-up procedures. In most protocols, the use of a fibrinolytic agent will be followed by the use of antiplatelet agents (aspirin, IIbIIIa blockers) and anticoagulants (heparin, hirudin, direct thrombin inhibitors), some of which require monitoring in standard fashion. The timing and dosage will depend on current protocols which are under continuous revision. It is usually considered safe to start anticoagulants when the fibrinogen concentration exceeds 0.05 g/l of plasma. If the fibrinogen concentration is 0.05 g/l and the prolongation of APTT does not exceed twice the base line clotting time, heparin treatment can be safely given with monitoring. This usually occurs 4–6 h after streptokinase and urokinase infusion and sooner after t-PA. However, after streptokinase infusion, occasional patients may show persistent hypofibrinogenaemia for up to 24 h. Such individuals must be monitored at 4-h intervals and not

given heparin and warfarin until their APTT has fallen to twice the baseline clotting time.

INVESTIGATION OF A PATIENT WHO BLEEDS WHILE ON THROMBOLYTIC AGENTS OR IMMEDIATELY AFTERWARDS

Haemorrhage is an inevitable risk associated with fibrinolytic therapy and may occur despite normal coagulation tests. When severe, bleeding will necessitate cessation of fibrinolysis and administration of aprotinin or tranexamic acid to inhibit its activity. Coagulation tests may guide replacement therapy with plasma or cryoprecipitate. The tests, the timing and the likely mechanism of bleeding are shown in Table 18.6.

Table 18.6 Investigation of a patient who is bleeding while on thrombolytic treatment

Timing	Test	Result	Comment
During infusion	TT or APTT	Very long	Hyperplasminaemia.
	Fibrinogen	Low	Stop infusion, transfuse FFP
Before heparin	TT or APTT	Very long	Hypofibrinogenaemia.
	Fibrinogen	Very low	DO NOT give heparin, transfuse FFP if necessary
While on heparin	APTT	Very long	
	a. Fibrinogen	Normal	Excess heparin, reduce dose
	Platelets	Normal	
	b. Fibrinogen	Low	Heparin given too soon*
	Platelets	Normal	
	c. Fibrinogen	Low	DIC, liver or renal disease.* Investigate
	Platelets	Low	

APTT, activated partial thromboplastin time; DIC, disseminated intravascular coagulation; FFP, fresh-frozen plasma; TT, thrombin time.
*Use anti-Xa assay to measure heparin concentration.

ANTI-PLATELET THERAPY

Many drugs inhibit platelet function in vitro but only a few have anti-platelet activity in acceptable doses. Each category of drugs has a different pharmacological action and requires different methods to demonstrate its effect on platelets. Anti-platelet agents are used in primary and secondary prevention of coronary heart disease, in unstable angina, in certain forms of cerebrovascular disease, to prevent thrombo-embolism associated with valvular disease and prosthetic heart valves, and to prevent thrombosis in arteriovenous shunts.

Haematologists are only exceptionally asked to monitor these aspects of anti-platelet therapy. Indeed, it is said that the advantage of these agents is that monitoring is unnecessary.

A proportion of patients with thrombocytosis or thrombocythaemia experience episodes of arterial thrombosis. Such patients are often given anti-platelet drugs and the effect of these drugs is sometimes monitored. Three techniques are available for monitoring: prolongation of the bleeding time (see p. 371), inhibition of platelet aggregation response to standard agonists (see p. 380) and normalization of platelet survival using ^{111}Indium-labelled platelets (p. 334). Such monitoring is usually tailored to the individual patient and the choice of test depends on the drug used, on the abnormalities detectable in the patient, and on the laboratory facilities available. Thus aspirin affects both bleeding time and platelet aggregation, whereas the effect of dipyridamole on platelet aggregation is unpredictable, and can only be shown reliably by measuring platelet survival. Platelet function analysers such as the PFA-100 can detect aspirin effect and may prove to be useful in future.[14]

REFERENCES

1 Hirsh J, Dalen JE, Anderson DR, et al 1998 Oral anticoagulants: mechanism of action, clinical effectiveness, and optimal therapeutic range. Chest 114:445s–469s.

2 World Health Organization 1999 Guidelines for thromboplastins and plasma used to control oral anticoagulant therapy. WHO Technical Report Series 889:64–93.

3 Kitchen S, Preston FE 1999 Standardization of prothrombin time for laboratory control of oral anticoagulant therapy. Seminars in Thrombosis and Hemostasis 25:17–25.

4 Poller L, Barrowcliffe TW, van den Besselaar AM, et al 1997 A simplified statistical method for local INR using linear regression. European Concerted Action on Anticoagulation. British Journal of Haematology 98:640–647.

5 British Committee for Standards in Haematology 1998 Guidelines on oral anticoagulation: third edition. British Journal of Haematology 101:374–387.

6 Hirsh J, Warkentin TE, Raschke R, et al 1998 Heparin and low-molecular-weight heparin: mechanisms of action, pharmacokinetics, dosing considerations, monitoring, efficacy, and safety Chest 114:489s–510s. [erratum published in Chest (1999) 115:1760].

7 Gray E, Heath AB, Mulloy B, et al 1995 A collaborative study of proposed European Pharmacopoeia reference preparations of low molecular mass heparin. Thrombosis and Haemostasis 74:893–899.

8 Popma JJ, Prpic R, Lansky AJ, et al 1998 Heparin dosing in patients undergoing coronary intervention. American Journal of Cardiology 82:19–24.

9 Sheridan D, Carter C, Kelton JG 1986 A diagnostic test for heparin-induced thrombocytopenia. Blood 67:27–30.

10 Warkentin TE 1999 Heparin-induced thrombocytopenia: a clinicopathologic syndrome. Thrombosis and Haemostasis 82:439–447.

11 Amiral J, Meyer D 1998 Heparin-induced thrombocytopenia: diagnostic tests and biological mechanisms. Baillières Clinical Haematology 11:447–460.

12 Collen D 1999 The plasminogen (fibrinolytic) system. Thrombosis and Haemostasis 82:259–270.

13 Ludlam CA, Bennett B, Fox KA, et al 1995 Guidelines for the use of thrombolytic therapy. Haemostasis and Thrombosis Task Force of the British Committee for Standards in Haematology. Blood Coagulation Fibrinolysis 6:273–85.

14 Homoncik M, Jilma B, Hergovich N, et al 2000 Monitoring of aspirin (ASA) pharmacodynamics with the platelet function analyzer PFA-100. Thrombosis and Haemostasis 83:316–321.

19

Blood cell antigens and antibodies: erythrocytes, platelets and granulocytes

S. M. Knowles

ERYTHROCYTES

RED CELL ANTIGENS

Since Landsteiner's discovery in 1901 that human blood groups existed, a vast body of serological, genetic and biochemical data on red cell (blood group) antigens has been accumulated. More recently, the biological functions of some of these antigens have been appreciated.

Twenty-five blood group systems have been described (Table 19.1). Each system is a series of red cell antigens, determined either by a single genetic locus or very closely linked loci. In addition to the blood group systems, there are 5 'collections' of antigens (e.g. Cost), which bring together other genetically, biochemically, or serologically related sets of antigens, and separate series of low-frequency (e.g. Rd) and high-frequency (e.g. Vel) antigens, which do not fit into any system or collection. A numerical catalogue of red cell antigens is being maintained by an International Society of Blood Transfusion (ISBT) Working Party.[1,2]

Apart from the ABO system, most of these antigens were detected by antibodies stimulated by transfusion or pregnancy.

Alternative forms of gene(s) coding for red cell antigens at a particular locus are called alleles and individuals may inherit identical or non-identical alleles. Most blood group genes have been assigned to specific chromosomes, e.g. ABO system on chromosome 9, Rh system on chromosome 1. The term genotype is used for the sum of the inherited alleles of a particular gene (e.g. AA, AO) and most red cell genes are expressed as co-dominant antigens, i.e. both genes are expressed in the heterozygote. The phenotype refers to the recognizable product of the alleles and there are many racial differences in the frequencies of red cell phenotypes, as shown in Table 19.2.

Table 19.1 Blood group systems recognized by the ISBT Working Party

System number	System name conventional	System symbol ISBT	Chromosomal location	Gene(s)
001	ABO	ABO	9q34.1-q34.2	ABO
002	MNS	MNS	4q28-q31	GPYA GPYB
003	P	PI	22q11.2-qter	P
004	Rh	RH	1p36.2-p34	RHD RHCE
005	Lutheran	LU	19q12-q13	LU
006	Kell	KEL	7q33	KEL
007	Lewis	LE	19p13.3	FUT3
008	Duffy	FY	1q22-q23	FY
009	Kidd	JK	18q11-q12	HUT11
010	Diego	DI	17q12-q21	SLC4A1
011	Yt	YT	7q22	ACHE
012	Xg	XG	Xp22.32	XG
013	Scianna	SC	1p36.2-p22.1	SC
014	Dombrock	DO	12p13.2-p12.1	DO
015	Colton	CO	7p14	AQP1
016	LW	LW	19p13.2-cen	LW
017	Chido/Rogers	CH/RG	6p21.3	C4A,C4B
018	H	H	19q13	FUT1
019	Kx	XK	Xp21.1	XK
020	Gerbich	GE	2q14-q21	GYPC
021	Cromer	CROM	1q32	DAF
022	Knops	KN	1q32	CR1
023	Indian	IN	11p13	CD44
024	Ok	OK	19pter-p13.2	OK
025	MER2	RAPH	11p15	MER2

Red cell antigens are determined either by carbohydrate or protein structures. Carbohydrate-defined antigens are indirect gene products (e.g. ABO, Lewis, P). The genes code for an intermediate product, usually an enzyme that creates the antigenic specificity by transferring sugar molecules onto the protein or lipid. Protein-defined antigens are direct gene products, and the specificity is determined by the inherited amino acid sequence and/or the conformation of the protein. Proteins carrying red cell antigens are inserted into the membrane in one of three ways: single pass, multipass, and linked to phosphotidylinositol (GPI-linked). Only a few red cell antigens are erythroid-specific (Rh, LW, Kell and MNSs), the remainder being expressed in many other tissues. The structure and functions of the membrane proteins and glycoproteins carrying blood group

Table 19.2 Frequencies of red cell phenotypes in US black and white populations

System	Phenotype	African American population (%)	US white population (%)
ABO	O	49	43.7
	A	26	41.7
	B	20.5	10.6
	AB	4.5	4
Lewis	Le (a–b–)	28.5	6
Rh	Dce	47.8	2.1
	DCcEe	4.2	13.4
	dce	5.6	14.6
	DCe	2.6	18.9
MNSs	S–,s+	68.1	45
	S+s+	24.5	44
	S+s–	5.9	11
	S–s–	1.5	Rare
Duffy	Fy (a–,b–)	63.7	Rare
	Fy (a–, b+)	18.8	34
	Fy (a+,b+)	2	44
	Fy (a+,b–)	15.5	17
Kidd	Jk (a+,b–)	50	27.5
	Jk (a+b+)	41.4	49.4
	Jk (a–b+)	8.6	23.1

antigens have been recently reviewed by Cartron et al[3] and Daniels.[4] An illustration of the putative functions of molecules containing blood group antigens is provided in Table 19.3.

The clinical importance of a blood group system depends upon the capacity of allo-antibodies (directed against the antigens not possessed by the individual) to cause destruction of transfused red cells, or to cross the placenta and give rise to haemolytic disease in the fetus or newborn. This in turn depends upon the frequency of the antigens and the allo-antibodies and the characteristics of the latter – thermal range, immunoglobulin class and ability to fix complement. On these criteria, the ABO and Rh systems are of major clinical importance. Anti-A and anti-B are naturally occurring and are capable of causing severe intravascular haemolysis after an incompatible transfusion. The RhD antigen is the most immunogenic red cell antigen after A and B, being capable of stimulating anti-D production after transfusion or pregnancy in the majority of RhD-negative individuals.

ABO SYSTEM

Discovery of the ABO system by Landsteiner in 1901 marked the beginning of safe blood transfusion. The ABO antigens, although most important in relation to transfusion, are also expressed on most endothelial and epithelial membranes and are important histocompatibility antigens.[5] Transplantation of ABO-incompatible solid organs increases the potential for hyperacute graft rejection. Major ABO-incompatible stem cell transplants (e.g. group A stem cells into a group O recipient) will provoke haemolysis, unless the donation is depleted of red cells.

ABO antigens and encoding genes (Table 19.4)

There are four main blood groups: A, B, AB and O. In the British Caucasian population, the frequency of group A is 42%, B 9%, AB 3% and O 46% but there is racial variation in these frequencies.[6] The epitopes of ABO antigens are determined by carbohydrates (sugars), which are linked either to polypeptides (forming glycoproteins) or to lipids (glycolipids).

Table 19.3 Putative functions of molecules containing blood group antigens

Class	Blood group system	Structure	Function
Transporter/channel	Kidd	Multipass GP	Urea transporter
	Colton	Aquaporin 1 Multipass CP	Water channel
	Diego	Band 3, multipass GP	Anion exchanger
Receptors	Duffy	DARC, multipass GP	Chemokine (*Plasmodium vivax* receptor)
	Indian	Single-pass GP	Hyaluronate receptor
Complement pathway	Chido/Rogers	Complement absorbed onto red cells	Complement component
	Cromer	DAF	Complement regulator
	Knops	Complement receptor 1	Complement regulator
Adhesion	LW	IgSF	Binds CD11/CD18 Integrins
Molecule	Lutheran	IgSF	? Laminin receptor
Enzyme	Yt	GPI-linked GP Acetylcholinesterase	Unknown on red cells
	Kell	Single-pass GP	? Endopeptidase
Structural protein	Gerbich	Glycophorins C and D Single-pass GP	Attachment to membrane skeleton

Table 19.4 ABO blood-group system

Blood group	Sub-group	Antigens on red cells	Antibodies in plasma
A	A_1	$A + A_1$	Anti-B
	A_2	A	(Anti-A_1)*
B	–	B	Anti-A, Anti-A_1
AB	A_1B	$A + A_1 + B$	None
	A_2B	A + B	(Anti-A_1)*
0	–	(H)***	Anti-A Anti-A_1 Anti-B Anti-A,B**

* Anti-A_1 found in 1–2% of A_2 subjects and 25–30% of A_2B subjects.
** Cross-reacting with both A and B cells.
*** The amount of H antigen is influenced by the ABO group; 0 cells contain most H and A_1B cells least. Anti-H may be found in occasional A_1 and A_1B subject (see text).

The expression of ABO antigens is controlled by three separate genetic loci: *ABO* located on chromosome 9, and *FUT1* (*H*) and *FUT2* (*Se*), both of which are located on chromosome 19. The genes from each locus are inherited in pairs as Mendelian dominants. Each gene codes for a different enzyme (glycosyltransferase) which attaches specific monosaccharides onto precursor disaccharide chains (Table 19.5). There are four types of disaccharide chains known to occur on red cells, other tissues and in secretions. The Type 1 disaccharide chain is found in plasma and secretions and is the substrate for the *FUT2* (*Se*) gene, whereas Types 2, 3 and 4 chains are only found on red cells

Table 19.5 Glycosyltransferases produced by genes encoding for antigens within the ABO, H and Lewis blood group systems

Gene	Allele	Transferase
FUT1	H	α-2-L-fucosyltransferase
	h	None
A	A	α-3-N-acetyl-D-galactosaminyltransferase
B	B	α-3-D-galactosyltransferase
0	0	None
FUT2	Se	α-2-L-fucosyltransferase
	se	None
FUT3	Le	α-3/4-L-fucosyltransferase
	le	None

and are the substrate for the *FUT1* (*H*) gene. It is likely that the *O* and *B* genes are mutations of the *A* gene. The *O* gene does not encode for the production of a functional enzyme; group O individuals commonly have a deletion at nucleotide 261 (the *O1* allele) which results in a frame-shift, premature termination of the translated polypeptide and the production of an enzyme with no catalytic activity. The *B* gene differs from *A* by consistent nucleotide substitutions.[7] The expression of A and B antigens is determined by the *H* and *Se* genes, which both give rise to glycosyltransferases that add L-fucose, producing the H antigen. The presence of an *A* or *B* gene (or both) results in the production of further glycosyltransferases which convert H substance into A and B antigens by the terminal addition of N-acetyl-D-galactosamine and D-galactose respectively (Fig. 19.1). Since the *O* gene produces an inactive transferase, H substance persists unchanged as group O. In the extremely rare Oh Bombay phenotype, the individual is homozygous for the *h* allele of *FUT1* and hence cannot form the H precursor of the A and B antigen. Their red cells type as group O but their plasma contains anti-H, in addition to anti-A, anti-B and anti-A,B which are all active at 37°C. As a consequence, individuals with an Oh Bombay phenotype can only be safely transfused with other Oh red cells.

Serologists have defined two common subgroups of the A antigen. Approximately 20% of group A and group AB individuals belong to group A_2 and group A_2B respectively, the remainder belonging to group A_1 and group A_1B. These subgroups arise as a result of inheritance of either the A^1 or A^2 alleles. The A_2 transferase is less efficient in transferring N-acetyl-D-galactosamine to available H antigen sites and cannot utilize Types 3 and 4 disaccharide chains. As a consequence, A_2 red cells have fewer A antigen sites than A_1 cells and the plasma of group A_2 and group A_2B individuals may also contain anti-A_1. The distinction between these subgroups is most conveniently made using the lectin *Dolichos biflorus* which only reacts with A_1 cells. The H antigen content of red cells depends on the ABO group and when assessed by agglutination reactions with anti-H, the strength of reaction tends to be graded $O > A_2 > A_2B > B > A_1 > A_1B$. Other subgroups of A are occasionally found (e.g. A_3, A_x) which are due to mutant forms of the glycosyltransferases produced by the A gene and are less efficient at transferring N-acetyl-D-galactosamine onto H substance.[7]

The A, B and H antigens are detectable early in fetal life, but are not fully developed on the red cells at birth. The number of antigen sites reaches 'adult' level at around 1 year of age and remains constant until old age when a slight reduction may occur.

Secretors and non-secretors (Table 19.6)
The ability to secrete A, B and H substances in water-soluble form is controlled by *FUT2* (dominant allele *Se*). In a Caucasian population, about 80% are secretors (genotype *SeSe or Sese*) and 20% non-secretors (genotype *sese*). Secretors have H substance in the saliva and other body fluids together with A and/or B substances depending on their blood group. Only traces of these substances are present in the secretions of non-secretors, although the antigens are expressed normally on their red cells and other tissues.

An individual's secretor status can be determined by testing for ABH substance in saliva (p. 453).

ABO system and disease
Group A individuals may rarely acquire a B antigen as a result of bacterial infection which results in the release of a deacetylase enzyme. This converts N-acetyl-D-galactosamine into α-galactosamine, which is similar to galactose, the immunodominant sugar of group B, thereby sometimes causing the red cells to appear to be group AB. In the original report, five out of seven of the patients had

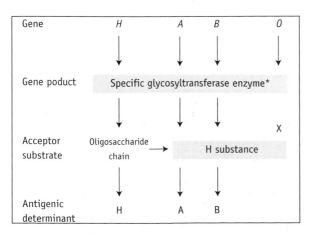

Fig. 19.1 Pathways from HAB blood-group genes to antigens. *Glycosyltransferase H transfers L-fucose; A transfers *N*-acetyl-D-galactosamine; B transfers D-galactose; 0 is inactive.

Table 19.6 Secretor status

	Genes	Blood group of red cells	ABH substance present in saliva	Incidence (%)
Secretors	SeSe or Sese	A B AB 0	A + H B + H A + B + H H	80
Non-secretors	sese	A, B, AB or 0	None	20

carcinoma of the gastrointestinal tract. Case reports attest to the danger of individuals with an acquired B antigen being transfused with AB red cells, resulting in a fatal haemolytic transfusion reaction following the production of hyperimmune anti-B.[8]

The inheritance of ABH antigens is also known to be weakly associated with predisposition to certain diseases. Group A individuals have 1.2 times the risk of developing carcinoma of the stomach than group O or B, group O individuals have 1.4 times the risk of developing peptic ulcer than non-group O and non-secretors of ABH have 1.5 times the risk of developing peptic ulcer than secretors.[9]

ABH antigens are also frequently more weakly expressed on the red cells of persons with leukaemia.

ABO antibodies
Anti-A and anti-B. ABO antibodies, in the absence of the corresponding antigens, appear during the first few months after birth, probably as a result of exposure to ABH antigen-like substances in the diet or the environment, i.e. they are 'naturally occurring' (Table 19.4). This allows for reverse (serum) grouping as a means of confirming the red cell phenotype.

The antibodies are a potential cause of dangerous haemolytic transfusion reactions if transfusions are given without regard to ABO compatibility. Anti-A and anti-B are always, to some extent, IgM. Although they react best at low temperatures, they are nevertheless potentially lytic at 37°C. Hyperimmune anti-A and anti-B occur less frequently, usually in response to transfusion or pregnancy, but they may also be formed following the injection of some toxoids and vaccines. They are predominantly of IgG class and are usually produced by group O and sometimes by group A_2 individuals. Hyperimmune IgG anti-A and/or anti-B from group O or group A_2 mothers may cross the placenta and cause haemolytic disease of the newborn (HDN). These antibodies react over a wide thermal range and are more effective haemolysins than the naturally occurring antibodies. Group O donors should always be screened for hyperimmune anti-A and anti-B antibodies which may cause haemolysis when group O platelets or whole blood are transfused to recipients with A and B phenotypes. Plasma-containing blood components from these 'dangerous' universal donors should be reserved for group O recipients.

Anti-A_1 and anti-H. Anti-A_1 reacts only with A_1 and A_1B cells and is occasionally found in the serum of group A_2 individuals (1–8%) and not uncommonly in the serum of group A_2B subjects (25–50%). However, anti-A_1 normally acts as a cold agglutinin and is very rarely reactive at 37°C, when it is only capable of limited red cell destruction. There have been a few reports of red cell haemolysis ascribed to anti-A_1 which some authors have questioned since, although the antibodies reacted only with A_1 red cells, no attempts were made to absorb them with A_2 cells, which would have revealed their anti-A specificity.

Anti-H reacts most strongly with group O and A_2 red cells and also normally acts as a cold agglutinin. A notable, but rare, exception is the anti-H that occurs in the Oh Bombay phenotype, which is an IgM antibody and causes lysis at 37°C (Table 19.4).

LEWIS SYSTEM
Lewis antigens and encoding genes
The Lewis antigens (Le^a and Le^b) are located on soluble glycosphingolipids found in saliva and plasma and are secondarily absorbed to the red cell membranes from the plasma.

The Le gene at the *FUT3 (LE)* locus is located on chromosome 19 and codes for a fucosyltransferase which acts on an adjacent sugar molecule to that acted on by the *Se* gene. Where *Se* and *Le* are present, the Le^b antigen is produced; where *Le* but not *Se* is present, Le^a is produced; and where *Le* is not present, neither Le^a nor Le^b is produced. After transfusion of red cells, donor red cells convert to the Lewis type of the recipient owing to the continuous exchange of glycosphingolipids between the plasma and red cell membrane.

Neonates have the phenotype Le(a-b-), since low levels of the fucosyltransferase are produced in the first 2 months of life.

Lewis antibodies

Lewis antibodies are naturally occurring and are usually IgM and complement binding. In vitro, their reactivity is enhanced with the use of enzyme-treated red cells, when lysis may occur. However, only rare examples of anti-Le^a, strictly reactive at 37°C, have given rise to haemolytic transfusion reactions and there is no good evidence that anti-Le^b has ever caused a haemolytic episode. Explanations for the relative lack of clinical significance include their thermal range, neutralization by Lewis antigens in the plasma of transfused blood, and the gradual elution of Lewis antigens from the donor red cells. Consequently, it is acceptable to provide red cells for transfusion which have not been typed as negative for the relevant Lewis antigen, but are compatible with the recipient plasma when the compatibility test is performed strictly at 37°C.

Lewis antibodies have not been implicated in haemolytic disease of the fetus or newborn. The role of Lewis in influencing the outcome of renal transplants is unclear.

THE P SYSTEM AND GLOBOSIDE COLLECTION
Antigens

The P$_1$ antigen of the P system and the P and P^k antigens of the globoside collection are related. Little is known of the genes involved or their products, but all are derived from the precursor, lactosyl ceramide dehexoside (CDH). Carbohydrate products related to the P system are widely distributed in nature.

Expression of P$_1$ varies considerably between individuals. One in 100 000 individuals is p (negative for P) and is resistant to parvovirus B19 infection.

Antibodies

Anti-P$_1$ is a common naturally occurring antibody of no clinical significance and red cells for transfusion can be provided which are crossmatch compatible at 37°C. Allo anti-P is also a naturally occurring antibody found in individuals with the rare P^k phenotype. Auto-anti-P is the specificity attributed to the Donath–Landsteiner antibody; it is a potent biphasic haemolysin, responsible for paroxysmal cold haemoglobinuria (PCH).

Anti-PP$_1$P^k is a naturally occurring high titre IgM or IgG antibody, and only found in individuals with the rare p phenotype. It is reactive at 37°C and is capable of causing intravascular haemolysis and HDN. It is also associated with abortion in early pregnancy.

RH SYSTEM (FORMERLY KNOWN AS RHESUS SYSTEM)

The Rh system was so named because the original antibody that was raised by injecting red cells of rhesus monkeys into rabbits and guinea pigs reacted with most human red cells. Although the original antibody (now called anti-LW) was subsequently shown to be different from anti-D, the Rh terminology has been retained for the human blood group system. The clinical importance of this system is due to the fact that RhD-negative individuals are easily stimulated to make anti-D if transfused with RhD-positive blood or, in the case of pregnant women, if exposed to RhD-positive fetal red cells which have crossed the placenta.

Rh antigens and encoding genes

This is a very complex system. At its simplest, it is convenient to classify individuals as RhD-positive or RhD-negative, depending on the presence of the RhD antigen. This is largely a preventive measure, to avoid transfusing an RhD-negative recipient with the cells expressing the RhD antigen, which is the most immunogenic red cell antigen after A and B. At a more comprehensive level, it is convenient to consider the Rh system as a gene complex which gives rise to various combinations of three alternative antigens, C or c, D or d and E or e, as originally suggested by Fisher. The d gene was thought to be amorphic without any corresponding antigen on the red cell. More recently it has been confirmed that the *RH* locus is on chromosome 1, and comprises two highly homologous very closely linked genes; *RHD* and *RHCE*, each with 10 exons. Each gene codes for a separate transmembrane protein with 417 residues and 12 putative transmembrane domains. The RhD and RhCE proteins differ at 35 residues. The *RHCE* gene has four main alleles; *CE*, *Ce*, *ce* and *cE*. Positions 103 and 226 on the CE polypeptide, situated in the external loops, determine the C/c (serine/proline) and E/e (proline/alanine) polymorphisms respectively. This concept of D and CcEe genes linked closely and transmitted together is consistent with the Fisher nomenclature.

In Caucasian, RhD-negative individuals, the *RHD* gene is deleted, whereas in black people and other populations, single point mutations, partial deletions or recombinations have been described. In individuals with a weak D antigen (D^u), there is a quantitative reduction in D antigen sites, believed to arise from an uncharacterized transcriptional defect. These individuals do not make anti-D antibodies following a D antigen challenge. Partial D individuals lack one or more epitopes of the D antigen, defined using panels of monoclonal reagents. D^{VI} is perhaps the most important partial D phenotype, as such individuals not infrequently make anti-D. Partial D phenotypes arise from DNA exchanges between *RHD* and *RHCE* genes and from other rearrangements. Comprehensive recent reviews of this system have been provided by Cartron & Agre,[10] Huang,[11] and Avent & Reid.[12]

The Rh haplotypes are named either by the component antigens (e.g. CDe; cde) or by a single shorthand symbol (e.g. R^1 = CDe; r = cde). Thus a person may inherit *CDe* (R^1) from one parent and *cde* from the other, and have the genotype *Cde/cde* (R^1r). The haplotypes in order of frequency and the corresponding shorthand notation are given in Table 19.7. Although two other nomenclatures are also used to describe the Rh system, namely, Wiener's Rh-Hr terminology and Rosenfield's numerical notation, the CDE nomenclature, derived from Fisher's original theory, is recommended by a World Health Organization Expert Committee[13] in the interest of simplicity and uniformity. The Rh antigens are defined by corresponding anti-sera, with the exception of 'anti-d' which does not exist. Consequently, the distinction between homozygous DD and the heterozygous Dd cannot be made by direct serological testing but may be resolved by informative

Table 19.7 The Rh haplotypes in order of frequency (Fisher nomenclature) and the corresponding short notations

Fisher	Short notations	Approximate frequency (%)
CDe	R^1	41
cde	r	39
cDE	R^2	14
cDe	R^0	3
C^wDe	R^{1w}	1
cdE	r″	1
Cde	r′	1
CDE	R^z	rare
CdE	r^y	rare

family studies. It is still routine practice to predict the genotype from the phenotype on the basis of probability tables for the various Rh genotypes in the population (Table 20.2, p. 478). However, in women with anti-D and a history of an infant affected by HDN, *RH* DNA typing has been in use since 1993 in prenatal testing for the fetal RhD status, to decide on the clinical management of the pregnancy. DNA typing requires less fetal tissue and can be performed earlier in pregnancy before the Rh proteins are expressed on red cells. Suitable sources include amniotic fluid (amniocytes), and trophoblastic cells (chorionic villi). In practice, Multiplex polymerase chain reaction (PCR) is used, involving more than two primer sets, to detect the different molecular bases for RhD negative phenotypes in non-Caucasians. *RH* DNA typing also has applications in paternity testing and forensic medicine.[14]

There are racial differences in the distribution of Rh antigens, e.g. RhD negativity is more common in Caucasians, (approximately 15%), whereas R^0 (cDe) is found in approximately 48% Afro-Americans but is uncommon (approximately 2%) in Caucasians. The Rh antigens are present only on red cells and are a structural part of the cell membrane. Complete absence of Rh antigens (Rh null phenotype) may be associated with a congenital haemolytic anaemia with spherocytes and stomatocytes in the blood film, increased osmotic fragility and increased cation transport.[15] This phenotype arises either as a result of homozygosity for a silent allele at the *RH* locus (the amorph type), or more commonly by homozygosity for an autosomal suppressor gene (X^0r), genetically independent of the *RH* locus (the regulator type). Rh antigens are well developed before birth and can be demonstrated on the red cells of very early fetuses.

Antibodies

Fisher's nomenclature is convenient when applied to Rh antibodies, and antibodies directed against all Rh antigens, except Rhd, have been described: namely, anti-D, anti-C, anti-c, anti-E and anti-e. Rh antigens are restricted to red cells and Rh antibodies are due to previous allo-immunization by previous pregnancy or transfusion, except for some naturally-occurring forms of anti-E and anti-C^W. Immune Rh antibodies are predominantly IgG (IgG1 and/or IgG3), but may have an IgM component. They react optimally at 37°C, do not bind complement and their detection is often enhanced by the use of enzyme-treated red cells. Haemolysis, when it occurs, is therefore extravascular and predominantly in the spleen.

Anti-D is the most important clinically; it may cause haemolytic transfusion reactions and was a common cause of fetal death resulting from HDN before the introduction of anti-D prophylaxis in 1969. Anti-D is accompanied by anti-C in 30% cases and anti-E in 2% cases.[16] Primary immunization following a transfusion of RhD positive cells becomes apparent within 2 to 5 months, but may not be detectable following exposure to a small dose of RhD-positive cells in pregnancy. However, a second exposure to RhD-positive cells in a subsequent pregnancy will provoke a prompt anamnestic or secondary immune response.

Of the non-D Rh antibodies, anti-c is most commonly found and can also give rise to severe haemolytic disease of the fetus and newborn. Anti-E is less common, whilst anti-C is rare in the absence of anti-D.

KELL AND Kx SYSTEMS
Antigens and encoding genes

Twenty-five antigens have been identified (K1–K25), but three very closely linked sets of alleles are clinically important; *K (KEL1)* and *k (KEL2)*; *Kp^a (KEL3)*, *Kp^b (KEL4)* and *Kp^c (KEL21)*; and *Js^a (KEL6)* and *Js^b (KEL7)*. These antigens are encoded by alleles at the *KEL* locus on chromosome 7, but their production also depends upon genes at the *KX* locus on the X chromosome. The K antigen is present in 9% of the English population. The Kp^b antigen has a high frequency in Caucasians; the Js^b antigen is universal in Caucasians and almost universal in black people.

The Kell protein is a single-pass glycoprotein, and is believed to be complexed by a disulphide bridge to the Kx protein, which is multipass with ten putative transmembrane domains. It has considerable sequence homology to other neutral endopeptidases.

In the McLeod phenotype, red cells lack Kx, and there is a marked decrease in all Kell antigens, an acanthocytic morphology and a compensated haemolytic anaemia. The McLeod syndrome is X-linked with slow progression to cardiomyopathy, skeletal muscle wasting and neurological defects.

Kell antibodies

Immune anti-K is the commonest antibody found outside the ABO and Rh systems. It is commonly IgG1 and occasionally complement binding. Other immune antibodies directed against Kell antigens are less common. The presence of some of these antibodies, such as anti-k, anti-Kp^b and anti-Js^b, may cause extensive difficulties in the selection of antigen-negative units for transfusion.

DUFFY (Fy) SYSTEM
Duffy (Fy) antigens and encoding genes

The *Fy* locus is on chromosome 1 and encodes a multipass protein with seven or nine putative transmembrane domains.

The locus has the following alleles: *Fy^a*, *Fy^b*, which code for the co-dominant Fy^a and Fy^b antigens respectively; *Fy^x* which is responsible for a weak Fy^b antigen; and *Fy*, responsible when homozygous for the Fy(a-b-) phenotype in black people. This *Fy* gene is identical to the *Fy^b* gene in its structural region but has a mutation in the promoter region, resulting in the lack of production of red cell Duffy glycoprotein.

The Fy glycoprotein (also known as Duffy Antigen Receptor for Chemokines, DARC) is a receptor for the CC and CXC classes of pro-inflammatory chemokines, and is expressed on vascular endothelial cells and Purkinje cells in the cerebellum, but its precise role as a potential scavenger of excess chemokines is unknown. The Fy glycoprotein is also a receptor for *Plasmodium vivax* and *P. knowlesi*.

Duffy (Fy) antibodies

Anti-Fy^a is much more common than anti-Fy^b, and all other Duffy antibodies are rare. They are predominantly IgG1 and are sometimes complement binding.

KIDD (Jk) SYSTEM
Kidd antigens and encoding genes

Genes at the *HUT11 (JK)* locus on chromosome 18 encode for a multipass protein, which carries both the Kidd antigens and the human erythroid urea transporter. The co-dominant alleles, *Jk^a* and *Jk^b*, produce a polymorphism on *HUT11* which differs by a single amino acid substitution at position 280 (Asp/Asn).

The Jk(a-b-) phenotype is very rare and caused by homozygous inheritance of the silent allele, *Jk*, at the *JK* locus or by inheritance of the dominant inhibitor gene *In (Jk)* unlinked to the *JK* locus. These Jk(a-b-) cells are resistant to lysis by solutions of urea and have a selective defect in urea transport.

Kidd antibodies

Anti-Jk^a is commoner than anti-Jk^b; both are usually IgG. Kidd antibodies are usually complement binding which is thought to be because most of them contain an IgG3 fraction. Anti-Jk3 is produced by individuals of the Jk(a-b-) phenotype.

Kidd antibodies can be difficult to detect, because they often show dosage (may only react with cells showing homozygous expressions of *Jk^a* or *Jk^b*), they fall to undetectable levels in plasma and they are often present in mixtures of allo-antibodies.

MNSs SYSTEM
MNSs antigens and encoding genes

GYPA and *GYPB* are closely linked genes on chromosome 4 and encode for glycophorin A (GPA) and glycophorin B (GPB), respectively. Both GPA and GPB are single-pass membrane sialoglycoproteins. *M* and *N* are alleles of *GYPA* (encoding for the M and N antigens on GPA) and *S* and *s* are alleles of *GPYB* (encoding for the S and s antigens on GPB). Many rare variants have been described owing to gene deletions, mutations and segmental exchanges.

The U antigen is found on the red cells of Caucasians and 99% of black people. U-negative individuals are, with rare exceptions, S-s- and lack GPB, or have an altered form of GPB.

MNSs antibodies

Anti-M is a relatively common antibody, which may be IgM or IgG. Rare examples are reactive at 37°C when they can give rise to haemolytic transfusion reactions. Anti-M very rarely gives rise to HDN.

Anti-N is uncommon and of no clinical significance.

Anti-S and anti-s are usually IgG; both have rarely been implicated in haemolytic transfusion reactions and HDN.

Anti-U is a rare immune antibody, usually containing an IgG1 component. It has been known to cause fatal haemolytic transfusion reactions and severe HDN.

OTHER BLOOD GROUP SYSTEMS
Lutheran system

The antigens in the Lutheran system are not well developed at birth and as a consequence there are no documented cases of clinically significant haemolytic disease owing to Lutheran antibodies.

Anti-Lu^a is uncommon and rarely of clinical significance. Anti-Lu^b has caused extravascular haemolysis.

Yt (cartwright) system

The antigens Yt^a and Yt^b are found on GPI-linked acetylcholinesterase. Some examples of anti-Yt^a have caused accelerated red cell destruction.

Colton system

The antigens Co^a and Co^b are carried on the water-transport protein, channel-forming integral protein (CHIP-1). Anti-Co^a and the rarer anti-Co^b are sometimes both clinically significant.

Dombrock system

The antigens include Do^a and Do^b and also include the high-incidence antigens Gy^a, Hy and Jo^a. Antibodies of this system are usually weak, but all should be considered as potentially significant.

Table 19.8 Antibody specificities related to the mechanism of immune haemolytic destruction

Blood group system	Intravascular haemolysis	Extravascular haemolysis
ABO,H	A, B, H	
Rh		All
Kell	K	K,k,Kp^a,Kp^b,Js^a,Js^b
Kidd	Jk^a	Jk^a,Jk^b,Jk^3
Duffy		Fy^a,Fy^b
MNS		M,S,s,U
Lutheran		Lu^b
Lewis	Le^a	
Cartwright		Yt^a
Colton		Co^a,Co^b
Dombrock		Do^a,Do^b

CLINICAL SIGNIFICANCE OF RED CELL ALLO-ANTIBODIES

The significance of the allo-antibodies described, with respect to the nature of the haemolytic transfusion reaction they produce, is provided in Table 19.8. The majority of haemolytic transfusion reactions however, are due to ABO incompatibility[17] as shown in Table 19.9.

Mollison et al[18] analysed the significance of blood group antigens other than those of the ABO system and RhD by looking at the prevalence of transfusion-induced red cell allo-antibodies, excluding anti-D, -CD and -DE (Table 19.10). Rh antibodies, mainly anti-c or anti-E, accounted for 53% of the total and anti-K and anti-Fy^a for a further 38%, leaving only about 9% for all other specificities. A similar distribution of the different red cell antibodies was found in a smaller group of patients who experienced immediate haemolytic transfusion reactions (HTR). On the other hand, the figures for delayed HTR showed a striking increase in the relative frequency of Jk antibodies which reflects the outlined characteristics of Jk antibodies.

Haemolytic disease of the fetus and newborn has not been associated with antibodies directed against Lewis antigens, and only very mild disease is produced by anti-Lu^a and anti-Lu^b. With these exceptions, all other IgG antibodies directed against antigens in the systems mentioned should be considered capable of causing haemolysis in this setting.

The significance of the many other blood group antigens not referred to in the text is summarized in Table 19.11. However, it should be noted that the antibodies listed are usually wholly or predominantly IgG and would be detectable in routine pre-transfusion testing using the indirect antiglobulin test (IAT).

It is difficult to find suitable blood for transfusion to a patient whose serum contains an antibody, such

Table 19.9 Fatal acute haemolytic transfusion reactions reported to the FDA between 1976 and 1985

Incompatibility	No. of deaths
O recipient and A red cells	80
O recipient and B/AB red cells	26
B recipient and A/AB red cells	12
A recipient and B red cells	6
O plasma to A/AB recipient	6
B plasma to AB recipient	1
Total ABO incompatibilities	**131**
Anti-K	5
Anti-E+K+P$_1$	1
Anti-Jk^b	1
Anti-Jk^a+Jk^b+Jk^3	1
Anti-Fy^a	1
Total non-ABO incompatibilities	**9**

Table 19.10 Relative frequency of immune red-cell allo-antibodies*

Patient group	No. studied	Blood group allo-antibodies (% of total)				
		Rh**	K	Fy	Jk	Other
Transfused (some pregnant)	5228	53.1	28.1	10.2	4.0	4.7
Immediate HTR†	142	42.2	30.3	18.3	8.5	0.7
Delayed HTR†	82	34.2	14.6	15.9	32.9	2.4

* Excluding antibodies of ABO, Lewis, P systems and anti-M and anti-N.
** Excluding anti-D (or -CD or -DE); almost all were anti-c or anti-E.
† Haemolytic transfusion reaction.
Adapted from Mollison PL, et al 1993 Blood transfusion in clinical medicine, 9th edn. Blackwell Scientific, Oxford, p 112, based on published data from several sources.

Table 19.11 'Minor' blood group antigens

Antigen	Antigen frequency (%) Caucasians	Assoc. HTR	Assoc. HDN	Comments
Di^a	0	Yes	Yes	Part of DI system. Di^a
Di^b	100	Yes	Yes	More common in American Indians and Orientals
Wr^a	<0.1	Yes	Yes	
Xg^a	65 (males) 88 (females)	Rarely	Rarely	Xg^a only antigen in system
Sc1	>99.9	No	No	3 antigens in SC system
Sc2	<0.1	No	Mild	
Ge2	100	Some	No	7 antigens in GE system
Ge3	>99.9	Some	No	
Cr^a	100	Some	No	10 antigens in CR system
Ch1	96	No	No	9 antigens in CH/RG systems,
Rg1	98	No	No	reside on C4
Kn^a	98	No	No	Belong to KN system of 5 antigens
McC^a	98	No	No	
Yk^a	92	No	No	
In^a	0.1	Yes	No	In^a has incidence of 4% in
In^b	99	Yes	No	Asian Indians
LW^a	100	Some	Mild	
JMH	>99.9	No	No	One of 901 series of high incidence antigens
Vel	>99.9	Yes	No	One of 901 series; Complement binding
Bg^a	approx 15	No	No	Corresponds HLA-B7, detectable on red cells

as anti-Vel, which has a specificity for a high-frequency antigen and which can cause severe haemolytic transfusion reactions. Autologous blood should be considered, and the compatibility of red cells from close relatives (particularly siblings) should be investigated. Antibodies such as anti-Kn^a are commonly found and not clinically important, but their presence may cause delay in the provision of blood until their specificity has been determined.

MECHANISMS OF IMMUNE DESTRUCTION OF RED CELLS[19]

Immune-mediated haemolysis of red cells depends upon:

1. The immunoglobulin class of the antibody and for all practical purposes, antibodies directed against red cell antigens are either IgM or IgG or both.
2. The ability of the antibody to bind complement.
3. Interaction with the reticuloendothelial system (mononuclear phagocytic (MP) system). The most important phagocyte participating in immune haemolysis is the macrophage, predominantly in the spleen.

The mechanism of immune haemolysis also determines the site of haemolysis:

a. *Intravascular haemolysis* owing to sequential binding of complement components (C1 through C9) cascade and the formation of the membrane attack complex (MAC; C5b678(9)$_n$). This is characteristic of IgM antibodies but some IgG antibodies can also act as haemolysins. Red cells are typically destroyed by intravascular complement lysis in ABO incompatible transfusion reactions (p. 484). Most other allo-immune red cell destruction is extravascular and mediated by the MP system.

Red cell auto-antibodies may also cause intravascular lysis, especially the IgG auto-antibody of PCH (p. 214) and some auto-antibodies of the cold haemagglutinin syndrome (CHAD) (p. 213). Complement-mediated intravascular lysis may also occur in drug-induced immune haemolysis (p. 216).

b. *Extravascular haemolysis* by the MP system is characteristic of IgG antibodies and occurs predominantly in the spleen. This is caused by non-complement binding IgG antibodies or those which bind sub-lytic amounts of complement. Macrophages have Fcγ receptors for cell-bound IgG, and sensitized red cells may be wholly phagocytosed or lose part of the membrane and return to the circulation as a microspherocyte. Spherocytes are less deformable and more readily trapped in the spleen than normal red cells; this shortens their life-span. In addition to Fc receptor mediated phagocytosis, antibody-dependent cell-mediated cytotoxicity (ADCC) may also contribute to cell damage during the close contact with splenic macrophages. Red cells are destroyed external to the monocyte membrane by lysosomal enzymes secreted by the monocyte.[20]

Complement components may enhance red cell destruction. Complement activation by some IgM and most IgG antibodies is not always complete and the red cell escapes intravascular lysis. The activation of complement stops at the C3 stage and, in these circumstances, complement can be detected on the red cell by the antiglobulin test using appropriate anti-complement reagents. The first activation product of C3 is membrane-bound C3b, which is constantly being broken down to C3bi. Red cells with these components on their surface adhere to phagocytes (monocytes, macrophages and granulocytes) which have complement receptors, CR1 (CD35) and CR3 (CD11b/CD18). These sensitized cells are rapidly sequestered in the liver because of its bulk of phagocytic cells (Küpffer) cells and large blood flow, but no engulfment occurs. When C3bi is cleaved, leaving only C3dg on the cell surface, the cells tagged with 'inactive' C3dg return to the circulation, as in CHAD. However, when IgG is also present on the cell surface, C3b enhances phagocytosis, and under these circumstances both liver and spleen are important sites of extravascular haemolysis. Hence, C3b and C3bi augment macrophage-mediated clearance of IgG-coated cells, and antibodies binding sub-lytic amounts of complement (e.g. Duffy and Kidd antibodies) often cause more rapid destruction and more marked symptoms than non-complement binding antibodies (e.g. Rh antibodies).

Macrophage activity is an important component of cell destruction and further study of cellular interactions at this stage of immune haemolysis may provide an explanation for the differing severity of haemolysis in patients with apparently similar antibodies. In vitro macrophage (monocyte) assays have been introduced to supplement conventional serological techniques in order to assess this aspect of immune haemolysis.[21]

Factors which may affect the interaction between sensitized cells and macrophages include:

1. *IgG subclass.* IgG1 and IgG3 antibodies have a higher binding affinity to mononuclear Fcγ receptors than IgG2 and IgG4 antibodies.
2. *Antigen density* affects the number of antibody molecules bound to the cell surface.
3. *Fluid-phase IgG.* Serum IgG concentration is a determinant of Fc-dependent MP function. Normal levels of IgG block the adherence of sensitized red cells to monocyte Fc receptors (particularly FcγR1) in vitro. Haemoconcentration within the splenic sinusoids is probably a major factor in minimizing this effect in vivo, which may explain why the spleen is about one hundred times more efficient at removing IgG-sensitized cells than the liver, in spite of the greater macrophage mass and higher blood flow of the latter organ.

    The initial effect of high-dose intravenous IgG is to cause blockade of macrophage FcγR. This reduces the immune clearance of antibody-coated cells, and has particular application in the management of auto-immune thrombocytopenia and post-transfusion purpura.
4. *Regulation of macrophage activity.* Cytokines are now known to be important in the upregulation of macrophage receptors. Interferon gamma enhances macrophage phagocytic activity by increasing the expression of FcγRI in vitro and in vivo and also activates FcγII without increasing the number of these receptors.[22]

    Interleukin-6 also enhances FcγRII activation and increased activity of the CR1 receptor occurs through the action of T-cell cytokines and through chemotactic agents released in the inflammatory response.[23] The increased levels of pro-inflammatory cytokines and other biological mediators and their effects upon the activity of the monocyte phagocytic system have been monitored in patients with systemic inflammatory response syndrome.[24] It is therefore possible that release of cytokines during viral and bacterial infections could, at least in part, trigger some episodes of auto-immune cell destruction.

The rate of immune destruction is therefore determined by antigen and antibody characteristics and the level of activation of the monocyte phagocytic system.

ANTIGEN–ANTIBODY REACTIONS

The red cell is a convenient marker for serological reactions. Agglutination or lysis (owing to complement action) is a visible indication (end-point) of an antigen-antibody reaction. The reaction occurs in two stages: in the first stage, the antibody binds to the red cell antigen (sensitization); the second stage involves agglutination (or lysis) of the sensitized cells.

The *first stage*, i.e. association of antibody with antigen (sensitization), is reversible and the strength of binding (equilibrium constant) depends on the 'exactness of fit' between antigen and antibody. This is influenced by:

1. *Temperature* – cold antibodies (usually IgM) generally bind best to the red cell at a low temperature, e.g. 4°C, whereas warm antibodies (usually IgG) bind most efficiently at body temperature, i.e. 37°C.
2. *pH* – there is relatively little change in antibody binding over the pH range 5.5–8.5, but to ensure comparable results, it is preferable to buffer the saline in which serum or cells are diluted to a fixed pH, usually 7.0. Some antibody elution techniques depend on altering the pH to below 4 or above 10.
3. *Ionic strength* of the medium – low ionic strength increases the rate of antibody binding. This is the basis of antibody detection tests using low ionic strength saline (LISS).

The *second stage* depends on various laboratory manipulations to promote agglutination or lysis of sensitized cells. The cell surface is negatively charged (mainly owing to sialic acid residues), which keeps individual cells apart; the minimum distance between red cells suspended in saline is about 18 nm. Agglutination is brought about by antibody cross-linking between cells. The span between antigen-binding sites on IgM molecules (30 nm) is sufficient to allow IgM antibodies to bridge between saline suspended red cells (after settling) and so cause agglutination. IgG molecules have a shorter span (15 nm) and are usually unable to agglutinate sensitized red cells suspended in saline; notwithstanding this, heavy IgG sensitization owing to high antigen density lowers intercellular repulsive forces and is able to promote agglutination in saline (e.g. IgG anti-A, anti-B). The agglutination of red cells coated by either IgM or IgG antibodies is enhanced by centrifugation. However, it is standard procedure to promote agglutination of IgG-sensitized red cells by:

a. Reducing intercellular distance by pre-treatment of red cells with protease enzymes, e.g. papain or bromelin, which reduce the surface charge of red cells (p. 445).
b. Adding polymers, e.g. albumin, although the mechanism by which albumin or other water-soluble polymers enhance agglutination is uncertain.
c. Bridging between sensitized cells with an antiglobulin reagent in the antiglobulin test (p. 448).

Some complement-binding antibodies (especially IgM) may cause lysis in vitro (without noticeable agglutination), which can be enhanced by the addition of fresh serum as a source of complement. On the other hand, complement activation may only proceed to the C3 stage; in these circumstances cell-bound C3 can be detected by the antiglobulin test using an appropriate anticomplement reagent (p. 449).

GENERAL POINTS OF QUALITY ASSURANCE WITHIN THE LABORATORY

It has long been appreciated that the test systems employed for routine pre-transfusion testing are of the utmost importance, since errors can and do lead to patient morbidity and mortality. It is therefore of little surprise that within the European Union (EU), as from July 2000, all reagents, calibrators and control materials for red cell typing and for determining the presence of 'irregular anti-erythrocytic antibodies' have been included

under the EU In-vitro Diagnostics (IVD) Medical Devices Directive.[25] In effect this means that by 2003, all reagents sold within the EU will have to display the CE mark to show that they conform to the agreed Common Technical Specifications (CTS). In each country, a Competent Authority will be able to withdraw or suspend certification of any reagent, depending upon the information received from its Notified Body which will perform batch release approval and monitor the performance of the manufacturer and the product.

The arrival of this Directive further reinforces the potential liabilities of an individual laboratory, which takes on the product liability of a manufacturer if reagents are made 'in-house' or if the manufacturer's recommended method is not strictly adhered to.

The majority of the following points are taken from the British Committee for Standards in Haematology (BCSH) guidelines[26] for pre-transfusion compatibility testing:

1. General aspects
a. The laboratory should document its Quality System, appropriate to its requirements.
b. Attention should be given to the sensible inclusion of internal controls in all the tests undertaken.
c. The laboratory should participate in External Quality Assessment exercises.
d. The laboratory should only make use of systems which have been validated against its documented requirements.
e. The laboratory should ensure that they have procedures to cover the failure of automated equipment and computer(s). The laboratory should develop procedures to build in checks for all critical points in transfusion testing, e.g. preserving the identity of patient samples, transcribing results.

2. Reagents
a. The head of the laboratory should refer to available specifications for reagents given by, e.g. the International Society of Blood Transfusion (ISBT), the American Association of Blood Banks (AABB) or the Guidelines for the Blood Transfusion Services.[27–29]
b. All reagents or systems should be used in accordance with the manufacturer's instructions.

Where this is not possible, the procedure should be validated in accordance with the BCSH Guidelines on evaluation, validation and implementation of new techniques for blood grouping, antibody screening and crossmatching.[30]

c. There should be a record of all batch numbers and expiry dates of all reagents used in the laboratory.

3. Techniques

a. All procedures used should be in accordance with recommended practice as outlined below.

b. It is essential that the antiglobulin technique chosen has been validated against the documented requirements of the laboratory and has been subjected to a thorough field trial before being introduced into the laboratory.[31]

c. All changes in techniques must be thoroughly validated in accordance with the BCSH Guidelines on evaluation, validation and implementation of new techniques before being introduced into routine use.

d. Written authorized standard operating procedures (SOPs) which cover all aspects of the laboratory work must be available and reviewed regularly.

e. The regular checking and maintenance of all laboratory equipment must be documented. In particular, there should be a documented quality assurance procedure for cell washers, e.g. using the National Institute of Biological Standards and Control (NIBSC) anti-D standard.[32]

4. Staff training and proficiency

a. There should be a documented programme for training laboratory staff which covers all SOPs in use and which fulfils the documented requirements of the laboratory.

b. Laboratory tasks should only be undertaken by appropriately trained staff.

c. There must be a documented programme for assessing staff proficiency, e.g. replicate testing for the IAT, which should include details of the action limits for retraining.[33]

5. Auditing and reviewing practice

a. There should be a system in place for documenting and reviewing all incidents of non-compliance with procedures.

b. The systems should enable a full audit trail of laboratory steps, including the original results, interpretations, authorizations, and all staff responsible for conducting each step.

c. A programme of independent audits should be conducted to assess compliance with documented 'in-house' procedures.

6. Health and safety

Whenever possible, reagents should be used that have been screened for HIV, HBV and HCV. All high-risk samples must be handled in accordance with the laboratory safety code.

GENERAL POINTS OF SEROLOGICAL TECHNIQUE

Serum versus plasma

Serum is preferred to plasma for the detection of red cell alloantibodies. Nevertheless, plasma is being used increasingly for convenience in microplate technology and in automated systems.

When plasma is used, complement is inactivated by the EDTA anticoagulant. This is relevant for the detection of some complement-binding antibodies, e.g. of Kidd specificity, that may be missed or give only weak reactions with anti-IgG in the routine antiglobulin test, but can be readily detected by anti-complement (p. 449). It is therefore essential, before using plasma, to optimize the sensitivity of techniques for detecting weak IgG antibodies and to validate the procedure (p. 449). For example, in antibody screening, increased sensitivity can be achieved by using panel cells with homozygous expression of selected antigens (p. 478).

Collection and storage of blood samples

Positive identification of the patient and careful labelling of blood samples are essential to avoid misidentification errors. Venous blood is desirable for blood-grouping purposes and 5–10 ml of blood should be taken and either allowed to clot at room temperature or anticoagulated with EDTA in a sterile glass tube. This will provide serum or plasma and red cells. If serum is required urgently, the specimen may be placed in a 37°C water-bath and centrifuged as soon as the clot can be seen to have started to retract.

Storage of sera or plasma

Great care must be taken to identify and label correctly any serum or plasma separated from the patient's original sample.

Whole blood samples will deteriorate over a period of time. Problems associated with storage include red cell lysis, loss of complement in the serum, decrease in potency of red cell antibodies, particularly IgM antibodies, and bacterial contamination. However, in the absence of evidence, it has been suggested that whole blood can be stored at room temperature for up to 48 h and up to 7 days at 4°C. It has also been recommended that laboratories evaluate the stability of weak antibodies before making local decisions for storage conditions. Patient's serum or plasma is best stored frozen at −20°C or lower in 1–2 ml volumes in glass or plastic vials. Repeated thawing of a sample is harmful. If the sera are stored at −20°C or below, no precautions are necessary with respect to sterility. Complement deteriorates rapidly on storage, but sera separated from blood as quickly as possible and stored at −20°C retain most of their complement activity for 1 to 2 weeks. For compatibility tests, samples of serum should be separated from the red cells as soon as possible and stored at −20°C until used, as the content of complement may be important for the detection of some antibodies.

Red cell suspensions

Normal ionic strength saline (NISS)

A 2–3% suspension of washed red cells in phosphate buffered saline (PBS), pH 7.0, is generally recommended. Cells suspended in NISS are routinely used for antibody titrations, but their use in routine pre-transfusion testing has declined over the last decade as observations from external quality assessment exercises have demonstrated that laboratories employing NISS have a significantly lower detection rate of antibodies than those employing other technologies.[34]

Low ionic strength saline (LISS)

It is known that the rate of association of antibodies with red cell antigens is enhanced by lowering the ionic strength of the medium in which the reactions take place. Hence, a major advantage of LISS is that the incubation period in the IAT (p. 450) can be shortened whilst maintaining or increasing sensitivity to the majority of red cell antibodies. The LISS solution can be made up in the laboratory (p. 604) or purchased commercially.

There was historical reluctance to use low ionic strength media in routine laboratory work for two reasons: first, non-specific agglutination may occur when NaCl concentrations <2 g/l (0.03 mol/l) are used, and second, complement components are bound to the red cells at low ionic strengths.

To avoid false-positives, the following rules should be followed:

a. Red cells resuspended in LISS and serum or plasma should be incubated together in equal volumes: 2 volumes of cells to 2 volumes of serum are recommended to ensure the optimal molarity in the test of the order of 0.09 mol. Doubling the serum to cell ratio (by halving the cell concentration from 3% to 1.5%) will enhance the detection of some antibodies, e.g. anti-K, that might otherwise be missed.[35]
b. The red cells should be washed in saline (×2) and then LISS (×1) before suspending in LISS at 1.5–2% cell suspension.
c. The working solution of LISS should be freshly made and kept at room temperature.
d. Centrifugation force and time should be optimal to give maximum sensitivity with freedom from false-positive or false-negative reactions (p. 450).

False-positive reactions may still infrequently occur with some sera/plasma. If plasma is used, subsequent serological work may be performed using NISS; if serum is used, anti-IgG should replace the polyspecific antiglobulin reagent.

REAGENT RED CELLS

Red cells of selected phenotypes are required for ABO and RhD grouping, Rh phenotyping, and antibody screening and identification (see Ch. 20). Such cells are available commercially or from Blood Transfusion Centres.

Use of enzyme-treated cells

Enzyme-treated red cells are useful reagents in the detection and investigation of auto- and allo-antibodies. Papain and bromelin are currently used for this purpose. Enzyme treatment is known to increase the avidity of both IgM and IgG antibodies. The receptors of some red cell antigens however, may be inactivated by enzyme treatment, e.g. M, N, S, Fy[b].

The most sensitive techniques are those using washed enzyme-pretreated red cells (two-stage) techniques which should match the performance of the spin tube LISS antiglobulin test (p. 450) One-stage mixtures and papain inhibitor techniques are relatively insensitive and are now not recommended. An ISBT/International Council for Standardization in Haematology (ICSH) protease enzyme standard and an agreed method for its use are available from listed centres.[27]

Low's method for the preparation of papain solution[36]

A 1% solution of papain is made as follows:

Grind 2 g of papain in a mortar in 100 ml of Sorensen's phosphate buffer, pH 5.4 (p. 606). Centrifuge for 10 min and add 10 ml of 0.5 mol/l cysteine hydrochloride to the supernatant to activate the enzyme. Dilute the solution to 200 ml with the phosphate buffer and incubate for 1 h at 37°C. Dispense the enzyme in small volumes (e.g. 0.1–0.2 ml); it will keep satisfactorily for many months at –20°C, but once a tube is unfrozen any of the solution not immediately used should be discarded.

The enzyme activity should be standardized using an azoalbumin assay,[37] as this will determine the incubation time for enzyme treatment of the cells. The enzyme preparation should also be compared with the ISBT/ICSH papain standard using the same batch of azoalbumin, and so serve as an 'in house' standard.[27]

Two-stage papain method[38]

Add 1 volume of 1% papain (activated as described above) to 9 volumes of Sorenson's phosphate buffer, pH 7.0 (p. 606) in a 10 × 75 mm glass tube. Incubate at 37°C equal volumes of the freshly diluted papain and packed washed red cells for a time which must be determined for each batch of papain depending on the azoalbumin activity; this is normally 15–30 min. After incubation, wash the cells in two changes of saline, pH 7.0, then dilute as required to 3% in NISS or 1.5% in LISS. For NISS tests, add 1 drop of NISS-suspended cells to 1 drop of serum. For LISS tests, add 2 drops of LISS-suspended cells to 2 drops of serum. Incubate for 15 min in a 37°C water-bath.

Preparation of bromelin solution[39]

Prepare a 0.5% solution by dissolving the bromelin powder in a mixture of 9 volumes of saline and 1 volume of Sorensen's phosphate buffer, pH 5.4 (p. 606). Store the solution in 0.5–1.0 ml volumes at –20°C, at which temperature it will keep for months. As preservatives, add 0.1% sodium azide and 0.5% Actidione (a fungicide). Add the bromelin, in the same way as papain is added in Low's technique, to the serum just before the addition of the red cells. There is no need to pretreat the red cells with the enzyme. Bromelin activity can be standardized by an azoalbumin assay as for papain.

Controls are particularly important when enzyme-treated cells are being used, and it must be established without question that the altered cells are reacting appropriately with sera of known antibody content. Only in this way can the potency of the enzyme and the method of enzyme treatment be checked. Enzyme-treated cells are compared with untreated cells in reactions with a positive control (0.25 iu/ml anti-D) and a negative control (AB serum or fresh compatible serum).

AGGLUTINATION OF RED CELLS BY ANTIBODY: A BASIC METHOD

Agglutination tests are usually carried out in tubes or microtitre plates, employing centrifugation or sedimentation. Slide tests are sometimes used for emergency ABO and RhD grouping (pp. 473 and 476). For microplate tests, see page 473.

Tube tests

Add 1 volume of a 2% red cell suspension to 1 volume of serum or serum dilution in a disposable plastic or glass tube. Mix well and leave undisturbed for the appropriate time (see below).

Tubes. For agglutination tests, use medium-sized (75 × 10 or 12 mm) disposable plastic or glass tubes. Similar tubes should be used for lysis tests when it is essential to have a relatively deep layer of serum to look through, if small amounts of lysis are to be detected. The level of the fluid must rise well above the concave bottom of the tubes.

Glass tubes should always be used if the contents are to be heated to 50°C or higher, or if organic solvents are being used. Glass tubes, however, are difficult to clean satisfactorily, particularly small bore tubes, and cleaning methods such as those given in the Appendix (p. 609) should be followed carefully.

Temperature and time of exposure of red cells to antibody

In blood-group serology, tube tests are generally done at 37°C and/or room temperature. There is some advantage in using a 20°C water-bath rather than relying on 'room temperature' which in different countries and seasons may vary from 15°C (or less) to 30°C (or more).

Sedimentation tube tests are usually read after 1–2 h have elapsed. Strong agglutination will, however, be obvious much sooner than this. In spin tube tests, agglutination can be read after only 5–10 min incubation if the cell-serum mixture is centrifuged.

Slide tests

Because of evaporation, slide tests must be read within about 5 min. Reagents which produce strong agglutination within 1–2 min are normally used for rapid ABO and RhD grouping. Since the results are read macroscopically, strong cell suspensions should be used (35–45% cells in their own serum or plasma) (see Fig. 19.2).

Reading results of tube tests

Only the strongest complete (C) grade of agglutination seems to be able to withstand a shake procedure without some degree of disruption which may downgrade the strength of reaction. The BCSH Blood Transfusion Task Force has therefore recommended the following reading procedure.[40]

(a) Microscopic reading

It is essential that a careful and standardized technique be followed. Lift the tube carefully from its rack without disturbing the button of sedimented cells. Holding the tube vertically, introduce a Pasteur pipette, with its tip cut at 90°. Carefully draw up a column of supernatant about 1 cm in length and then, without introducing an air bubble, draw up a 1–2 mm column of red cells by placing the tip of the pipette in the button of red cells. Gently expel the supernatant and cells on to a slide over an area of about 2 × 1 cm. It is import-

ant not to overload the suspension with cells, and the method described above achieves this.

A scheme of scoring the results is given in Table 19.12.

(b) Macroscopic reading

A gentle agitation tip-and-roll 'macroscopic' method is recommended. It is possible to read agglutination tests macroscopically with the aid of a hand reading-glass or concave mirror, but it is then difficult to distinguish reactions weaker than + (microscopic reading) from the normal slight granular appearance of unagglutinated red cells in suspension. Macroscopic reading thus gives lower titration values than does microscopic reading, but the former is recommended. Follow the system of scoring in Table 19.12.

A good idea of the presence or absence of agglutination can often be obtained by inspection of the deposit of sedimented cells: a perfectly

Table 19.12 Scoring of results in red cell agglutination tests

Symbol	Agglutination score*	Description
4+ or C (complete)	12	Cell button remains in one clump, macroscopically visible
3+	10	Cell button dislodges into several large clumps, macroscopically visible
2+	8	Cell button dislodges into many small clumps, macroscopically visible
1+	5	Cell button dislodges into finely granular clumps, macroscopically just visible
(+) or w (weak)	3	Cell button dislodges into fine granules, only visible microscopically**
–	0	Negative result – all cells free and evenly distributed

* Titration scores are the summation of the agglutination scores at each dilution.
** May be further classified depending on the number of cells in the clumps, e.g. clumps of 12–20 cells (score 3); 8–10 cells (score 2); 4–6 cells (score 1) – this is the minimum agglutination that should be considered positive.

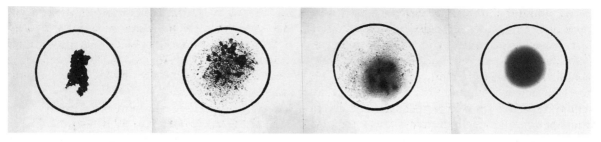

Fig. 19.2 Macroscopic appearances of agglutination in round-bottom tubes or hollow tiles. Agglutination is shown by various degrees of 'graininess'; in the absence of agglutination, the sedimented cells appear as a smooth round button, as on the extreme right.

smooth round button suggests no agglutination whilst agglutination is shown by varying degrees of irregularity, 'graininess' or dispersion of the deposit (Fig. 19.2).

DEMONSTRATION OF LYSIS

Many blood-group antibodies lyse red cells under suitable conditions in the presence of complement. This is particularly true of anti-A and anti-B, anti-P, anti-Le^a and Le^b, anti-PP$_1$P^k (anti-Tj^a) and certain auto-antibodies (p. 212). If it is necessary to add fresh complement, this should be mixed with the serum being tested before the addition of red cells. Otherwise, agglutination occurs and could block complement access. Lysis should be looked for at the end of the incubation period before the tubes are centrifuged, if the cells have sedimented sufficiently; lysis may be scored semi-quantitatively after centrifuging the suspensions and comparing the colour of the supernatant with that of the control.

If the occurrence of lysis is of interest, then the final volume of the cell-serum suspension has to be greater than is required for the reading of agglutination. 75 × 10 or 12 mm tubes should be used and the level of the cell-serum suspension must rise well above the concave bottom of the tubes.

In testing for lytic activity, a high concentration of complement may be required. Therefore, in contrast to tests for agglutination, it is advantageous to use a stronger red cell suspension (*c* 5%).

Lysis tests are usually carried out at 37°C, but with cold antibodies a lower temperature, e.g. 20°C or 30°C, would be appropriate, depending on the upper thermal range of activity of the anti-

body, or, in the case of the Donath–Landsteiner antibody, 0°C followed by 37°C (p. 214).

With certain antibodies the pH of the cell-serum suspension affects the occurrence of lysis. In these, optimal pH is 6.5–6.8.

Controls

It is necessary to be sure that any lysis observed is not artefactual, i.e. that lysis is brought about by the serum under test and not by the serum added as complement, and that the added complement is potent. A complement control (no test serum) is thus necessary and also a control using a serum known to contain a lytic antibody.

In lysis tests, great care should be taken to deliver the cell suspension directly into the serum. If the cell suspension comes into contact with the side of the tube and starts to dry, this in itself will lead to lysis.

ANTIGLOBULIN TEST

The antiglobulin test (Coombs test) was introduced by Coombs, Mourant and Race in 1945[41] as a method for detecting 'incomplete' Rh antibodies, i.e. IgG antibodies capable of sensitizing red cells, but incapable of causing agglutination of the same cells suspended in saline, as opposed to 'complete' IgM antibodies which do agglutinate saline-suspended red cells.

Direct and indirect antiglobulin tests can be carried out. In the *direct* antiglobulin test (DAT), the patient's cells, after careful washing, are tested for sensitization which has occured in vivo; in the *indirect* antiglobulin test (IAT), normal red cells are incubated with a serum suspected of containing an antibody and subsequently tested, after washing, for in vitro bound antibody.

The antiglobulin test is probably the most important test in the serologist's repertoire. The DAT is used to demonstrate in vivo attachment of antibodies to red cells, as in auto-immune haemolytic anaemia (p. 206), allo-immune HDN (p. 487); and allo-immune haemolysis following an incompatible transfusion (p. 484). The IAT has wide application in blood transfusion serology, including antibody screening and identification and crossmatching.

Antiglobulin reagents

(a) Polyspecific (broad-spectrum) reagents
The majority of red cell antibodies are non-complement-binding IgG; anti-IgG is therefore an essential component of any polyspecific reagent. Anti-IgA is not required as IgG antibodies of the same specificity always occur in the presence of IgA antibodies. Anti-IgM is also not required because clinically significant IgM allo-antibodies that do not cause agglutination in saline are much more easily detected by the complement they bind.

Anti-complement has also traditionally been considered essential; namely anti-C3c and anti-C3d. However, if plasma is used, only anti-IgG is necessary as EDTA prevents complement activation. In addition, it seems that most, if not all, antibodies detected by the C3-anti-C3 reaction in normal ionic strength tests, can be detected with anti-IgG in polybrene, polyethylene glycol (PEG) and LISS. Laboratories using techniques other than NISS have adopted the use of anti-IgG alone, supported by changes to guidelines from the AABB in 1990 and from the BCSH in 1996. Nevertheless, the BCSH guidelines stress the importance of having screening cells with homozygous expression of Jk[a] before deciding to use anti-IgG rather than a polyspecific antiglobulin reagent. Anti-C3 will certainly be required for direct antiglobulin tests for the diagnosis of auto-immune haemolytic anaemia.

(b) Monospecific reagents
These can be prepared against the heavy chains of IgG, IgM and IgA and are referred to as anti-γ, anti-μ, and anti-α; antibodies against IgG subclasses are also available. Specific antibodies against the complement components C4 and C3 and C3 breakdown products can be prepared as mentioned above.

The main clinical application of these monospecific reagents is to define the immunochemical characteristics of antibodies. This is relevant to the mechanisms of in vivo cell destruction and, in the case of IgG, the subclasses have different biological properties (p. 442).

Quality control of antiglobulin reagents
The quality control of antiglobulin reagents must always be carried out by the exact technique by which they are to be used. All reagents should be used according to the manufacturer's instructions, unless appropriately standardized for other methods.

An ISBT/ICSH freeze-dried reference reagent is available for evaluating either polyspecific anti-human globulin reagents or those containing their separate monospecific components.[28] The validation of a new antiglobulin reagent should assess the following qualities of the reagent:

1. *Specificity.* The reagent should only agglutinate red cells sensitized with antibodies and/or coated with significant levels of complement components.
2. *Potency of anti-IgG* by serological titration.
3. *Specificity and potency of anti-complement antibodies.* A polyspecific reagent should contain anti-C3c and anti-C3d at controlled levels to avoid false-positive reactions or a suitable potent monoclonal anti-C3d (e.g. BRIC-8). It should contain little or no anti-C4. The assessment of these qualities requires red cells specifically coated with C3b, Cb3i, C3d and C4. Details of the procedures recommended for the preparation of such cells have been published by an ISBT/ICSH Working Party.[42]

It is appreciated that some hospital blood banks will be unable to evaluate an antiglobulin reagent as comprehensively as outlined above. They should, however, carry out the following minimal assessment of all new antiglobulin reagents:

1. Test the antiglobulin reagent for freedom from false-positives by simulated crossmatch tests:
   a. Test for excess anti-C3d by incubating fresh serum at 37°C by NISS and LISS tests with six ABO compatible cells from CPD-A1 donor unit segments (10–30 days old). This is a critical test for false positives owing to

C3d uptake by stored blood which is further augmented by incubation with fresh serum.

b. Tests for contaminating red cell antibodies (against washed A_1, B and O cells) must be negative.

Only proceed further if the antiglobulin reagent passes the above tests.

2. Compare the antiglobulin reagent with the current reagent using a selection of weak antibodies. These antibodies may be selected from those encountered in routine work or can be obtained from a Transfusion Centre or Reference Laboratory. Store such antibodies in small volumes at 4°C for repeated tests.

3. Dilute a weak IgG anti-D (0.8 iu/ml), as used for routine antiglobulin test controls, from undiluted (neat) to 1 in 16 and sensitize R_1r red cells with each dilution of anti-D. These sensitized cells (washed × 4) should then be tested with neat to 1 in 8 dilutions of the antiglobulin reagents. The antiglobulin reagent should not show prozones by immediate spin tests using 2 volumes of antiglobulin per test. The potency of the test antiglobulin should at least match the current antiglobulin reagent.

The ISBT/ICSH antiglobulin reference reagent can be used to calibrate an 'in-house' antiglobulin reagent for use as a routine standard.

The quality control of Ig class and subclass specific antiglobulin reagents, while following the above general principles, is more complex. Details of the appropriate techniques are beyond the scope of this chapter and the reader should consult the review by Engelfriet et al.[43]

Recommended antiglobulin test procedure

A spin tube technique is recommended for the routine antiglobulin test and the procedure described here is based on BCSH *Guidelines for Compatibility Testing in Hospital Blood Banks.*[26,40] Reliable performance depends on the correct procedure at each stage of the test and appropriate quality control measures.

The test should be carried out in glass tubes (75 × 10 or 12 mm). Plastic tubes are not recommended as they may adsorb IgG which could neutralize anti-IgG of the antiglobulin reagent.

1. *Sensitize red cells* (not relevant to the direct test) by using the following serum:cell ratios:

a. For NISS, use at least 2 volumes of serum (preferably 4) and 1 volume of a 3% suspension of red cells washed (×3) and suspended in phosphate buffered saline (PBS) or 0.15 mol/l NaCl (p. 606).

b. For LISS, use 2 volumes of serum and 2 volumes of a 1.5% suspension of red cells washed (× 2) in PBS or 0.15 mol/l NaCl and once in LISS and then suspended in LISS (p. 604).

c. For commercial low ionic strength additive solutions, the manufacturer's instructions must be followed.

As the volume of 'a drop' varies according to the type of pipette or dropper bottle, a measured or known drop volume should be used to ensure that appropriate serum:cell ratios are maintained.

Mix the reactants by shaking, the incubate at 37°C, preferably in a water-bath, for a minimum period of 15 min for LISS tests and 45 min for NISS tests.

2. *Wash the test cells* four times with a minimum of 3 ml of saline per wash. Vigorous injection of saline is necessary to resuspend the cells and achieve adequate mixing. As much of the supernatant as possible should be removed after each wash to achieve maximum dilution of residual serum.

3. *Add 2 volumes of a suitable antiglobulin reagent* to each test tube and centrifuge without delay after thorough mixing. The combinations of centrifugal force (RCF) and time for spin-tube tests are as follows:

RCF (g)	100	200–220	500	1000
Time (s)	60	25–30	15	8–10

4. *Read agglutination* as previously described (p. 447).

5. *Quality control of the test* should be monitored by:

a. An IgG anti-D diluted to give 1+ or 2+ reactions with Rh D positive (R_1r) cells as a *positive control.*

b. An inert group AB serum with the same RhD positive cells as a *negative control*; this is not essential as most tests are negative.

c. *The addition of sensitized cells to all negative tests.* This is widely used to detect neutralization of the antiglobulin reagent owing to incomplete removal of serum by the wash step. The value of this test as a control depends on the strength of reaction of the sensitized cells. Appropriate control cells sensitized with IgG anti-D should give a 3+ reaction when tested directly with the antiglobulin reagent and should still be positive (if the reagent is potent) when added to negative tests, but downgraded (1+ or 2+) owing to the 'pooled-cell' effect of the non-sensitized cells. The reaction will of course be negative if the antiglobulin has been neutralized by residual serum.

The production of satisfactory antiglobulin control cells can be achieved by limiting the level of anti-D sensitization to that which gives a negative test in the presence of 1 in 1000 parts serum in saline.[40]

The suitability of the antiglobulin control cells can be checked as follows:

i.   Prepare two tubes (10 × 75 mm) with 1 volume of 3% unsensitized cells; wash four times.
ii. Add 2 volumes of antiglobulin to each of the tubes, mix well, spin and read the tubes to confirm the tests are negative.
iii. Add 1 volume of 1 in 1000 serum in saline to one tube and 1 volume of saline as a control to the other tube. Mix and incubate for 1 min at RT.
iv. Add 1 volume of control cells to each tube, mix, spin and read the tests.

The test containing 1 in 1000 serum in saline should be negative and the control tube should give at least 2+ reaction. A negative reaction with the control tube suggests a washing deficiency and demands corrective action. If an automated cell-washing centrifuge is used, the washing efficiency should be checked: see *Quality Control of Cell Washing Centrifuges.*[32,40]

New technology for antibody detection by the antiglobulin test

New techniques have emerged that have a simpler reading phase than the manually read spin-tube IAT. These are of two main types: solid phase red cell adherence methods[44] and column agglutination techniques.[45] Before the introduction of a new technique, it is essential to remember that val-idation and routine test trials must be performed by competent workers who are fully familiar with the new system, and that it should be carried out strictly according to the manufacturer's instructions.[30] A well-performed spin-tube IAT, as described above, is the standard against which any new system should be compared.

Solid phase red cell adherence methods involve systems in which known red cells, which may also be sensitized, are immobilized on a solid matrix. In the method referenced, ABO and RhD typing plates are prepared by immobilizing A_1, B and RhD-positive red cells to chemically modified U-bottom strips. The cells are then exposed to the appropriate antibody and the sensitized red cell monolayers are then dried. The unknown test cells are added and the plates are centrifuged after incubation. In a positive reaction, the cells spread over the surface of the well since they have adhered to the bound antibody. In a negative reaction, there is no adherence and the cells form a small button in the centre of the well when the plates are centrifuged.

For reverse typing and antibody screening, A_1, B and O screening cell monolayers are prepared and dried. The test serum is added and if antibodies to any of the immobilized antigens are present, they attach to the monolayer. The tests are read by the addition of A_1B cells that are coated with anti-IgG.

Solid phase methods are highly suited for automated reading by passing a light beam through the well at a point at which it will not be interrupted by the button of cells in a negative test, but will be dispersed by the layer of red cells spread across the well in a positive test.

Column agglutination techniques. In these methods, very small volumes of serum and cells are mixed in a reservoir at the top of a narrow column that contains either a dextran gel* or glass beads.** The columns with the integral reservoirs are supplied in card or cassette form respectively. After a suitable incubation period, the cards/cassettes containing the tests are spun in a centrifuge in which the axis of the column is strictly in line with the centrifugal force. The red cells, but not the medium in which they are suspended, enter the column. Agglutinated

*DiaMed, AG, Switzerland
** Bio Vue, Ortho-Clinical Diagnostics, New Jersey

red cells are trapped at the top of the column, unagglutinated red cells form a pellet at the bottom of the column (see Fig. 20.4, p. 480).

The columns can also contain an antiglobulin reagent for performing. DATs or IATs. Since, during centrifugation, the red cells but not the suspending fluid pass through the gel, the red cells do not have to be washed before coming into contact with the antiglobulin reagent. The columns can also include an antibody, e.g. anti-D, for cell typing. Antigen positive cells are agglutinated and trapped in the upper portion of the column.

The advantages of column agglutination technology are as follows:

1. Ease of use and reading, and can theoretically be performed by relatively unskilled staff.
2. Less chance of aerosol contamination from infected samples, since no cell washing before IATs.
3. The cards can be kept for up to 24 h, enabling the results to be reviewed by experienced staff
4. Ease of automation and positive sample identification.

However, the technology is expensive and its performance does not always compare favourably with the standard LISS-IAT in experienced hands (see Ch. 20).

Assessment of individual worker performance
It is recommended that all staff (including 'on-call' staff who do not routinely work in the blood bank) should be assessed at regular intervals. A procedure based on 'blind' replicate antiglobulin tests may be used for this purpose.[33,40]

The procedure is as follows:

1. A low titre (8–16) IgG anti-D, as used for the control of the antiglobulin test, should be titrated against OR^1r or pooled O RhD-positive cells to find the dilution of anti-D that gives 1+ or 2+ sensitized cells (most workers use around 0.3 iu/ml). A standard BCSH– NIBSC anti-D reference reagent $(95/784)$[46] is available for this purpose (available from NIBSC, PO Box 1193, Potters Bar, Herts EN6 3QG, UK).
2. A batch of sensitized cells is prepared, e.g. by incubating 16 ml of the selected anti-D dilution with 8 ml of 3% washed OR^1 red cells at 37°C for 45 min.

3. Twelve tubes are labelled for blind tests by another person. One volume of 3% 1+ or 2+ sensitized cells and 2 volumes of group AB inert serum (to simulate the volumes of serum used in routine tests) are placed in nine random tubes, and then 1 volume of unsensitized cells + 2 volumes of group-AB inert serum are placed in the remaining tubes. The position of the various tests is recorded.
4. The cells are washed thoroughly four times, antiglobulin is added and the tubes are spun and read.
5. The number of false-negative (and false-positive) results are recorded for each worker and analysed in relation to reading and/or washing technique. It is advisable to give immediate tuition to any workers with washing or reading test faults, followed by further blind replicate trials to demonstrate improvement in procedure and to restore confidence.

Titration of antibodies
A method for preparing primary dilutions of serum and subsequent antibody titration is illustrated in Figure 19.3.

External quality assessment exercises have demonstrated the wide range of titres reported for a single sample, reflecting the differing sensitivities of technologies in use, and have also highlighted the lack of reproducibility.[47] The following points are taken from an addendum to the BCSH guidelines.[48]

Preparation of serial dilutions of patient's or other sera

1. All dilutions and titrations should be made using calibrated pipettes and a separate tip for each step.
2. The diluent should be buffered saline, pH 7.0, for agglutination tests; or for lysis tests undiluted ABO-compatible fresh normal human serum acidified so that the pH of the cell-serum mixture is c 6.8. The normal serum serves as a source of complement.
3. Tube sizes and assay volumes should be chosen to permit thorough mixing of the dilutions.
4. When assaying high-titre samples, an initial dilution should be made to reduce the number of doubling serial transfers to less than 10. A sufficient range of dilutions should be chosen

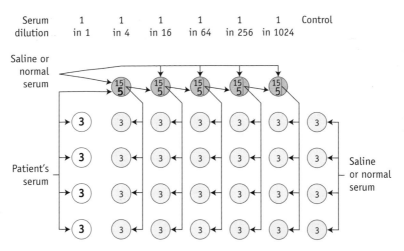

Fig. 19.3 Diagram illustrating method of preparing four sets of four-fold dilutions of a serum. The large circles at the top represent the large tubes in which the primary dilutions are made; the smaller circles represent the tubes in which the titrations are carried out. The figures represent drops or volumes. The patient's neat serum is indicated by the bold type.

to ensure that two negative results can be observed.

5. The end-point should be macroscopic and well defined. The use of visual comparator aids should be considered where possible.

6. Wherever possible, each sample should be tested in parallel with the previous sample.

7. Titrations should be repeated if there is more than a one-tube difference in the titres obtained from sequential samples.

Addition of red cell suspensions to dilutions of serum

It is conventional to add 1 volume of red cell suspension to 1 volume of serum or serum dilution. This means that each antibody dilution, and

hence the 'final' titre, will be twice that of the original serum dilution. Since red cell antigen expression varies with the source and age of the sample, wherever possible, the same cell sample should be used.

ABH SUBSTANCE SECRETION

In the majority of the population, substances with the appropriate A, B and H antigenic activity are distributed widely in saliva and all body fluids, controlled by a regulator secretor gene (Se) which is inherited independently of ABH genes. Only about 20% of people are non-secretors. An individual's secretor status can be determined by testing saliva. A method for this is described in the 8th edition (p. 467).

PLATELET AND GRANULOCYTES

PLATELET AND GRANULOCYTE ALLO-ANTIGEN SYSTEMS

Platelet and granulocyte allo-antigens may be exclusive to each cell type (cell-specific) or shared with other cells. The currently recognized human platelet antigens (HPA) and human neutrophil antigens (HNA) are shown in Tables 19.13–19.15.[49–51] The historical nomenclature for granulocyte antigens used the letter N to indicate neutrophil specificity, and has been retained, although it is

recognized that many studies used granulocytes rather than pure neutrophils and many 'neutrophil specific' antibodies can also target granulocyte precursors. In the HPA nomenclature, HPA-1, -2, -3,-4 and -5 were designated as separate diallelic allo-antigen systems. The high-frequency allele of a system was designated with the letter a and the low-frequency allele with the letter b. However this system is difficult to reconcile with recent molecular genetic knowledge which suggests that each new base exchange does not constitute a

Table 19.13 Molecular genetics of human platelet antigens (HPA)

Antigen	Synonym	Glycoprotein location	Nucleotide substitution	Aminoacid substitution
HPA-1a	Zw^a, Pl^{A1}	GPIIIa	T$_{196}$	Leu$_{33}$
HPA-1b	Zw^b, Pl^{A2}		C$_{196}$	Pro$_{33}$
HPA-2a	Ko^b	GPIbα	C$_{524}$	Thr$_{145}$
HPA-2b	Ko^a Sib^a		T$_{524}$	Met$_{145}$
HPA-3a	Bak^a, Lek^a	GPIIb	T$_{2622}$	Ile$_{843}$
HPA-3b	Bak^b		G$_{2622}$	Ser$_{843}$
HPA-4a	Yuk^b, Pen^a	GPIIIa	G$_{526}$	Arg$_{143}$
HPA-4b	Yuk^a, Pen^b		A$_{526}$	Gln$_{143}$
HPA-5a	Br^b, Zav^b	GPIa	G$_{1648}$	Glu$_{505}$
HPA-5b	Br^a, Zav^a, Hc^a		A$_{1648}$	Lys$_{505}$
HPA-6bW	Ca^a, Tu^a	GPIIIa	A$_{1564}$ G$_{1564}$	Gln$_{489}$ Arg$_{489}$
HPA-7bW	Mo^a	GPIIIa	G$_{1317}$ C$_{1317}$	Ala$_{407}$ Pro$_{407}$
HPA-8bW	Sr^a	GPIIIa	T$_{2004}$ C$_{2004}$	Cys$_{636}$ Arg$_{636}$
HPA-9bW	Max^a	GPIIb	A$_{2603}$ G$_{2603}$	Met$_{837}$ Val$_{837}$
HPA-10bW	La^a	GPIIIa	A$_{281}$ G$_{281}$	Gln$_{62}$ Arg$_{62}$
HPA-11bW	Gro^a	GPIIIa	A$_{1996}$ G$_{1996}$	His$_{633}$ Arg$_{633}$
HPA-12bW	Iy^a	GPIbβ	A$_{141}$ G$_{141}$	Glu$_{15}$ Gly$_{15}$
HPA-13bW	Sit^a	GPIa	T$_{2531}$ C$_{2531}$	Met$_{799}$ Thr$_{799}$
HPA-	Oe^a	GPIIIa		
HPA-	Va^a	GPIIIa		
HPA-	Pe^a	GPIbα		

GP, Glycoprotein location of epitopes

new diallelic allo-antigen system but rather defines a single allele that expresses a single new epitope. Currently, eight different GPIIIa alleles have been found in the human gene pool, three allelic variants have been described for GPIa and GPIIb and two allelic variants have been found for the GPIbα and GPIbβ subunits. A database of human platelet antigens is available at the NIBSC website.* Of the shared antigens, the HLA system is the most important clinically; only class 1 antigens (HLA-A, -B, and to a lesser extent -C) are expressed on platelets and granulocytes. ABH

---

* (*http://www.nibsc.ac.uk*)

Table 19.14 Human platelet antigen frequencies (%) in different populations

Antigen	Dutch	Finns	American Caucasian	Japanese	Korean
HPA-1a	97.9	99.0	98.0	100.0	99.5
HPA-1b	28.8	26.5	20.0	0.3	2.0
HPA-2a	100.0	99.0	97.0	99.2	99.0
HPA-2b	13.5	16.5	15.0	19.7	14.0
HPA-3a	81.0	83.5	88.0	85.1	82.5
HPA-3b	69.8	66.5	54.0	66.2	71.5
HPA-4a	100.0		100.0	100.0	100.0
HPA-4b	0.0		0.0	2.0	2.0
HPA-5a	100.0	99.5	98.0	99.0	100.0
HPA-5b	19.7	10.0	21.0	7.0	4.5
HPA-6a		100.0		99.7	100.0
HPA-6b		2.4		4.8	4.0

Table 19.15 The human neutrophil antigen (HNA) systems

Antigen system	Antigen	Location	Acronym	Caucasian phenotype frequency (%)
HNA-1	HNA-1a	FcγRIIIb	NA1	58
	HNA-1b	FcγRIIIb	NA2	88
	HNA-1c	FcγRIIIb	SH	5
HNA-2	HNA-2a	gp50–64	NB1	97
HNA-3	HNA-3a	gp70–95	5b	97
HNA-4	HNA-4a	CD11b	MART	99
HNA-5	HNA-5a	CD11a	OND	96

antigens are also expressed on platelets (in part absorbed from the plasma), but cannot be demonstrated on granulocytes.

CLINICAL SIGNIFICANCE OF PLATELET AND GRANULOCYTE ANTIBODIES

Platelet and granulocyte antibodies may be classified on the basis of the antigenic stimulus, e.g. allo-, iso-, auto- and drug-induced antibodies.

(a) Allo-antibodies

Allo-immunization to platelet and granulocyte antigens is most commonly due to transfusion or pregnancy. The associated clinical problems depend on the specificity of the antibody, which determines the target cell involved. Cell-specific allo-antibodies are associated with well-defined clinical conditions which are summarized in Tables 19.16 and 19.17.

Allo-immune fetal and neonatal thrombocytopenia are commonly caused by anti-HPA-1a, and less frequently by anti-HPA-5b. The chance of HPA-1a allo-immunization is strongly associated with maternal HLA class-II DRB3*0101 (DR52a) type.[52] Partners should be offered HPA genotyping and if heterozygous, with a severely affected

Table 19.16 Clinical significance of platelet-specific allo-antibodies[112]

1. Neonatal allo-immune thrombocytopenia
2. Post-transfusion purpura
3. Refractoriness to platelet transfusion Usually due to HLA antibodies

Table 19.17 Clinical significance of granulocyte-specific allo-antibodies[113–115]

1. Neonatal allo-immune neutropenia
2. Febrile reactions following transfusion (HLA antibodies also involved)
3. Transfusion-related acute lung injury (TRALI) (transfusion of high-titre antibody)
4. Poor survival and function of transfused granulocytes (HLA antibodies also involved)
5. Auto-immune neutropenia – some auto-antibodies have allospecificity for HNA system antigens.

previous child, fetal HPA grouping should be considered in the first trimester of the next pregnancy, using amniocyte DNA. There is some evidence that severe thrombocytopenia is associated with a third trimester anti-HPA-1a titre >32, using monoclonal antibody immobilization of platelet antigens (MAIPA)[53] (see below). Potential strategies for routine antenatal screening and the acceptability and cost-effective of such a programme are discussed in several recent publications.[53,54]

Post-transfusion purpura is most commonly caused by anti-HPA-1a, but can be associated with HPA antibodies with other specificities against HPA-1b, HPA-2b, HPA-3a, HPA-3b, HPA-4a, HPA-5b.[55]

Immunological refractoriness to platelet transfusions is usually due to anti-HLA antibodies. However, in multitransfused patients with HLA-immunization, up to 25% may also have anti-HPA antibodies.[56,57]

(b) Isoantibodies

Rarely, after blood transfusion or pregnancy, patients with type I Glanzmann's disease make antibodies which react with platelet glycoprotein (GP) IIb/IIIa not present on their own platelets but present on normal platelets, i.e. isotypic determinants.[58–61] Similarly, patients with Bernard–Soulier syndrome may make antibodies against isotypic determinants on GP Ib/V/IX not present on their own platelets.[62] This may present a serious clinical problem because no compatible donor platelets can be found to treat severe bleeding episodes.

(c) Auto-antibodies

Auto-immune thrombocytopenia may be idiopathic or secondary in association with other conditions. Demonstration of a platelet auto-antibody is not mandatory; even with the most suitable techniques now available, platelet auto-antibodies remain elusive in a variable proportion (10–20%) of patients. The autoreactive antibodies target epitopes on certain glycoproteins. In 30–40% of patients these are directed against epitopes on the $\alpha IIb\beta 3$ integrin heterodimer, platelet glycoprotein (GP) IIb/IIIa (CD41) and in 30–40% against the von Willebrand receptor or complex GpIbα/GPIbβ/IX (CD42).[63–66]

In the diagnosis of auto-immune thrombocytopenia it is important to consider and exclude three other immunological conditions:

1. *Post-transfusion purpura (PTP)* – a blood transfusion within 2 weeks will suggest this possibility.[55]
2. *Drug-induced immune thrombocytopenia* – a drug history is essential. Heparin-induced thrombocytopenia (HIT) is the most frequent drug-induced thrombocytopenia and can be confirmed by the demonstration of antibodies to the heparin/platelet factor 4 (PF4) complex by ELISA.[67]
3. *Pseudo-thrombocytopenia* – the patient has an EDTA-dependent platelet antibody which is active only in vitro. The antibody (IgG and/or IgM) reacts with hidden (cryptic) antigens on platelet GP IIb/IIIa, which are exposed owing to confirmational changes in the complex caused by the removal of Ca^{2+} by EDTA.[68] The antibody causes platelet agglutination in the EDTA blood sample associated with large platelet clumps on the blood film or platelet satellitism around neutrophils, both of which lead to a falsely low platelet count.

Auto-immune neutropenia may be idiopathic or secondary. Idiopathic auto-immune neutropenia is more common in infants than in adults, in whom it is usually associated with other disorders which have in common a postulated imbalance of the immune system.[69] However it is the least well studied of the auto-immune cytopenias, because it is rare and performing granulocyte assays is difficult, lengthy, labour-intensive and expensive.

Granulocyte auto-antibodies (which are usually IgG) are unusual in that they often have well-defined specificity for allo-antigens, especially NA1 or NA2.[70] These auto-antibodies may suppress granulocyte precursors in the bone marrow and cause more severe neutropenia. The investigation of suspected auto-immune neutropenia should, when possible, include granulocyte immunology and clonal assays (e.g. CFU-GM) on bone marrow precursors as target cells.

(d) Drug-induced antibodies

Drug-induced antibodies may cause selective haemolytic anaemia (p. 216), thrombocytopenia or neutropenia, or various combinations of these in the same patient.[71,72]

A drug may cause an immune cytopenia by stimulating production of either an *auto-antibody* (which reacts directly with the target cell independently of the drug itself) or a *drug-dependent antibody* which destroys the target cell by reacting with a drug-membrane complex on the target cell.[73] Laboratory tests may demonstrate both types of antibody in some patients.[74]

DEMONSTRATION OF PLATELET AND GRANULOCYTE ANTIBODIES

No single method will detect all types of platelet and granulocyte antibodies equally well. In practice, it is useful to have a basic screening method that will detect most commonly occurring antibodies, both cell-bound (direct test) and in serum (indirect test), and to supplement this with other selected methods for demonstrating particular properties of an antibody and for measuring the amount of cell-bound antibody.

The various techniques used over the last decade by participants in Australasian Platelet Workshops are shown in Table 19.18.[75]

(a) Allo-antibodies

Reports of recent national and international workshops make it possible to formulate guidelines for *platelet immunological tests*. The basic procedure for demonstrating platelet allo-antibodies should include:

(i) A platelet test for platelet-reactive antibodies
The ISBT/ICSH Working Party on Platelet Serology[76] recommended the platelet suspension

Table 19.18 Changing patterns shown in number of participants using various platelet immunology techniques in the Australasian Platelet Workshops between 1989 and 1998

Technique	1989	1992	1995	1998
PIFT microscopic	5	4	1	2
PIFT flow cytometric	3	5	5	7
ELISA	5	2	0	0
SPRCA	3	5	10	8
Chroloquine or acid HLA removal	3	12	11	9
Western immunoblot	3	1	0	0
MAIPA or MACE	0	4	4	6
DNA-based genotype of panel	0	0	7	8
No. of participants	14	17	15	14

PIFT, platelet immunofluorescence test; ELISA, enzyme-linked immunosorbent assay; SPRCA, solid-phase red cell adherence; MAIPA, monoclonal antibody immobilization of platelet antigens; MACE, modified antigen capture ELISA.

immunofluorescence test[77] as the standard for assessment of other platelet antibody techniques.

It is important to combine a sensitive binding assay, such as the platelet immunofluorescence test (PIFT), with an antigen-capture method, such as the MAIPA[78], to increase the chance of detecting weak antibodies or those that react with relatively few antigen sites.

(ii) A lymphocyte test for detecting HLA antibodies

As HLA antibodies also react with platelets, a lymphocyte cytotoxicity and/or ELISA assay should be included in the basic antibody screening procedure.

(iii) Tests to differentiate platelet-specific from HLA antibodies

The MAIPA technique using appropriate monoclonal antibodies is particularly useful for resolving mixtures of platelet-reactive antibodies (p. 463). The chloroquine-'stripping' technique to inactivate HLA Class 1 molecules on platelets[79] is also helpful in this respect (p. 463). Conventional serological techniques (e.g. differential reactions with a panel of normal lymphocytes and platelets; differential absorption of HLA antibodies) can also be used to differentiate cell-specific and HLA antibodies, but these are less suitable for rapid screening than the choroquine- 'stripping' technique.

Further characterization of platelet-specific antibodies will require referral to a reference laboratory. Identification of allospecificity should be carried out as for red cell antibodies by reaction with a selected genotyped panel of group O platelets, preferably with reference to the patient's platelet genotype.

An important consideration in platelet serology is the occasional occurrence of antibodies against hidden (cryptic) antigens of the GP IIb/IIIa complex which are exposed by EDTA and paraformaldehyde (PFA) fixation.[80] These antibodies, which are only active in vitro, are unpredictable, but when suspected can be avoided by using unfixed test platelets from citrated blood.

The detection and identification of granulocyte allo-antibodies should be left to experienced reference laboratories, but follow a similar schedule with the use of monoclonal antibody immobilization of granulocyte antigens (MAIGA)[81,82] or adsorption of the sera with pooled platelets to differentiate between granulocyte-specific and HLA antibodies.

(b) Auto-antibodies

The detection of auto-antibodies and drug-induced antibodies requires special consideration.

It can be misleading, when looking for platelet (or granulocyte) auto-antibodies, only to test the patient's serum against normal platelets (granulocytes), as positive reactions may be due to the presence of allo-antibodies (e.g. HLA or cell-specific) induced by previous transfusion or pregnancy. It is important to show that an auto-antibody in the patient's serum reacts with the patient's own cells. Ideally a DAT (e.g. PIFT) should be performed, before treatment is given, to detect antibody bound in vivo. Where a severe cytopenia exists, it may not be possible to harvest enough cells for the test; nevertheless, serum samples should be stored at −20°C and tested retrospectively against the patient's cells when the peripheral platelet (or neutrophil) count has increased in response to treatment.

A major interest in platelet auto-immunity has been the quantitative measurement of platelet-associated immunoglobulins as an indication of in vivo sensitization. A criticism of these quantitative methods is that they detect not only platelet auto-antibody, but also Ig non-specifically trapped or bound to platelets and platelet fragments,[83] and are therefore generally non-specific in the diagnosis of auto-immune thrombocytopenia.[84] It is now more customary to use the direct PIFT,[85,86] using flow cytometry. The patient's platelets are incubated with isotype specific FITC-labelled conjugates (anti-IgG, anti-IgM and anti-IgA) and the test reported as positive when the fluorescence intensity is > mean + 2SD when compared with the results obtained with pooled (10 or more) normal donor platelet suspensions. In a study of 75 patients with ITP, using microscopy rather than flow cytometry, von dem Borne et al[87] found a weak positive (± to +) direct PIFT in 60% of patients and strong reactions (++ to ++++) in only 26% of patients. In the same study, the indirect PIFT was positive with the patient's serum in 66% of cases who had a positive direct PIFT, and positive with an ether eluate of the patient's platelets in 94% of the same cases. While these results may be a reflection of the relative insensitivity of the method, they may also be due to a low-affinity antibody that is easily eluted during the assay procedure,[83] or indicate an alternative immune mechanism for thrombocytopenia in some cases.

The immunoglobulin (Ig) class of platelet auto-antibodies is similar in idiopathic and secondary auto-immune thrombocytopenia; mostly it is IgG (92%), but often (also) IgM (42%), and sometimes (also) IgA (9%).[87] All IgG subclasses occur, but IgG1 and/or IgG3 are the most frequent.

A combination of the granulocyte immuno-fluorescence test (GIFT)[88] and the granulocyte agglutination test (GAT)[89] provides the most effective means of granulocyte antibody detection. However, immune complexes and aggregates in a patient's serum can still cause false-positive results. This can cause a problem for sera from adult patients with secondary auto-immune neutrope-nia, which should also be investigated for immune complexes (e.g. Clq-enzyme-linked immuno-sorbent assay). The granulocyte chemilumines-cence test (GLCT)[90] is relatively insensitive to the presence of immune complexes when inactivated serum is used, but is unable to detect antibodies of the IgM. Several reviews provide an appraisal of the techniques available for detecting granulocyte-specific antibodies and antigens.[91,92]

(c) Drug-induced antibodies

The serological investigation of drug-induced immune thrombocytopenia (neutropenia) follows the same pattern as for haemolytic anaemia (p. 216), with the exception that it is not always possible to collect enough cells to test at the nadir of thrombocytopenia or neutropenia. The follow-ing blood samples are therefore necessary:

1. *Acute phase blood sample* when the cell count is at the nadir. If there are too few cells to test for cell-bound antibody and complement at this time, it is necessary to test the acute phase serum against the patient's cells during remission. These tests will demonstrate the immune basis of the cytopenia.

If the patient's acute phase serum is tested against *normal* donor cells, it is essential to take account of positive reactions owing to HLA or cell-specific allo-antibody in the patient's serum. Furthermore, negative results with normal donor cells may be due to absence of the antigen for the particular drug-dependent antibody, e.g. owing to genetic restriction of the antigen concerned.[93]

2. *Subsequent samples after stopping the drug.* Ideally, sampling should be done when the drug has been eliminated and the antibody is still detectable. Tests using this sample with and without the drug in the assay system are necessary to demonstrate the part played by the drug in causing the immune cytopenia. The drug may be added directly to the assay system (and included in the wash solution) or the cells may be pretreated with the drug. For some drugs, a metabolite and not the native drug is the appropriate antigen for testing; in these cases an 'ex vivo' drug antigen from urine or plasma may be used.[94]

METHODS OF DEMONSTRATING ANTIBODIES

The basic immunofluorescent antiglobulin method and the MAIPA assay will be described in detail. Only brief mention will be made of other methods.

THE IMMUNOFLUORESCENT ANTIGLOBULIN METHODS

The immunofluorescent antiglobulin methods are based on the conventional antiglobulin technique (p. 448) and are suitable for platelet,[77] granulo-cyte[88] and lymphocyte[95] serology. The PIFT and GIFT* are described in detail in this chapter.

These tests can either be read by direct exami-nation of a cell suspension using fluorescence microscopy, or by flow cytometry. These tests can detect allo-, auto- and drug-induced antibodies and by using appropriate monospecific antiglobu-lin reagents can determine the Ig class and subclass of the antibody and cell-bound complement com-ponents. Both tests can be used with chloroquine-treated cells to differentiate cell-specific from HLA antibodies.[96]

Patient's and screening panel cells

Platelets and granulocytes are prepared from venous blood taken into 5% (w/v) Na_2 EDTA in water (9 volumes blood:1 volume anticoagulant).

Screening panel cells should be obtained from group O donors for platelet serology to avoid posi-tive reactions owing to anti-A and anti-B, but this is not necessary for granulocyte serology as A and B antigens cannot be demonstrated on granulocytes.

---

* Fison Ltd, Loughborough, UK.

If a patient's serum must be tested with ABO-incompatible platelets, anti-A and/or anti-B can be absorbed with corresponding red cells or A or B substance.

The best results are obtained with the freshest cell preparations, but some delay is tolerable (see below). Neutrophils are more susceptible to storage damage than platelets; cells should be fixed (see below) on the day of collection, but serology may be delayed to the following day. Platelets are more resilient and an anticoagulated blood sample may be satisfactory for testing for up to 2 days at ambient temperature (c 20°C). Once fixed, platelets may be kept for up to 3 to 4 days at 4°C before serological testing. For longer storage, platelet-rich plasma may be kept at –40°C for at least 2 months; however, there is some membrane damage after recovery of frozen platelets, which causes increased background fluorescence that may limit the sensitivity of the test.[97,98] For longer-term storage a cryoprotectant, e.g. DMSO, may be used.[98]

Patient's serum

Serum from clotted venous blood should be heated at 56°C for 30 min to inactivate complement, and stored in 1–2 ml volumes (to avoid repeated thawing of a stock) at –40°C.

Control sera

Negative control serum is prepared from a pool of 10 sera from normal group AB male donors who have never been transfused. *Positive control* sera containing platelet-specific antibodies (e.g. anti-HPA-1a), granulocyte-specific antibodies, or multi-specific HLA antibodies should be obtained from reference centres.

Eluate from patient's sensitized cells

Elution is important to confirm the antibody nature of cell-bound immunoglobulin and to determine the specificity of antibodies. This applies especially when no antibody is demonstrable in the patient's serum, which often occurs in patients with auto-immune thrombocytopenia and neutropenia.

Elution by lowering the pH of the medium, by ether (or DMSO) and by heating to 56°C, has been used.[99] For routine platelet serology, ether elution for platelet auto-antibodies or heating to

56°C for platelet-specific allo-antibodies is most convenient.

Heat eluate. Incubate platelets or granulocytes suspended in 0.5 ml of 0.2% bovine serum albumin (BSA) in PBS for 60 min at 56°C. Centrifuge and remove the supernatant which contains the eluted antibody.

Ether eluate. Mix washed packed platelets from 50 ml of EDTA blood with one part of PBS/BSA (0.2%) and two parts of ether, by vigorous shaking for 2 min. Incubate the mixture for 30 min at 37°C in a water-bath with repeated shaking. After centrifugation (2800 g, 10 min), three layers are present, consisting of ether, stroma and the eluate. Pipette off the eluate with a Pasteur pipette and test it in the indirect PIFT with normal donor platelets as described for serum.

Platelet preparation

1. Prepare platelet-rich plasma (PRP) by centrifugation of anticoagulated blood (200 g, 10 min).
2. Wash the platelets × 3 (2500 g, 5 min) in PBS/EDTA buffer (8.37 g of Na_2 EDTA dissolved in 2.5 litres of phosphate buffered saline, pH 7.2); resuspend the platelets thoroughly each time.
3. Fix the platelets in 3 ml of 1% paraformaldehyde (PFA) solution for 5 min at room temperature. (A stock solution of PFA is prepared by dissolving 4 g of PFA (BDH) in 100 ml of PBS by heating to 70°C with occasional mixing. Add 1 mol/l NaOH dropwise with continuous mixing until the solution clears. This 4% stock solution may be stored at 4°C protected from light for several months. Prepare a 1% PFA working solution by adding 1 volume of the 4% PFA stock solution to 3 volumes of PBS and by correcting the pH if necessary to 7.2–7.4 with 1 mol/l HCl.)

Wash the platelets twice as before and resuspend in PBS/EDTA buffer at a concentration of $250–500 \times 10^9/l$ for use in the PIFT.

Granulocyte preparation

1. Mix anticoagulated blood or blood retained from platelet preparation after removal of PRP

(and made up to its original volume with PBS) with 2 ml of Dextran solution per 10 ml of blood (Dextran 150 injection BP in 5% dextrose).* Incubate this mixture at 37°C for 30 min at an angle of about 45° to accelerate red cell sedimentation, and then remove the leucocyte-rich supernatant (LRS).

2. Granulocytes can be separated by double density sedimentation (Fig. 19.4). The LRS is underlayered with 2 ml of lymphocyte separating medium (LSM) (LSM = Ficoll-hypaque sp gr 1.077) which is then underlayered with 2 ml of mono-poly resolving medium (MPRM) (MPRM = Ficoll-hypaque sp gr 1.114).* The density gradient tube is then centrifuged at 2500 *g* for 5 min. Granulocytes form an opaque layer at the LSM/MPRM interface

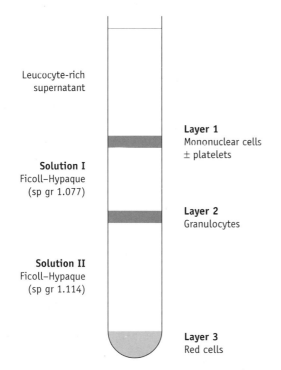

Leucocyte-rich supernatant

Layer 1
Mononuclear cells
± platelets

Solution I
Ficoll–Hypaque
(sp gr 1.077)

Layer 2
Granulocytes

Solution II
Ficoll–Hypaque
(sp gr 1.114)

Layer 3
Red cells

Fig. 19.4 Double density separation of lymphocytes and granulocytes. A leucocyte-rich supernatant is underlayered with Ficoll–Hypaque with a specific gravity of 1.077 (Solution 1) and 1.114 (Solution 2) and then centrifuged at 2500 *g* for 5 min. Lymphocytes concentrate in layer 1, granulocytes in layer 2.

* Both LSM and MPRM supplied by Flow Laboratories Ltd.

from which they are harvested by careful pipetting (microscopic examination shows that the cells from this layer are predominantly neutrophil polymorphs). Lymphocytes can similarly be harvested from the plasma/LSM interface, e.g. for use in the lymphocyte immunofluorescence test (LIFT).[95]

3. Wash the granulocytes three times at 400 *g* for 5 min) in PBS/BSA buffer (PBS pH 7.2 with 0.2% BSA).

4. Fix the granulocytes in 3 ml of 1% PFA for 5 min at room temperature.

5. Wash the granulocytes twice as before, and resuspend in PBS/BSA buffer at a concentration of about $10 \times 10^9/l$ for use in the GIFT.

PLATELET AND GRANULOCYTE IMMUNOFLUORESCENCE TESTS

The serological methods for testing platelets and granulocytes in the suspension immunofluorescence test are similar, except that platelets are washed throughout in PBS/EDTA buffer, and granulocytes in PBS/BSA buffer. A flow diagram of the PIFT is shown in Figure 19.5.

Fluorescein-isothiocyanate (FITC)-labelled antiglobulin reagents are used as follows: anti-Ig (polyspecific), anti-IgG, anti-IgM and anti-C3. $F(ab)_2$ fragments of these reagents should be used to minimize non-specific membrane fluorescence owing to Fc receptor binding, which is a particular problem with granulocytes. The optimal dilution for each reagent should be determined by chequerboard titration. Centrifuge the FITC conjugates at 2500 *g* for 10 min before use to remove fluorescent debris and reduce background fluorescence.

Positive and negative controls (as described above) should be included with each batch of tests.

Indirect test

1. In plastic precipitin tubes (7 × 50 mm), mix 0.1 ml of serum and 0.1 ml of the appropriate cell suspension, as prepared above. (The method can also be adapted for use with microtitre plates which has the advantage of using smaller volumes.)

2. Incubate for 30 min at 37°C (for IgG and C3 tests) and at room temperature (for IgM tests). For C3 tests *only*, sediment cells (1000 *g*, 5 min), remove the supernatant and resuspend

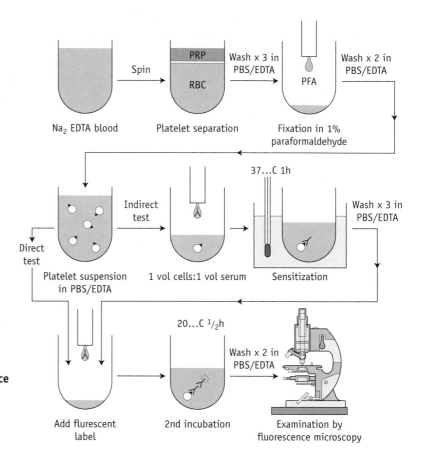

Fig. 19.5 Platelet immunofluorescence test. PRP, platelet-rich plasma; PBS, phosphate buffered saline; PFA, paraformaldehyde; RBC, red blood cells.

the cell button in 0.1 ml of freshly thawed human serum as a source of complement. Incubate for 30 min at 37°C.

3. Wash the cells three times at 1000 g, for 5 min with appropriate buffer – PBS/EDTA for platelets, PBS/BSA for granulocytes; decant the final supernatant. This and subsequent steps are common for both the *indirect* test (i.e. patient's serum with donor cells) and the *direct* test (i.e. patient's own cells to detect in vivo sensitization).

4. Add the fluorescent antiglobulin reagent (0.1 ml of the appropriate dilution determined by chequerboard-titration), mix with the cell button and leave at room temperature for 30 min in the dark.

5. Wash twice as before, and remove the supernatant.

6. Mix 0.5 ml of glycerol–PBS (3 volumes glycerol: 1 volume PBS) with the cell button and mount on a glass slide under a cover-slip.

7. Examine microscopically using ×40 objective and epifluorescent UV illumination.

Scoring results

Reactions in the PIFT and GIFT may be scored on a scale from negative (–) through graded positives + to + + + +. Although subjective, this method of scoring in experienced hands can produce semi-quantitative results in the PIFT.[100]

In general, normal platelets and granulocytes incubated with AB serum do not fluoresce after incubation with an appropriately diluted FITC antiglobulin reagent. Sometimes the negative control may show weak fluorescence (up to two fluorescing points on some cells): in these cases, the test result is classified as positive only if it is clearly stronger than the negative control (AB serum). Stronger fluorescence in the negative control should raise doubts about the performance of the test.

Use of flow cytometry

With simplification of flow cytometers and improved software, more platelet reference laboratories are using them for primary analysis in

PIFT, since sensitivity is improved. Nevertheless, platelets are more difficult to work with flow cytometrically than other cells, and particular attention has to be paid to prevent aggregation, and to ensure single cell suspensions. Presence of platelet particles and debris may also cause confusion. The technical considerations of applying flow cytometry to platelet work are the subject of several recent reviews.[85,86]

CHLOROQUINE TREATMENT OF PLATELETS AND GRANULOCYTES[79,101]

Platelets for chloroquine (Cq) treatment should be prepared from fresh blood or blood stored overnight at 4°C; granulocytes are suitable only if freshly prepared. An important consideration is the extent of chloroquine-induced cell membrane damage, which is minimal with fresh cells.

1. Cells are prepared as already described. Two-thirds of the cells are treated with chloroquine; the remaining one-third is not treated. After washing, and before PFA fixation, the cell button is incubated with 4–5 ml of chloroquine diphosphate in PBS (200 mg/ml, pH adjusted to 5.0 with 1 mol/l NaOH) for 2 h at room temperature with occasional mixing, or overnight at 4°C without mixing, if this is more convenient for the laboratory routine.
2. Wash three times in the appropriate buffer and fix in 1% PFA as previously described. Cell clumping during washing may be a problem after chloroquine treatment, especially with granulocytes; cell clumps should be dispersed by repeated gentle aspiration with a Pasteur pipette. The final cell suspension for serological testing should be prepared as previously described.

When reading the test under fluorescence microscopy, it is important to recognize and allow for any fluorescence owing to chloroquine-induced cell damage, which is more likely to occur with granulocytes than platelets. Damaged cells are easily recognized by bright homogeneous fluorescence. Such cells should be excluded from assessment; only cells showing obvious punctuate fluorescence should be considered positive.

Chloroquine-treated cells were tested initially in the fluorescent antiglobulin method, but they may also be used in enzyme and radionuclide-labelled antigen methods.

Interpretation of results with chloroquine-treated cells

Typical results with HLA and cell-specific antibodies are shown in Table 19.19. If a serum, which has been shown to contain HLA antibodies by LCT and/or LIFT, gives equal or stronger reactions with chloroquine-treated cells than with untreated cells, then a cell-specific antibody is also present. The Second Canadian Workshop on Platelet Serology[97] concluded that a weaker reaction with chloroquine-treated platelets should be interpreted with caution; this could indicate residual HLA reactivity, especially in the presence of high-titre multispecific HLA antibodies. If a platelet-specific antibody is nevertheless still suspected, other methods should be used to confirm this, e.g. MAIPA using appropriate monoclonal antibodies for capture (see below).

Similar caution should be observed in interpreting the GIFT results with chloroquine-treated cells.

MAIPA ASSAY

The principle of the MAIPA assay is shown in Figure 19.6. The test is based on the use of monoclonal antibodies, such as anti-IIb/IIIa, anti-Ib/IX,

Table 19.19 Platelet and granulocyte antibody reactions using cells prepared with and without treatment with chloroquine

Sera	Untreated cells		Chloroquine-treated cells	
	Platelets	Granulocytes	Platelets	Granulocytes
Negative	–	–	–	–
Multispecific HLA antibodies	+++	++	–	–
Granulocyte-specific antibody	–	++	–	+++
Platelet-specific antibody	+++	–	+++	–

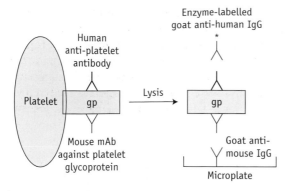

Fig. 19.6 Monoclonal antibody immobilization of platelet antigens (MAIPA): principle of the method. gp, platelet membrane glycoprotein; mAb, monoclonal antibody.

anti-Ia/IIa, anti-HLA class I, to 'capture' specific platelet membrane glycoproteins. The availability of appropriate monoclonal antibodies has led to the wider clinical application of this method.[78] The same principle can be used with granulocytes, depending on the availability of appropriate monoclonal antibodies.[78,102]

The following assay protocol was developed from the original method described by Kiefel.[78,103]

1. Prepare platelets as for the PIFT (p. 460) except that PFA fixation is omitted.
2. Resuspend a pellet of $50–100 \times 10^6$ platelets in 30 μl of human serum or plasma to be tested and incubate at 37°C for 30 min in a U-well microplate.
3. Wash platelets ×2 in PBS/EDTA buffer (p. 460); resuspend the platelets in 30 μl of mouse monoclonal antibody (anti-Gp IIb/IIIa, Ia/IIa, Ib/IX or HLA at 20 μg/ml), and incubate at 37°C for 30 min.
4. Wash platelets ×2 in PBS/EDTA buffer, lyse by the addition of 100 μl of Tris buffered saline (TBS) containing 0.5% Nonidet P-40 and leave at 4°C for 30 min.
5. Transfer the platelet lysate to a 2-ml conical tube and centrifuge at 11 600 g for 30 min at 4°C to remove particulate matter.
6. Dilute 60 μl of the resulting supernatant with 180 μl of TBS wash buffer (0.5% Nonidet P-40, 0.05% Tween 20 and 0.5 mmol CaCl$_2$).
   Transfer 100 μl of diluted platelet lysate, in duplicate, to a flat-well microplate previously coated with goat anti-mouse IgG.* Leave at 4°C for 90 min.
7. Wash the microplate well ×4 with 200 μl of TBS wash buffer and then add 100 μl of alkaline phosphatase-labelled anti-human IgG (Jackson, code 109–055–008) diluted 1:4000 in TBS wash buffer.
   Leave at 4°C for a further 90 min, then wash the wells ×4 with TBS wash buffer and add 100 μl of substrate solution (1 mg/ml p-nitrophenyl phosphate in diethanolamine buffer, pH 9.8) to each well.
8. Measure the resulting colour change at 30 min using a dual wavelength spectrometer (e.g. Bio-Rad model 450).

Express results as the mean absorbance at 405 nm of duplicate tests minus the mean of eight blanks containing TBS wash buffer instead of platelet lysate.

Use pooled AB serum as a negative control.

OTHER METHODS

Several other methods have been developed for the detection of platelet antibodies.

Solid-phase red cell adherence (SPRCA) techniques, (some commercially available) evolved as alternatives to the microscopic reading initially required for the PIFT. These assays combine traditional red cell serology technology with platelet serology. Platelets are captured on microtitre wells, test antibodies are applied, and, after washing and addition of anti-human globulin, platelet or HLA allo-antibody binding is detected using tanned sheep red cells[104] or anti-D sensitized RhD positive red cells.[105] SPRCA are robust, sensitive tests that lend themselves to automation, and the chloroquine treatment of platelets can be used effectively to screen out HLA antibodies.

GTI PakPlus is a platelet antibody kit based upon an ELISA principle**. Microwells coated

---

* The microplate is prepared by adding to each well 100 μl of goat anti-mouse IgG (Sera-Lab, code SBA 1030–01) at 3 μg/ml in carbonate coating buffer, pH 9.6. Leave the plate to stand overnight at 4°C. Next morning, wash the plate ×4 with TBS wash buffer. Leave the last wash supernatant for 30 min to 'block' non-specific protein adsorption to the plastic and then decant.

** Quest Biomedical, Solihull B90 2EL (UK)

with platelet glycoproteins or HLA class I antigens are incubated with test serum. After incubation, followed by washing to remove unbound proteins, any antibody bound to the microwell is detected using an alkaline-phosphatase-conjugated anti-human globulin reagent (anti-GAM or anti-IgG) and the appropriate substrate. Results are considered positive when the ratio of the mean absorbance of the test sample to that of the OD of the normal control sera is 2.0 or more.[106]

With respect to testing for granulocyte antibodies when working with the GIFT or GAT, elucidation of the allo-antibody requires panels of typed granulocytes which cannot be preserved for more than a few hours. A technique has recently been reported which uses extracted granulocyte antigens coated onto U-well Terasaki plates and a micro-mixed passive haemagglutination test. Patient's serum and appropriate controls (sera known to contain granulocyte-specific antibodies, monoclonal antibodies, e.g. anti-CD16 and anti-NA1 and sera from normal donors) are added to the wells and following incubation and washing, indicator blood cells are added (sheep RBC coated with antihuman IgG and anti-mouse IgG). If successful on a large scale, such a technique, together with molecular characterization of the antigens, could make granulocyte immunology more readily available in reference laboratories.[107]

MOLECULAR GENOTYPING OF PLATELET ALLO-ANTIGENS

The application of DNA technology for platelet genotyping is based on the knowledge that the platelet antigen systems are due to single DNA base changes which lead to single amino acid polymorphisms in the platelet membrane glycoproteins (see Table 19.13).

Molecular genotyping involves amplification of the relevant segments of genomic DNA from any nucleated cell by the polymerase chain reaction (PCR) in combination with sequence-specific primers[108] or by allele-specific restriction enzyme analysis[109] or allele-specific oligonucleotide dotblot hybridization.[110]

Of the variety of PCR-based techniques available, the PCR with sequence-specific primers (PCR–SSP) is the most widely used in the UK[111] for the determination of HPA-1 to 5. Molecular

genotyping has now been accepted to be an essential part of confirming the specificity assigned to platelet allo-antibodies, as well as allowing the investigation of patients with severe thrombocytopenia and making possible the determination of the fetal platelet genotype in early pregnancy to assess the risk of allo-immune thrombocytopenia.

REFERENCES

1 Daniels GL, Anstee DJ, Cartron JP 1995 Blood group terminology 1995: From the ISBT Working Party on Terminology for Red Cell Surface Antigens. Vox Sanguinis 69:265–279.

2 Daniels GL, Anstee DJ, Cartron JP 1999 Terminology for red cell surface antigens. Vox Sanguinis 77:52–57.

3 Cartron JP, Bailly P, Le Van Kim C 1998 Insights into the structure and function of membrane polypeptides carrying blood group antigens. Vox Sanguinis 74 (Suppl. 2):29–64.

4 Daniels G 1999 Functional aspects of red cell antigens. Blood Reviews 13:14–35.

5 Eastlund T 1998 The histo-blood group ABO system and tissue transplantation. Transfusion 38:975–988.

6 Mourant AE, Kopec AC, Domaniewska-Sobczak K 1976 The distribution of the human blood groups and other biochemical polymorphisms, 2nd edn. Oxford University Press, Oxford.

7 Yamamoto F 1995 Molecular genetics of the ABO histo-blood group system. Vox Sanguinis 69:1–7.

8 Garratty G, Arndt P, Co S 1993 Fatal ABO haemolytic transfusion reaction resulting from acquired B antigen only detectable by some monoclonal grouping reagents. Transfusion 33 (Suppl. 47S).

9 Garratty G 1996 Association of blood groups and disease: do blood group antigens and antibodies have a biological role? History and Philosophy of the Life Sciences 18:321–344.

10 Cartron JP, Agre P 1993 Rh blood group antigens: protein and gene structure. Seminars in Hematology 30:193–208.

11 Huang CH 1997 Molecular insights into the Rh protein family and associated antigens. Current Opinion in Haematology 4:94–103.

12 Avent ND, Reid ME 2000 The Rh blood group system: a review. Blood 95:375–387.

13 World Health Organization (WHO) 1977 Twenty-eighth Report of WHO Expert Committee on Biological Standardization. Technical Report Series 610. WHO, Geneva.

14 Avent ND 1998 Antenatal grouping of the blood groups of the fetus. Vox Sanguinis 74: (Suppl. 2):365–374.

15 Nash R, Shojania AM 1987 Hematological aspects of Rh deficiency syndrome: a case report and review of the literature. American Journal of Haematology 24:267–275.

16 Medical Research Council 1954 The Rh blood groups and their clinical effects. Memorandum Medical Research Council, London, 27.

17 Sazama K 1990 Reports of 355 transfusion-associated deaths: 1976 through 1985. Transfusion 30:583–590.

18 Mollison PL, Engelfriet CP, Contreras M 1997 Blood transfusion in clinical medicine, 10th edn. Blackwell Scientific, Oxford, p 89.

19 Engelfriet CP 1992 The immune destruction of red cells. Transfusion Medicine 2:1.

20 Horsewood P, Kelton JG 1994 Macrophage-mediated cell destruction. In: Garratty G (ed) Immunobiology of transfusion medicine. Marcel Dekker, New York, p 434–464.

21 Zupanska BA 1994 Cellular bioassays and their use in predicting the clinical significance of antibodies. In: Garratty G (ed) Immunobiology of transfusion medicine. Marcel Dekker, New York, p 465–492.

22 Guyre PM, Miller R 1983 Recombinant immune interferon increases immunoglobulin G Fc receptors on cultured human mononuclear phagocytes. Journal of Clinical Investigation 72:393–397.

23 Griffin JA, Griffin FM 1979 Augmentation of macrophage complement receptor function in vitro. Journal of Experimental Medicine 150:653–675.

24 Volk HD, Reinke P, Krausch D 1996 Monocyte deactivation–rationale for a new therapeutic strategy in sepsis. Intensive Care Medicine 22:S474–S481.

25 In-vitro diagnostics IVD Medical Devices Directive 1998 Official Journal of the European Communities (7.12.98) 1331.

26 British Committee for Standards in Haematology 1996 Guidelines for pre-transfusion compatibility testing in blood transfusion laboratories. Transfusion Medicine 6:273–283.

27 Scott ML, Voak D, Phillips P 1994 Review of the problems involved in using enzymes in blood group serology – provision of freeze-dried ICSH/ISBT protease enzyme and anti-D reference standards. Vox Sanguinis 67:89–98.

28 Case J, Ford DS, Chung A 1999 International reference reagents: antihuman globulin. Vox Sanguinis 77:121–127.

29 Department of Health 1998 Guidelines for the blood transfusion services in the United Kingdom, 4th edn. HMSO, London.

30 British Committee for Standards in Haematology 1995 Recommendations for the evaluation, validation and implementation of new techniques for blood grouping antibody screening and crossmatching. Transfusion Medicine 5:145–150.

31 Voak D 1992 Validation of new technology for antibody detection by antiglobulin tests. Transfusion Medicine 2:177.

32 Phillips PK, Voak D, Whitton CM, et al 1993 BCSH–NIBSC anti-D reference reagent for antiglobulin tests: the in-house assessment of red cell washing centrifuges and of operator variability in the detection of weak macroscopic agglutination. Transfusion Medicine 3:143.

33 Voak D, Downie DM, Moore BPL 1988 Replicate tests for the detection and correction of errors in anti-human globulin AHG tests: optimum conditions and quality control. Haematologia 2:3–16.

34 Knowles S, Milkins CE, Chapman JF 2001 UK NEQAS BTLP; trends in proficiency over the last 15 years. Transfusion Medicine (in press).

35 Voak D, Downie DM, Haigh T, et al 1982 Improved antiglobulin tests to detect difficult antibodies: detection of anti-Kell by LISS. Medical Laboratory Sciences 39:363.

36 Löw B 1955 A practical method using papain and incomplete Rh-antibodies in routine Rh blood-grouping. Vox Sanguinis 5(OS):94.

37 Scott ML, Voak D, Downie DM 1988 Optimum enzyme activity in blood grouping and a new technique for antibody detection: an explanation for the poor performance of the one-stage mix technique. Medical Laboratory Sciences 45:7.

38 Scott ML, Phillips PK 1987 A sensitive two-stage papain technique without cell washing. Vox Sanguinis 52:67.

39 Pirofsky B 1959 The use of bromelin in establishing a standard cross-match. American Journal of Clinical Pathology 32:350.

40 British Committee for Standards in Haematology 1991 Standard haematology practice (Roberts B, ed.) Blackwell Scientific, Oxford, p 150.

41 Coombs RRA, Mourant AE, Race RR 1945 A new test of the detection of weak and 'incomplete' Rh agglutinins. British Journal of Experimental Pathology 26:255.

42 Voak D, Downie DM, Moore PBL, et al 1986 Anti-human globulin reagent specification: the European and ISBT/ICSH view. Biotest Bulletin 1:7.

43 Engelfriet CP, Overbeeke MAM, Voak D 1987 The antiglobulin test, Coombs test and the red cell. In: Cash JD (ed) Progress in transfusion medicine. Churchill Livingstone, Edinburgh, vol 2, p 74–98.

44 Sinor LT 1992 Advances in solid-phase red cell adherence methods and transfusion serology. Transfusion Medicine Reviews 6:26–31.

45 Lapierre Y, Rigel D, Adams J, et al 1990 The gel test: a new way to detect red cell antigen–antibody reactions. Transfusion 30:109.

46 Phillips P, Voak D, Downie M 1998 New reference reagent for the quality assurance of anti-D antibody detection. Transfusion Medicine 8:225–230.

47 O'Hagan J, Milkins CE, Chapman JF, et al 1997 Antibody titres – results of a UK NEQAS BGS exercise and accompanying questionnaire. Transfusion Medicine 7: Suppl. 1.

48 British Committee for Standards in Haematology 1999 Addendum for guidelines for blood grouping and red cell antibody testing during pregnancy. Transfusion Medicine 9:99.

49 Santoso S 1998 Human platelet-specific alloantigens: update. Vox Sanguinis 74 (Suppl. 2):249–253.

50 Bux J, von dem Borne AEG, de Haas L 1999 ISBT Working Party on Platelet and Granulocyte Serology, Granulocyte Antigen Working Party: Nomenclature of granulocyte alloantigens. Vox Sanguinis 77:251.

51 Lucas GF, Metcalfe P 2000 Platelet and granulocyte polymorphisms. Transfusion Medicine 10:157–174.

52 Decary F, L'Abbe D, Tremblay L, et al 1991 The immune response to the HPA-1a antigen: association with HLA-DRw52a. Transfusion Medicine 1:55.

53 Williamson LW, Hackett G, Rennie J, et al 1998 The natural history of fetomaternal alloimmunization to the platelet-specific antigen HPA-1a PI[AI] Zw[a] as determined by antenatal screening. Blood 92:2280–2287.

54 Flug F, Karpatkin M, Karpatkin S 1994 Should all pregnant women be tested for their platelet PLA Zw HPA-1 phenotype? British Journal of Haematology 86:1–5.

55 Mueller-Eckhardt C, Kroll H, Kiefel V, et al 1991 European PTP study group: Post-transfusion purpura. Platelet immunology: fundamental and clinical aspects. (Kaplan-Gouet C, Schlegel N, Salmon C, McGregor J, eds.) INSERM/John Libbey Eurotext.

56 Schnaidt M, Northoff H, Wernet D 1996 Frequency and specificity of platelet-specific allo-antibodies in HLA-immunized haematologic-oncologic patients. Transfusion Medicine 6:111–114.

57 Kurz M, Hildegard G, Hocker P, et al 1996 Specificities of anti-platelet antibodies in multitransfused patients with haemato-oncological disorders. British Journal of Haematology 95:564–569.

58 Bierling P, Fromont P, Elbez A, et al 1988 Early immunization against platelet glycoprotein IIIa in a new born Glanzmann type I patient. Vox Sanguinis 55:109.

59 Brown CH, Weisberg RJ, Natelson EA, et al 1975 Glanzmann's thrombasthenia: assessment of the response to platelet transfusion. Transfusion 15:124.

60 Ribera A, Martin-Vega C, Pico M, et al 1988 Sensitization against platelet antigens in Glanzmann disease. Abstract XX, Congress of the International Society of Blood Transfusion in Association with British Blood Transfusion Society (BBTS), Manchester, p 240.

61 Van Leeuwen EF, von dem Borne AEGKr, Von Riesz LE, et al 1981 Absence of platelet specific alloantigens in Glanzmann's thrombasthenia. Blood 57:49.

62 Degos L, Tobelem G, Lethielliux P, et al 1977 A molecular defect in platelets of patients with Bernard–Soulier syndrome. Blood 50:899.

63 Van Leeuwen EF, Helmerhorst FM, Engelfriet CP, et al 1982 Specificity of auto-antibodies in autoimmune thrombocytopenia. Blood 59:23–26.

64 Fujisawa K, Tani P, O'Toole TE, et al 1992 Different specificities of platelet-associated and plasma auto-antibodies to platelet GPIIb–IIIa in patients with chronic immune thrombocytopenic purpura. Blood 79:1441–1446.

65 Fujisawa K, Tani P, McMillan R 1993 Platelet-associated antibody to glycoproteinIIb/IIIa from chronic immune thrombocytopenic purpura patients often binds to divalent cation-dependent antigens. Blood 81:1284–1289.

66 Hou M, Stockelberg D, Kutti J, et al 1995 Glycoprotein IIb/IIIa autoantigenic repertoire in chronic idiopathic thrombocytopenic purpura. British Journal of Haematology 91:971–975.

67 Kelton JG, Sheridan DP, Santos AV, et al 1988 Heparin-induced thrombocytopenia: laboratory studies. Blood 72:925–930.

68 Pegels JG, Bruynes ECE, Engelfriet CP, et al 1982 Pseudothrombocytopenia: an immunologic study on platelet antibodies dependent on ethylene diamine tetra-acetate. Blood 59:157.

69 Shastri KA, Logue GL 1993 Autoimmune neutropenia. Blood 81:1984.

70 McCullough J, Clay ME, Thompson HW 1987 Autoimmune granulocytopenia. Baillière's Clinical Immunology and Allergy 1:303.

71 Bux J, Mueller-Eckhardt C 1992 Autoimmune neutropenia. Seminars in Hematology 29:45.

72 Mueller-Eckhardt C 1987 Drug-induced immune thrombocytopenia. Baillière's Clinical Immunology and Allergy 1:369.

73 Mueller-Eckhardt C, Salama A 1990 Drug-induced immune cytopenias: a unifying pathogenetic concept with special emphasis on the role of drug metabolities. Transfusion Medicine Reviews 4:69.

74 Salama A, Schutz B, Kiefel V, et al 1989 Immune-mediated agranulocytosis related to drugs and their metabolites: mode of sensitization and heterogeneity of antibodies. British Journal of Haematology 72:127.

75 Minchinton RM 2000 What can we learn from National and International Platelet Serology Workshops? Transfusion Medicine Reviews 14:74–83.

76 Metcalfe P, Waters AH 1990 Report on the fourth ISBT/ICSH platelet serology workshop. Vox Sanguinis 58:170–175.

77 Von dem Borne AEGKr, Verheught FWA, Oosterhof F, et al 1978 A simple immunofluorescence test for the detection of platelet antibodies. British Journal of Haematology 39:195.

78 Kiefel V 1992 The MAIPA assay and its applications in immunohaematology. Transfusion Medicine 2:181.

79 Nordhagen R, Flaathen ST 1985 Chloroquine removal of HLA antigens from platelets for the platelet immunofluorescence test. Vox Sanguinis 48:156.

80 von dem Borne AEGKr, van der Lelie J, Vos JJE, et al 1986 Antibodies against crypt antigens of platelets. Characterisation and significance for the serologist. Current Studies in Hematology and Blood Transfusion 52:33. Karger, Basel.

81 Bux J, Kober B, Kiefel V, et al 1993 Analysis of granulocyte-reactive antibodies using an immunoassay based upon monoclonal-antibody-specific immobilization of granulocyte antigens. Transfusion Medicine 3:157–162.

82 Minchinton RM, Noonan K, Johnson TJ 1997 Examining technical aspects of the monoclonal antibody immobilization of granulocyte antigen assay. Vox Sanguinis 73:87–92.

83 Shulman NR, Leissinger CA, Hotchkiss AJ, et al 1982 The non-specific nature of platelet associated IgG. Transactions of the Association of American Physicians 95:213.

84 Von dem Borne AEGKr 1987 Autoimmune thrombocytopenia. Baillière's Clinical Immunology and Allergy 1:269.

85 Goodall AH, Macey MG 1994 Platelet-associated molecules and immunoglobulins. In: Macey MR (ed) Flow cytometry – clinical applications. Blackwell Scientific, London, p 148–191.

86 Ault KA 1988 Flow cytometric measurement of platelet-associated immunoglobulin. Pathology and Immunopathology Research 7:395–408.

87 Von dem Borne AEGKr, Vos JJJE, van der Lelie J, et al 1986 Clinical significance of positive platelet immunofluorescence test in thrombocytopenia. British Journal of Haematology 64:767.

88 Verheugt FWA, von dem Borne AEGKr, Decary F, et al 1977 The detection of granulocyte allo-antibodies with an indirect immunofluorescence test. British Journal of Haematology 36:533–544.

89 McCullough J, Clay ME, Press C, et al 1988 Granulocyte serology. A clinical and laboratory guide. ACSP, Chicago IL.

90 Lucas GF 1994 Prospective evaluation of the chemiluminescence test for the detection of granulocyte antibodies: comparison with the immunofluorescence test. Vox Sanguinis 66:141–147.

91 Bux J 1996 Challenges in the determination of clinically significant granulocyte antibodies and antigens. Transfusion Medicine Reviews 10:222–232.

92 Stroncek DF 1997 Granulocyte immunology: is there a need to know? Transfusion 37:886–888.

93 Claas FHJ, Langerak J, de Beer LL 1981 Drug-induced antibodies: interaction of the drug with a polymorphic platelet antigen. Tissue Antigens 17:64.

94 Salama A, Mueller-Eckhardt C, Kissel K, et al 1984 Ex vivo antigen preparation for the serological detection of drug-dependent antibodies in immune haemolytic anaemias. British Journal of Haematology 58:525.

95 Decary F, Vermeulen A, Engelfriet CP 1975 A look at HLA antisera in the indirect immunofluorescence technique LIFT. In: Histocompatibility testing. Munksgaard, Copenhagen, p 380.

96 Metcalfe P, Minchinton RM, Murphy MF, et al 1985 Use of chloroquine-treated granulocytes and platelets in the diagnosis of immune cytopenias. Vox Sanguinis 49:340.

97 Decary F 1988 Report on the second Canadian workshop on platelet serology. Current Studies in Hematology and Blood Transfusion 54:1. Karger, Basel.

98 Helmerhorst FM, Ten Boerge ML, van der Plas-
    van Dalen C, et al 1984 Platelet freezing for
    serological purposes with and without a
    cryopreservative. Vox Sanguinis 46:318.

99 Helmerhorst FM, van Oss CJ, Bruynes ECE, et al
    1982 Elution of granulocyte and platelet
    antibodies. Vox Sanguinis 43:196.

100 Vos JJE, Huisman JG, Winkel IN, et al 1987
    Quantification of platelet-bound allo-antibodies
    by radioimmunoassay: a study on some variables.
    Vox Sanguinis 53:108.

101 Minchinton RM, Waters AH 1984 Chloroquine
    stripping of HLA antigens from neutrophils
    without removal of neutrophil specific antigens.
    British Journal of Haematology 57:703.

102 Metcalfe P, Waters AH 1992 Location of the
    granulocyte-specific antigen LAN on the Fc-
    receptor III. Transfusion Medicine 2:283.

103 Kiefel V, Santoso S, Weisheit M, et al 1987
    Monoclonal antibody specific immobilization of
    platelet antigens MAIPA: a new tool for the
    identification of platelet-reactive antibodies.
    Blood 70:1722.

104 Shibata Y, Juji T, Nishizawa Y, et al 1981
    Detection of platelet antibodies by a newly
    developed mixed agglutination with platelets. Vox
    Sanguinis 41:25–31.

105 Lown JA, Ivey JG 1991 Evaluation of solid phase
    red cell adherence technique for platelet antibody
    screening. Transfusion Medicine 1:163–167.

106 Lucas GF, Rogers SE 1999 Evaluation of an
    enzyme-linked immunosorbent assay kit GTI
    PakPlus® for the detection of antibodies against
    human platelet antigens. Transfusion Medicine
    9:63–67.

107 Araki N, Nose Y, Kohsaki M, et al 1999 Anti-
    granulocyte antibody screening with extracted
    granulocyte antigens by a micro-mixed passive
    haemagglutination method. Vox Sanguinis
    77:44–51.

108 Metcalfe P, Waters AH 1993 HPA-1 typing by
    PCR amplification with sequence-specific primers
    PCR-SSP: a rapid and simple technique. British
    Journal of Haematology 85:227.

109 Simsek S, Faber NM, Bleeker PM, et al 1993
    Determination of human platelet antigen
    frequencies in the Dutch population by
    immunophenotyping and DNA allele-specific
    restriction enzyme analysis. Blood 81:835.

110 McFarland JG, Aster RH, Bussel JB, et al 1991
    Prenatal diagnosis of neonatal alloimmune
    thrombocytopenia using allele-specific
    oligonucleotide probes. Blood 78:2276.

111 Cavanagh G, Dunn A, Chapman CE, et al 1997
    HPA genotyping by PCR sequence specific
    priming PCR-SSP: a streamlined method for
    rapid routine investigations. Transfusion Medicine
    7:41–45.

112 von dem Borne AEGKr, Ouwehand WH 1989
    Immunology of platelet disorders. Bailliere's
    Clinical Haematology 2:749.

113 Engelfriet CP, Tetteroo PAT, van der Veen JPW,
    et al 1984 Granulocyte-specific antigens and
    methods for their detection. In: Advances in
    immunobiology: blood cell antigens and bone
    marrow transplanatation. Liss, New York, p. 121.

114 McCullough J 1985 The clinical significance of
    granulocyte antibodies and in vivo studies of the
    fate of granulocytes. In: Garratty G (ed) Current
    concepts in transfusion therapy. American
    Association of Blood Banks, Arlington, VA, p 125.

115 Minchinton RM, Waters AH 1984 The occurrence
    and significance of neutrophil antibodies. British
    Journal of Haematology 56:521.

20

Laboratory aspects of blood transfusion

S. M. Knowles

The effective development and maintenance of satisfactory standards of transfusion medicine practice require an organization-wide approach and adoption of a quality assurance system. In the absence of a quality infrastructure, errors will abound in this process. Haemovigilance reports confirm that the majority of life-threatening haemolytic reactions (owing to ABO incompatibility) are caused by errors occurring outside the transfusion laboratory,[1,2,3] and all groups of staff administering blood should be trained in accordance with appropriate procedures.[4]

Safe and efficient blood transfusion practice also depends on accurate documentation and the elimination of clerical errors within the laboratory (see British Committee for Standards in Haematology (BCSH) *Guidelines on Hospital Blood Bank*

Documentation and Procedures[5a] and BCSH *Guidelines on Hospital Blood Bank Computing*,[5b,6] consideration of the patient's clinical history, particularly with respect to previous transfusions, pregnancy and drugs and a satisfactory pre-transfusion testing procedure to ensure donor-recipient compatibility are essential. The principles of quality assurance within the laboratory, which underpin every test undertaken, are provided in Chapter 24.

This chapter is primarily concerned with pre-transfusion compatibility testing and follows the BCSH *Guidelines for Pre-transfusion Compatibility Procedures in Blood Transfusion Laboratories*.[5c,7] It also includes sections on antenatal antibody screening, investigation of allo-immune haemolytic disease of the fetus and newborn (HDN) and investigation of transfusion reactions.

PRE-TRANSFUSION COMPATIBILITY TESTING

A satisfactory compatibility procedure should include:

1. ABO and RhD grouping of the patient

2. Antibody screening of the patient, or the mother in the case of neonatal transfusion, to detect the presence of clinically significant antibodies. In the event of a positive antibody screen, antibody

identification should be undertaken to assist the selection of compatible blood.

3. A computer or manual check of records to compare current and historical findings. (These three elements constitute a group/type and screen.)

4. Donor red cell selection and crossmatching.

TO CROSSMATCH OR NOT TO CROSSMATCH?

The serological crossmatch, and in particular the antiglobulin phase has been traditionally regarded as the ultimate check of ABO incompatibility. However, in recent years, serological crossmatching has been abbreviated to an 'immediate spin' technique and some hospitals have eliminated all serological crossmatching for certain categories of patient and rely entirely on computer issue of red cells.

The BCSH *Guidelines for Pre-transfusion Compatibility Procedures in Blood Transfusion Laboratories*[7] and the American Association of Blood Banks (AABB) *Standards for Blood Banks and Transfusion Services*[8] emphasize the fundamental requirements and the validation which should be undertaken, prior to omitting the antiglobulin phase of the crossmatch and before instigating computer issue.

DOCUMENTATION

The safety of blood transfusion depends on accurate patient and sample identification at all stages, starting with taking the blood sample from the patient for compatibility testing and ending with the transfusion of compatible blood. In the UK Serious Hazards of Transfusion Report 1998–1999, mis-identification of the patient or sample outside the laboratory was responsible for 53% instances when the wrong blood was given to a patient.[3]

The use of computers in the laboratory can also help to eliminate errors,[5b,6] by making historical records accessible at the time of pre-transfusion testing.

BLOOD SAMPLES

Immediately on receipt of the blood sample, laboratory staff should confirm that it is appropriately labelled and that the information on the sample and request form is identical. The BCSH guidelines require a minimum patient identification of family name, first name, date of birth and hospital/accident and emergency department number. Samples received from trauma or unconscious accident and emergency patients are unlikely to be fully identified, but there should be at least one unique identifier and the sex of the patient. If these requirements are not met, group O blood should be issued until a suitably labelled sample is available. Pre-menopausal females should receive O RhD-negative units.

If the patient has been transfused within the last month, the sample should be taken as close as possible to the following transfusion, to ensure that newly developed antibodies are detected. Patients who are being repeatedly transfused should be retested every 72 h.

Great care must be taken to identify and label correctly any serum or plasma separated from the patient's original blood sample; the serum or plasma should be stored at or below −20°C.

ABO AND RhD GROUPING

These must be performed by an approved technique with appropriate controls. Before use, all new batches of grouping reagents should be checked for reliability by the techniques used in the laboratory. Grouping reagents should be stored according to the manufacturer's instructions.

ABO GROUPING

Correct interpretation of the patient's ABO group requires confirmation, whenever possible, by tests on the patient's serum or plasma (except for newborn infants up to 4 months of age in whom naturally occurring anti-A and anti-B are normally absent). Ideally, cell and serum or plasma grouping should be carried out by different workers who then check each other's results. Where this is not feasible, the distinct tasks can be separated, e.g. separating the documentation of the reaction patterns from the final interpretation.

Reagents

Anti-A, anti-B and anti-A,B reagents were traditionally used for cell grouping tests. The anti-A,B reagent (group O serum) acted as an additional check on red cells which were agglutinated by anti-A or anti-B, and detected weaker A or B antigens. Conventional polyclonal reagents have been replaced by superior anti-A and anti-B monoclonal reagents,[9] and there is now no requirement to continue to use anti-A,B or A+B in ABO grouping.

The monoclonal reagents should contain EDTA (0.1 mol/l pH 7.1–7.3) to prevent haemolysis they should be used in the presence of fresh patient's serum, as these potent IgM antibodies are strong haemolysins in the presence of complement.

Methods

ABO grouping may be carried out by tube or slide methods or in microplates. The reader is referred to the BCSH *Guidelines on Microplate Technology.*[5d]

Tube methods

Spin-tube methods have replaced sedimentation tube methods.

Spin-tube tests may be performed in 75×10 or 12 mm glass or plastic tubes. Immediate spin tests may be used in an emergency, whereas routine tests are usually left for 15 min at room temperature ($c20°C$) before centrifugation. For details of spin force (RCF) and time, see p. 609. Equal volumes (1 drop from either a commercial reagent dropper or a Pasteur pipette) of liquid reagents or serum/plasma and 2% cell suspensions are used.

The patient's red cells (diluted in phosphate buffered saline, PBS) should be tested against monoclonal anti-A and anti-B grouping reagents.

The patient's serum or plasma should be tested against A_1 and B reagent red cells (reverse grouping). In addition, the serum or plasma should also be tested against either the patient's own cells or group O cells, i.e. a negative control to exclude reactions with A and B cells owing to cold agglutinins in the patient's sample other than anti-A or anti-B. To prevent misinterpretation of results owing to haemolysis where serum is used, it is recommended that the diluent for resuspension of reverse grouping cells contains EDTA (see below).

Mix the suspensions by tapping the tubes and leave them undisturbed for 15 min. Agglutination should be read as described on p. 447.

Any discrepancy between the results of the red cell grouping and the reverse grouping should be investigated further, and any repeat tests should involve cells taken from the original sample rather than the prepared suspension. Reverse grouping is not carried out for infants under 4 months of age as the corresponding antibodies are normally absent.

EDTA for diluents. Stock solution: prepare a 0.1 mol/l solution of EDTA (di-potassium salt) in distilled water. Adjust the pH to 7.0 using 5 mol/l NaOH. Working solution: mix 1 volume of stock solution with 9 volumes of saline or low ionic strength saline (LISS). Check the pH and adjust to 7.0 if necessary.

Controls

Positive and negative controls must be included with every test or batch of tests. The anti-A reagent should be tested against group A (positive control) and B (negative control) cells, and the anti-B reagent against group B (positive control) and group A (negative control) cells.

Slide method

In an emergency, ABO grouping may be carried out rapidly on slides or tiles. The method is satisfactory if potent grouping reagents are used (see p. 447). An immediate spin-tube test is preferable.

Microplate method

ABO and RhD grouping may be carried out on one U-well plate if monoclonal reagents are used. The layout of the plate is as shown in Figure 20.1.

Using a commercial reagent dropper or Pasteur pipette, add 1 volume of antiserum to each well of the appropriate row (D–H).

Add 1 volume of 2% patient's cells in PBS to these rows and the auto control row (C).

Add 1 volume of patient's serum or plasma to the A and B cell rows and the auto control (C) row, followed by 1 volume of 2% A and B cells in PBS.

Add the control cells as indicated. Anti-D controls are incorporated in the ABO control cells, e.g. Arr, Brr and OR^1r.

Mix on a microplate shaker. Leave the microplate at room temperature (20°C) for 15 min, then centrifuge at 700 rpm for 1 min.

The plate can be read by one of two methods – streaming (microplate set at an angle) or agitation. Automated microplate readers may also be used.[10]

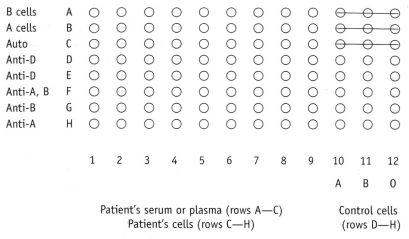

		1	2	3	4	5	6	7	8	9	10	11	12
B cells	A	○	○	○	○	○	○	○	○	○	○	○	○
A cells	B	○	○	○	○	○	○	○	○	○	○	○	○
Auto	C	○	○	○	○	○	○	○	○	○	○	○	○
Anti-D	D	○	○	○	○	○	○	○	○	○	○	○	○
Anti-D	E	○	○	○	○	○	○	○	○	○	○	○	○
Anti-A, B	F	○	○	○	○	○	○	○	○	○	○	○	○
Anti-B	G	○	○	○	○	○	○	○	○	○	○	○	○
Anti-A	H	○	○	○	○	○	○	○	○	○	○	○	○

A   B   0

Patient's serum or plasma (rows A—C)   Control cells
Patient's cells (rows C—H)   (rows D—H)

Fig. 20.1 Microplate layout for ABO and RhD grouping. The patient's serum or plasma is added to rows A–C for ABO reverse grouping and the auto control (C). The patient's cells are added to rows C–H for ABO and RhD cell grouping and the auto control (C). The ABO control cells (rows D–H) incorporate controls for the two anti-D reagents, e.g. Arr, Brr, OR¹r.

CAUSES OF DISCREPANCIES IN ABO GROUPING

Before any tests are read the controls must show that the reagents are working correctly.

(a) False-positive results

(i) Rouleaux formation

Marked rouleaux formation can simulate true agglutination (Figs 20.2 and 20.3). In reverse grouping the two can be distinguished by repeating

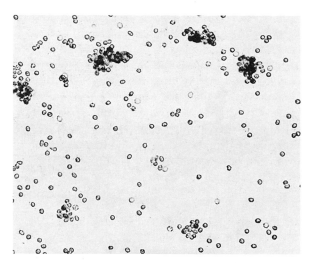

Fig. 20.3 Photomicrograph of a suspension of red cells in serum, showing weak agglutination The small agglutinates are more irregularly distributed than the rouleaux and vary more in size. There are also more free cells.

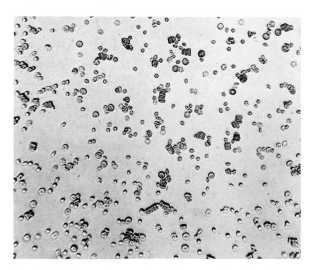

Fig. 20.2 Photomicrograph of a suspension of red cells in serum, showing a minor degree of rouleaux formation. The numerous small rouleaux are characteristically relatively evenly spaced throughout the field and do not vary greatly in size.

the test using the serum diluted 1 in 2 or 1 in 4 in saline. Rouleaux should disappear; agglutination will hardly be affected. If rouleaux are apparent in red cell grouping tests, the tests should be repeated after washing the patient's red cells thoroughly.

(ii) Auto-immune haemolytic anaemia

Cold agglutinins will cause auto-agglutination and apparent panagglutination, if active at room temperature. If this is suspected, the reverse grouping test should be repeated at 37°C, at which temperature the auto-agglutination control should be negative. Any anti-A and/or anti-B present in the patient's serum will, however, still react. The patient's red cells should be washed several times in warm (37°C) saline and the cell grouping repeated.

There is no problem with warm IgG autoantibodies when monoclonal reagents are used.

(b) False-negative reactions in ABO grouping

1. Failure of agglutination or weak reactions are usually due to impotent sera. Loss of potency results if sera are carelessly left at room temperature or stored frozen in large volumes so that repeated freezing and thawing are required. The controls should be carefully checked.
2. Failure to add the grouping reagents will cause false results; the use of coloured reagents – blue for anti-A, yellow for anti-B – is a check for this error.
3. In reverse grouping tests, false-negative results may be recorded if lysis is not recognized as a positive result. All reverse grouping tubes should be carefully inspected for lysis and its presence recorded before attempting microscopic reading of agglutination. To avoid lysis, reverse grouping cells should be diluted in an EDTA solution.

(c) Mixed-field reactions

These may be due to:

1. The previous transfusion of group O cells to group A or B recipients.
2. An earlier incompatible transfusion.
3. An ABO-incompatible bone-marrow transplant.
4. A permanent dual population of cells, which may be the first indication of blood-group chimerism.

RhD GROUPING

This is usually performed at the same time as ABO grouping to minimize clerical errors that may arise through repeated handling of patients' samples. Each sample should be tested in duplicate, at least for first-time patients, as there is no counterpart of 'reverse grouping', as in ABO grouping.

Reagents

The availability of high-titre monoclonal IgM anti-D reagents[9] has made it possible to use the same techniques as for ABO grouping. These reagents work equally well at room temperature (c 20°C) and at 37°C and are reliable for emergency D grouping by immediate spin-tube techniques as described for ABO grouping. In the UK, guidelines[7] recommend that reagents should be selected which do not detect D^{VI}; a partial D with the fewest epitopes and theoretically, the greatest propensity to form anti-D.

Non-potentiated monoclonal reagents should be used in preference to potentiated reagents which do not cause agglutination in saline unless potentiators (e.g. polyethylene glycol) have been added to the diluent. These potentiated anti-D reagents must be used strictly according to the manufacturer's instructions and an additional reagent or diluent control must be included. The diluent control is essential to demonstrate that the diluent itself does not promote agglutination of the patient's cells, as might occur with red cells already coated with immunoglobulin owing to in vivo sensitization.

All anti-D grouping reagents should be checked by the method used in the laboratory for specificity with *positive* (OR^1r or OR^1R^2) and *negative* (Orr or Or′r) controls. Additional controls are necessary for polyclonal reagents to confirm the *absorption* of any contaminating anti-A (using A_1rr cells) and anti-B (using Brr cells). Before a new batch of reagent is introduced, it should be evaluated in parallel with the reagent in current use.

Methods

Slide, tube and microplate methods may be used as for ABO grouping.

Tube method

Working in sequence for ABO and D grouping provides for efficient batch testing.

Add 1 volume of anti-D to each tube of the anti-D row of each rack.

Then add 1 volume of the 2% red cell suspension to each tube.

The tests are mixed, incubated and read, as described for ABO tests.

Microplate method

ABO and RhD grouping are usually carried out in one microplate using monoclonal reagents (Fig. 20.1).

Controls

Controls and tests should be set up in one operation. Each batch of tests should include *positive* (R_1r or R_1R_2) and *negative* (rr) controls. Each test sample must have an *auto*-control (own cells and own serum).

Emergency RhD grouping

Spin-tube method

For emergency D grouping, use the spin-tube method and centrifuge the tubes at $150\,g$ for 1 min either immediately or after incubation, depending on the time available.

Slide method

Monoclonal anti-D reagents are available that agglutinate D-positive cells within a few minutes. The manufacturer's instructions must be followed (see also p. 473).

For both methods it is essential to use potent anti-D reagents and to include positive and negative controls.

False-positive results in RhD grouping

Misclassification of an RhD-negative patient as RhD-positive could lead to the transfusion of RhD-positive blood. Resultant anti-D sensitization could have potentially harmful clinical consequences, especially for RhD-negative girls or women of child-bearing age (see also p. 477).

False-positive results may occur for the following main reasons:

1. Red cells may already be coated with immunoglobulin owing to in vivo sensitization. For this reason, antiglobulin and enzyme techniques should not be used for routine RhD grouping. Furthermore, direct agglutination tests with potentiated anti-D reagents should include an appropriate diluent control to exclude false-positive results.
2. A polyclonal anti-D grouping reagent may contain a contaminating antibody which has not been adequately absorbed, e.g. contaminating anti-A or anti-B, or anti-C (leading to a false-positive result in a D-negative C-positive patient). This type of false-positive result may occur when reagents have not been adequately controlled for the method in use or when the reagent manufacturer's instructions have not been followed.
3. Bacterial contamination of reagents may also cause false-positive agglutination.

Clinical significance of D variant phenotypes.

Discrepant results in RhD grouping with different anti-D reagents may indicate a serious reagent fault (e.g. contaminating antibody as discussed above), but are usually caused by weak D phenotypes which have fewer D antigen sites than normal (called D^u).[9] The incidence of weak D is c 0.7%, if selected by an IgM monoclonal anti-D at suitable dilution, e.g. MAD-2.

In clinical practice, if the serological reactions with standard methods are weak or there is a discrepancy in the reactions obtained using two reagents, the patient should be grouped as RhD-negative. This 'error' will be of no clinical consequence, since the transfusion of RhD-negative blood will be compatible with respect to the D antigen. Similarly, a weak D pregnant woman, misclassified as RhD-negative, will not be harmed serologically by prophylactic IgG anti-D. Nothing is to be gained by further testing of RhD-negative patients by other techniques, e.g. antiglobulin or enzyme methods, to detect possible weak D; a more important consideration is the risk of false-positive results with such methods, as indicated above.

In the routine grouping of blood donors at transfusion centres, only some weak D samples will be misclassified as RhD-negative; the incidence varies, but can be reduced to as low as 0.23% by the sensitive automated methods now being used.[11a] The clinical consequences will not be serious since weak D red cells are thought to be unlikely to undergo accelerated destruction if transfused to an immunized patient; moreover, weak D red cells are thought to be poorly immunogenic and unlikely to provoke a primary immune response in an RhD-negative recipient.[11a]

In addition to weak D antigens (D^u), there are rare RhD-positive individuals who lack some of the epitopes of the complex D antigen (partial Ds). Polyclonal reagents (being the product of several B-cell clones and containing a mixture of antibodies recognizing different epitopes on the same antigen) react with the whole D antigen, but monoclonal reagents are directed against specific epitopes and may give negative results with partial D red cells if the antibody is directed against the missing epitopes. Category D^{VI} individuals possess the fewest D epitopes and are most likely to be immunized by transfusion of RhD-positive red cells; making an antibody against the epitopes they lack. Similarly, a partial D mother may be immunized by a normal fetal D antigen, and this could cause RhD haemolytic disease of the newborn (HDN).[12]

Rh PHENOTYPING

Reagents for determining the Rh phenotype are available commercially. It is essential to follow the manufacturer's instructions in doing the tests. The following specificities are required: anti-D, anti-C + C^w, anti-E, anti-c and anti-e.

It is essential to use a panel of cells of known genotypes as controls. Cells that are heterozygous for the antigen under test are used as positive controls; cells that do not have the antigen under test are used as negative controls. If polyclonal reagents are being used, absorption controls, i.e. cells which do not express the antigen under test but would be agglutinated by the most common contaminants, should be included as indicated in Table 20.1. Reagent 'diluent' controls should be set up if potentiated reagents are being used and as instructed by the manufacturer.

GROUPING IN ANTENATAL WORK

Pregnant women must be grouped for ABO and RhD and this should be done early in pregnancy as a routine.

Table 20.1 Genotypes of the red cells to use as controls for Rh grouping sera

Antiserum	Negative control	Positive control	Absorption control
Anti-D	Cde/cde	CDe/cde	A$_1$ B cde/cde
Anti-C	cDE/cDE	CDe/cDE	A$_1$ B cde/cde
Anti-E	cDe/cde	CDe/cDE	A$_1$ B cde/cde
Anti-c	CDe/CDe	CDe/cDE	A$_1$ B CDe/CDe or A$_1$ + B, both CDe/CDe
Anti-e	cDE/cDE	cDE/cde	A$_1$ B cDE/cDE or A$_1$ + B, both cDE/cDE

Accuracy in RhD grouping of antenatal samples is particularly important as RhD-negative women erroneously grouped as RhD positive carry the risk of:

1. Being transfused with RhD-positive blood and consequently being sensitized to the RhD antigen which could result in severe HDN in subsequent pregnancies.
2. Not receiving prophylactic anti-D immunoglobulin, with the same potential consequences as (1).

All pregnant women, whether RhD-negative or RhD-positive, should be screened for antibodies other than anti-D. Although HDN owing to anti-D is the most severe form of the disease, anti-c and anti-K can give rise to significant haemolysis in utero, sufficient to cause intrauterine death and to warrant intervention during pregnancy. Other IgG antibodies, e.g. anti-E, anti-Ce, anti-Fy^a and anti-Jk^a, uncommonly give rise to fetal haemolysis of sufficient severity to merit antenatal intervention.

The UK guidelines also recommend that all pregnant women are grouped for a second time, between 28 and 36 weeks' gestation.[13]

The paternal blood group phenotype should be determined in all cases where the mother has a clinically significant allo-antibody. If the paternal red cells lack the corresponding antigen, the baby is not at risk. However, caution is advised, as the assumed parent may not be the biological father of the fetus!

It is useful to predict whether the partner of an RhD-negative woman with anti-D is homozygous or heterozygous for the D antigen. This is essential to forecast the chances of the couple having children affected by RhD HDN.

No antisera against the 'd' antigen are available as the 'd' antigen is amorphic. Because of the lack of an 'anti-d' serum, the zygosity of the D antigen is usually predicted from the results of tests with anti-C, anti-c, anti-E and anti-e sera, and from tables of the likelihood of the homo-or heterozygous association of D with the other Rh antigens. These tables have been compiled for different racial groups. It is important, therefore, to tell the specialist laboratory the racial origin of the patient.

Table 20.2 gives the results of testing samples of RhD-positive red cells from an English population with anti-D and four other anti-Rh antisera, and

Table 20.2 Probability of Rh D-positive genotypes in terms of homozygosity (D/D) or heterozygosity (D/d) in an English population

Reaction with anti-					Probable genotype	% of total giving these results	Next most probable	% of total giving these results	Relative frequency of heterozygous:homozygous amongst samples giving these results
D	C	c	E	e					
+	+	+	−		$R^1r(D/d)$	94	$R^1R^0(D/D)$	6	15:1
+	+	−	−		$R^1R^1(D/D)$	96	$R^1r'(D/d)$	4	1:21
+	+	+	+		$R^1R^2(D/D)$	88	$R^1r''(D/d)$	8	1:8
+	−	+	+	+	$R^2r(D/d)$	93	$R^2R^0(D/D)$	6	15:1
+	−	+	+	−	$R^2R^2(D/D)$	86	$R^2r''(D/d)$	14	1:6
+	−	+	−		$R^0r(D/d)$	97	$R^0R^0(D/D)$	3	30:1
+	+	−	+		$R^1R^2(D/D)$	97	$R^2r'(D/d)$	2	1:41

the interpretation of the data in terms of D homozygosity and heterozygosity for the common and not so common genotypes. The relative frequencies in the last column apply to a random population. They are applicable to RhD-positive partners of RhD-negative women in general, but RhD-positive fathers of children who have had RhD HDN are a selected rather than a random population. The chances of such a father provisionally called 'heterozygous' being in reality homozygous for the D antigen becomes more likely with every child that is affected. However, as the genetic basis of the common D groups is now known, *RH* DNA typing of both the father and fetus provides the better alternative for predicting the potential for HDN.[14]

GROUPING FOR PATIENTS WITH HAEMOGLOBINOPATHIES

In patients with haemoglobinopathies, who are likely to require long-term transfusion support, it is advisable to perform an extended red cell phenotype before they are transfused. Phenotyping should include Rh antigens, K, Jk^a, Jk^b, Fy^a, Fy^b and MNSs. This information can then be used to help investigate the specificities of any allo-antibodies formed as a result of repeated transfusions.

ANTIBODY SCREENING

In parallel with determining the ABO and RhD groups, all patients should be screened for unexpected allo-antibodies, i.e. other than anti-A and anti-B. This facilitates the selection of suitable blood for a patient requiring transfusion.

The patient's serum or plasma should be tested against at least two red cell suspensions, used separately and *not* pooled. The screening cells must be group O and should encompass the common antigens of the ethnic population. In the UK, the screening cells should express, as a minimum, the following antigens: C,c, D, E, e, M, N, S, s, P_1, K, k, Le^a, Le^b, Fy^a, Fy^b, Jk^a, Jk^b.[7,15] At least one cell must have the stronger D antigen combination R_2.

It is also desirable, to have apparent homozygous expression of the following antigens, in the stated order of priority; D, c, Fy^a, Jk^a, Jk^b, S, s, Fy^b, because heterozygous red cells may fail to detect antibodies that would react positively with homozygous cells. In practice, 95% of hospitals in the UK use three or four screening cells which together guarantee homozygous expression of the relevant antigens (Table 20.3).[16] The majority of UK hospitals that have abolished the routine use of an indirect antiglobulin test (IAT) crossmatch also select cells which express C^w and Kp^a.

Screening cells are available commercially or from Blood Transfusion Centres.

Table 20.3 Selection of units for patients with red cell allo-antibodies

Specificity	Clinical significance	Selection of units
Rh antibodies (reactive in IAT)	Yes	Antigen negative
Kell antibodies	Yes	Antigen negative
Duffy antibodies	Yes	Antigen negative
Kidd antibodies	Yes	Antigen negative
Anti-S,-s	Yes	Antigen negative
Anti-A$_1$, -P$_1$, -N	Rarely	IAT crossmatch Compatible 37°C
Anti-M	Rarely	IAT crossmatch Compatible 37°C
Anti-M reactive at 37°C	Sometimes	Antigen negative
Anti-Le^a, anti-Le^{a+b}	Rarely	IAT crossmatch Compatible 37°C
Anti-Le^b	No	Not clinically significant and can be ignored
High-titre low-avidity antibodies (HTLA)	Unlikely	Seek advice from Transfusion Centre
Antibodies against low/high frequency antigens	Depends on specificity	Seek advice from Transfusion Centre

The antibody screening procedure is designed to detect antibodies of clinical significance. No single test will detect all blood-group antibodies, but since antiglobulin methods can detect almost all clinically significant antibodies, it is acceptable to use an IAT for pre-transfusion antibody screening without any additional screening techniques provided that the following conditions are met:

1. The laboratory has implemented a documented programme for assessment of worker proficiency in the IAT method.
2. The laboratory has implemented a documented programme of replicate testing to assure the efficacy of cell washers.
3. The IAT method has been properly validated against the documented requirements of the laboratory.
4. The laboratory has performed consistently well in external quality assessment exercises using different workers and the IAT method in use.

In a retrospective study of 10 000 patients,[17] 35 samples were found to contain antibodies reacting with ficin-treated cells which were not demonstrable in a LISS-IAT. However only one patient with an anti-c reactive only with enzyme-treated cells suffered a delayed haemolytic transfusion reaction.

UK guidelines specifically recommend the use of red cells suspended in LISS, which has been shown in repeated external quality assessment exercises to provide significantly better antibody detection rates than normal ionic strength saline (NISS).

Each batch of antibody screens should be controlled with a weak anti-D serum, standardized against a pool of R$_1$r cells. Although reagent red cells are validated by the manufacturer to ensure antigen stability under the storage conditions given in the package insert, many laboratories prudently also include a weak anti-Fy^a or anti-S with each batch of tests to ensure that there is no deterioration of screening cells during their shelf life.

New techniques, e.g. column agglutination technology[18] (Fig. 20.4) and solid phase,[19] which have simpler reading phases and are suitable for automation, are being introduced for routine antibody

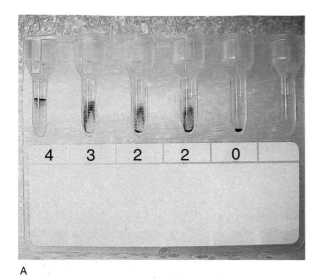

A

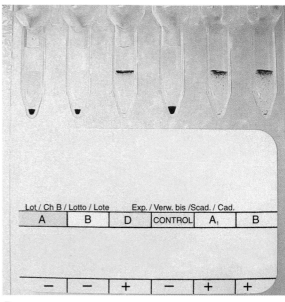

B

Fig. 20.4 Column agglutination technology.
(A) Antibody screening. (B) Blood grouping: O RhD+.

screening. A fully automated screening IAT method,[20] including positive sample identification at the sampling and reading stages, provides a valuable additional security check if a single antibody screening method is used. It should be recognized that non-automated methods are more prone to human error.

Although column agglutination technology has many advantages and in most instances has comparable sensitivity in detecting unexpected antibodies to a LISS–IAT technique, and can improve detection if there is under performance of the LISS–IAT, it has been shown to be less sensitive in detecting weak ABO and Kidd antibodies.[16,21–23]

ANTIBODY IDENTIFICATION

A positive result in the antibody screen should be followed by antibody identification. The serum or plasma under investigation is normally tested against a panel of eight or more group O red cell samples of known antigen composition, using as a starting point, the test method(s) with which the antibody was initially detected. Inclusion of the patient's own red cells is helpful in distinguishing between an auto-antibody and one directed against a high-frequency antigen. The specificity of an antibody can only be assigned when it is reactive with at least two examples of reagent red cells carrying the antigen and non-reactive with at least two examples of red cells lacking the antigen. Additional antibodies may be present in a serum and it is essential that the presence of additional clinically significant antibodies is not overlooked. This can only be achieved by testing the serum

against additional red cell samples negative for the apparent specificity but positive for other antigens to which clinically significant antibodies may arise. It is therefore essential to know the phenotype of the autologous red cells to predict the specificities of additional antibodies that might be present. When phenotyping patient's red cells, a reagent control or AB serum control should be incorporated, used by the same technique as the phenotyping serum. A positive direct antiglobulin test (DAT) will invalidate test results.

Although it is commonplace to use an IAT technique in isolation for antibody screening, the use of additional techniques is essential to determine the immunochemical properties of an antibody, which can assist in the resolution of mixtures of antibodies. If the antibody is clearly cold-reacting and causing direct agglutination in saline at 20°C or

25°C, but is inactive at 37°C, it is not likely to be anti-D; but it might well be anti-P_1 or anti-Le^a. IgG antibodies are usually not active in saline tests and are best detected in IATs (exceptions are anti-A, anti-B, anti-M and anti-N because the reactive red cells have a very high antigen density). Also, as papain destroys M, N, S and Fy^a antigens, but enhances the reactivity of anti-Rh antibodies, the inclusion of an enzyme test helps to sort out these antibody specificities. It is also important to note that antibodies directed against M, N, S and s, Duffy and Kidd antigens also show dosage effect, i.e. they react better with cells having apparent homozygous rather than heterozygous expression of the antigen.

The UK specifications for suitable red cells for use in antibody identification can be summarized as follows:

1. The panel should permit confident identification of those clinically significant allo-antibodies which are most frequently encountered, e.g. anti-D, anti-E, anti-c, anti-K and anti-Fy^a.
2. A distinct pattern of reactivity should be apparent for each of the commonly encountered allo-antibodies.
3. The antigenic profile of the reagent red cells should, as far as possible, permit assignment of specificity in test sera containing more than one commonly encountered allo-antibody, e.g. anti-D+K.
4. Minimum red cell characteristics are: (i) one individual should be R^1R^1 and one $R^{1w} R^1$. Between them, these two individuals should express the antigens: K, k, Fy^a, Fy^b, Jk^a, Jk^b, S, s; (ii) one individual should be R_2R_2 and one r′r; (iii) a minimum of four individuals should lack the Rh antigens C and D. One of these individuals should be K+ and one should be E+. Between them, these individuals should exhibit apparent homozygous expression of: c, k, Fy^a, Fy^b, Jk^a, Jk^b, S, s.

CROSSMATCHING

The function of the crossmatch is to prevent the transfusion of incompatible red cell units which will have a reduced survival and provoke a haemolytic transfusion reaction. This is most serious when there is ABO incompatibility and, in particular, when A or B cells are transfused into a group O person. The procedure may include serological tests or electronic blood issue.

There are two approaches:

1. Follow a 'group, antibody screen and save' policy; or
2. Crossmatch all patients who may need a transfusion.

GROUP, ANTIBODY SCREEN AND SAVE PROCEDURE

This is ideal for operative procedures where blood is often not required, but where it has been customary to have compatible blood on standby. This may be co-ordinated with a maximum blood ordering schedule for planned surgical operations.[5e] The patient's blood is ABO and RhD grouped and screened for red cell allo-antibodies and if the antibody screen is negative, the patient's sample is retained and blood may be provided when required on the basis of an immediate spin crossmatch or it may be issued electronically.

However several requirements must be met before abolishing an IAT crossmatch, (i.e. relying entirely on an immediate spin technique) and additional security is required before considering electronic issue of red cells.

IMMEDIATE SPIN CROSSMATCH

The purpose of this technique is to detect ABO incompatibility. However, it is known that incompatibilities between A_2B donor red cells and group B patient sera are not consistently detected with this technique.[24,25] Of more concern is the potential failure of agglutination with potent ABO antibodies, on account of rapid complement fixation, with bound C1 interfering with agglutination.[26] For this reason, and also to prevent lysis interfering with the interpretation of tests, red cells should be resuspended in EDTA-saline (see above).

Incubate (c 20°C) equal volumes of a 2% donor cell suspension and the patient's serum or plasma for 2–5 min. The donor red cells should be suspended in EDTA-saline if serum is being used.

Centrifuge at 100 *g* for 1 min (see p. 450) and inspect for agglutination.

UK guidelines[58] state that the immediate spin crossmatch must not be used alone:

(i) if the patient's serum/plasma contains or has been known to contain clinically significant antibodies;
(ii) if the antibody screen does not conform to the recommendations given above;
(iii) if ABO grouping reveals macroscopically undetectable anti-A or anti-B, (except in group AB patients);
(iv) if the patient has had an ABO incompatible solid organ transplant and is being transfused within 3 months of the transplant;
(v) except in emergency situations.

ELECTRONIC BLOOD ISSUE

This is an alternative to the immediate spin crossmatch for ensuring the issue of ABO-compatible units. Although there are some differences between the AABB standards[8] and the BCSH guidelines,[7] both contain the following essential elements:

1. The computer contains logic to prevent assignment and release of ABO incompatible blood.
2. No clinically significant antibodies are detected in the recipient's serum/plasma and there is no record of previous detection of such antibodies.
3. There are concordant results of at least two determinations of the recipient's ABO type on record, one of which is from a current sample.
4. Critical elements of the system have been validated on-site.

The BCSH guidelines, unlike the AABB standards, do not require the donor units to be regrouped, if the supplying Transfusion Service will provide written verification of the accuracy of the donor unit label. However, the former guidelines strongly recommend the use of automated patient ABO and RhD grouping procedures, with positive sample identification and electronic transfer of the results to the computer. The BCSH guidelines also require that the computer software directs the process, as opposed to manual procedures, and will not permit the issue of blood if there is only one ABO and RhD group on file, will not display the historical results of the patient until current typing is complete and will not allow the issue of blood if the current blood group does not match the historical record.

Electronic issue of red cells has been in place in several countries for more than a decade and has been proven to be clinically safe, provided that the recommendations given are rigidly adhered to.[27-29]

ROUTINE CROSSMATCHING

This consists of testing the patient's serum or plasma against donor red cells by:

1. Direct agglutination test in NISS or LISS (i.e. an immediate spin). The test can be read in the tube after gentle agitation over a ×5 or ×6 magnification illuminated mirror, and incorporated with (2) as one-tube procedure.
2. IAT using a minimum incubation 15-min LISS test or a 45-min NISS test. The incubation temperature should be 37°C using a water-bath or warmed block (air incubators are less reliable).

Spin-tube or microplate techniques may be used.

The IAT crossmatch should always be used in the circumstances noted in the section on the immediate spin crossmatch. When antibody identification has revealed clinically significant antibodies, antigen-negative units should be selected for crossmatch by IAT. For antibodies unlikely to be of clinical significance, e.g. anti-P_1, anti-Le^a, it is acceptable to issue units which are crossmatch compatible in an IAT performed strictly at 37°C, i.e. when both serum and cells have been pre-warmed (see Table 20.3).

The argument for routinely retaining an IAT crossmatch surrounds the failure to identify antibodies directed against low frequency antigens in the antibody screen.[30] However there is abundant evidence over the last two decades that the likelihood of missing a clinically significant antibody is in the order of 1 in 17 000 and that the usual outcome of this event is limited to a shortened red cell survival.[31-33] However, the decision to abolish the routine use of an IAT crossmatch should only be considered when the antibody screen, particularly in the IAT meets the requirements given above.[5c]

EMERGENCY BLOOD ISSUE (WHERE TIME DOES NOT PERMIT FULL COMPATIBILITY TESTING)

A blood sample should be obtained from the patient before the administration of intravenous colloids, such as Dextran and hydroxethyl-starch (HES), which may cause troublesome red cell aggregation in serological testing.

Laboratories that use LISS for routine work are well placed to meet urgent compatibility requests. However, where laboratories use NISS routinely, it is not recommended that they change to LISS tests for emergency techniques.

Patients should be ABO and RhD grouped by rapid techniques and group-compatible blood should be issued. Exclude ABO incompatibility by an immediate spin crossmatch. If this procedure is followed, it should seldom be necessary to have to resort to issuing group O RhD-negative blood. Should this need arise, only previously group-checked units should be issued, unless the suppliers have indicated their confidence in the validity of their donor unit labelling. Furthermore, this should be changed to blood of the patient's own group as soon as possible to avoid subsequent confusion over ABO grouping.

An antibody screen should be performed as soon as possible and if positive, both antibody identification and retrospective crossmatching should be undertaken with the pre-transfusion sample. Any incompatible units must be immediately withdrawn from issue.

If a massive transfusion has been given, in which the number of units transfused in 24 h exceeds the recipient's blood volume, compatibility testing may be reduced to an immediate spin crossmatch.

Donor units that have issued without conducting the routine pre-transfusion compatibility procedures should be clearly labelled, e.g. 'Selected for patient …, but *not* crossmatched'.

SPECIAL TRANSFUSION SITUATIONS

There are some situations where the provision of compatible blood requires special consideration.

COMPATIBILITY TESTS IN NEWBORN INFANTS

For infants under 4 months, both baby and maternal blood samples should be ABO and RhD grouped, the maternal serum screened for unexpected antibodies, and a DAT done on the baby's cells.

If a maternal antibody screen is negative and the baby's DAT is negative, blood of the same ABO and D group as the infant may be issued without crossmatching, even after repeated small volume transfusions. Recent studies indicate that infants under the age of 4 months do not make red cell allo-antibodies even after multiple small volume transfusions.[34]

If the infant is suffering from HDN, or if unexpected antibodies are detected in the maternal serum, it is important to use the maternal serum for compatibility testing. This may dictate the use of group O blood, and if the infant is not group O, care should be taken to ensure that donor units have low titre anti-A and anti-B (i.e. <32). If ABO HDN is suspected, group O blood of low titre anti-A and anti-B should be used. An alternative to low titre group O blood is O cells reconstituted in one-third volume of AB plasma. It should be noted that compatible red cells from adult group A or B donors should not be used, as adult red cells will almost certainly have more A and B antigen sites than the infant's own red cells and are likely to undergo more rapid destruction by the residual maternal anti-A or anti-B. In the event of an exchange transfusion, plasma-reduced (Hct <0.6) cytomegalovirus (CMV)-seronegative blood, which is 5 days old or less, is indicated. Irradiation to 25 Gy is not mandatory in the UK, unless the infant has received an intra-uterine transfusion, but all units are leucodepleted and K-negative.[35]

COMPATIBILITY TESTS FOR INTRA-UTERINE TRANSFUSION

Blood for an intra-uterine transfusion should be tested for compatibility with the mother's serum. It should be group O and RhD-negative (except, for example, when the mother is RhD-positive and has made antibodies other than anti-D or anti-D mixtures). K-negative blood should also be used.[36] Compatibility tests for subsequent transfusions must be repeated every time using fresh maternal serum, for the manipulations of intra-uterine transfusions are not uncommonly followed by the escape of donor cells into the maternal circulation which could lead to the formation of antibodies of a new specificity. It is essential to repeat the antibody identification on each fresh sample of the mother's serum to identify any new allo-antibodies formed.

Blood for intra-uterine transfusion should be less than 5 days old. It should be CMV seronegative, have a Hct >0.75, be irradiated to a minimum of 25 Gy[37] to avoid graft-versus-host disease and transfused within 24 h of irradiation. Plasma-reduced blood or washed red cells suspended in saline should be used.

COMPATIBILITY TESTS IN PATIENTS RECEIVING TRANSFUSIONS AT CLOSE INTERVALS

Allo-antibodies may develop quickly following a transfusion early in a series. It is important, therefore, to obtain a fresh sample of serum from the recipient before each transfusion if they are separated by an interval of 3 days or longer; while if the patient is receiving daily transfusions, only blood that is likely to be used in the 3 days following the collection of the serum should be crossmatched. It is advisable to do a DAT on the patient's red cells each time, as antibodies that have formed may be adsorbed to incompatible cells and not be present in the serum.

COMPATIBILITY TESTS IN AUTO-IMMUNE HAEMOLYTIC ANAEMIA (AIHA)

(a) Warm-type AIHA

ABO grouping is usually straightforward, but antibody coating on the patient's red cells can cause false-positive RhD grouping results unless saline-reacting monoclonal IgM anti-D reagents are used.

The problem here is that the auto-antibody almost always reacts with all donor blood samples, so that no crossmatch-compatible blood can be found. In this situation it is essential to exclude any incompatibility owing to the simultaneous presence of allo-antibodies stimulated by previous transfusion or pregnancy. Recent reports indicate that allo-antibodies may be present in up to 40% of cases, the most frequent being anti-C and anti-K.[38,39] It is therefore helpful to determine the patient's Rh phenotype and K type (at least) before transfusions are started, so that donor-compatible blood can be selected. Monoclonal reagents should be used when phenotyping the patient's red cells to avoid false-positive reactions owing to cell-bound autoantibody.

Useful advice on the detection of allo-antibodies in the presence of an autoantibody, which can be quite difficult, has been given by Petz & Garratty[40] (see also p. 209).

(b) Cold-type AIHA

Cold agglutinins cause blood grouping and antibody screening problems (p. 474). Even if agglutination is avoided by performing these tests strictly at 37°C, complement binding may cause false-positive results in the antiglobulin test during antibody screening and crossmatching. Useful advice on compatibility testing in the presence of cold agglutinins is given by Petz & Garratty.[40]

INVESTIGATION OF A HAEMOLYTIC TRANSFUSION REACTION

Donor-recipient compatibility for ABO taking account of clinically significant allo-antibodies in the recipient, is essential to ensure normal survival of transfused red cells and to avoid the harmful effects of a haemolytic transfusion reaction. The mechanism of haemolysis depends on the Ig class of the antibody and its ability to fix complement. This also determines the site of haemolysis.

Haemolytic transfusion reactions (HTR) may be acute (intravascular or extravascular) or delayed (mainly extravascular).

(A) ACUTE INTRAVASCULAR HAEMOLYSIS

Acute intravascular haemolysis is potentially fatal and is usually due to ABO incompatibility resulting

Table 20.4 Investigation of a haemolytic transfusion reaction

I. **Check for haemolysis**
  (i)   Examine patient's plasma and urine for haemoglobin
  (ii) Blood film may show spherocytosis, agglutination or erythrophagocytosis
  (iii) Biochemical evidence, including bilirubin and haptoglobin levels

II. **Check for incompatibility**
  (a) *Clerical causes*
      An identification error will indicate the type of incompatibility
  (b) *Serological causes*
      (i)   Repeat ABO and RhD group of patient (pre- and post-transfusion) and donor units
      (ii) Screen patient's serum (pre- and post-transfusion for red cell antibodies)
      (iii) Repeat cross-match with pre- and post-transfusion serum
      (iv) Direct antiglobulin test (pre- and post-transfusion samples)
      (v)   When direct antiglobulin test is positive, elute the antibody from the cells

III. **Check for disseminated intravascular coagulation (DIC)**
  (i)   Blood film (red cell fragmentation)
  (ii) Platelet count
  (iii) Coagulation screen

IV. **Check for bacterial infection**
  Gram stain and culture donor blood

V. **Check for baseline renal function**
  Urea/creatinine and electrolytes

from a misidentification error. This is an acute emergency, in which prompt diagnosis and treatment can be life saving. At the first suspicion of reaction, the transfusion must be stopped, as the severity of the clinical consequences depends partly on the volume of red cells transfused to the patient. The laboratory performing the pre-transfusion compatibility testing must be notified immediately.

Diagnosis depends on demonstrating haemolysis in the patient and incompatibility between the donor and the patient (Table 20.4). Patient identification and the donor unit compatibility label should be rechecked at the bedside. As clerical errors involving one patient may involve others crossmatched at the same time, it is essential to check the samples, donor units and documentation of all crossmatches done at that time. Differential diagnosis from other conditions causing a similar clinical presentation is also important, the most serious being the transfusion of infected blood (Table 20.5).

Serological investigations
Specimens required:

1. Pre-transfusion serum and red cells of the patient.

Table 20.5 Differential diagnosis of acute haemolytic transfusion reaction

Red cell incompatibility

Transfusion of infected blood

Other causes of haemolysis:
  (i)   Post-operative infection (e.g. clostridial septicaemia)
  (ii) Infusion of hypotonic solutions (including hypotonic dialysis)
  (iii) Haemolytic anaemia (e.g. PNH)

Transfusion of lysed red cells:
  (i)   Thermal damage (pre-transfusion heating or freezing)
  (ii) Mechanical damage (e.g. extracorporeal machines, excessive infusion pressure and/or small bore needle)
  (iii) Addition of drugs or intravenous fluids
  (iv) Donor red cell enzyme deficiency

2. Post-transfusion serum and red cells of the patient.
3. The donor unit involved, together with the giving set and any other donor units transfused.
4. Urine from the patient for the first 24 h after the reaction. This will be dark, owing to the

presence of haemoglobin in the case of intravascular haemolysis.

Serological tests

1. Confirm the ABO and RhD groups of the patient's pre- and post-transfusion samples and the donor units.
2. Perform a DAT on the patient's pre- and post-transfusion washed red cells: a negative DAT post-transfusion does not exclude a severe haemolytic reaction. In the event of a positive DAT, elution of the antibody may aid identification, or confirm the specificities identified in the serum in cases of non-ABO incompatibility.
3. Repeat the crossmatch tests of donor's red cells with patient's serum, using pre- and post-transfusion samples.
4. Screen the donor plasma and the patient's pre- and post-transfusion serum samples for unexpected antibodies.
5. If the donor was group O and the patient group A or B, then titre the anti-A and anti-B levels in the donor plasma, as high titres (>64) are found in 'dangerous group O donors'.

Haematological tests

1. Blood count – including platelet and reticulocyte counts.
2. Blood film – spherocytosis, red cell agglutinates and possibly some fragmentation.
3. Coagulation screen, including fibrinogen assay and a test for fibrin degradation products.

Disseminated intravascular coagulation (DIC) is a feature of intravascular HTR and the transfusion of infected blood; severe DIC is a bad prognostic sign.

Bacteriological tests

Inspect the donor unit(s) for any obvious haemolysis. The donor blood unit(s) and giving set should be tested by culturing the remaining blood at 4°C, 20°C and 37°C and by Gram stain and smear examination.

Biochemical tests

The patient's post-transfusion serum should be inspected for haemolysis, tested for free haemoglobin and haptoglobin and bilirubin levels esti-

mated, and the results compared with those of the pre-transfusion sample. Urea/creatinine and electrolytes should also be estimated to obtain baseline information on renal function.

If the above testing does not indicate a HTR or infected blood, other possible causes of an adverse immunological but non-haemolytic reaction, e.g. leucocyte antibodies, allergic reactions to plasma proteins should be taken into consideration when selecting blood for further transfusions.

(B) ACUTE EXTRAVASCULAR HAEMOLYSIS

Acute extravascular haemolysis is a feature of IgG antibodies that do not cause complement lysis, e.g. anti-D. This is a less severe haemolytic reaction. The main clinical features are fever, sometimes with rigors, and an inadequate haemoglobin response to the transfusion that cannot be explained by blood loss; jaundice may occur, but haemoglobinuria is not common. These reactions are not commonly seen because of improved pre-transfusion antibody screening and crossmatching procedures. Serological diagnosis should follow the procedure set out (in A) above.

(C) DELAYED HAEMOLYTIC TRANSFUSION REACTIONS

Delayed HTRs may occur in patients allo-immunized by previous pregnancy or transfusion. The antibody titre is too low to be detected in the pre-transfusion compatibility testing, but after re-exposure to the incompatible antigen, a secondary (anamnestic) immune response occurs. IgG antibodies are made and the transfused red cells are destroyed. Kidd antibodies are often implicated in delayed HTRs, since they can be difficult to detect; showing dosage, falling rapidly to undetectable levels after stimulation and being frequently present in a combination of antibodies.

Haemolysis is usually extravascular, and typically the patient develops anaemia, fever, jaundice and sometimes haemoglobinuria about 1 week after transfusion. The clinical picture may resemble an auto-immune or drug-induced immune haemolytic anaemia with a positive DAT (in this case owing to allo-antibody on the donor cells), spherocytosis and reticulocytosis. However, the history of a preceding transfusion should suggest the correct diagnosis. Serological diagnosis should follow the outline provided in (A) above. However it should be noted that the antibody may not be immediately apparent in the post-transfusion serum although it may be eluted from the red cells. If the immediate post-transfusion sample is inconclusive, then a repeat sample should be taken 10 days later, to allow for an increase in antibody titre. More sensitive techniques may have to be employed to detect the antibody and since a significant proportion of these reactions[1] involve more than one allo-antibody, it is important that the panels used for red cell identitation have sufficient cells of appropriate phenotypes to exclude additional specificities. There is usually no need for further action in most cases as the process is self-limiting. Many delayed HTRs of this type almost certainly go undetected.

HAEMOLYTIC DISEASE OF THE NEWBORN

HDN is an immune haemolytic anaemia affecting the fetus and newborn infant. It occurs when maternal allo-antibody to fetal red cell antigens crosses the placenta and causes haemolysis of fetal red cells. As IgG is the only immunoglobulin transferred across the placenta, only red cell antibodies of this class are a potential cause of HDN. Anti-D causes the most severe form of HDN. However, the success of anti-D prophylaxis has reduced the number of cases of RhD HDN; consequently the relative proportion of cases due to other antibodies has increased, notably anti-c, and anti-K, but almost every other red cell IgG antibody has been reported as a cause of HDN. ABO HDN is considered separately as a number of special factors combine to protect the fetus from the effects of ABO incompatibility. For a more detailed discussion of HDN the reader is referred to the review by Bowman et al[41] and the textbook by Mollison et al.[11b]

ANTENATAL SEROLOGY

Maternal ABO and RhD grouping and antibody titration or quantification are the basis of any system for the prediction and management of HDN. Protocols for antenatal screening vary from country to country but also depend on the presence and specificity on an antibody capable of causing haemolytic disease status, and obstetric history of HDN.

The following recommendations are based upon the BCSH guidelines:[13]

1. All pregnant women, (RhD-positive and RhD-negative) should be ABO and RhD grouped and have an antibody screen performed at booking and again, between 28 and 36 weeks of pregnancy.
2. Pregnant women with anti-D-, anti-c- and K-related antibodies should be tested monthly until 28 weeks and 2 weekly thereafter. Testing should consist of titration and/or quantification.
3. Pregnant women with other clinically significant antibodies detected at booking, should have titrations performed at booking and these should be repeated at 28 weeks.
4. All pregnant women who have a previous history of HDN or who have a significant increase in anti-D-, anti-c- or K-related antibodies whilst being monitored in pregnancy should be referred to a specialist centre for further assessment of the need for antenatal intervention.
5. Pregnant women who have antibodies of other specificities, capable of giving rise to HDN and which demonstrate a significant rise in titre over the course of pregnancy should have their condition discussed with the obstetrician. It is now appreciated that a trend in titration scores rather than an individual level is more predictive of an affected fetus.

ANTIBODY TITRATIONS DURING PREGNANCY

It was historically accepted that antibody titres of 32 or greater were more likely to cause HDN.[42] However these data were collected using NISS tube techniques in a single institution and cannot be extrapolated to the current range of available IAT technologies, e.g. column agglutination technology and solid phase microplate, with differing sensitivities. The BCSH have as a consequence[43] recently recommended that the National Institute of Biological Standards and Controls (NIBSC) anti-D standard should be used to validate the consistency of individual laboratory techniques and to act as a comparator. Hence, laboratories should ensure that the titres obtained with the anti-D standard are always within one doubling dilution, when it is used as an internal control. Laboratories can use the titre obtained with the anti-D standard as a means of inter-laboratory comparison, when transferring patient care.

Titrations performed in pregnancy should always be performed in parallel with the previous sample. Rise in titres of more than one doubling dilution should always be monitored in conjunction with the obstetricians.

Antenatal assessment of severity of RhD HDN

The role of the serologist is to carry out serial antibody measurements on sensitized women to determine the titre or concentration (μg/ml plasma) of the antibody. Individual laboratories should work closely with local obstetricians to establish the clinical significance of their own titration results.

Automated quantitative measurement of the amount of anti-D (iu or μg/ml) defines the fetal risk more accurately,[44] as also may the antibody-dependent cell-mediated cytotoxicity (ADCC) assay used as a model of in vivo haemolysis in the fetus.[45] The place of cellular assays in the in vitro testing to predict the severity of HDN has been subject to several reviews.[46] However, further essential information regarding management depends on amniotic fluid spectrophotometry[47] and on direct fetal blood sampling by ultrasound-guided cordocentesis.[48] The last procedure provides not only direct diagnostic information, but also a new approach to fetal therapy by direct fetal intravascular transfusion.[49,50]

The declining incidence of severe RhD HDN and the increasingly specialized management of severely affected pregnancies have meant that these women are now being referred to specialist centres dealing with this condition.

Tests on maternal and cord blood at delivery

It should be standard practice to collect an adequate sample (e.g. 20 ml) of cord blood (both EDTA and clotted specimens) for serological studies, as subsequent (small) samples from the baby may not be enough for all the necessary tests to be carried out. There should be an agreed local procedure for labelling mother's and baby's samples to avoid identification errors.

The following tests should be carried out on all RhD-negative mothers and their babies:

(a) Tests on cord blood

1. ABO and RhD grouping.
2. DAT (if positive, test the mother's serum against a cell panel to identify the antibody).
3. Haemoglobin concentration.
4. Bilirubin concentration (Rh D positive babies).

(b) Tests on maternal blood

1. Repeat ABO and RhD grouping.
2. Repeat antibody screen (in case anti-D sensitization has occurred in a previously unsensitized woman).
3. Kleihauer test for detection and subsequent quantification of fetomaternal haemorrhage, if the cord blood groups as RhD positive. This governs the dose of anti-D immunoglobulin to be given to the mother to avoid sensitization (see below).

The above tests should also be carried out on the cord blood of all babies born to mothers with antibodies other than anti-D.

Anti-D prophylaxis

The dose of anti-D given to RhD-negative women delivering an RhD-positive infant depends on the size of the fetomaternal haemorrhage initially determined by the Kleihauer technique and preferably, if greater than 4 ml, confirmed by flow cytometric analysis. The Kleihauer technique depends on the Hb F of fetal red cells resisting acid elution to a greater extent than the Hb A of maternal red cells. When the treated eluted maternal blood film is stained with eosin, the cells stain dark pink, whereas the maternal cells appear as pale 'ghosts' (see p. 276). The Kleihauer testing is invalid in women with high levels of Hb F as a result of hereditary persistence of fetal haemoglobin. In these circumstances quantification of fetomaternal haemorrhage requires flow cytometric analysis (see below)

The following recommendations are adapted from the BCSH guidelines.[51] Using a ×10 objective, scan 25 fields for the presence of fetal cells. If no fetal cells are seen, the fetomaternal haemorrhage (FMH) can be reported as <4 ml of fetal cells and no further anti-D is needed. If fetal cells are detected, it is recommended that fetal cells are expressed as a proportion of adult cells with a minimum of 6000 cells being counted using a ×40 objective. This method is aided by use of a Miller Square disc or equivalent.

The calculation of the volume of FMH is based upon the work of Mollison[52] which assumed that the maternal cell volume is 1800 ml, fetal cells are 22% larger than maternal cells and only 92% of fetal cells stain darkly. The feto-maternal haemorrhage should be calculated as follows:

Uncorrected volume of bleed =

$$\frac{1800 \times \text{fetal cells counted (F)}}{\text{Adult cells counted (A)}}$$

Corrected for fetal volume (1.22) =

$$(1800 \times \frac{F}{A}) \times 1.22 = J$$

Corrected for staining efficiency (1.09) = J × 1.09 = fetomaternal haemorrhage

Details of flow cytometric quantitation using labelled anti-human IgG or anti-HbF are described elsewhere.[51,53]

The administration of an adequate dose of anti-D to prevent maternal sensitization is the responsibility of the clinician in charge of the patient.

The following procedure is recommended:

(a) After delivery

1. To avoid the situation where anti-D is sometimes withheld because a report on the baby's RhD group has not been received, all RhD-negative women should be given a *standard* intramuscular dose of anti-D (500 iu) within 72 h of delivery, unless the baby is known to be RhD-negative.
2. On the basis of the Kleihauer test, *extra* anti-D may be indicated to cover a larger fetomaternal leakage of red cells.

(b) During pregnancy

1. Following abortion before 20 weeks a standard dose of 250 IU should be given; after 20 weeks, give 500 IU or more, based on the Kleihauer count.

2. Following obstetric manipulations (e.g. amniocentesis, version) and antepartum haemorrhage (APH) give 500 IU of anti-D or more, based on the Kleihauer count.

Prophylactic anti-D is also given routinely in the third trimester in some countries.[54,55]

ABO HAEMOLYTIC DISEASE OF THE NEWBORN

This is considered separately, as a number of special factors combine to protect the fetus from the effects of ABO incompatibility. For practical purposes, only group O individuals make high titres of IgG anti-A and anti-B. Therefore only A and B infants of group O mothers are at risk from ABO HDN. Although 15% of births are susceptible, only about 1% are affected; even then, the condition is usually mild and very rarely severe enough to need exchange transfusion. Two mechanisms protect the fetus against anti-A and anti-B: one is the relative weakness of A and B antigens on fetal red cells; the other is the widespread distribution of A and B glycoproteins in fetal fluids and tissues, which diverts much of the maternal IgG antibody away from the fetal red cell 'target'.

ABO HDN may be seen in the first incompatible pregnancy. This is unlike anti-D HDN, where immunization usually takes place at the end of the first pregnancy, the first child thus being unaffected.

Serological investigation

ABO haemolytic disease is difficult to diagnose, especially in Caucasians, as the DAT may be negative or weak even in a case of severe haemolytic disease. Furthermore, anti-A or anti-B is normally present in the mother's serum and special tests are needed to demonstrate a high titre of IgG anti-A or anti-B in the presence of IgM anti-A or anti-B.

In cases of suspected ABO HDN the main features are:[56]

1. It is almost always confined to infants of group O mothers as there is more IgG anti-A and anti-B in group O than in group B or group A mothers.
2. As anti-A and anti-B are always present in group O mothers, evidence for ABO HDN depends on demonstrating a high titre of IgG anti-A or anti-B, e.g. by treating the mother's serum with

2-mercapto-ethanol (2-ME) or dithiothreitol (DTT) to distinguish between IgG and IgM antibodies (for method, see p. 215).

3. The DAT on cord blood may be weak or negative; the latter at least excludes any other serological incompatibility. This probably reflects the low A and B antigen density on the red cells of newborn infants.

4. The simplest evidence for the occurrence of ABO haemolytic disease is obtained by testing the serum of the cord blood sample for incompatible anti-A or anti-B by the antiglobulin method with adult A_1, B and O cells. If the baby is group A, the important test is with the A_1 cells which will be positive in ABO HDN. A strong reaction with B cells will always occur with a group A baby. The test with O cells should be negative, but if positive, it indicates the presence of a further antibody as a possible contributory or major cause of the disease, especially if the DAT is strongly positive. Similarly, if the baby is group B the critical test is with adult B cells; a strong reaction will also be found with A_1 cells, but this will not harm the baby's B cells.

   Note. If the blood sample from the baby is not taken until the time of crisis of the disease, usually about 2 to 3 days after delivery, the serological tests may be negative because most, if not all, of the maternal anti-A or anti-B will have been absorbed in the destruction of the baby's red cells.

5. The best diagnostic test of ABO HDN is to prepare a heat eluate from the baby's red cells (from the cord blood sample), and test it (together with the last wash supernatant as a control) by the antiglobulin method with adult A_1, B and O cells. In some cases, reactions occur with both A_1 and B cells owing to anti-A,B cross-reacting antibodies, but most severe cases of ABO HDN involve separate specific anti-A or anti-B antibodies. The tests with O cells and the last wash control should be negative.

Antenatal prediction

Antenatal prediction of ABO HDN is not essential for medical management, as there is time to observe the baby after birth and to treat according to the severity of the condition. Nevertheless, a baby is likely to be more severely affected if the maternal IgG anti-A (-B) titre is greater than 128.[57]

Acknowledgements
The author wishes to thank Mrs Clare Milkins FIMLS for advice in the preparation of this chapter and, with great respect, to again pay tribute to the late Eleanor Lloyd, FIMLS, who was her mentor and a co-author of a previous edition.

REFERENCES

1 Sazama K 1990 Reports of 355 transfusion-associated deaths: 1976 through 1985. Transfusion 30:583–590.

2 Linden JV, Paul B, Dressler KP 1992 A report of 104 transfusion errors in New York State. Transfusion 32:601–606.

3 Serious hazards of transfusion (SHOT) annual reports. Royal College of Pathologists, UK, 1996–1999.

4 Murphy MF, Atterbury CLJ, Chapman JF, et al 1999 The administration of blood components and the management of transfused patients. Transfusion Medicine 9:227–238.

5 British Committee for Standards in Haematology 1991 Standard haematology practice. (Roberts B, ed.) Blackwell Scientific, Oxford, (a) p 128, (b) p 139, (c) p 150, (d) p 164, (e) p 189.

6 British Committee for Standards in Haematology 2000 Guidelines for blood bank computing. Transfusion Medicine 10 307–314.

7 British Committee for Standards in Haematology 1996 Guidelines for pre-transfusion compatibility procedures in blood transfusion laboratories. Transfusion Medicine 6:273–283.

8 American Association of Blood Banks 2000 Standards for blood banks and transfusion services, 20th edn. (Widmann F, ed.) American Association of Blood Banks, Bethesda, MD.

9 Voak D 1990 Monoclonal antibodies as blood grouping reagents. Baillière's Clinical Haematology 3:219.

10 Whitrow W, Ross DW 1990 Automation in blood grouping: impact of microplate technology. Baillière's Clinical Haematology 3:255.

11 Mollison PL, Engelfriet CP, Contreras M 1997 Blood transfusion in clinical medicine, 10th edn. Blackwell Scientific, Oxford, (a) p 155, (b) p 390.

12 Issitt PD, Anstee DJ 1998 Applied blood group serology, 4th edn. Montgomery Scientific Publications, Durham, USA.

13 British Committee for Standards in Haematology 1996 Guidelines for blood grouping and red cell antibody testing during pregnancy. Transfusion Medicine 6:71–74.

14 Vent ND 1998 Antenatal genotyping of the blood groups of the fetus. Vox Sanguinis 74 (Suppl. 2):365–374.

15 Department of Health 1998 Guidelines for the Blood Transfusion Services in the United Kingdom, 4th edn. HMSO, London.

16 Knowles SM, Milkins CE, Chapman JF, et al 2001 UK NEQAS (BTLP); trends in proficiency over the last 15 years. Transfusion Medicine (in press).

17 Issitt PD, Combs MR, Bredehoeft SJ, et al 1993 Lack of clinical significance of 'enzyme-only' red cell alloantibodies. Transfusion 33:284–293.

18 Reis KJ, Chachowski R, Cupido A 1993 Column agglutination technology: the antiglobulin test. Transfusion 33:639–643.

19 Sinor LT 1992 Advances in solid-phase red cell adherence methods and transfusion serology. Transfusion Medicine Reviews VI (1):26–31.

20 Morelati F, Revelli N, Maffei LM 1998 Evaluation of a new automated instrument for pretransfusion testing. Transfusion 38: 959–965.

21 Pinkerton PH, Chan R, Ward J 1993 An evaluation of a gel technique for antibody screening compared with conventional tube method. Transfusion Medicine 3:201–205.

22 Pinkerton PH, Chan R, Ward J 1993 Sensitivity of column agglutination technology in detecting unexpected red cell antibodies. Transfusion Medicine 3:275–279.

23 Phillips P, Voak D, Knowles SM, et al 1997 An explanation and the clinical significance of the failure of microcolumn tests to detect weak ABO and other antibodies. Transfusion Medicine 7:47–53.

24 Berry-Dortch S, Woodside CH, Boral LI 1985 Limitations of the immediate spin crossmatch when used for detecting ABO incompatibility. Transfusion 22:176–178.

25 Meyer EA, Shulman IA 1989 The sensitivity and specificity of the immediate spin crossmatch. Transfusion 29:99–102.

26 Judd WJ, Steiner EA, O'Donnell DB 1989 Discrepancies in reverse ABO typing due to prozone. How safe is the immediate spin crossmatch? Transfusion 28:334–338.

27 Butch SH, Judd WJ, Steiner EA 1994 Electronic verification of donor-recipient compatibility: the computer crossmatch. Transfusion 37:960–964.

28 Georgsen J, Jensen F, Jeppeson S 1997 Transfusion service of the county of Funen. Organisational and economic aspects of restucturing. Ugeskrift for Laeger 159:1758–1762.

29 Fwenburg J, Hogman CF, Cassemar B 1997 Computerised delivery control – a useful and safe complement to the type and screen compatibility testing. Vox Sanguinis 72:162–168.

30 Bove JR, Cedergren B, Davey RJ 1982 International Forum; do you think the crossmatch with donor red cells can be omitted when the serum of a patient has been tested for the presence of red cell alloantibodies with a cell panel? Vox Sanguinis 43:151–168.

31 Boral LI, Henry JB 1977 The type and screen: a safe alternative and supplement in selected surgical procedures. Transfusion 17:163–168.

32 Garratty G 1986 Abbreviated pretransfusion testing. Transfusion 26:217–219.

33 Oberman HA, Barnes BA, Friedman BA 1978 The risk of abbreviating the major crossmatch in urgent or massive surgery. Transfusion 18:137–141.

34 Ludvigsen CW Jr, Swanson JL, Thompson TR, et al 1987 The failure of neonates to form red blood cell alloantibodies in response to multiple transfusions. American Journal of Clinical Pathology 87:250.

35 British Committee for Standards in Haematology 2001 Guidelines for the use of blood and blood products in neonates and older children. Transfusion Medicine (in preparation).

36 Bowman JM 1990 Treatment options for the fetus with allo-immune hemolytic disease. Transfusion Medicine Reviews 4:191.

37 British Committee for Standards in Haematology 1996 Guidelines on gamma-irradiation of blood components for the prevention of transfusion-associated graft-versus-host disease. Transfusion Medicine 6:261–271.

38 Laine ML, Beattie KM 1985 Frequency of alloantibodies accompanying autoantibodies. Transfusion 25:545.

39 Wallhermfechtel MA, Polk BA, Chaplain H 1984 Alloimmunisation in patients with warm autoantibodies. A retrospective study employing three donor alloabsorptions to aid antibody detection. Transfusion 24:482.

40 Petz LD, Garratty G 1980 Acquired immune hemolytic anemias. Churchill Livingstone, New York.

41 Bowman JM, Pollock JM, Biggins KR 1988 Antenatal studies and the management of hemolytic disease of the newborn. Methods in Hematology 17:163.

42 Udd WJ, Luban NLC, Ness PM 1990 Prenatal and perinatal haematology: recommendations for serological management of the fetus, newborn infant, and obstetric patient. Transfusion 30:175–183.

43 British Committee for Standards in Haematology 1999 Addendum for guidelines for blood grouping and red cell antibody testing in pregnancy. Transfusion Medicine 9:99.

44 Bowell PJ, Wainscoat JS, Peto TEA, et al 1982 Maternal anti-D concentrations and outcome in rhesus haemolytic disease of the newborn. British Medical Journal 285:327.

45 Hadley AG, Garner SF, Taverner JM 1993 Autoanalyzer quantification, monocyte-mediated cytotoxicity and chemiluminescence assays for predicting the severity of haemolytic disease of the newborn. Transfusion Medicine 3:195.

46 Hadley AG 1998 A comparison of in vitro tests for predicting the severity of haemolytic disease of the fetus and newborn. Vox Sanguinis 74 (Suppl. 2):375–383.

47 Liley AW 1961 Liquor amnii analysis in management of pregnancy complicated by rhesus immunization. American Journal of Obstetrics and Gynecology 82:1359.

48 Daffos F, Capella-Pavlovsky M, Forestier F 1985 Fetal blood sampling during pregnancy with use of a needle guided by ultrasound; a study of 606 consecutive cases. American Journal of Obstetrics and Gynaecology 153:655.

49 Grannum PA, Copel JA, Plaxe SC, et al 1986 In utero exchange transfusion by direct intravascular injection in severe erythroblastosis fetalis. New England Journal of Medicine 314:1431.

50 Nicolaides KH, Soothill PW, Rodeck CH, et al 1986 Rh disease: intravascular fetal blood transfusion by cordocentesis. Fetal Therapy 1:185.

51 British Committee for Standards in Haematology 1999 The estimation of feto-maternal haemorrhage. Transfusion Medicine 9:87–92.

52 Mollison PL 1972 Quantitation of transplacental haemorrhage. British Medical Journal 3:31–34.

53 Kumpel BL 2000 Quantification of anti-D and fetomaternal haemorrhage by flow cytometry. Transfusion 40:6–9.

54 Bowman JM 1985 Controversies in Rh prophylaxis: who needs Rh immune globulin and when should it be given? American Journal of Obstetrics and Gynecology 151:289.

55 British Committee for Standards in Haematology 1999 Recommendations for the use of anti-D immunoglobulin for Rh prophylaxis. Transfusion Medicine 9:93–97.

56 Voak D, Bowley CC 1969 A detailed serological study on the prediction and diagnosis of ABO haemolytic disease of the newborn (ABO HD). Vox Sanguinis 17:321.

57 Bowley CC, Voak D 1971 What is the optimal serological analysis of haemolytic disease of the newborn due to ABO incompatibility? International Forum. Vox Sanguinis 20:183.

58 British Committee for Standards in Haematology 1996 Guidelines for pre-transfusion compatibility procedures in blood transfusion laboratories. Transfusion Medicine 6:273–283.

21

Molecular techniques
Tom Vulliamy & Jaspal Kaeda

INTRODUCTION TO THE ANALYSIS OF DNA

DNA analysis is playing an increasingly important role in refining haematological diagnosis and determining treatment. Information for the construction of proteins is encoded in its four bases adenine(A), cytosine(C), guanine(G) and thymine(T) that lie along the sugar-phosphate backbone of the DNA molecule. The points listed below should help in the understanding of the methods described.

1. The DNA found in the nucleus of all eukaryotic cells is a double-stranded molecule.

2. The two strands are held together by hydrogen bonds that form specifically between A and T residues and between G and C residues.

3. Because of this, the sequence of bases on one strand of the DNA molecule (say TAGGCTAG) has only one possible partner on the other strand (ATCCGATC). These sequences are called complementary.

4. The strands have a polarity; one end is called the 5′ end, the other is the 3′ end. The two strands run in opposite directions, i.e. they are antiparallel.

The ability to manipulate DNA as recombinant molecules followed from the discovery of bacterial DNA modifying enzymes such as restriction enzymes. These are endonucleases that cut DNA molecules wherever there is a short specific sequence of bases. More than 100 different restriction enzymes are now commercially available. Using these enzymes it is possible to cut the genetic material found in human nuclei – the human genome – into specific fragments of a manageable size. With the necessary DNA-modifying enzymes, these restriction fragments can be inserted into cloning vectors such as plasmids or cosmids. Bacteria that host these vectors can be isolated as colonies and subsequently propagated indefinitely.

In this way, genes can be isolated as cloned recombinant DNA molecules and their DNA sequence established. The cloning and complete sequencing of the human genome is now at an advanced stage, with the recent publication of the sequence of the first human chromosome.[1] Expressed sequences, cloned as cDNAs, are known for a large proportion of human genes. This dramatic increase in sequence information over recent years has been made accessible through parallel developments in computing technology. The ability to amplify specific DNA fragments from small amounts of starting material by the polymerase chain reaction (PCR)[2] has revolutionized many aspects of DNA analysis. Since this technique is relatively simple, rapid, inexpensive and requires only some basic pieces of laboratory equipment, it has opened up molecular genetics, permitting access to molecular diagnosis away from specialist centres.

As a result, there has been a vast expansion in the application of DNA-based methods in diagnosis, and many alternative protocols have become available: a comprehensive laboratory manual describing the techniques of molecular biology runs to three volumes.[3] Guidelines from the American Association for Molecular Pathology address the choice and development of appropriate diagnostic assays, quality control and validation and implementation of molecular diagnostic tests.[4] In this chapter, applications of PCR in a diagnostic haematology laboratory are described. For the reasons just mentioned, PCR analysis has largely superseded the technique of Southern blot analysis, but there are situations in which the latter is still appropriate, and it will therefore also be described.

EXTRACTION OF DNA

DNA can be extracted from any blood or tissue sample. The quality and quantity of the DNA obtained will vary depending on the size, age and cell count of the sample. As a rule, 5 ml of blood in EDTA, ACD or preservative-free heparin will suffice (see p. 5). The DNA is extracted from all nucleated cells and is called genomic DNA.

In the nucleus, the DNA is tightly associated with many different proteins as chromatin. It is important to remove these as well as other cellular proteins in order to extract the DNA. This is achieved through the use of organic solvents or salt precipitation. An aqueous solution of DNA is obtained from which the DNA is further purified by ethanol precipitation. The method which is described in Appendix A yields DNA that is of sufficiently high quality for all routine analysis.[5]

A number of DNA extraction kits are now commercially available. These can significantly reduce the amount of time required for DNA extraction, bypass the use of organic solvents, and provide good quality control of the reagents used. However, the use of kits in all aspects of molecular biology may inhibit the development of improvements.[3]

THE POLYMERASE CHAIN REACTION

Development of the PCR[2] has had a dramatic impact on the study and analysis of nucleic acids. Through the use of a thermostable DNA polymerase, Taq polymerase extracted from the bacterium *Thermus aquaticus*, PCR results in the amplification of a specific DNA fragment such that it can be visualized by ethidium bromide staining on an agarose gel. The procedure takes only a few hours, does not require the use of radionucleotides, and requires only a very small amount of starting material.

Principle

A DNA polymerase will synthesize the complementary strand of a DNA template in vitro. A stretch of double-stranded DNA is required for the synthesis to be initiated. This double-stranded sequence can be generated by annealing an oligonucleotide (oligo), which is a short single-stranded DNA molecule usually between 17 and 22 bases in length, to a single-stranded DNA template. These oligos, which are synthesized in vitro, will prime the DNA synthesis and are therefore referred to as primers.

In the PCR, at least two oligos are used. One primes the synthesis of DNA in the forward direction, or along the coding strand of the DNA, while the other primes DNA synthesis in the reverse direction, or along the non-coding strand. The other components of the reaction are the DNA template from which the DNA fragment will be amplified, the four deoxynucleotide triphosphates (dATP, dTTP, dCTP and dGTP) required as the building blocks of the DNA that is to be synthesized, the necessary buffer and the thermostable DNA polymerase, or *Taq* polymerase.

The first step of the reaction is to denature the template DNA by heating the reaction mixture to 95°C. The reaction is then cooled to a temperature, usually between 50°C and 65°C, that permits the annealing of the oligos to the DNA template, but only at their specific complementary sequences. The temperature is then raised to 72°C, at which temperature the *Taq* polymerase efficiently synthesizes DNA, extending from the oligo in a 5′ to 3′ direction. Cyclical repetition of the denaturing, annealing and extension steps, by simply changing the temperature of the reaction in an automated heating block, results in exponential amplification of the DNA that lies between the two oligos (Fig. 21.1).

The specificity of the DNA fragment that is amplified is therefore determined by the sequences of the oligos used. A sequence of 17 base pairs (bp) is theoretically unique in the human genome and so oligos of this length and above will anneal at only one specific place on a template of genomic DNA. One general requirement of the PCR is therefore some knowledge of the DNA sequence of the gene that is to be amplified. The relative positioning of the two oligos is another important consideration. They must prime DNA synthesis in opposite directions, but pointing towards one another. There is also an upper limit to the distance apart that the oligos can be placed; fragments of several kilobase pairs (kb) in length can be amplified, but the process is most efficient for fragments of several hundred bp.

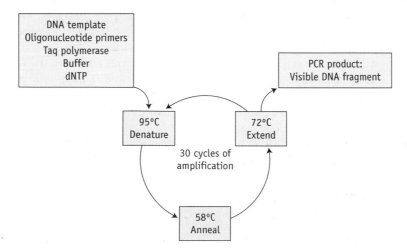

Fig. 21.1 The polymerase chain reaction. Cyclical repetition of three temperatures for denaturing, annealing and extending DNA respectively gives rise to an exponential amplification of a DNA fragment between two primer sequences directing DNA synthesis on opposite strands of the DNA template.

Reagents and methods

See Appendix B, page 512.

Problems and interpretation

If the amplification has been successful, a discrete fragment of the expected size is seen in an ethidium-bromide-stained agarose gel in all samples, except where a blank control is loaded. If a product is seen in the blank control, then one of the solutions has been contaminated. In this case, the experiment and all the working solutions must be discarded, and the micropipettes must be cleaned.

The absence of a fragment in all tracks indicates that the PCR has failed. This could be due to a number of reasons, the most obvious being the poor quality or omission of one of the essential reagents. The reaction may also fail if the magnesium concentration is too low, or the annealing temperature is too high. DNA quality is often one of the major reasons for failure. If one particular DNA sample repeatedly fails to amplify, then the sample should be re-extracted with phenol and chloroform, and re-precipitated in 1/10 volume of 5 mol/l ammonium acetate and 2.5 volumes of ethanol (see DNA extraction protocol p. 510). Another problem is the presence of non-specific fragments or just a smear of amplified product. This can occur if the magnesium concentration is too high, or the annealing temperature is too low.

ANALYSIS OF PCR PRODUCTS

THE PRESENCE OR ABSENCE OF A PCR PRODUCT

PCR products are most commonly and conveniently visualized by agarose gel electrophoresis. If appropriate primers and controls are included in an experiment, the actual presence of a product can be highly informative. With the development of automated analysis of PCR proceeding fast, this +/– reading of a reaction is likely to be of increasing importance.

THE AMPLIFICATION REFRACTORY MUTATION SYSTEM (ARMS)
Principle

Point mutations and small insertions or deletions can be identified directly by the presence or absence of a PCR product using allele-specific primers.[6,7] Two different oligos are used that differ only at the site of the mutation (the ARMS primers) with the mismatch distinguishing the normal and mutant base located at the 3′ end of the oligo. In a PCR, an oligo with a mismatch at its 3′ end will fail to prime the extension step of the reaction. Each test sample is amplified in two separate reactions containing either a mutant ARMS primer or a normal ARMS primer. The mutant primer will prime amplification together with one common primer from DNA with this mutation, but not from a normal DNA. A normal primer will do the opposite. To increase the instability of the 3′ end mismatch, and so ensure the failure of the amplification, it is sometimes necessary to introduce a second nucleotide mismatch three or four bases from the 3′ end of both oligos. A second pair of unrelated primers at distance from the ARMS primers is included in each reaction as internal control, to demonstrate that efficient amplification has occurred. This is essential because a failure of the ARMS primer to amplify is interpreted as a significant result and must not be due to suboptimal reaction conditions.

Interpretation

In all the samples, apart from the blank control, the fragment produced by amplification with the internal control primers must be seen. If this is the case, then the presence or absence of a mutation is simply determined by the presence or absence of the expected fragment produced by amplification with the mutant ARMS primer and the common primer. The presence or absence of the normal allele is determined in the same way in the reaction that includes the normal ARMS primer. In this way, heterozygous, homozygous normal and homozygous mutant individuals can be distinguished. An example of this analysis in the diagnosis of a β-thalassaemia mutation is given on page 498.

Gap-PCR

Large deletions can be detected by Gap-PCR. Primers located 5′ and 3′ to the breakpoints of a deletion will be too far apart on the normal chromosome to generate a fragment in a standard PCR. When the deletion is present, these primers will be brought together enabling them to give rise to a product. An example of this is given for the detection of deletions in α^0-thalassaemia on page 500.

By the same principle, primers can be brought together by chromosomal translocation, giving rise to a diagnostic product. Breakpoints may be clustered over too large a region for genomic DNA to be used in these instances. However, leukaemic translocations can also give rise to transcribed fusion genes. Primers from different genes are then juxtaposed in a hybrid mRNA molecule and can give rise to an RT–PCR product. An example of this is given in the analysis of minimal residual disease in chronic myeloid leukaemia (CML) on page 502.

THE SIZE OF THE PCR PRODUCT

Principle
Deletions and insertions can be identified simply, after agarose gel electrophoresis, when their size significantly alters that of the PCR product. An example of this analysis is given for a β-thalassaemia mutation on page 499.

A higher resolution of fragment sizes is obtained after polyacrylamide gel electrophoresis. This is particularly appropriate in the analysis of short tandem repeat (STR) sequences that can be highly variable in length and therefore useful as genetic markers of different individuals. A high-resolution gel is also used in PCR analysis of immunoglobulin and T-cell receptor gene rearrangement in the diagnosis of lymphoproliferative disorders described on page 504. A modification of this technique, running the denatured PCR products in a non-denaturing gel, enables the migration of single-stranded fragments to be determined. In these gels, their migration depends not only on their size but also on their sequence since fragments with different sequences fold in different ways and the secondary structure formed affects their mobility. This is the basis of the single-strand conformation polymorphism (SSCP) technique which is commonly used to locate point mutations and can also be employed in gene rearrangement studies.

Reagents and methods
See Appendix C, page 514.

RESTRICTION ENZYME DIGESTION
Principle
Restriction enzymes (RE) cleave DNA at short specific sequences. Since many RE are available, it is not uncommon for a single point mutation to coincidentally create or destroy an RE recognition sequence. If this is the case, digestion of the appropriate PCR product prior to agarose gel eletrophoresis enables the mutation to be identified. A difference in the size of the restriction fragments seen in normal and mutant samples can be predicted from a restriction map of the amplified fragment and the site of the mutation that changes a restriction site. The observed fragments should be consistent with either the mutant or the normal pattern. An example is shown on page 499 in the diagnosis of the sickle-cell mutation.

Even when a mutation docs not itself create or destroy an RE site, this method can be applied if one of the primer sequences is modified. In this technique that has been called the amplification created restriction enzyme site (ACRES), one or two deliberate mismatches are introduced in to one primer, 2 to 5 bases from its 3′ end, which is then located immediately adjacent to the site of the mutation. These mismatches will be incorporated into the PCR product and can be designed such that an RE site is created in the presence of either the normal or the mutant base at the appropriate site. Cleavage with that enzyme will then distinguish mutant from normal sequences. An example of this analysis is shown for factor V Leiden (FVL) mutation on page 501.

Method
See Appendix D, page 515.

ALLELE-SPECIFIC OLIGONUCLEOTIDE HYBRIDIZATION (ASOH)
Principle
Under appropriate conditions, short oligonucleotide probes will hybridize to their exact complementary sequence, but not to a sequence where there is even a single base mismatch.[8] A pair of oligos are therefore used to test for the presence of

a point mutation: a mutant oligo complementary to the mutant sequence and a normal oligo complementary to the normal sequence, with the sequence difference placed near the centre of each oligo.

The stability of the duplex formed between the oligo and the target DNA being tested (the product of a PCR reaction) depends on the temperature, the base composition and length of the oligo and the ionic strength of the washing solution. For ASOH studies, an empirical formula has been derived for the dissociation temperature (Td), the temperature at which half of the duplexes are dissociated. This value is used as a guideline; the exact temperature at which only perfect base pairing is maintained is usually determined by trial and error. The method is described in specialized laboratory manuals.[3]

Interpretation

The oligos should hybridize to their exact complementary DNA sequence, such that the mutant oligo gives a signal with a homozygous mutant control but not with a normal control. When this is the case, the interpretation of the result is straightforward; a positive signal from a particular oligo indicates the presence of that allele in the test sample. Heterozygotes and homozygotes are distinguished by using the mutant and normal oligos in tandem.

If there is no significant difference in the intensity of the radioactive signal seen in the control samples, a further wash of the filters at a higher temperature (e.g. Td + 2°C) may be necessary. A problem with the method is that it is relatively time-consuming, and care has to be taken in establishing the correct washing condition for each oligo. Non-radioactive probes, with detection systems involving horseradish peroxidase, are now quite widely used in this procedure.[9]

This technique has been modified such that the allele specific oligonucleotides are immobilized on the nylon membrane and the patient-specific PCR product is used as the probe – the reverse dot blot procedure.[10] This allows for several different mutations to be analyzed simultaneously and has proved particularly useful in the diagnosis of β-thalassaemia mutations.[11]

INVESTIGATION OF HAEMOGLOBINOPATHIES

SICKLE-CELL DISEASE

The presence of a sickle-cell gene can be determined by haemoglobin cellulose acetate electrophoresis or a sickling test. However, there are occasions when it is beneficial to make this diagnosis by DNA analysis, e.g. in prenatal diagnosis, which can be performed at 10 weeks of pregnancy, or when HbS β-thalassaemia is suspected, or in confirming the diagnosis of sickle-cell anaemia in a neonate. For the type of specimens collected for prenatal diagnosis, refer to page 270.

The sickle-cell mutation in codon 6 of the β globin gene (GAG → GTG) results in the loss of a Bsu36 I (or Mst II, Sau I, OxaN I, or Dde I) restriction enzyme site that is present in the normal gene.[12] It is therefore possible to detect the mutation directly by restriction enzyme analysis of a DNA fragment generated by the PCR. A pair of primers are used to amplify exons 1 and 2 of the β globin gene, and the products of the PCR are digested with Bsu36 I. The loss of a Bsu36 I site in the sickle-cell gene gives rise to an abnormally large restriction fragment that is not seen in normal individuals (Fig. 21.2).

β THALASSAEMIA

The ethnic groups with the highest incidence of β-thalassaemia are the Mediterranean populations, Asian Indians, Chinese and Africans. Although over 100 β-thalassaemia mutations are known,[13] each of these groups has its own subset of mutations, so that as few as five different mutations may account for more than 90% of the affected individuals in a population. This makes the direct detection of β-thalassaemia mutations a reasonable possibility and it has become the method of choice where it is most important – in prenatal diagnosis.[14]

The majority of mutations causing β-thalassaemia are point mutations affecting the coding sequence,

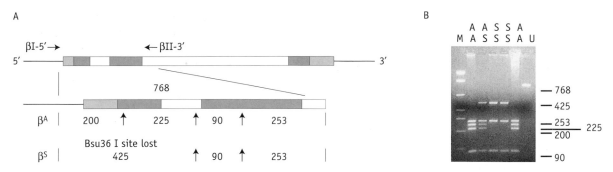

Fig. 21.2   Detection of the sickle-cell mutation. (A) A sketch of the β globin gene shows the position of the primers used to amplify a 768 bp fragment in a PCR. The sequence of β I–5′ is 5′TAAGCCAGTGCCAGAAAGAGCC3′ and that of β II-3′ is 5′CATTCGTCTGTTTCCCATTCTA3′. Maps of the Bsu36 I restriction sites and the fragment sizes from βA and βS genes are shown below. (B) An ethidium-bromide-stained minigel illustrates the fragment sizes generated by Bsu36 I digestion of the PCR product from normal (A/A), sickle-cell trait (A/S) and sickle-cell anaemia (S/S) individuals, along with the undigested amplified fragment (U) and the molecular size marker (M).

splice sites or promoter of the β globin gene. Favoured methods for their detection are either ARMS or reverse dot blot analysis. Larger deletions can be identified directly from the size of the amplified product. If the mutation is not known, it may be identified by sequence analysis.

Example 1: the 619 bp deletion
Using primers that flank this common deletion mutation, the size of the product of the PCR is directly informative (Fig. 21.3). A small fragment of 224 bp is seen when the deletion is present, compared to the 843 bp fragment derived from the normal chromosome. This pair of primers can

also be used as internal controls for the PCR when using ARMS primers.

Example 2: the 41/42 frameshift mutation
In this diagnosis, the presence or absence of the product generated by the ARMS oligos and the common primer determine the genotype of the test individual. An example of this is shown in Figure 21.4. All individuals have amplified with the control primers (upper band) and the normal primer (lower band, lanes 6 to 9). Two have also amplified with the mutant primer (lanes 3 and 4): these two individuals are therefore heterozygous for the 41/42 frameshift mutation.

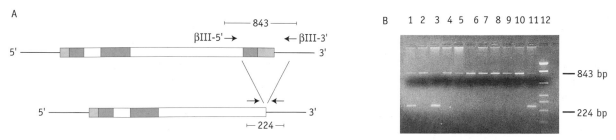

Fig. 21.3   Detection of a 619 bp deletion using the PCR. (A) A sketch of the normal β globin gene and the deleted gene shows the location of the primers (arrows) used to amplify across this deletion. The sequence of β III–5′ is 5′ACAGTGATAATTTCTGGGTT 3′ and that of β III-3′ is 5′TAAGCAAGAGAACTGAGTGG3′. (B) A minigel shows the expected 843 bp fragment yielded by the two primers from a normal β globin gene in all lanes, and the 224 bp fragment derived from a deleted gene in individuals who are heterozygous for the mutation in lanes 1, 3, and 11.

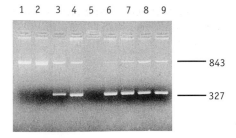

Fig. 21.4 Diagnosis of the 41/42 (-TTCT) frameshift mutation using ARMS. The gel shows the 843 bp fragment generated by the internal control primers (β III-5′ and β III-3′) in all lanes, except lane 5 which is the blank control. Four DNA samples are tested with the mutant ARMS primer (5′GTCTACCCTTGGACCCAGAGGTTGA3′) in combination with the common primer (5′CATTCGTCTGTTTCCCATTCTA3′) in lanes 1–4, and with the normal ARMS primer (5′GTCTACCCTTGGACCCAGAGGTTCTT3′) in combination with the common primer in lanes 6–9. The presence of a 327 bp product in lanes 3 and 4 and lanes 6–9 indicates that the individuals in lanes 3 and 4 are heterozygous for the 41/42 frameshift mutation, while individuals 1 and 2 are normal with respect to this mutation.

α THALASSAEMIA

Several PCR-based methods for the detection of the common α^+-thalassaemia deletions have been described.[15,16] However, some laboratories have found these difficult to implement and Southern blot analysis is still widely used in their diagnosis (see p. 506).

The most common large α^0-thalassaemia deletions can be identified by Gap–PCR.[17,18] In these reactions, PCR buffer II is used and dimethyl-sulphoxide (DMSO) is added to a final concentration of 10% (see Appendix B, p. 512). Three primers are included in each reaction, two of which flank the breakpoints of the deletion and one of which is just inside the deleted region, giving a product from the normal chromosome. The fragment generated by these primers across the deletion breakpoint is different in size to the fragment generated from the normal chromosome. The primers that flank the deletion breakpoint are too far apart to generate a fragment from the normal chromosome in the PCR. Only when these are brought closer together as a result of the deletion can a fragment be produced. Primer sequences used in this analysis are given in Table 21.1 and an

Table 21.1 Primers used in Gap–PCR analysis of α^0-thalassaemia

Deletion	Primer name	Sequence, 5′→3′
$--^{SEA}$	5′SEA	CTCTGTGTTCTCAGTATTGGAG
	3′SEAN	TGAAGAGCCTGCAGGACCAGTCA
	3′SEA	ATATATGGGTCTGGAAGTGTATC
$--^{MED}$	5′MED	ACAGTCACTCCTGAGGCCAGTC
	5′MEDN	TACAGCAGAGTGAGTGCTGCAT
	3′MED	GGAGAAGTAGGTCTTCGTGGC
$--(\alpha)^{20.5}$	5′-$(\alpha)^{20.5}$	GGCAAGCTGGTGGTGTTACACA
	C1	TGGAGGGTGGAGACGTCCTG
	3′α1	CCATGCTGGCACGTTTCTGAGG
$--^{FIL}$	F1	CTGCCCTTCACACCTCAGACA
	F2	GCAATCTTGGCTCACTGCAGG
	F3	GAAATGGTATTCTCAAGGTGACAC

example of their application in the diagnosis of the—^{SEA} deletion is shown in Figure 21.5.

Recently, a single tube multiplex PCR reaction has been described that identifies the six most frequently observed determinants of α-thalassaemia, including the α^0 and α^+ deletions.[19]

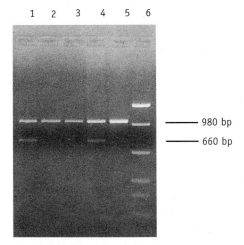

Fig. 21.5 Detection of South-east Asian α^0-thalassaemia (--^{SEA}) by Gap–PCR. The sequence of the primers used (5′SEA, 3′SEAN and 3′SEA) are shown in Table 21.1. A normal fragment of 980 bp is generated by the primers 5′SEA and 3′SEAN in all lanes, except lane 6 which is a molecular weight marker. The primers 5′SEA and 3′SEA generate a smaller fragment of 660 bp, which is seen in lanes 1 and 4; these individuals are heterozygous for the deletion.

More than 30 non-deletional forms of α-thalassaemia have been described. Of these, Hb Constant Spring and the α-thal-2(-5nt) genes are relatively common in East Asian and Mediterranean populations respectively. These can be detected by ASOH, ARMS, or restriction enzyme digestion following PCR amplification of the specific α globin gene.[20]

DISORDERS OF COAGULATION

THROMBOPHILIA (See Ch. 17)

Considerable advances have been made in our understanding of the genetic risk factors found in patients with venous thromboembolism (VTE).[21] Among these are the diverse mutations causing protein C, protein S and antithrombin deficiency. A raised factor VIII level is also a risk factor for VTE, but the genetic determinants of this are unclear. Homozygosity for the common C677T mutation of the methylenetetrahydrofolate reductase gene, which gives rise to a thermolabile variant of this protein, has been reported to be a risk factor for VTE. However, other studies have not supported this claim.[22]

A point mutation in the 3'UTR of the prothrombin gene associated with elevated protein levels has been identified as a genetic risk factor for VTE.[23] It is most commonly detected by ACRES using a mutagenic primer that creates a Hind III site in combination with the G20210A mutation. On its own, however, this mutation does not appear to be a major risk factor[24] and routine testing may not be warranted. The most common of the known genetic risk factors for VTE is a resistance to the anticoagulant effect of activated protein C caused by the Arg506Gln substitution in factor V (FVL).[25]

Method

A variety of different methods have been used to detect this mutation, mostly employing the fact that it creates an Mnl I restriction enzyme site. Since this enzyme is relatively expensive and using limited amounts may give rise to partial digestion, we have adapted a primer sequence to create a Taq I site – and example of the ACRES technique.

PCR is performed as in Appendix B, using buffer III and an $MgCl_2$ concentration of 2.0 mmol/l. The forward primer is 5'GTAAGAGCAGAT-CCCTGGACAGtC3', with the deliberate mismatch shown in lower case. The reverse primer is 5'TGTTATCACACTGGTGCTAA3'. The normal sequence of the gene at the position of the mutation is AGGCGA, altered to AGGCAA in FVL. The last 4 bases of the mutagenic oligo (AGtC) will create a Taq I site (TCGA) in the normal gene (AGtCGA), which will not be present in the FVL gene (AGtCAA). The PCR product is digested with Taq I at 65°C as described in Appendix D.

Interpretation

The primer pair gives rise to a fragment of 180 bp; after *Taq* I cleavage, the normal gene (1691G) gives rise to fragments of 157 bp and 23 bp while the mutant gene (1691A) remains uncut at 180 bp. Although the 23 bp fragment is not easily detected, the 157 bp and 180 bp fragments are clearly resolved on a 3% agarose gel (Fig. 21.6). When only the smaller fragment is seen, the sample is normal (1691 G/G); when both the smaller and larger fragments are seen, the sample is heterozygous for FVL (1691 A/G); when only the larger fragment is seen, the sample is homozygous for FVL (1691 A/A). Since the latter is seen as an

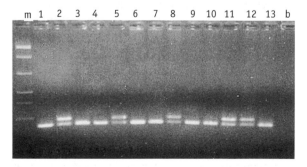

Fig. 21.6 Detection of the factor V Leiden (FVL) mutation using ACRES. PCR products generated using one mismatch-containing primer are digested with Taq I prior to agarose gel electrophoresis as described in the text. Heterozygotes for the FVL mutation are identified in lanes 2, 5, 8, 11 and 12. The other subjects are normal. m is the molecular weight size marker and b is the blank control.

uncut PCR product, this result is always confirmed by repetition. The Taq I enzyme is relatively robust, and partial digestion – the only potential pitfall in this analysis – is avoided by using a significant excess of enzyme.

BLEEDING DISORDERS (See Ch. 16)

Diverse mutations underlie haemophilia A and haemophilia B, and these are usually only identified in each family through SSCP and DNA sequence analysis in specialized laboratories. It may still be relevant to determine carrier status and offer prenatal diagnosis through genetic linkage analysis. Problems with this include the number of sporadic cases, lack of informative markers, unavailable family members and the possibility of recombination.

Of particular diagnostic significance is the fact that from between one-third and one-half of all patients with severe haemophilia A have a large genomic inversion mutation involving recombination between a region in intron 22 of the factor VIII gene and telomeric homologous sequences.[26] These inversions are readily detected by Southern blot analysis using the p482.6 probe[27] to Bcl I digests of genomic DNA. A method has also recently been described using long-distance PCR enabling identification of these deletion mutations in a single tube reaction.[28]

LEUKAEMIA AND LYMPHOMA

TRANSLOCATIONS AND MINIMAL RESIDUAL DISEASE (MRD)

The accurate characterization of haematological malignancies at the chromosomal and molecular level has advanced greatly in recent years and now makes an important contribution to initial treatment decisions. For example, a large number of patients with acute leukaemia, CML and lymphomas have specific chromosomal lesions known to be associated with particularly favourable or unfavourable prognoses and the proportion of such patients with defined chromosomal lesions is increasing. Usually the presence of these cytogenetic abnormalities can be confirmed by molecular biology techniques and in some cases the latter may be more informative than cytogenetics.

The Philadelphia (Ph) chromosome (22q-) present in 95% of cases of CML may be identified by routine cytogenetic studies; its presence can be confirmed by demonstrating the presence of the *BCR–ABL* fusion gene by RT–PCR. The Ph chromosome may also be found in 25% and 5% of adult and childhood acute lymphoblastic leukaemia (ALL) respectively,[29] where it is associated with relatively poor prognosis and indicates the need for a more aggressive therapy. Patients suspected of CML or a myeloproliferative disorder should be tested for *BCR–ABL* for definitive diagnosis. To optimize clinical management, patients with ALL should also be tested for *BCR–ABL*.

Small cleaved lymphoid cells are observed in a number of conditions with different treatments and prognoses. In such cases, detection of a translocation involving *BCL-1* is commonly associated with mantle cell lymphoma, t(11;14), whereas identification of *BCL-2* involvement implies a follicular lymphoma, t(14;18).[30] The former is much more aggressive with poor prognosis, thus requiring a more intensive treatment. Translocations associated with lymphomas usually lead to the deregulation of a normal gene, for example t(14;18) places the *BCL-2* gene adjacent to the IgH gene, leading to deregulation of the former. In contrast, the leukaemia-associated translocations often give rise to a chimeric gene that is transcribed, e.g. t(15;17) which yields a novel *PML/RAR-α* fusion gene.[31]

Frequently, the breakpoints within the translocation are too widely distributed to allow direct amplification of DNA by PCR. In such cases, the mRNA from the fusion gene can be reverse transcribed using reverse transcriptase (RT) to yield cDNA which can than be amplified by PCR. In addition, RT–PCR is an exquisitely sensitive tool which has been exploited in the detection of residual disease. This is illustrated by BCR–ABL fusion gene and has enabled a better assessment of the response of individual patients to therapy and has thus allowed the evaluation of treatment protocols on groups of patients. Quantitation of residual disease, i.e. determining the number of BCR–ABL transcripts by competitive PCR has been described.[32]

BCR–ABL RT–PCR

Principle and interpretation

The *BCR–ABL* analysis is performed by two-stage reverse transcriptase–polymerase chain reaction (RT–PCR). The RNA extracted from nucleated cells is reverse transcribed by reverse transcriptase to generate coding or complementary DNA (cDNA) using random primers 6 bp long or hexamers. Following the RT step, the samples are subjected to multiplex PCR, to test for the presence or absence of *BCR–ABL*.[33] Multiplex PCR is similar to conventional PCR, but includes more than one pair of primers in a single PCR test. This strategy enables the detection of all the known *BCR–ABL* transcripts. The most commonly observed transcripts are b3a2, b2a2 and e1a2, giving rise to 385, 310 and 481 bp amplicons respectively (Fig. 21.7).

In addition to *BCR–ABL*, the normal BCR gene is co-amplified yielding a 808 bp amplicon. The co-amplification of BCR is an indication of the quality of RNA and the efficiency of cDNA synthesis. Absence of any fragments indicates failure of the procedure. The latter is often due to an aged sample, i.e. over 72 hours old. For RT–PCR analysis, the sample should be processed to lysate stage (see nuclear lysate preparation (p. 516)) within 48 h of collection. In addition, the BCR fragment is often not observed in diagnostic samples where the *BCR–ABL* is preferentially amplified.

If *BCR–ABL* is undetectable by multiplex PCR in follow-up samples from patients undergoing therapy, the cDNA is tested at higher level of sensitivity by nested PCR.[34] Nested PCR enables the detection of one leukaemic cell in a background of 10^5 to 10^6 normal cells. The choice of primers for nested PCR is dependent on the type of transcript detected by multiplex PCR at presentation. The primers for b3a2 and b2a2 are the same; however, for e1a2 transcript a different set of primers is

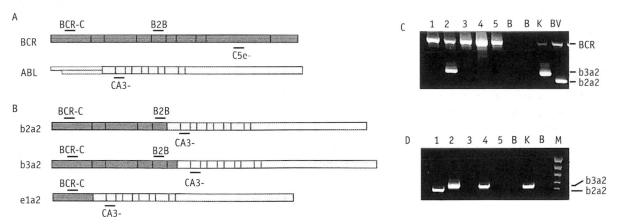

Fig. 21.7   Detection of minimal residual disease in chronic myeloid leukaemia (CML) by RT–PCR.
(A) Diagrammatic representation of the processed exons of the BCR and ABL genes together with the relative position of the B2B and C5e– primers used to co-amplify BCR in the multiplex PCR. (B) Commonly observed BCR–ABL derivatives, b2a2 and b3a2 which give rise to p210 BCR–ABL and e1a2 which gives rise to p190 BCR–ABL. The relative positions of the primers used to amplify the chimeric transcripts by multiplex PCR are shown. (C) A 2.0% agarose gel containing ethidium bromide through which amplicons generated by multiplex PCR using cDNA from 5 patients (lanes 1 to 5) were electrophorezed. The co-amplified normal BCR fragment, 808 bp in length, is seen in all samples except for the lanes containing the blank controls (B). The diagnostic sample from a patient with suspected CML, in lane 2, revealed a fragment corresponding to the b3a2 BCR–ABL transcript, 385 bp in length, in addition to the BCR amplicon. BCR–ABL is not detectable in lanes 1, 3, 4 and 5 containing follow-up samples from patients following stem-cell transplant (SCT). (D) The cDNA of these individuals was subjected to nested PCR to exclude residual disease. This reveals BCR–ABL transcripts, b3a2 (385 bp) and b2a2 (310 bp) in lanes 1 and 4, previously undetectable by the less sensitive multiplex PCR. However, BCR–ABL is not detectable in lanes 3 and 5, implying these samples are from patients in molecular remission post-SCT. B, blank controls; K (K562-b3a2) and BV (BV173-b2a2), positive controls; M, molecular size marker.

used. The nested PCR yields fragments of 385 bp (b3a2), 310 bp (b2a2) or 481 bp (e1a2) in length. Generally, diagnostic samples are not subjected to nested PCR if *BCR–ABL* is undetectable by multiplex PCR. Its detection is compatible with molecular relapse.

Reagents and methods
See Appendix E, page 516.

THE LYMPHOPROLIFERATIVE DISORDERS

The vast majority of lymphoproliferative disorders can be readily diagnosed using cytochemical and immunological techniques as described in Chapters 13 and 14. However, in monitoring residual disease and in certain cases where the diagnosis is ambiguous, genetic techniques may be useful.[30,35] Examples include cases of controversial lineage, lymphomas in which the histology is ambiguous and occult lymphomas. DNA analysis may also help in determining whether a lymphocytosis is monoclonal, oligoclonal or polyclonal. Translocations do occur in these disorders, and may be employed in monitoring disease as described for CML above. However, the most commonly used markers, because they are more universally applicable, are the rearranged immunoglobulin (Ig) and T-cell receptor (TCR) genes.

Principle
This analysis is possible because the Ig and TCR genes undergo a rearrangement during the normal differentiation of B and T lymphocytes respectively, but not during differentiation of other cells. This rearrangement results in a unique fusion of variable diversity and joining (VDJ) segments, interdigitated by random nucleotide insertion or deletion. The sequence and length of the DNA at these sites of recombination are therefore characteristic of any particular lymphocyte clone. Traditionally, this rearrangement has been detected by Southern blot analysis, described on page 518. More recently, because of its simplicity and potential sensitivity, the PCR has been used to amplify across this rearrangement. A polyclonal population of cells will give rise to a ladder of various fragment sizes; however, if one clone becomes abnormally large, a discrete fragment size will begin to dominate the products of the PCR – the basis of the so-called 'fingerprinting' method for the diagnosis of lymphoproliferative disorders.[36] This analysis can be refined by using SSCP gels in which the sequence as well as the size of the amplified product determines its mobility. To gain further sensitivity in following disease, the product of a 'clonal' amplification can be sequenced to derive a clone-specific sequence at the site of rearrangement. This sequence can then be used for the design of clone-specific oligonucleotide probes or primers that can be used in ASOH or ARMS procedures. This methodology has been used to monitor minimal residual disease in lymphoproliferative disorders,[37,38] but is very labour intensive and requires a specialist laboratory.

Method: immunoglobulin gene rearrangement
To study Ig gene rearrangement, the locus of choice is the heavy chain gene. The simplest procedure is to use one primer derived from a consensus sequence within framework 3 of each variable segment of the gene, and one primer from the joining segment. These are FR3: 5'CCGAGGACACGGC(CT)(CG)TGTATTA3' and JH: 5'ACCTGAGGAGACGGTGACCAGGGT3'. Amplification is performed in PCR buffer I with 1.5 mmol/l $MgCl_2$ and an annealing temperature of 55°C. The products of this reaction are in the order of 120 bp, and can be visualized as either a smear or discrete band in thick agarose gels. However, a better resolution is obtained when the products are resolved on a 6% denaturing polyacrylamide gel (see Appendix C, p. 514). They can be visualized by autoradiography if a trace of $[\alpha^{32}P]dCTP$ is included in the PCR reaction or through silver staining.[39] With access to an automated fragment analyser (e.g. the Applied Biosystems DNA Sequencer), this method is easily converted by attaching a fluorescent label to the JH primer and reading the peaks of fluorescence as an 'electrophoretogram'.

A more comprehensive analysis is obtained using the JH primer as above, but in conjunction with a different primer derived from a consensus sequence of the framework 1 region for each family of variable segments. These primers are:

VH1 5'CCTCAGTGAAGGTCTCCTGCAAGG3'
VH2 5'GAGTCTGGTCCTGCGCTGGTGAAA3'
VH3 5'GGTCCCTGAGACTCTCCTGTGCA3'

VH4 5′TTCGGA(GC)ACCCTGTCCCTCACCT3′
VH5 5′AGGTGAAAAAGCCCGGGGAGTCT3′
VH6 5′CCTGTGCCATCTCCGGGGACAGTG3′

PCR buffer II is used in conjunction with DMSO in these PCR reactions, with an annealing temperature of 62°C and including a radioactive trace as above. Again, the products, at about 320 bp, can be visualized after electrophoresis on 6% denaturing polyacrylamide gels or on an automated fluorescence analyser.

Interpretation

Because of the variable number of nucleotides either removed or added at the point of joining of VDJ segments of the immunoglobulin heavy chain gene, the distance between V segment and J segment primers will alter accordingly. For the gene to be functional, the reading frame must be maintained and therefore variations in length are in multiples of three base pairs. The polyclonal population of B cells therefore gives rise to a characteristic 'ladder', with peak intensity observed at the median length at its centre. If one B-cell clone is abnormally large, it will give rise to a disproportionately intense band at the size (and using a V primer from the appropriate family, if these are employed) corresponding to its VDJ length. At presentation of a B-cell malignancy, this band may be the only one visible, confirming the presence of an abnormal B-cell clone. Subsequently, an abnormal intensity of this fragment size in the background of a ladder can be used to monitor the disease.

There are two main problems that can be encountered in this analysis. The first is that the consensus V primers may not amplify all V segments perfectly because of variations in sequence. This is particularly true of the framework 3 primer. Second, the evolution of a B-cell clone or the emergence of other subclones during the course of the disease, may result in the fragment size (and family) being followed to change and therefore be missed.

Method: T-cell receptor gene rearrangement

The choice of locus for PCR analysis of the TCR gene rearrangement is the TCR gamma locus as it is rearranged in the vast majority of T-cell clones and does not have the complexity of the TCR beta locus, which has 24 different V segment families. Amplification of DNA around the joining region of the TCR gamma gene is performed in a similar way to that described above for the IgH locus, using a consensus primer for the joining segment (JγC) and one for each of the four variable segment families (Vγ1–4). The primer sequences are as follows:

JγC: 5′CAACAAGTGTTGTTCCAC3′
Vγ1: 5′TGCAGCCAGTCAGAAATCTTCC3′
Vγ2: 5′TGCAGGTCACCTAGAGCAACCT3′
Vγ3: 5′AGCAGTTCCAGCTATCCATTTCC3′
Vγ4: 5′TGCAATTGCACTTGGGCAGTTG3′

Standard PCR amplification conditions can be employed using these primer combinations, and analysis is again performed on acrylamide gels (Appendix C, p. 514).

Interpretation

As in the analysis of the immunoglobulin heavy chain gene, discrete bands of amplified product are obtained from clonal T-cell populations, while smears are obtained from polyclonal populations, in this case differing by only one base pair, since non-productive rearrangements are present. A greater resolution can be obtained in SSCP gels in which fragment mobility is determined by sequence as well as by size. Products from a polyclonal population have a great variety of sequences and after denaturing, they do not easily re-anneal to give the double-stranded product, but migrate as a long smear of single-stranded products. If an abnormally large T-cell clone is present, many copies of the same product are present which will re-anneal to give a double-stranded fragment, and also show up as discrete single-stranded fragments (Fig. 21.8).

GLUCOSE-6-PHOSPHATE DEHYDROGENASE DEFICIENCY (See Ch. 10)

Most of the polymorphic variants of glucose-6-phosphate dehydrogenase (G6PD) that are associated with acute haemolysis have been defined at the molecular level and it may be important to distinguish these from a G6PD-deficient variant that is the cause of chronic haemolysis. Since it is an

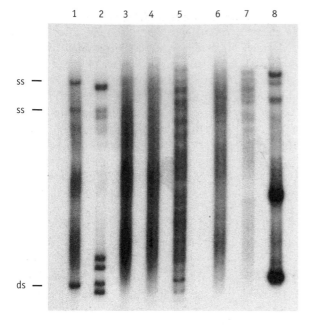

ss —

ss —

ds —

Fig. 21.8   SSCP analysis of TCR γ-chain gene rearrangement. Electrophoresis of denatured radiolabelled PCR products in a native 6% polyacrylamide gel, visualized by autoradiography. Discrete single- (ss) and double- (ds) stranded fragments, indicating the presence of abnormal T-cell clones, are seen in lanes 1, 2, and 8 from patients with hypereosinophilia, cutaneous T-cell lymphoma, and a γδ lymphoma respectively. Polyclonal smears of single-stranded fragments are seen in lanes 3, 4 and 6 and multiple single-stranded fragments against a background smear are seen in lanes 5 and 7 indicating an oligoclonal expansion of T-cell clones.

X-linked disorder, it may be difficult to identify heterozygous females, in whom levels of enzyme activity may vary from reduced to normal. This is particularly important in female relatives of men with chronic haemolytic anaemia caused by G6PD deficiency. Furthermore, G6PD deficiency can be masked by reticulocytosis in individuals with acute haemolysis and in neonates.

In such cases, it may be beneficial to test for a G6PD-deficient variant by DNA analysis. Although more than 100 G6PD mutations have now been described,[40] some of the most common deficient variants are readily diagnosed by restriction enzyme digestion of the appropriate PCR products. For example, the G6PD Mediterranean mutation creates an Mbo II site in exon 6, and the two mutations found in G6PD A- create an Nla III site in exon 4 and a Fok I site in exon 5 of the G6PD gene.

SOUTHERN BLOT ANALYSIS

This technique is used for the detection of specific sequences among DNA fragments separated by gel electrophoresis.[41] The size of a specific DNA fragment from a particular individual can therefore be determined by its mobility.

Principle

The digestion of human genomic DNA with a restriction enzyme that recognizes a six base-pair sequence yields fragments that can be conveniently separated according to size by electrophoresis in an agarose gel. Good resolution is obtained in the size range of about 500 bp to about 20 kb. DNA is negatively charged in a neutral buffer; smaller fragments migrate faster towards the anode than larger fragments.

A specific DNA fragment is detected using a labelled probe. The probe is usually a purified DNA fragment which can be labelled to a high specific activity with a radionucleotide. The specificity of DNA–DNA base pairing means that, in the appropriate conditions, the denatured probe will only hybridize to its perfectly complementary sequence among the digested DNA fragments. The location of the signal seen after autoradiography allows the size of the DNA fragment to be determined with reference to a size marker run on the gel.

The agarose gel in which the DNA fragments are resolved is not a suitable matrix for this hybridization. After denaturing the fragments by immersing the gel in alkali, they are transferred to a nylon membrane by capillary action; this is a Southern blot.

Reagents and methods
See Appendix F, page 518.

DNA probes
Any piece of DNA can be used as a probe, from total genomic DNA to a short oligonucleotide. The only requirements are that there is a sufficient amount of DNA (more than 20 ng) and it can be labelled. Probes that are in regular use are typically DNA fragments between a few hundred bp and a few kb in length, which have been cloned into a plasmid vector. Many plasmids have been specifically engineered to enable the efficient propagation of these DNA fragments as cloned recombinant molecules in *Escherichia coli*.

It is beyond the scope of this chapter to go into the details of how these clones are produced. Those that are described in this chapter are all freely available from the laboratories in which they were first isolated. With any probe, it is important to obtain the following information in order to use it properly:

1. whether the fragment is derived from genomic DNA or cDNA
2. which vector the fragment has been cloned into
3. the restriction enzymes that were used in the cloning, and those that can be used to release the DNA fragment (or insert) from the vector
4. the size of the insert
5. a restriction map of the region of DNA from which the probe is derived.

Probes will usually be sent out as plasmid DNA or bacterial strains harbouring the recombinant plasmid. They may also be obtained from commercial companies in a form in which they are ready to use. Protocols for the transformation of competent *E. coli* with plasmid DNA and the large-scale preparation of plasmid DNA from liquid cultures of *E. coli* are to be found in specialist laboratory manuals.[3] The preparation of the insert from plasmid DNA and a recommended method for labelling the insert with $[\alpha^{32}P]dCTP$ are described in Appendix G (p. 520).

DIAGNOSIS OF α-THALASSAEMIA BY SOUTHERN BLOT ANALYSIS

The α-thalassaemias, which are mostly caused by gene deletions,[42] can be identified readily by Southern blot analysis. Since this technique allows the detection of multiple deletions in one reaction, it often remains the method of choice.[43] The clinically significant α°-thalassaemias are caused by large deletions that remove both of the α globin genes from one chromosome, and therefore go undetected when an α globin gene probe is used. In the most common of these, the South-East Asian ($-^{SEA}$) and Mediterranean ($-^{MED}$) forms, the deletions extend from within the ζ globin genes to the region of the α globin 3′ hypervariable region (HVR). The resulting disruption of the ζ globin genes can be detected using a ζ globin gene probe. Since the deletions of the common α^{+}-thalassaemias also disrupt fragments around the ζ globin locus, this is the probe of choice in screening for α-thalassaemia. The most commonly used probe is a 1.8 kb Sac I ζ_1 genomic fragment[44] that will hybridize to both the ζ_1 and ζ_2 genes.

Interpretation
The different fragment sizes seen in the most common α-thalassaemia deletions by different probes in various restriction digests are shown in Table 21.2. The most informative of these is the hybridization of the ζ globin probe to a Bgl II digest.

Other larger, but less common deletions, such as $-^{FIL}$ and $-^{THAI}$, remove both the α and ζ globin genes and therefore go undetected when these genes are used as probes. Flanking probes have to be used instead. Alternatively, these can be detected by Gap–PCR in their identification as described earlier. Another problem in this analysis is that the non-deletional forms of α-thalassaemia will also go undetected.

Attention must be paid to the presence of a hypervariable region between the two ζ globin genes (inter-ζ HVR)[45] which is highly polymorphic in both normal and α-thalassaemic individuals. In addition, there is a rare polymorphic Bgl II site between the ζ_2 and α_2 globin genes which splits the 12.6 kb fragment into 5.2 kb and 7.4 kb fragments (the latter is not seen by the ζ globin probe). Variation can also be observed resulting from the triplication or the deletion of one of the ζ globin genes.

Comments
Unlike the β-thalassaemias, α-thalassaemias are not easily diagnosed using routine haematological

Table 21.2 Restriction enzyme (RE) fragment sizes in common α globin gene deletions

Probe	RE	Genotype				
		αα	$-\alpha^{3.7}$	$-\alpha^{4.2}$	$_{-}{-}^{SEA}$	$_{-}{-}^{MED}$
α	BamH I	14.0	10.3	9.8	–	–
	EcoR I	23.0	19.3	18.8	–	–
	Bgl II	12.6; 7.4	16.0	8.4; 7.4	–	–
ζ	BamH I	10.8; 5.7	10.8; 5.7	10.8; 5.7	20.0	5.9
	EcoR I	23.0; 4.8	19.3; 4.8	18.8; 4.8	17.2; 4.8	4.8
	Bgl II	12.6	16.0	8.4	10.5	13.9
		9.5–12.5*	9.5–12.5*	9.5–12.5*	9.5–12.5*	9.5–12.5*

*Range of normal fragment sizes is due to the inter-ζ HVR. Fragment sizes given in kb.

techniques. The diagnosis of α-thalassaemia is often made following exclusion of β-thalassaemia and/or iron deficiency. Since the vast majority of cases of α-thalassaemia are of the clinically benign type (i.e. α^+-thalassaemia), it is debatable whether molecular analysis is justified in order to reach a definitive diagnosis in these individuals. However, it is essential that individuals with α°-thalassaemia are identified and, if it is appropriate, are investigated at the molecular level. This is particularly relevant if prenatal diagnosis is to be offered to a couple who are at risk of having a hydropic fetus, where there is an increased risk of maternal death at delivery. Guidelines derived from the UK experience as to how and when DNA analysis should be implemented have recently been proposed.[46]

DIAGNOSIS OF LYMPHOPROLIFERATIVE DISORDERS BY SOUTHERN BLOT ANALYSIS

Principle

Southern blot analysis can be used to detect rearrangement of the Ig and TCR genes since this process results in a change in the restriction fragments seen at the joining region of these loci. The rearranged fragments from any one clone are only detected when it represents an abnormally large proportion of the cells in the population being studied, as it will in a clonal lymphoproliferative disorder. In a polyclonal population, each of the many different rearranged fragments that are present, which are derived from the large number of different clones, will be below the level of detection by this method. In this situation only the germ line fragments will be seen. The most infor-

mative probes used in gene rearrangement studies are the JH probe,[47] for the joining region of the Ig heavy chain gene, and the Cβ probe,[48] for the constant region of the TCR β-chain gene.

Interpretation

The detection of a rearranged fragment with a TCR or Ig gene probe that is different in size to the germ line fragments indicates the presence of an abnormal lymphocyte clone. In all cases, it is important to corroborate the findings seen with one restriction enzyme by seeing the same pattern with another enzyme. Some examples that illustrate these general points, as well as problems encountered in this analysis, are shown in Figures 21.9 and 21.10. Figure 21.9A shows the detection of an abnormal B-cell clone in a patient with chronic lymphoblastic leukaemia (CLL). Using the JH probe to Hind III and Bgl II digests, only a single germ line fragment is seen in the control sample. In the patient, two additional rearranged bands of roughly equal intensity are seen representing two rearranged alleles in the clone. The relative intensity of these bands to the germ line band shows that the clone represents a large proportion of the mononuclear cells in peripheral blood, from where the DNA was extracted.

Figure 21.9B shows the hybridization of the JH probe to Bgl II digests of DNA from the peripheral blood of a patient with a lymphocytosis (lane 1), CLL (lane 2) and cold agglutinins (lane 3). In lane 1, only a germ line fragment is seen, demonstrating that the lymphocytosis is not due to a clonal expansion of B cells. In lane 2, two rearranged alleles from the abnormal B-cell clone

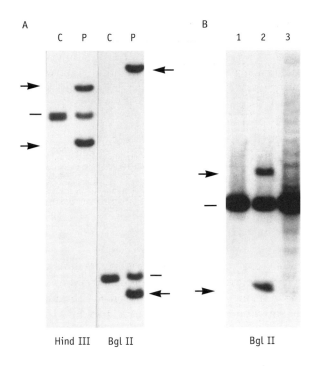

Hind III   Bgl II   Bgl II

Fig. 21.9   Southern blot analysis of IgH gene rearrangement. Hybridization of the JH probe to genomic DNA is visualized by autoradiography. Dashes to the left and right of each panel indicate the position of the germ line fragments. The arrows point to the rearranged fragments. C, control sample; P, patient sample. The restriction enzymes used are shown beneath each panel. For explanations, see text.

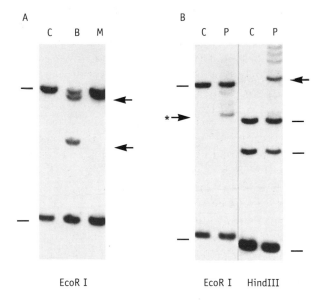

EcoR I   EcoR I   HindIII

Fig. 21.10   Southern blot analysis of TCR gene rearrangement. Hybridization of the Cβ probe to genomic DNA is visualized by autoradiography. Markings are as for Figure 21.9 *Fragments generated by partial digestion. B, peripheral blood sample; M, bone marrow sample. For explanations, see text.

are detected. In lane 3, there are clearly a number of faint rearranged bands detected in addition to the germ line fragment. The significance of this pattern is not altogether clear and it has been called an oligoclonal expansion of B-cell clones.

In Figure 21.10A, two germ line fragments are seen with the Cβ probe in an EcoR I digest of DNA extracted from a control sample. Two

rearranged bands are seen in DNA extracted from peripheral blood mononuclear cells (B) and a bone marrow aspirate (M) of a patient with pure red cell aplasia. These bands are strong in the blood sample, indicating the presence of a relatively large abnormal T-cell clone, but much weaker in the bone marrow aspirate where the clone represents a smaller proportion of the total cell population.

In Figure 21.10B, additional bands are seen with the Cβ probe in the same patient in both Hind III and EcoR I digests. In this case, however, it is very likely that these bands do not represent gene rearrangement, but partial digestion. The Hind III and EcoR I sites at $C\beta_2$ are particularly resistant to digestion in suboptimal conditions. This results in additional fragments of 13 kb in Hind III digests and 8 kb in EcoR I digests. Additional larger faint bands are also seen in this patient, which is again indicative of incomplete digestion. These partial fragments will be the same size in all the different samples in which they are seen, while genuine rearranged fragments will almost invariably be of a different size in different patients. Partial digestion is a problem encountered with the JH probe as well, but again the fragments generated are of a consistent size.

Problems

Two major problems in this analysis are poor film quality and partial digestion. The latter has been illustrated and is relatively easy to identify. Poor film quality is the more frustrating, as the sensitivity of this technique depends on obtaining good signals against a low background. At their best, these gene rearrangement studies can detect clones that represent as little as 2–5% of the total cell population.

As with all Southern blot analysis, a reasonable amount (at least 30 μg) of high-quality DNA is required. Although this is not usually a problem with blood or marrow samples, it can be a major problem in dealing with small tissue biopsies. This is one of the principal reasons for establishing PCR-based methods for the study of gene rearrangements.

There are also problems intrinsic to the method itself. These include the time taken to perform the analysis, the experience required to obtain consistently high-quality autoradiographs and the use of a radionuclide, which is still the only way to obtain the strength of signal required in this procedure.

APPENDICES: TECHNICAL METHODS

APPENDIX A: EXTRACTION OF GENOMIC DNA

Reagents

General note. For all the buffers and solutions described in this chapter, it is recommended that reagents of the highest grade available and double distilled deionized water are used throughout.

Stock solutions

NaCl 5 mol/l. Weigh 146.1 g of NaCl into a beaker and make up the volume to 500 ml with water; stir until dissolved.

Tris-HCl, 1 mol/l, pH 8.5. Dissolve 60.5 g of Trizma base (tris(hydroxy)methylaminomethane) in 350 ml water; add concentrated HCl until the pH falls to 8.5; make up to 500 ml with water.

Tris-HCl, 1 mol/l, pH 7.4. Prepare as for above but reduce the pH to 7.4 with HCl.

NaOH, 5 mol/l. Add 200 g of NaOH to 800 ml water and stir until dissolved; make up to 1 litre with water.

Ethylenediamine tetra-acetic acid (EDTA), 0.5 mol/l, pH 8.0. Weigh 93 g of EDTA disodium salt (dihydrate) and add to 400 ml of water; stir until most of it has dissolved. Add 0.5 mol/l NaOH until the pH rises to 8.0, when the rest of the solid should go into solution. Make up to 500 ml with water.

Phosphate-buffered saline (PBS), pH 7.3. See page 606 for preparation.

Nonidet P-40 (NP40), 10%. Add 10 ml of NP40 to 90 ml water and mix well.

Sodium dodecyl sulphate (SDS, lauryl sulphate), 20%. Weigh 100 g of SDS and add to 350 ml of water. Stir and heat to 65°C until it is in solution and top up to 500 ml with water. **Caution.** SDS is a respiratory irritant: wear a face mask and weigh out in a fume hood.

Working solutions

PBS + 0.1% NP40. Add 5 ml of 10% NP40 to 495 ml of PBS.

Ten times concentrated (10×) lysis buffer. Mix 60 ml of 5 mol/l NaCl, 20 ml of 0.5 mol/l

EDTA, 10 ml of 1 mol/l Tris pH 7.4 and 10 ml of water to give 100 ml of 3 mol/l NaCl, 100 mmol/l EDTA, 100 mmol/l Tris.

Lysis solution.   Prepare an appropriate amount of this solution fresh every time; for 50 ml weigh 21 g of urea (7 mol/l), add 5 ml of 10× lysis buffer and make up to a final volume of 50 ml with water.

Chloroform/isoamyl alcohol (24:1).   Add 20 ml of isoamyl alcohol to 480 ml of chloroform.

Ethanol 70%.   Add 30 ml of water to 70 ml of absolute ethanol.

TE (10 mmol/l Tris, 1 mmol/l EDTA).   Add 5 ml of 1 mol/l Tris pH 7.4 and 1 ml of 0.5 mol/l Na_2 EDTA to 494 ml water.

TE equilibrated phenol.   The condition of the phenol is crucial to the quality of the DNA obtained. DNA is soluble in acidic water-saturated phenol, and so it is necessary to equilibrate it to a neutral pH.

1. Take 500 ml of water-saturated phenol. Prepare 500 ml of 0.5 mol/l Tris pH 8.5, add 150 ml of this to the phenol and mix by inversion for 2–3 min. Leave to stand until the aqueous and organic phases have separated.
2. Remove and discard the upper aqueous layer. Add another 125 ml of 0.5 mol/l Tris, mix, stand and remove the aqueous layer as before and then repeat.
3. To the remaining 100 ml of 0.5 mol/l Tris, add 400 ml of water to give 500 ml of 0.1 mol/l Tris. Add 150 ml of this to the phenol, and then mix, stand and remove as above. Repeat two more times.
4. To the remaining 50 ml of 0.1 mol/l Tris add 449 ml of water and 1 ml of 0.5 mol/l EDTA to give 500 ml of TE. Add, mix, stand and remove this in three stages as before. The phenol will have reduced in volume during this procedure, but is now TE equilibrated and ready for use.

Method

1. Freeze an anticoagulated blood sample at –20°C. EDTA, ACD or preservative-free heparin are all suitable anticoagulants. It is convenient to collect the blood in a tube that can be centrifuged, such as a disposable plastic 30 ml universal container. Any sample size from 2 to 20 ml will be satisfactory. Blood can be shipped at room temperature to a reference laboratory, preferably within a few days of taking it. The sample can be stored at –20°C for several weeks; storage for longer periods is better at –80°C.
2. Thaw the blood and centrifuge at 700 *g* for 15 min. Carefully pour off the supernatant. The pellet is hard to see at this stage, and may be quite loose.
3. Resuspend the pellet in 1–2 ml of PBS + 0.1% NP40 by mixing up and down in a wide bore standard plastic transfer pipette. Top up the suspension to the original volume with PBS + 0.1% NP40.
4. Centrifuge again at 700 *g* for 15 min and pour off the supernatant. If necessary, repeat until the pellet has lost most of its red colour.
5. Add 2 to 3 drops of lysis solution. Break up the pellet into this solution using a non-wettable sterile stick (e.g. a plastic disposable bacterial inoculating loop) or a clean siliconized glass rod. The solution will become viscous. Make it as homogeneous as possible.
6. Add successive 0.5 ml volumes of the lysis solution, mixing each time, until the viscosity is such that the solution can be pipetted up and down without difficulty. The final volume will depend on the size, nature and quality of the blood sample. For 10 ml of freshly frozen normal blood, use 2–3 ml of lysis solution.
7. Add 1/10 volume of 20% SDS. Mix gently with a transfer pipette and incubate at 37°C for a minimum of 15 min. The samples can be left overnight at this stage.
8. Transfer the sample to a capped polypropylene tube. Add an equal volume of chloroform/isoamyl alcohol and an equal volume of phenol. Mix gently by inversion for 5 min. Centrifuge at 1300 *g* for 15 min.
9. Transfer the upper aqueous phase to a new polypropylene tube. Leave behind the white protein interface and the organic phase. This may be difficult if the solution is too viscous, in which case further dilution with lysis solution is necessary.
10. Repeat steps 8 and 9 at least once more and continue until the interface is clear. Add an equal volume of chloroform/isoamyl alcohol and mix gently by inversion for 5 min. Centrifuge as before

and again transfer the aqueous phase to a universal or capped 10 ml tube.

11. Add 2.5 volumes of absolute ethanol. Mix the solution by inverting the tube several times. The DNA should precipitate as a 'cotton wool' ball. Using a micropipette tip, transfer the DNA to a microcentrifuge tube containing 1 ml of 70% ethanol.

12. Centrifuge in a microcentrifuge at 12 000 g for 5 min. Pour off the residual ethanol, and remove all of this with a micropipette.

13. Leave to dry on the bench for 10 min.

14. Add 50–500 µl of TE depending on the size of the pellet. Aim to have a DNA concentration of approximately 0.5 mg/ml. Leave to resuspend for at least one night. Mix gently by flicking the tube; never vortex. The DNA can be stored for long periods at 4°C or frozen at −20°C.

Extraction of DNA from other sources

For the analysis of immunoglobulin and T-cell receptor gene rearrangements, it is necessary to enrich a peripheral blood sample for lymphocytes prior to DNA extraction. This is achieved through the separation of mononuclear cells on Ficoll/ Hypaque (or Lymphoprep). After washing the cell pellet in PBS, lysis and DNA extraction can proceed as from step 5 above.

DNA is extracted from bone marrow aspirates in the same way as from peripheral blood, except that before freezing they are diluted in at least 5 volumes of PBS.

Tissue biopsies vary greatly in nature, size and cell content and, as a result, so does the quality and quantity of DNA obtained from them. To obtain sufficient quantities of high molecular weight DNA for Southern blot analysis the biopsy must be several mm³ in size and fresh frozen. If such a biopsy is available, sufficient cells can be obtained by mechanically disrupting it into PBS firstly by chopping finely with a clean blade and then breaking it up with the blunt end of a 5 ml syringe plunger. The suspension is centrifuged to obtain a pellet, from which DNA is extracted as above (from step 5). For smaller biopsies, it is better to treat the sample with proteinase K prior to extraction as follows:

1. Place the tissue in 700 µl of 50 mmol/l Tris-HCl pH 8.0, 100 mmol/l NaCl, 1% (w/v) SDS containing 100 µg/ml proteinase K.

2. Cut up the tissue with a fine pair of scissors, and incubate at 50°C overnight.

3. Proceed with phenol/chloroform extraction and DNA precipitation as from step 8 above.

Determining the DNA concentration

Take 5 µl of the DNA solution and dilute into 245 µl of water. Mix well by vortexing. (This DNA is to be discarded and can therefore be treated in this way.) Read the absorbance (A) in a spectrometer at 260 nm against a water blank. An A of 1.0 is obtained from a solution of DNA at a concentration of 50 µg/ml. Therefore, multiply the A reading obtained by 2500 to get the concentration of the original DNA solution in µg/ml. The ratio of the A_{260} to the A_{280} gives an indication as to the purity of the DNA solution. This ratio should be in the range 1.7–2.0.

APPENDIX B: PCR

Reagents

Taq polymerase and oligonucleotide primers. These can be purchased from a variety of different companies. The oligos are usually 18–22 bases in length.

PCR buffers: these are usually supplied along with the Taq polymerase. Three different buffers can be prepared as follows:

- *10× PCR buffer I:* 100 mmol/l Tris-HCl pH 8.3, 500 mmol/l KCl, 15 mmol/l MgCl₂, 0.1% (w/v) gelatin, 0.5% (v/v) NP40 and 0.5% (v/v) Tween 20.
- *10× PCR buffer II:* 670 mmol/l Tris pH 8.8, 166 mmol/l (NH₄)₂SO₄, 25 mmol/l MgCl₂, 670 µmol/l Na₂ EDTA, 1.6 mg/ml BSA and 100 mmol/l β-mercapto-ethanol. This buffer is used in conjunction with 10% DMSO in the final reaction mixture.
- *10 × PCR buffer III:* 750 mmol/l Tris pH 8.8, 200 mmol/l (NH₄)₂SO₄, 0.1% (v/v) Tween 20. A solution of 25 mmol/l MgCl₂ is also prepared and added separately to the PCR reaction.

dNTP, 10 mmol/l. Take 10 µl of 100 mmol/l dATP, 10 µl of 100 mmol/l dTTP, 10 µl of 100 mmol/l dCTP, 10 µl of 100 mmol/l dGTP and 60 µl of water to make a 100 µl of 10 mmol/l dNTP

Dimethylsulphoxide (DMSO).

Agarose, Type II medium electro-endosmosis.

10× Tris-borate-EDTA (TBE) buffer: add 216 g of Trizma base, 18.6 g of EDTA and 110 g of orthoboric acid to 1600 ml water, dissolve and top up to 2 l; dilute 1 in 20 for use as 0.5× TBE buffer.

Ethidium bromide, 10 mg/ml. Dissolve 1 g of ethidium bromide in 100 ml of water, and keep in brown or foil-wrapped bottle. **Caution.** Ethidium bromide is a known teratogen; wear a face mask and handle with double gloves.

Tracking dye. Weigh 15 g of Ficoll (type 400), 0.25 g of bromophenol blue and 0.25 g of xylene cyanol. Make up to 100 ml with water, cover and mix by inversion; it will take quite a considerable amount of mixing to get the solution homogeneous. Dispense into aliquots.

Method

Optimal conditions for the reaction have to be derived empirically, with the magnesium concentration and annealing temperature being the most important parameters.[49] The choice of buffer depends on the enzyme being used, and the company will usually supply the most appropriate one. For genes with a high GC content, buffer II (above) in combination with 10% DMSO may give better amplification. In most cases, a 25 µl reaction volume suffices, although 50 µl should be used if it is necessary to check whether the amplification has been successful prior to one subsequent manipulation. A blank control should always be included (i.e. a reaction without any template) in order to control for contamination. If the blank control yields a product, the analysis is invalidated. A DNA sample that is known to amplify can also be included and this sample may then be used as a normal or positive control.

The risk of contamination cannot be overemphasized. It can be minimized by using plugged tips and having dedicated micropipettes and areas for each step of the analysis. The optimum cycling conditions need to be determined for each thermocycler. Specificity is often improved by 'hot start' PCR. This is achieved by setting up all the PCR tests on wet ice and transferring the tubes to the thermocycler on it reaching 96°C. In preparing a group of reactions, pipetting errors can be minimized by making a pre-mix solution which can be dispensed into microcentrifuge tubes containing the DNA template. When a particular PCR is to be performed repetitively over a period of time, it is helpful to prepare a large volume (10 ml) of the reaction mixture (without DNA or *Taq* polymerase), aliquot it and store at –20°C.

1. Prepare a PCR mixture for ten reactions (with a final volume of 50 µl for each DNA sample) as follows:

Stock solution	Vol (µl)	Final concentration
10× PCR buffer	50	1×
10 mmol/l dNTP	10	0.2 mmol/l
Primer (1) 20 µmol/l	10	0.4 µmol/l
Primer (2) 20 µmol/l	10	0.4 µmol/l
Taq polymerase 5 u/ml	2	0.02 u/ml
Water	408	
Final volume	490	

Add the *Taq* polymerase last, mix well and pulse-spin in a microcentrifuge to bring down the contents of the tube.

Note. For some PCR reactions and in using PCR buffer III above, appropriate volumes of 25 mmol/l $MgCl_2$ should be added: the correct final concentration, usually between 1.5 mmol/l and 3.0 mmol/l, should be determined empirically for each primer pair. Adjust the volume of water to compensate for this.

2. Put 1 µl of template DNA at approximately 0.5 mg/ml into each of nine 0.5 ml microcentrifuge tubes and 1 µl of double distilled water into the tenth tube. Aliquot 49 µl of the mix prepared above in to each tube.

3. Overlay the mixture with 50 µl of light paraffin oil and place the tubes in a PCR machine, programmed for the following conditions: an initial step of 5 min at 94°C and then 30 cycles of 58°C for 1 min, 72°C for 1 min and 94°C for 1 min in sequence followed by a final extension step at 72°C for 10 min. These conditions are suitable for many primer pairs, although some will require different annealing temperatures, or longer extension times.

4. While the PCR program is running, a 1.5% agarose mini-gel is prepared: add 0.75 g of agarose to 50 ml of 0.5× TBE buffer and heat until completely dissolved. Add 2 µl of ethidium bromide (10 mg/ml), allow the agarose to cool slightly and pour with the appropriate comb in position.

5. To check if the amplification has been successful, add 1 µl of tracking dye to a 10 µl aliquot of the PCR reaction mixture, being careful not to pipette the mineral oil overlaying the PCR reaction.

6. Load the gel and run at a constant voltage of 100 V for 1 h in 0.5× TBE buffer. A molecular size marker should be included to establish the size of the amplified fragment; these are commercially available. The marker used in this chapter is the plasmid pEMBL 8 digested with Taq I and Pvu II to yield fragments of 1443, 1008, 613, 357, 278, 193 and 108 bp.

7. Visualize the DNA on a UV transilluminator and, if required, take a photograph.

Modifications and developments

The procedure described above is a guideline for setting up and checking a standard PCR amplification. As the test dictates, modifications can be employed such as:

Radiolabelling: a PCR can be labelled with ^{32}P by adding 0.1 µl of $[\alpha^{32}P]dCTP$ per tube to the reaction mixture.

Multiplex: more than one fragment can be amplified in the same tube, simply by adding in further primer pairs. It is important that the different pairs all work equally well under the same conditions.

Nested PCR: successive rounds of amplification using two pairs of primers, the second pair, located within the sequence amplified by the first, allows products to be generated from as little as a single cell.

Long-range amplification: fragments upwards of 10 kb can now be generated by PCR using modified polymerases.

Automation: high-throughput PCR amplification is being achieved through the use of robots and 96-well plate technology.

Real-time PCR: oligonucleotide probes, with a fluorescent and quencher group at their 5′ and 3′ end respectively, are hydrolysed during PCR by the 5′ nuclease activity of the Taq polymerase. This results in a release of fluorescence proportional to the accumulation of PCR product and can be directly measured during the course of a reaction using the Applied Biosystems (ABI) Prism 7700 sequence detector. The 5′ nuclease assay can also be used in allelic discrimination owing to the inefficient cleavage of fluorogenic probes that contain a single base mismatch.

Automated fragment analysis: the method of gel electrophoresis is modified for the detection of fluorescently labelled PCR products on DNA fragment analysers (e.g. the ABI 373 DNA sequencer).

APPENDIX C: POLYACRYLAMIDE GEL ELECTROPHORESIS

Equipment and reagents

A vertical gel electrophoresis tank with appropriate plates, combs and spacers.

A slab gel dryer with vacuum pump.
40% (w/v) acrylamide solution.

Caution: Acrylamide is a potent neurotoxin.

2% (w/v) bis-acrylamide solution.
Glycerol.
Urea (ultrapure).
10% (w/v) ammonium persulphate.
TEMED.
10 × TBE buffer (see Appendix B).
Formamide dye: to 10 ml deionized formamide, add 10 mg xylene cyanol FF, 10 mg bromophenol blue and 200 µl 0.5 mol/l EDTA.

Method

The following procedure describes the preparation of a large, thin (34 cm × 40 cm × 0.4 mm) 6% denaturing polyacrylamide gel.

1. Clean the glass plates thoroughly with detergent and a scourer. Rinse well and dry. Swab the larger plate with 100% ethanol. Treat one surface of the smaller plate with a siliconizing solution or a non-toxic gel coating solution (e.g. Gel Slick from FMC), by applying a few ml and buffing dry with a paper towel. Assemble the gel using spacers, bulldog clips and electrical tape around the bottom of the gel. Ensure that the gaskets closely abut the smaller plate.

2. Mix 12 ml 40% acrylamide, 12 ml 2% bis-acrylamide, 8 ml 10×TBE, 36.8 g urea and adjust the volume to 80 ml with dd H_2O. Add 500 µl of 10% ammonium persulphate and 50 µl of TEMED, mix and pour the solution slowly between the glass plates using a 50 ml syringe. When full, insert an inverted sharks tooth comb

(smooth surface downward) no more than 6 mm into the gel. Leave to polymerize.

3. Remove the electrical tape and bulldog clips and place the gel in the electrophoresis tank. Fill the top and bottom chambers with 1×TBE. Remove the comb and flush the surface of the gel with TBE buffer using a syringe and bent needle. Clean and invert the comb and insert it between the plates until the teeth just indent the surface of the gel.

4. Mix 1–4 µl of the radiolabelled PCR product with 6 µl of formamide dye. Heat at 95°C for 5 min. Snap chill on wet ice. Flush out each well using TBE buffer and load 5 µl of each sample between the teeth. Run the gel at 40–60 V until the appropriate resolution has been obtained. (As a guide, the bromophenol blue and xylene cyanol will co-migrate with 25 bp and 105 bp DNA fragments respectively in a 6% denaturing polyacrylamide gel).

5. Disconnect the power supply, remove the plates and place them on a flat surface. Pull one of the spacers out from between the plates. Insert a metal spatula or a fine plastic wedge horizontally into the gap between the plates at the bottom corner where the spacer was. Lift the smaller siliconized plate off the gel. Cut a piece of 3 MM Whatman paper so that it is slightly larger than the gel area, and lay it down onto the gel. Return the smaller plate over the Whatman paper, apply gentle pressure and invert the plates. Carefully pull up the larger plate, ensuring that the gel sticks to the Whatman paper. Cover the gel with cling film (e.g. Saran Wrap) and trim all the edges.

6. Dry the gel under vacuum at 80°C for about 1 h. Peel off the Saran Wrap and expose the gel to X-ray film overnight at –80°C to obtain an autoradiograph.

For SSCP analysis, a non-denaturing gel is used. The procedure is the same as described above, but the composition of the gel is different. The following gel mix can be used for a large gel run overnight at 8–12 mA in a cool (20–22°C) laboratory: 12 ml 40% acrylamide, 2.4 ml 2% bis-acrylamide, 4 ml glycerol, 8 ml 10× TBE, 53.6 ml H_2O. Variations are often introduced in order to increase the chances of observing aberrant mobilities (or shifts) of mutant DNA strands. These include altering the content of the gel such as the % of glycerol, the % of the acrylamide and the acrylamide:bis-acrylamide ratio used, as well as variations in the temperature and speed of electrophoresis.

As an alternative to using ^{32}P-labelled PCR reactions, it is possible to visualize the DNA products in these polyacrylamide gels by silver staining using a method such as that described below.

Silver staining of DNA in polyacrylamide gels (courtesy of Dr P. Goncalves)

1. Dismantle the gel and fix it by soaking it in 100 ml of 10% acetic acid for 20 min at room temperature, preferably on a shaking platform.

2. Pour off the acetic acid and keep it. Wash the gel with water, three times for 2 min.

3. Incubate for 30 min at room temperature with a silver nitrate reagent composed of 0.1 g silver nitrate, 150 µl 37% (v/v) formaldehyde and water to a final volume of 100 ml.

4. Pour off and wash for 30 s with water.

5. Add 100 ml of a sodium carbonate reagent: make 200 ml 3% (w/v) Na_2CO_3 and just prior to use add 300 µl 37% (v/v) formaldheyde and 40 µl 10 mg/ml sodium thiosulphate. Incubate with agitation until the bands begin to appear.

6. Pour off and add the remaining 100 ml of the sodium carbonate solution. When the bands are clearly visible, pour off this solution and stop the reaction by adding back the 100 ml 10% acetic acid that was kept from step 2.

APPENDIX D: RESTRICTION ENZYME DIGESTION OF PCR PRODUCTS

Reagents

A number of companies now supply a comprehensive list of restriction enzymes (RE), but they may vary greatly in their cost. Those that are in regular use are generally quite cheap compared with the more specialized enzymes that are used only occasionally and which may be 10 to 100 times more expensive. RE buffers are now almost always supplied with each RE. Buffer compositions are always given, and will vary from enzyme to enzyme. Many commonly used REs cut perfectly well in a single 'universal' buffer. This is prepared using the following stock solutions:

Tris-acetate, 2 mol/l, pH 7.5. Dissolve 24.2 g of Trizma base in 60 ml of water, adjust the pH to 7.5 with glacial acetic acid and make up to 100 ml.

Potassium acetate, 2 mol/l. Weigh out 19.62 g, make up to 100 ml with water and dissolve.

Magnesium acetate, 2 mol/l. Weigh out 42.89 g, make up to 100 ml with water and dissolve.

BSA fraction V (molecular biology grade), 20 mg/ml.

Dithiothreitol (DTT), 0.5 mol/l. Weigh out 0.771 g, make up to 10 ml with water, dissolve and store at –20°C.

Spermidine (N-(3-aminopropyl)-1, 4-butane-diamine), 1 mol/l. Weigh out 1.273 g, make up to 10 ml with water, dissolve and store at –20°C.

10× RE buffer. For a 10-times concentrated buffer, prepare a solution that is 300 mmol/l Tris-acetate pH 7.5, 660 mmol/l potassium acetate, 100 mmol/l magnesium acetate, 1 mg/ml BSA, 10 mmol/l DTT and 30 mmol/l spermidine; aliquot into microcentrifuge tubes and store at –20°C.

Method

1. Transfer 30 µl of the amplified product to another microcentrifuge tube, being careful not to transfer any of the mineral oil. Add 4 µl of 10× restriction enzyme buffer, 4.5 µl of double distilled water and 2–5 units of the appropriate restriction enzyme (usually 0.5 µl), giving a final volume of 40 µl.

2. Incubate at 37°C (or other temperature as specified by the manufacturer) for a minimum of 4 h. In preparing more than one digestion with the same restriction enzyme, sufficient buffer, enzyme and water can be pre-mixed and dispensed into microcentrifuge tubes before adding 30 ml of the PCR product.

3. Pour a 3.0% agarose mini gel in a taped casting tray with the appropriate comb. The gel is made up of 1:1 mixture of type II medium electro-endosmosis agarose and Nusieve agarose (from FMC Bioproducts), i.e. 0.75 g of agarose and 0.75 g of Nusieve agarose in 50 ml of half-strength (0.5×) TBE buffer (see Appendix B).

4. After the incubation period, add 3 µl of tracking dye to the digests and load the samples on to the gel. The electrophoresis is continued until a clear separation of all the expected fragments is achieved, which may be checked at intervals by placing the gel on a UV transilluminator.

APPENDIX E: RT–PCR

Reagents

Ten-times concentrated (10×) red cell lysis buffer (RCLB). For 3 litres, weigh 248.7 g of NH$_4$Cl (1.55 mol/l), 30.03 g of KHCO$_3$ (0.1 mol/l), add 6 ml of 0.5 mol/l EDTA (0.1 mmol/l) pH 7.4 and make up to 3 litres with sterile water and store at 4°C.

RCLB. Make 500 ml of 10× RCLB up to 5 litres with sterile water and cool to 4°C. Adjust the working solution pH to 7.4 with HCl, and store at 4°C.

1 mol/l citrate, pH 7.0. Neutralize 1 mol/l trisodium citrate with 1 mol/l citric acid.

Sodium acetate. 3 mol/l sodium acetate is adjusted to pH 5.2 with glacial acetic acid.

Guanidinium thiocynate (GTC). As GTC is highly toxic, it is advisable to use the entire amount as purchased from the manufacturer, rather than weighing a required amount. Thus, with 1 kg of GTC add 21.15 ml of 0.5 mol/l EDTA (5.0 mmol/l) pH 8.0, 52.87 ml of 1 mol/l citrate pH 7.0, 35.25 ml of 30% sarcosyl (0.5%) and make up to 2.115 litres with sterile water. Store this solution in 50 ml aliquots. Add 7.1 µl of β-mercapto-ethanol per ml of GTC immediately before use.

Solutions for the cDNA mix:
5 mg/ml random hexamer primers: reconstitute 50 U pdN$_6$ (Pharmacia) with 539 µl of sterile water and add 21 µl 0.5 mol/l KCl.
5× RT-buffer (usually supplied) with M-MLV reverse transcriptase (RT): 0.25 mol/l Tris-HCl, pH 8.3, 0.375 mmol/l KCl, 15 mmol/l MgCl$_2$.
25 mM dNTP stock: mix an equal volume of ultrapure 100 mmol/l dATP, dCTP, dGTP and dTTP 0.1 M dithiothreitol. (DTT) usually supplied with M-MLV RT.

cDNA mix: to 428 µl of 5× RT-buffer, add the following, 21.5 µl of DTT, 85.5 µl of 25 mmol/l dNTPs, 45 µl of 5 mg/ml random hexamers and make up to 1000 µl with sterile water.

The composition for the multiplex and nested PCR mixes are given in Table 21.3, including the optimum MgCl$_2$ concentration for each mix as well as the primers used in the different PCR reactions.

Methods

Nuclear lysate preparation

1. Either blood or bone marrow aspirate can be analyzed for MRD in CML although bone marrow aspirates are preferred for ALL MRD studies. Centrifuge the anticoagulated peripheral blood sample at 700 g for 15 min. Bone marrow

Table 21.3 Composition of PCR mixes used in the amplification of BCR–ABL

	Multiplex PCR	Nested PCR			
		p210		p190	
		1st step	2nd step	1st step	2nd Step
PCR buffer (×10)	1.2×	1.25×	1.0×	1.25×	1.0×
MgCl$_2$ (mmol/l)	1.8	3.125	1.75	2.25	1.75
dNTP (µmol/l)	240	250	200	250	200
Primer 1 (µmol/l)	C5e– (0.6)	NB1 + (0.625)	CA3– (0.5)	BCR 1+ (0.625)	CA3– (0.5)
Primer 2 (µmol/l)	CA3– (0.6)	Abl3– (0.625)	B2A (0.5)	Ab13– (0.625)	E1N+ (0.5)
Primer 3 (µmol/l)	B2B (0.6)				
Primer 4 (µmol/l)	BCR-C (0.6)				

Primer sequences are as follows:

BCR1+: 5′ GAACTCGCAACAGTCCTTCGAC 3′
BCR-C: 5′ ACCGCATGTTCCGGGACAAAAG 3′
*C5e–: 5′ ataggaTCCTTTGCAACCGGGTCTGAA 3′
NB1+: 5′ GAGCGTGCAGAGTGGAGGGAGAACA 3′
Ab13–: 5′ GGTACCAGGAGTGTTTCTCCAGACTG 3′
B2A: 5′ TTCAGAAGCTTCTCCCTGACAT 3′
CA3–: 5′ TGTTGACTGGCGTGATGTAGTTGCTTGG 3′
E1N+: 5′ AGATCTGGCCCAACGATGACGA 3′

*Lower case letters represent changes introduced to create restriction enzyme recognition sites.

aspirates can be dealt with in the same way as buffy coats by proceeding directly to step 4 below.

2. Carefully remove and discard the plasma taking care not to disturb the buffy coat.

3. Using a sterile plastic pasteur pipette, collect the buffy coat and transfer it to a 50 ml polypropylene tube. It is not necessary to collect all of the buffy coat layer if the white cell count is >50 × 10^9/l.

4. To lyse the contaminating red cells, resuspend the buffy coat in ice cold RCLB to a final volume of 50 ml and vortex for a few seconds. The suspension is then incubated on wet ice for 10 min, inverting the tube occasionally.

5. Centrifuge again at 700 *g* for 10 min and discard the supernatant by inverting the tube, taking care not to lose the nuclear pellet.

6. Repeat steps 4 and 5 until the nuclear pellet is void of pink-red colour. Usually two washes with RCLB are sufficient.

7. Wash the nuclear pellet once with 20–30 ml PBS by spinning at 700 *g* for 10 min.

8. Resuspend the nuclear-pellet in 1–2 ml GTC containing β-mercapatoethanol. Homogenize the suspension by passing it through a 2 ml syringe and 21 G needle repeatedly until it loses its viscosity, i.e. the DNA is degraded. In some cases, it may be necessary to add more GTC.

9. The lysate can now be stored at –20°C or –70°C for several years.

RNA extraction

There are several protocols, including commercially available kits yielding RNA of varying qualities. The protocol described below, originally described by Chomczynski & Sacchi,[50] can easily be applied in a clinical laboratory.

1. Add 50 µl of 2M NaOAc pH 4.0 to 500 µl of GTC lysate in a 1.5 ml mircocentrifuge tube and vortex briefly.

2. Add 500 µl of un-neutralized water saturated phenol and 100 µl of chloroform. Vortex the mixture for 10 s and transfer to wet ice for 20 min.

3. Centrifuge at 12 000 *g* for 30 min at 4°C.

4. After centrifugation, two-distinct layers should be clearly discernible; if not, add a further 50 ml of chloroform. Vortex for 10 s and

centrifuge again for 30 min at 4°C. Transfer the upper aqueous layer to another 1.5 ml microcentrifuge tube, taking care not to disturb the interface.

5. Add an equal volume of propan-2-ol (isopropanol), cap the tube and mix by inverting, and incubate at –20°C for 2 h or overnight.

6. Spin in microcentrifuge for 30 min at 4°C and discard the supernatant, taking care not to lose the pellet which may be hard to see.

7. Wash the pellet in 1 ml of 80% ethanol. Do not mix. Centrifuge directly for 30 min at 4°C, and discard the supernatant. Re-centrifuge briefly to collect the residual ethanol and discard using a micropipette.

8. Air dry the pellet for 10 min and reconstitute in 20–40 μl of sterile water. The RNA must be stored at –70°C. However, immediate reverse transcription is the preferred option.

cDNA synthesis

1. Incubate 19 μl of RNA in 1.5 ml microcentrifuge tube (approximately 20 μg) at 65°C for 10 min. This is to denature the RNA which readily forms secondary structures, reducing the efficiency of the reverse transcriptase. Centrifuge at 12 000 g briefly to collect the condensation to the bottom of the tube. Transfer the tube to wet ice.

2. On the wet ice, add 21 μl of cDNA mix containing 300 u M-MLV reverse transcriptase and 30 u of RNasin.

3. Incubate the mixture at 37°C for 2 h. When using gene specific primers in this reaction, the temperature should be increased to 42°C.

4. Terminate the reaction by incubating the mixture at 65°C for 10 min. cDNA can be stored at –20°C.

Multiplex PCR

Add 2 μl of cDNA to 20 μl of multiplex PCR mix (see Table 21.3); add 0.5 u of Taq polymerase. Overlay with one drop of mineral oil and amplify using conditions as described in Appendix B (p. 512). The products are eletrophorezed through 2.0% agarose gel containing ethidium bromide.

Nested PCR

1. Add 5 μl cDNA to 20 μl first step PCR mix (see Table 21.3) and add 0.75 u Taq polymerase. Overlay with mineral oil and amplify. The PCR cycling conditions used as in Appendix B except that the annealing temperature is set at 68°C for 25 s.

2. Transfer 1 μl of the PCR products from the first step to 19 μl of the second step PCR mix (see Table 21.3). Overlay with one drop of mineral oil and amplify using an annealing temperature of 64°C for 50 s. The PCR products are eletrophorezed through 2.0% agarose gel containing ethidium bromide. The procedure for nested PCR is the same as for p210 (b3a2 and b2a2) and p190 (e1a2).

APPENDIX F: SOUTHERN BLOT ANALYSIS

Reagents

Restriction enzyme buffer
See Appendix D (p. 515)

40× Tris-acetate-EDTA (TAE) buffer. To 1600 ml water, add 387.2 g of Trizma base, 29.6 g of EDTA and 92 ml of glacial acetic acid. Stir to dissolve and bring the pH to 7.4 with acetic acid. Top up the solution to 2 litres with water. Dilute 1 in 40 for use.

Ethidium bromide, 10 mg/ml. See Appendix B (p. 512).

Tracking dye. See Appendix B.

Denaturation solution, 1.5 mol/l NaCl, 0.5 mol/l NaOH. Prepare this solution fresh every time by weighing 44 g of NaCl, making up to 450 ml with water and adding 50 ml of 5 mol/l NaOH.

20× standard sodium citrate (SSC). Add 351 g of NaCl and 176.5 g of sodium citrate (trisodium salt) to 1600 ml of water and stir to dissolve. Bring the pH to 7.0 with a very small amount of citric acid (anydrous free acid) and make up to 2 litres.

100× Denhardt's solution. Weigh 10 g of Ficoll (type 400), 10 g of polyvinylpyrrolidone and 10 g of BSA (fraction V, 96–99% purity) and make up to 500 ml with water. Dissolve and freeze at –20°C in 50 ml aliquots.

Carrier DNA, 10 mg/ml. Dissolve 1 g of salmon sperm DNA in 100 ml of water by heating to 65°C and leaving for several hours. Aliquot into 20 ml fractions and sonicate until the viscosity is reduced such that the solution can be pipetted with ease. Boil for 20 min and freeze at –20°C.

20% SDS. See Appendix A.

Hybridization solution, 6× SSC, 2× Denhardt's solution, 0.1 mg/ml carrier DNA and 1% SDS.

For 100 ml, take 62 ml of water and add 30 ml of 20× SSC, 2 ml of 100× Denhardt's solution, 1 ml of 10 mg/ml carrier DNA and 5 ml of 20% SDS.

Agarose. Type II medium electro-endosmosis.

Whatman paper. Large sheets of 17 MM and 3 MM paper.

Nylon membrane or filter. A selection of different hybridization membranes are commercially available. Always check the manufacturer's recommendations for their use.

Methods

Restriction enzyme digestion

For the digestion of genomic DNA, it is necessary to take into account the following points:

1. 5–10 μg of DNA are required to obtain a good signal from a Southern blot.
2. Restriction enzymes are usually sold at a concentration of around 10 u/μl. The unit is defined as the amount of enzyme that will cut 1 μg of cloned DNA in 1 h at the appropriate temperature.
3. A 4–6 fold excess of enzyme is used to ensure the complete digestion of genomic DNA, and the digestion is allowed to continue for at least 6 h.
4. The volume of enzyme added must be less than 10% of the final reaction volume, in order to avoid non-specific digestion. Attempt to keep the reaction volume below that of the well in the agarose gel (see below) into which the digested DNA solution will be loaded.

A typical-reaction mixture is set up in a 1.5 μl microcentrifuge tube as follows:

10 × RE-buffer	7 μl
Water	38 μl
Genomic DNA (0.5 mg/ml)	20 μl
RE (10 u/μl)	5 μl

The components are added in the order they are listed above. The suspension is mixed by a flicking of the tube, the contents are centrifuged to the bottom of the tube by a pulse centrifugation, and incubated at 37°C, or other appropriate temperature.

Agarose gel electrophoresis

A large horizontal-bed electrophoresis tank is required, with the appropriate gel casting tray and combs. Good resolution of DNA fragments from 20 samples can be obtained in a gel that is 20 × 24 cm. The % agarose of the gel depends on the size of the DNA fragments to be resolved; for most purposes described in this chapter a 0.8% gel is suitable.

1. Add 3.2 g of agarose to 400 ml of 1× TAE buffer in a 1 litre flask. Melt the agarose by boiling either in a microwave oven or in a saucepan of water over a Bunsen burner. Ensure the agarose is fully dissolved and well mixed in.
2. Cool to 55°C in a water-bath, add 10 μl of 10 mg/ml ethidium bromide, mix and pour on to the casting tray that has been taped up appropriately and has a comb to form wells in place. Remove any bubbles, and allow to set at room temperature.
3. To the completed restriction enzyme digests, add 1/10 volume of tracking dye and load into the gel, with the wells nearest the cathode so that the DNA runs towards the anode. Include a track with a size marker: 2.5 μg of λ bacteriophage DNA cut with the restriction enzyme Hind III in 40 μl of water with 4 μl of tracking dye is the standard marker used, and gives fragments of approximately 23, 9.6, 6.4, 4.5, 2.3, 2.0 and 0.56 kb.
4. Run the electrophoresis overnight, or until the bromophenol blue dye reaches the end of the gel.

Southern transfer

1. Remove the gel from the tank on its support into a tray containing TAE buffer. Photograph the gel on a transilluminator under UV illumination. Cut off the bottom right-hand corner of the gel for orientation.
2. Pour off the TAE and add 500 ml of denaturation solution. Leave for 40 min, preferably on a gently rocking platform.
3. Cut three pieces of 3 MM Whatman paper and one sheet of nylon hybridization transfer membrane to the size of the gel.
4. According to the instructions of the manufacturer of the nylon membrane, it may be necessary to neutralize the gel prior to transfer. This is done by immersing the gel in 500 ml of 1.0 mol/l Tris pH 8.0, 1.5 mol/l NaCl for 40 min.
5. Prepare the transfer apparatus as follows: pour 500 ml of 20× SSC into a tray. Place a glass plate over the tray to act as a bridge; this plate

should be larger than the size of the gel. Cut a piece of 17 MM Whatman paper to cover the plate and pass down into the 20× SSC to act as a wick. Wet it with the 20× SSC by first passing it under the bridge.

6. Place the gel on to the wick. Carefully lay on the nylon membrane (or filter). Cover the rest of the platform, all around the gel, with cling film. Do not leave any air bubbles between wick and gel or gel and filter.

7. One at a time, wet the three pieces of 3 MM Whatman paper in the denaturing solution and lay them on to the nylon filter. Roll out any bubbles that may be trapped using a graduated pipette.

8. Lay on a stack of paper towels about 10 cm high, unfolded to the size of the gel for the first 1 cm. Then place over the paper stack a glass plate and a weight (about 200 ml of water in a 500 ml bottle is convenient) so that good contact is maintained between the different layers of the blot. Leave overnight.

9. Remove the weight, the paper towels and Whatman papers. Mark the origins on the nylon filter with a pen and cut the corner for orientation.

10. Remove the filter and rinse in two changes of 200 ml of 3× SSC to remove traces of alkali and reduce the salt concentration. Dry the filter to dampness on a piece of Whatman paper.

11. Bake the filter in an oven at 80°C for 2 h to fix the DNA to the filter.

Hybridization and autoradiography

1. Prepare 50 ml of the hybridization solution and prewarm it at 65°C.

2. Place the filter in a thick polythene bag and seal close to the filter around three edges.

3. Pour in 40 ml of the hybridization solution. Remove all the air bubbles from the bag by rolling a pipette along the outside of it, taking care not to lose the solution, and seal the bag at a distance of about 10 cm from the fourth edge of the filter.

4. Leave at 65°C for at least 4 h for prehybridization.

5. Label the probe DNA with $[\alpha^{32}P]dCTP$ as described below. Boil it for 5–10 min in 0.5 ml carrier DNA and place immediately into ice.

6. Cut open the bag, leaving a gap between the filter and the opening and pour off the prehybridization solution. Pour in 5–10 ml of the hybridization solution, depending on the size of the filter;

10 ml is sufficient for a filter of 20 × 22 cm; for smaller filters, the volume should be reduced accordingly.

7. Add the probe to the hybridization solution and push out most of the air. Seal at the edge of the bag. Roll the radioactive air bubbles into the space between the filter and the edge using a pipette as before, leaving the hybridization solution around the filter, and seal close to the filter.

8. Leave overnight at 65°C.

9. Pre-warm the following washing solutions at 65°C: 500 ml of 3× SSC + 0.1% SDS (made from 422.5 ml of water, 75 ml of 20× SSC and 2.5 ml of 20% SDS); 1 litre 2× SSC + 0.1% SDS (895 ml of water, 100 ml of 20× SSC and 5 ml of 20% SDS); 1 litre of 0.2×SSC + 0.01% SDS (prepared by diluting the previous solution 1:10 with water).

10. Cut open the hybridization bag and pour off the solution. **Caution.** Carefully dispose of the radioactivity according to local regulations (see p. 316). Remove the filter and immediately plunge it into the 3' SSC. Leave for about 5 min to rinse away most of the radioactivity.

11. Pour off the 3× SSC and pour on 500 ml of the 2× SSC solution. Leave at 65°C for 20 min.

12. Repeat this wash in 2× SSC and then do two further 20 min washes in the 0.2×SSC solution, all at 65°C.

13. Remove the filter and dry to dampness on 3 MM Whatman paper.

14. Wrap the filter in cling film with a fluorescent orientation marker, and expose to X-ray film for at least one night at −80°C in a cassette with intensifying screens.

15. Develop the film, mark the position of the origins and orientation of the filter, and examine the position of the hybridizing signal with reference to the photograph taken of the gel. The size of the bands seen can be estimated by comparison with the λ Hind III marker on the gel: on semilogarithmic paper, plot the distance travelled by the marker fragments on the linear scale against their size on the log scale to give a standard curve.

APPENDIX G: DNA PROBES

Plasmid insert purification

The DNA fragment to be labelled can be purified away from the vector DNA, in which it is cloned, by size separation on an agarose gel and subsequent elution of the insert from the agarose.

Reagents
Plasmid DNA.

10× RE-buffer and restriction enzyme(s). See Appendix D (p. 515).

Tris-borate-EDTA (TBE) buffer. See Appendix B (p. 513).

Ultrapure (low melting) agarose.

Sodium acetate, 3 mol/l, pH 5.2. Dissolve 40.8 *g* of sodium acetate. $3H_2O$ in 80 ml of water, and adjust the pH to 5.2 with glacial acetic acid. Make up the volume to 100 ml with water.

Dialysis tubing. Boil strips of tubing in 2% sodium bicarbonate, 1 mmol/l EDTA for 10 min. Rinse well with water and then boil for 10 min in water. Store at 4°C.

Sephadex G50. Swell the Sephadex G50 powder in an excess volume of water overnight; take off the water that is above the beads and replace with TE (see p. 511). Mix up the beads, allow them to settle, remove the TE; repeat twice.

Method
1. Digest 5–10 μg of the plasmid with 20–40 u of the appropriate RE in RE-buffer and sufficient water such that the volume of enzyme is less than 10% of the final volume.

2. Pour a medium-sized 1% agarose gel in 0.5× TBE-buffer, and load the digested DNA into a wide (3 cm) well. Carry out electrophoresis until the insert resolves from the vector DNA fragment.

3. On a UV transilluminator, cut out a gel slice containing the insert.

4. Put the gel slice lengthways into a strip of dialysis tubing that has been rinsed well with water, clipped at one end and filled with 0.5× TBE-buffer. Empty out most of the TBE-buffer, leaving only enough to cover the gel slice, and clip the other end of the tubing without leaving any air bubbles.

5. Replace into the electrophoresis tank and continue the current for another 2–4 h with the gel slice toward the negative terminal.

6. Reverse the current for 30 s.

7. Open the dialysis bag and transfer the buffer in 400 μl aliquots into 1.5 ml microcentrifuge tubes, add 40 μl of 3 mol/l sodium acetate and 1 ml of absolute ethanol and freeze on dry ice for 30 min or at −20°C overnight.

8. Centrifuge at 12 000 g in a microcentrifuge for 5 min, pour off the supernatant, centrifuge again for a few seconds, remove all the remaining ethanol with a micropipette and allow to dry on the bench with the cap open.

9. Resuspend in a total of 50 μl of water, pool and load onto a G50 spinning column as described below.

G50 spin column
1. Plug an empty 1 ml syringe with a pinch of polymer wool; fill completely with TE equilibrated G50 Sephadex and allow the beads to settle.

2. Place the syringe in a 10 ml centrifuge tube so that the wings of the syringe hold it on to the rim of the tube and there is a void space between the end of the syringe and the bottom of the tube.

3. Centrifuge for 30 s at 400 *g*; the beads will pack down to about 0.9 ml. Fill the tube to the top with TE and centrifuge again for 30 s at 400 *g*.

4. Pour away the TE if this has risen above the bottom of the syringe, add two drops of TE to the top of the column and centrifuge for 4 min at 400 *g*.

5. Take out the column, pour the TE out of the centrifuge tube and drop a 0.5 ml microcentrifuge tube without its cap into the 10 ml tube.

6. Replace the column and, if necessary, support the microcentrifuge tube so that the end of the syringe sits inside it. Load the DNA solution on to the top of the G50 column and centrifuge for 4 min at 400 *g*; collect the eluate from the column from the microcentrifuge tube.

7. To assess the amount of insert DNA recovered, load a small aliquot (2 μl) on to an agarose minigel and compare the intensity of ethidium bromide staining against a known standard.

Labelling a DNA fragment with ^{32}P
There are several different ways of labelling a DNA fragment. The one that is preferred for generating probes of high specific activity for use in Southern blotting is called random priming.[51]

Principle
The DNA fragment to be labelled is denatured in the presence of short random oligonucleotides (6 or 9 bp in length), made of all the possible sequence combinations. As the DNA cools, these oligos anneal to the DNA along its length and act

as primers for DNA synthesis by the Klenow fragment of DNA polymerase using the DNA fragment as a template and the four deoxy-nucleotide triphosphates (dNTPs) as building blocks. This synthesis is carried out in the presence of a radio-labelled nucleotide (usually $[\alpha^{32}P]dCTP$) so that the copies of the DNA fragment are made radioactive. Unincorporated nucleotides are removed from the DNA, which is then boiled again before use as a probe so that the labelled single-stranded DNA molecules can hybridize to their complementary sequences in the target DNA.

Method

To obtain efficient incorporation of the labelled nucleotide and generate probes with a sufficiently high specific activity for use in genomic Southern hybridization experiments, a labelling kit is recommended. The Megaprime labelling system from Amersham can consistently yield probes with a specific activity greater than 5×10^8 cpm/mg DNA. The method is clearly described in a booklet that accompanies the kit.

Non-radioactive labelling

A number of non-radioactive labelling systems are now available. The advantages of working without hazardous radioisotopes are obvious, and probes can be obtained that will detect single copy genes in a standard Southern blot analysis. An additional advantage is that labelled probes can be stored at $-20°C$ for significant periods of time (at least 3 months), while ^{32}P-labelled probes decay rapidly and need to be freshly prepared each time they are used. However, the sensitivity of a ^{32}P-labelled probe, exposed to X-ray film for 10 to 14 days, is greater than any non-radioactive method.

The principle of these non-radioactive labelling systems is the same as described above in that random priming is used to generate a labelled DNA fragment. The difference is that instead of a ^{32}P-labelled nucleotide, other labels are utilized such as fluorescein-dUTP. Detection of the hybridization involves horseradish peroxidase conjugated antibodies and colour or luminescent visualization of bound antibody.

GLOSSARY (Courtesy of Professor Lucio Luzzatto)

Alleles. Alternate forms of a gene found at a particular locus, e.g. β^A, β^S and β^{thal}. There may be many different alleles in a population, but two at the most in one individual.

Base pair (bp). A single pairing of the nucleotides A with T or G with C in a DNA double helix (in RNA, A pairs with U).

cDNA. A DNA molecule complementary to an RNA molecule, usually synthesized in vitro by the enzyme reverse transcriptase (RT).

Clone, cellular. The progeny of a single cell. Cells belonging to the same clone are referred to as a monoclonal cell population.

Clone, molecular. A large number of identical DNA molecules, usually obtained by propagation of a single plasmid or bacteriophage molecule in bacteria.

Codon. A triplet of nucleotides that codes for an amino acid or termination signal.

Deletion. A mutation caused by the removal of a sequence of DNA, with the regions on either side being joined together.

Exon. A segment of a gene that codes for protein.

Gene. The unit of inheritance. In biochemical terms, a gene specifies the structure of a protein, which is the gene product. In molecular terms, a gene is a stretch of DNA that is transcribed in one block, a transcription unit.

Genomic clone. A molecular clone consisting of a portion of cellular DNA.

Genotype. The genetic constitution of an individual.

Heterozygote. An individual with two different alleles at a particular locus.

Hybridization. The pairing of complementary RNA or DNA strands to give an RNA–DNA hybrid or a DNA duplex.

Intron. A segment of a gene that is transcribed but is removed in the mature messenger RNA and therefore does not code for protein.

Linkage. The co-inheritance of genes as a result of their neighbouring location on the same chromosome.

Locus. The position on a chromosome where a particular gene is located.

Mutation. A particular change in the sequence of genomic DNA.

Northern blotting. A technique for transferring RNA from an agarose gel to a nitrocellulose or nylon filter on which it can be recognized by a suitable probe.

Oligonucleotide (Oligo). A short single-stranded DNA molecule, usually synthesized in vitro.

Phenotype. The appearance of an individual person or cell. In relation to a particular genetic character, the phenotype reflects the genotype conferring that character plus the effects of the environment.

Plasmid. An autonomously replicating extra-chromosomal circular DNA molecule, e.g. pBR322 and pUC19.

Point mutation. A change of a single base pair in DNA.

Polymerase chain reaction (PCR). A technique for amplifying an individual DNA sequence in vitro. The reaction is primed by using specific oligonucleotides.

Primers. Oligonucleotides used to initiate DNA synthesis in vitro by the enzyme DNA polymerase.

Probe. A fragment of DNA that can be used to hybridize to a specific DNA sequence or RNA molecule.

Recombinant DNA. Any DNA molecule constructed artificially by bringing together DNA segments of different origin.

Restriction enzymes. Enzymes that recognize short DNA sequences (usually 4 or 6 base pairs) and cut the DNA wherever those sequences are found (e.g. BamH I, Bgl II, EcoR I, Hind III, Pst I and Sac I). These sequences are called restriction sites.

Southern blotting. The procedure for transferring denatured DNA from an agarose gel to a nitrocellulose or nylon filter, where it can be recognized by an appropriate probe.

Vector. A DNA molecule capable of replication and specifically engineered to facilitate the cloning of another DNA molecule of interest.

ABBREVIATIONS

ACRES	amplification created restriction enzyme site	kb	kilobase pairs
ARMS	amplification refractory mutation system	PCR	polymerase chain reaction
ASOH	allele-specific oligonucleotide hybridization	RE	restriction enzyme
		RT	reverse transcriptase
bp	base pair	SDS	sodium dodecyl sulphate
CTP	cytosine triphosphate	SSC	standard sodium citrate
DNA	deoxyribonucleic acid	SSCP	single-strand conformation polymorphism
FVL	factor V Leiden	TAE	Tris acetate EDTA buffer
HVR	hypervariable region	TBE	Tris borate EDTA buffer
Ig	immunoglobulin	TCR	T-cell receptor
		TE	Tris EDTA buffer

REFERENCES

1 Dunham I, Shimizu N, Roe BA, et al 1999 The DNA sequence of human chromosome 22. Nature 402:489–495.

2 Saiki RK, Gelfand DH, Stoffel S, et al 1988 Primer-directed enzymatic amplification of DNA with a thermostable DNA polymerase. Science 239:487–491.

3 Sambrook J, Fritsch EF, Maniatis T 1989 Molecular cloning. A laboratory manual, 2nd edn. Cold Spring Harbor Laboratory Press, Cold Spring Harbor.

4 Association for Molecular Pathology statement. 1999 Recommendations for in-house development and operation of molecular diagnostic tests. American Journal of Clinical Pathology 111:449–463.

5 Sykes BC 1983 DNA in heritable disease. Lancet ii:787–788.

6 Newton CR, Graham A, Heptinstall LE, et al 1989 Analysis of any point mutation in DNA. The amplification refractory mutation system (ARMS). Nucleic Acids Research 17:2503–2516.

7 Old JM, Varawalla NY, Weatherall DJ 1990 Rapid detection and prenatal diagnosis of β-thalassaemia:

studies in Indian and Cypriot populations in the U.K. Lancet 336:834–837.

8 Wallace RB, Shaffer J, Murphy RF, et al 1979 Hybridization of synthetic oligodeoxyribonucleotides to PhiX174 DNA: the effect of single base pair mismatch. Nucleic Acids Research 6:3543–3547.

9 Saiki RK, Chang CA, Levenson CH, et al 1988 Diagnosis of sickle cell anemia and beta-thalassemia with enzymatically amplified DNA and non-radioactive allele specific oligonucleotide probes. New England Journal of Medicine 319:537–541.

10 Kawasaki E, Saiki R, Erlich H 1993 Genetic analysis using polymerase chain reaction-amplified DNA and immobilized oligonucleotide probes: reverse dot-blot typing. Methods in Enzymology 218:369–381.

11 Old J 1996 Haemoglobinopathies. Prenatal Diagnosis 16:1181–1186.

12 Orkin SH, Little PF, Kazazian HH Jr, et al 1982 Improved detection of the sickle mutation by DNA analysis. New England Journal of Medicine 307:32–36.

13 Huisman TH, Carver MF 1998 The beta- and delta-thalassemia repository (9th edn; Part I). Hemoglobin 22:169–195.

14 Cao A, Rosatelli R 1993 Screening and prenatal diagnosis of the haemoglobinopathies. Baillière's Clinical Haematology 6:263–286.

15 Dode C, Krishnamoorthy R, Lamb J, et al 1993 Rapid analysis of -alpha 3.7 thalassaemia and alpha alpha alpha anti 3.7 triplication by enzymatic amplification analysis. British Journal of Haematology 83:105–111.

16 Chang JG, Liu TC, Chiou SS, et al 1994 Rapid detection of -alpha(4.2) deletion of alpha-thalassemia-2 by polymerase chain-reaction. Annals of Hematology 69:205–209.

17 Bowden DK, Vickers MA, Higgs DR 1992 A PCR-based strategy to detect the common severe determinants of a thalassaemia. British Journal of Haematology 81:104–108.

18 Eng B, Patterson M, Borys S, et al 2000 PCR-based diagnosis of the Filipino (--FIL) and Thai (--THAI) alpha-thalassemia-1 deletions. American Journal of Hematology 63:54–56.

19 Chong SS, Boehm CD, Higgs DR, et al 2000 Single-tube multiplex-PCR screen for common deletional determinants of alpha-thalassemia. Blood 95:360–362.

20 Traeger-Synodinos J, Kanavakis E, Tzetis M, et al 1993 Characterization of nondeletion alpha-thalassemia mutations in the Greek population. American Journal of Hematology 44:162–167.

21 Cumming AM, Shiach CR 1999 The investigation and management of inherited thrombophilia. Clinical and Laboratory Haematology 21:77–92.

22 Kluijtmans LA, den Heijer M, Reitsma PH, et al 1998 Thermolabile methylenetetrahydrofolate reductase and factor V Leiden in the riks of deep-vein thrombosis. Thrombosis and Haemostasis 79:254–258.

23 Poort SR, Rosendaal FR, Reitsma PH, et al 1996 A common genetic variation in the 3'-untranslated region of the prothrombin gene is associated with elevated plasma prothrombin levels and an increase in venous thrombosis. Blood 88:3698–3703.

24 van der Meer FJ, Koster T, Vandenbroucke JP, et al 1997 The Leiden thrombophilia study (LETS). Thrombosis and Haemostasis 78:631–635.

25 Bertina RM, Koeleman BP, Koster T, et al 1994 Mutation in blood coagulation factor V associated with resistance to activated protein C. Nature 369:64–67.

26 Lakich D, Kazazian HH Jr, Antonarakis SE, et al 1993 Inversions disrupting the factor VIII gene are a common cause of severe haemophilia A. Nature Genetics 5:236–241.

27 Wion KL, Tuddenham EGD, Lawn R 1986 A new polymorphism in the factor VIII gene for prenatal diagnosis of haemophilia A. Nucleic Acids Research 14:4535–4542.

28 Liu Q, Nozari G, Sommer SS 1998 Single-tube polymerase chain reaction for rapid diagnosis of the inversion hotspot of mutation in hemophilia A. Blood 92:1458–1459.

29 Secker-Walker LM, Craig JM, Hawkins JM, et al 1991 Philadelphia-positive acute lymphoblastic leukaemia in adults: age distribution. BCR-breakpoint and prognostic significance. Leukaemia 5:196–199.

30 Macintyre EA, Delabesse E 1999 Molecular approaches to the diagnosis and evaluation of lymphoid malignancies. Seminars in Hematology 36:373–389.

31 Biondi A, Rambaldi A, Pandolfi PP, et al 1992 Molecular monitoring of the myl/retinoic acid receptor-α fusion gene in acute promyelocytic leukaemia by polymerase chain reaction. Blood 80:492–497.

32 Cross NCP, Lin F, Chase A, et al 1993 Competitive polymerase chain reaction to estimate the number of BCR-ABL transcripts in chronic myeloid leukaemia patients after bone marrow transplantation. Blood 82:1929–1936.

33 Cross NCP, Melo JV, Lin F, et al 1994 An optimised multiplex polymerase chain reaction for

detection of BCR-ABL fusion mRNAs in haematological disorders. Leukaemia 8:186–189.

34 Lin F, Goldman JM, Cross NCP 1994 A comparison of the sensitivity of blood and bone marrow for the detection of minimal residual disease in chronic myeloid leukaemia. British Journal of Haematology 86:683–685.

35 Foroni L, Harrison CJ, Hoffbrand AV, et al 1999 Investigation of minimal residual disease in childhood and adult acute lymphoblastic leukaemia by molecular analysis. British Journal of Haematology 105:7–24.

36 Deane M, Norton JD 1990 Detection of immunoglobulin gene rearrangement in B lymphoid malignancies by polymerase chain reaction gene amplification. British Journal of Haematology 74:251–256.

37 Cave H, van der Werff ten Bosch J, Suciu S, et al 1998 Clinical significance of minimal residual disease in childhood acute lymphoblastic leukemia. New England Journal of Medicine 339:591–598.

38 van Dongen JJ, Seriu T, Panzer-Grumayer ER, et al 1998 Prognostic value of minimal residual disease in acute lymphoblastic leukaemia in childhood. Lancet 352:1731–1738.

39 Bassam BJ, Caetano-Anolles G, Gresshoff PM 1991 Fast and sensitive silver staining of DNA in polyacrylamide gels. Annals of Biochemistry 196:80–83.

40 Vulliamy T, Luzzatto L, Hirono A, et al 1997 Hematologically important mutations: glucose-6-phosphate dehydrogenase. Blood Cells Molecules and Disease 23:302–313.

41 Southern E 1975 Detection of specific sequences using DNA fragments separated by gel electrophoresis. Journal of Molecular Biology 98:503–509.

42 Higgs DR 1993 Alpha-thalassaemia. Baillière's Clinical Haematology 6:117–150.

43 Kattamis AC, Camaschella C, Sivera P, et al 1996 Human alpha-thalassemia syndromes: detection of molecular defects. American Journal of Hematology 53:81–91.

44 Nicholls RD, Fischel-Ghodsian N, Higgs DR 1987 Recombination at the human α globin gene cluster: sequence features and topological constraints. Cell 49:369–378.

45 Goodbourn SEY, Higgs DR, Clegg JB, et al 1983 Molecular basis of length polymorphism in the human z globin gene complex. Proceedings of the National Academy of Sciences U.S.A. 80:5022–5026.

46 Bain BJ, Chapman C 1998 A survey of current United Kingdom practice for antenatal screening for inherited disorders of globin chain synthesis. UK Forum for Haemoglobin Disorders. Journal of Clinical Pathology 51:382–389.

47 Flanagan JC, Rabbits TH 1982 Arrangement of human immunoglobulin heavy chain constant region genes implies evolutionary duplication of a segment containing γ, ε and α genes. Nature 300:709–713.

48 Sims JE, Tunnacliffe A, Smith WJ, et al 1984 Complexity of human T-cell antigen receptor β-chain constant and variable region genes. Nature 312:541–545.

49 Harris S, Jones DB 1997 Optimisation of the polymerase chain reaction. British Journal of Biomedical Science 54:166–173.

50 Chomczynski P, Sacchi N 1987 Single step method of RNA isolation by acid guanidinium thiocyanate-phenol-chloroform extraction. Annals of Biochemistry 162:156–159.

51 Feinberg AP, Vogelstein B 1984 A technique for radiolabelling DNA restriction endonuclease fragments to high specific activity. Annals of Biochemistry 137:266–267.

22

Miscellaneous tests

S. Mitchell Lewis

TESTS FOR THE ACUTE PHASE RESPONSE

Inflammatory response to tissue injury (the acute phase response) includes alteration in serum protein concentration, especially increases in fibrinogen, serum amyloid A protein (SAA) and C-reactive protein (CRP), and decrease in albumin. The changes occur in acute infection, during active phases of chronic inflammation and following injury.

Measurement of the acute phase response is a helpful indicator of the presence and extent of inflammation or tissue damage, and response to treatment. Tests include estimation of CRP and measurement of the erythrocyte sedimentation rate (ESR) and plasma viscosity. There has been much debate on the relative value of these tests.[1,2]

Kits are available for CRP assay which are sensitive and fairly precise; small rises in serum levels can often be detected before any clinical features become apparent, whilst as a tissue-damaging process resolves the serum level rapidly decreases towards the normal range. The ESR is slower to respond to acute disease activity and it is insensitive to small changes in the disease activity. It is less specific as it is also influenced by anaemia which may be present in inflammatory disease; but this may be an advantage for a screening test of acute phase response as the various acute phase proteins respond differently in different clinical conditions. Measurement of plasma viscosity has an advantage over ESR in that it is not affected by anaemia and is less dependent on age and sex variable. However, it requires sophisticated equipment which is dependent on power supply, whereas ESR is a simple cheap test which is suitable for point-of-care (near patient) testing away from a laboratory.

ERYTHROCYTE SEDIMENTATION RATE

The method for measuring the ESR which has been recommended by the International Council for Standardization in Haematology[3] and also by various national authorities[4] is based on that of Westergren.[5] In this, diluted blood is sedimented in an open-ended glass tube of 30 cm length mounted vertically on a stand. To make the test more reproducible, a standardized method has been proposed in which EDTA blood is used and its packed cell volume (PCV) is adjusted to 0.35. This is, however, too laborious for routine use. Because of the biohazard risk of blood contamination inherent in using open-ended tubes, it is now recommended that, where possible, a closed system be used in routine practice.[6] Several automated closed systems are now available, e.g. Sediscan (Becton Dickinson), Sedimatic (AnalysInstrument), Starrsed (R & R Mechatronics), Test I System (SIRE). These use either blood collected in special evacuated tubes containing citrate or EDTA blood which is taken up through a piercable cap and then automatically diluted in the system or undiluted EDTA blood. Biohazard risk is also reduced in the manual method by using a closed system which circumvents transfer of the blood collection into the sedimentation tube by hand, e.g. Seditainer (Becton Dickinson); Sediplus (Sarstedt).

Westergren method

The recommended tube is a straight glass tube 30 cm in length and not less than 2.55 mm in diameter. The bore must be uniform to within 5% throughout. A scale graduated in mm extends over the lower 20 cm. The tube must be clean and dry and kept free from dust.

After use, it should be thoroughly washed in tap water, then rinsed with acetone and allowed to dry before being re-used. Specially made racks with adjustable levelling screws are available for holding the sedimentation tubes firmly in an exactly vertical position. The rack must be constructed so that there will be no leakage of the blood from the tube. It is conventional to set up sedimentation-rate tests at room temperature (18–25°C). Sedimentation is normally accelerated as the temperature rises and if the test is to be carried out at a higher ambient temperature, a normal range should be established for that temperature. Exceptionally, when high-thermal-amplitude cold agglutinins are present, sedimentation becomes noticeably less rapid as the temperature is raised towards 37°C.

109 mmol/l trisodium citrate (32 g/l $Na_3Ca6H_5O_7.2H_2O$) is used as the anticoagulant diluent solution. It is filtered through a micropore filter (0.22 μm) into a sterile bottle. It can be stored for several months at 4°C but must be discarded if it becomes turbid through the growth of moulds. The test is performed on venous blood diluted accurately in the proportion of 1 volume of citrate to 4 volumes of blood. The usual practice is to collect the blood directly into the citrate solution. The test should then be carried out within 4 h of collecting the blood, although a delay of up to 6 h is permissible provided that the blood is kept at 4°C. The test can be carried out equally well with blood anticoagulated with EDTA within 24 h if the specimen is kept at 4°C, provided that 1 volume of 109 mmol/l (32 g/l) trisodium citrate is added to 4 volumes of blood immediately before the test is performed.

Mix the blood sample thoroughly and then draw it up into the Westergren tube to the 200 mm mark by means of a teat or a mechanical device; mouth suction should never be used. Place the tube exactly vertical and leave undisturbed for exactly 60 min, free from vibrations and draughts, and not exposed to direct sunlight. Then read to the nearest 1 mm the height of the clear plasma above the upper limit of the column of sedimenting cells. The result is expressed as ESR = X mm in 1 h. A poor delineation of the upper layer of red cells may sometimes occur, especially when there is a high reticulocyte count.

Range in health

The mean values and the upper limit for 95% of normal adults are given in Table 22.1. There is a progressive increase with age, but above 70 years it is difficult to define a strictly healthy population for determining normal values.

In the newborn, the ESR is usually low. In childhood and adolescence, it is the same as for normal men with no differences between boys and girls.

Modified methods

A number of variations have been developed, especially for automated methods and closed systems. Whenever a different method is planned, a preliminary test should be carried out in order to check precision and to compare results with those obtained by the standardized method described below.

Table 22.1 ESR ranges in health

Age (years)	95% upper limit
Men	
17–50	10
51–60	12
61–70	14
>70	c30
Women	
17–50	12
51–60	19
61–70	20
>70	c35

Length of tube. The overall length of the tube is not a critical dimension for the test provided that it fits firmly in an appropriate holding device. The tube must, however, be long enough to ensure that packing of the cells does not start before the test has been completed.

Plastic tubes. A number of plastic materials – e.g. polypropylene and polycarbonate – are possible substitutes for glass in Westergren tubes. Nevertheless, not all plastics have similar properties and it must be demonstrated that the results with the chosen tubes are reproducible and comparable with those obtained with the standard method.

Disposable glass tubes. These should be supplied clean and dry and ready for use. It is necessary to show that neither the tube material nor the manufacturer's cleaning process affects the ESR.

Capillary method. Short tubes of narrower bore than in the standard tube are available mainly for tests on infants. Sedimentation is slower in these tubes and it is necessary to establish normal ranges or a correction factor to convert results to the equivalent ESR by the standard Westergren method.

Time. Sedimentation is measured after aggregation has occurred and before the cells start to pack (see p. 530), usually at 18–24 min. From the rate during this time period the sedimentation which would have occurred at 60 min is derived and converted to the conventional ESR equivalent by an algorithm.[7]

Sloping tube. Red cells sediment more quickly when streaming down the wall of a sloped tube. This phenomenon has been incorporated into an automated system in which the end-point is read after 20 min with the tube held at an angle of 18° from the vertical. This has been shown to give results comparable to the conventional method.[8]

ICSH STANDARDIZED METHOD[3]

This is intended to provide a reference method for verifying the reliability of any modification of the test. It is carried out on EDTA blood not diluted in citrate, using Westergren tubes as described above. Select ten blood samples with PCV 0.30–0.36 and, if possible, with ESRs in a wide range between 15 and 105 mm; if necessary, adjust the PCV to within the required range by centrifuging the specimens, removing an appropriate amount of plasma or red cells and then resuspending the cells by thorough mixing.

Immediately before filling the ESR tube, mix the specimen by at least eight complete inversions. Measure the ESR on each specimen (undiluted) by the standardized Westergren method.

Correct the reading for lack of dilution as follows:

Corrected ESR (mm in 1 h) =
(undiluted ESR × 0.86) − 12.

At the same time, carry out the ESR by the method which is to be verified on aliquots of the same specimens or on blood collected separately from the same subjects in accordance with specified requirements, e.g. directly into tubes containing citrate.

The modified method is satisfactory if 95% of results are within the limits given in Table 22.2. However, as the ESR may be affected by several uncontrolled variables, the reference method cannot be used as a calibrator to adjust the measurements that are obtained. Thus, if the new method gives disparate readings, it will be necessary to establish a normal range specifically for the method.

Quality control

The standardized method can also be used as a quality control procedure for the routine tests. Select one blood sample with a PCV between 0.30

Table 22.2 ESR values (mm) for verification of comparability of working (routine) method with ICSH standardized method

Standardized method*	Working method limits**	Standardized method*	Working method limits**	Standardized method*	Working method limits**
15	3–13	45	18–37	75	40–68
16	4–14	46	18–38	76	40–69
17	4–15	47	19–38	77	41–70
18	4–15	48	20–39	78	42–71
19	5–16	49	20–40	79	43–72
20	5–17	50	21–41	80	44–73
21	6–17	51	22–42	81	45–74
22	6–18	52	22–43	82	45–76
23	6–19	53	23–44	83	46–77
24	7–19	54	24–45	84	47–78
25	7–20	55	24–46	85	48–79
26	8–21	56	25–47	86	49–80
27	8–21	57	26–48	87	50–82
28	9–22	58	26–49	88	51–83
29	9–23	59	27–50	89	52–84
30	10–24	60	28–51	90	53–85
31	10–25	61	29–52	91	53–86
32	11–25	62	29–53	92	54–88
33	11–26	63	30–54	93	55–89
34	12–27	64	31–56	94	56–90
35	12–28	65	32–57	95	57–91
36	13–29	66	32–58	96	58–93
37	13–30	67	33–59	97	59–94
38	14–30	68	34–60	98	60–95
39	14–31	69	35–61	99	61–96
40	15–32	70	35–62	100	62–98
41	15–33	71	36–63	101	63–99
42	16–34	72	37–64	102	64–100
43	17–35	73	38–65	103	65–101
44	17–36	74	39–66	104	66–103
				105	67–104

*Standardized method: EDTA anticoagulated but undiluted whole blood of haematocrit of 0.35 or less.
**Working method: 4 volumes EDTA blood plus 1 volume citrate diluent. The values incorporate a correction for dilution of blood by citrate in the working method. Proposed working method valid if 95% of results are within indicated limits. (reproduced with permission from the *Journal of Clinical Pathology*[3])

and 0.36 and perform the ESR by the routine method and by the standardized method as described above. Apply the formula to obtain the corrected ESR for the undiluted sample.

The test is satisfactorily controlled if the results by the routine method do not differ from those obtained by the ICSH standardized method by more than the limits shown in Table 22.2.

This procedure may be too laborious for routine use; instead, a stabilized whole blood preparation is now available* which appears to be suitable as a daily control for use with different automated systems.[9]

Mechanism of erythrocyte sedimentation
The phenomenon of erythrocyte sedimentation has been investigated exhaustively.[1,10]

The rate of fall of the red cells is influenced by a number of interreacting factors. Basically, it depends upon the difference in specific gravity

---

*ESR-Chex (Streck Laboratory).

between red cells and plasma, but it is influenced very greatly by the extent to which the red cells form rouleaux, which sediment more rapidly than single cells. Other factors which affect sedimentation include the ratio of red cells to plasma, i.e. the PCV, the plasma viscosity, the verticality or otherwise of the sedimentation tube, the bore of the tube and the dilution, if any, of the blood.

The all-important rouleaux formation and redcell clumping are mainly controlled by the concentrations of fibrinogen and other acute-phase proteins, e.g. haptoglobin, ceruloplasmin, α_1 acidglycoprotein, α_1 antitrypsin and C-reactive protein. Rouleaux formation is also enhanced by the immunoglobulins. It is retarded by albumin. Defibrinated blood normally sediments extremely slowly, not more than 1 mm in 1 h, unless the serum-globulin concentration is raised or there is an unusually high globulin:albumin ratio.

Anaemia, by altering the ratio of red cells to plasma, encourages rouleaux formation and accelerates sedimentation. In anaemia, too, cellular factors may affect sedimentation. Thus in iron-deficiency anaemia, a reduction in the intrinsic ability of the red cells to sediment may compensate for the accelerating effect of an increased proportion of plasma.

Sedimentation can be observed to take place in three stages: a preliminary stage of at least a few minutes during which time rouleaux occur and aggregates form; then a period in which the sinking of the aggregates takes place at approximately a constant speed; and finally a phase during which the rate of sedimentation slows as the aggregated cells pack at the bottom of the tube. It is obvious that the longer the tube used, the longer the second period can last and the greater the sedimentation rate may appear to be. This is an advantage of the Westergren tube. With a shorter tube, e.g. a Wintrobe tube, packing may start before an hour has elapsed.

Significance of the measurement of the erythrocyte sedimentation rate in clinical medicine

Although the ESR is a non-specific phenomenon, its measurement is clinically useful in disorders associated with an increased production of acute-phase proteins. In rheumatoid arthritis or tuberculosis, it provides an index of progress of the disease, and it is of value in diagnosis of temporal arteritis and polymyalgia rheumatica. It is also useful as a screening test in the routine examination of patients. An elevated ESR occurs as an early feature in myocardial infarction.[11] Although a normal ESR cannot be taken to exclude the presence of organic disease, the fact remains that the vast majority of acute or chronic infections and most neoplastic and degenerative diseases are associated with changes in the plasma proteins which lead to an acceleration of sedimentation. It is not helpful in countries where chronic disease is rife. The ESR is higher in women than in men, and correlates with sex differences in fibrinogen levels.[12] An increase in fibrinogen occurs in normal pregnancy, resulting in increased red cell aggregation and elevated sedimentation.[13] The ESR is influenced by age, stage of the menstrual cycle and drugs (e.g. corticosteroids, contraceptive pills); it is especially low (0–1 mm) in polycythaemia, hypofibrinogenaemia and congestive cardiac failure, and when there are abnormalities of the red cells such as poikilocytosis, spherocytosis or sickle cells. C-reactive protein is markedly increased at high altitude with concomitant increase in ESR.[73]

PLASMA VISCOSITY

The ESR and plasma viscosity in general increase in parallel.[1] Plasma viscosity is, however, primarily dependent on the concentration of plasma proteins, especially fibrinogen, and it is not affected by anaemia. Change in viscosity seems to reflect the clinical severity of disease more closely than does the ESR.[14,15] Also, changes in the ESR may lag behind changes in plasma viscosity by 24–48 h.[14]

There are several types of viscometer; these are based on three principles:[1,15]

1. The rotational viscometer in which shear stress is determined at different shear rates.
2. The rolling ball viscometer in which the rate of rolling of a metal ball is measured in a tilted tube filled with plasma and calibrated with fluids of known viscosity.
3. The capillary viscometer in which comparison is made of the flow rate of plasma and distilled water under equal pressure and constant temperature through capillary tubes of equal bore and length. The results are expressed as viscosity of plasma relative to that of water.

Most reports of clinical studies have been based on the capillary viscometer. It requires only 0.3–0.5 ml of plasma, obtained from EDTA blood. Results are highly reproducible (CV 1%); they are, however, very sensitive to changes in temperature. The test is usually performed at 25°C although some workers recommend 37°C;[16] in either case, the temperature should be closely controlled, with a variation of less than ±0.5°C.

Precision is also affected by the way the plasma sample has been obtained and prepared; the formation of a fibrin clot will invalidate the test. Venous blood should be collected with minimum stasis into EDTA (1.2 mg/ml) and, as soon as possible, centrifuged in a stoppered tube at 3000 *g* for 5 min to obtain clear plasma. After separation, the plasma, if sterile, can be stored in a stoppered tube at room temperature (not in a refrigerator) for up to 1 week without change in its viscosity.

The actual test should be carried out as described in the instruction manual for the particular instrument used.

Reference values[1,16]

Normal plasma has a viscosity of 1.16–1.33 (mean 1.24) mPa/s* at 37°C; 1.50–1.72 (mean 1.60) mPa/s at 25°C. Plasma viscosity is lower in the newborn (0.98–1.25 mPa/s at 37°C), rising to adult values by the 3rd year; it is slightly higher in old age. There are no significant differences in plasma viscosity between men and women, or in pregnancy. It is remarkably constant in health, with little or no diurnal variation, and it is not affected by exercise. A change of only 0.03–0.05 mPa/s is thus likely to be clinically significant.

WHOLE BLOOD VISCOSITY

The viscosity of blood reflects its rheological properties; it is influenced by PCV, plasma viscosity, red cell aggregation and red cell deformability. It is especially sensitive to PCV, with which it is closely correlated. Its measurement has, however, limited clinical value as it does not take account of the interaction of the red cells with blood vessels which greatly influences blood flow in vivo. Guidelines for measuring blood viscosity and red cell deformability by standardized methods have been published.[17]

Rotational and capillary viscometers are suitable for measuring blood viscosity. Deformability can be measured by recording the rate at which red cells in suspension pass through a filter with pores 3–5 μm in diameter.

TESTS FOR HETEROPHILE ANTIBODIES IN HUMAN SERUM: THE PAUL–BUNNELL TEST FOR THE DIAGNOSIS OF INFECTIOUS MONONUCLEOSIS

Infectious mononucleosis (IM) is caused by Epstein–Barr virus (EBV). Every infected cell contains viral capsid antigens (VCA) which give rise to specific heterophile antibodies. Before this identity was known, Paul & Bunnell[18] demonstrated them as agglutinins directed against sheep red cells; they are, in fact, not specific for sheep red cells but also react with horse and ox, but not human, red cells. They are IgM (19S) globulins which are immunologically related to, but distinct from, antibodies which occur in response to Forssman antigens in serum sickness, in some leukaemias and lymphomas[19,20] and also, in low titre, in healthy individuals. In these non-IM conditions, the antibody can be absorbed out by guinea-pig cells.

For the diagnosis of IM, it is necessary to demonstrate that the antibody present has the characters of the Paul–Bunnell antibody, i.e. it is absorbed by ox red cells but not by guinea-pig kidney. This is the basis of the absorption tests for IM. Although sheep red cells have been widely used to demonstrate the Paul–Bunnell antibody, horse red cells give even better results.[21] Either type of cell, preserved by formalin, can be used in screening tests; however, the preserved cells are less able to detect low-titre antibodies than are fresh horse cells.

A SLIDE SCREENING TEST FOR INFECTIOUS MONONUCLEOSIS

Reagents

Sera. Patient's serum (fresh or inactivated by heating at 56°C for 30 min), and positive and negative control sera.

Red cell suspension. 20% suspension of horse blood in 109 mmol/l (32 g/l) trisodium citrate.

---

*If expressed in poise (P), 1 cP = 1 mPa/s.

Before use, the suspension must be well mixed by repeated inversion. For the screening test, it is unnecessary to wash the cells.

Guinea-pig kidney emulsion. See page 535.

10% autoclaved ox red suspension. See page 535.

Method[22]

Place 1 large drop (approximately 30 μl) of guinea-pig kidney emulsion and 1 large drop of ox-cell suspension on two adjacent squares on an opal glass tile. Add 1 drop of patient or control serum adjacent to each. Deliver 10 μl of horse-blood suspension to the corner of each square, by means of a micropipette avoiding contact with the drops in the squares. With a wooden applicator stick, mix the reagents (guinea-pig kidney emulsion or ox-cell suspension, serum and horse-blood suspension) and then examine with the naked eye for agglutination, using oblique light at an angle over a dark background. Negative and positive serum controls should always be set up at the same time. The appearances are shown in Figure 22.1.

Interpretation

Positive. Agglutination is stronger in the square containing guinea-pig kidney emulsion than in the square containing ox-cell suspension.

Negative. Agglutination is absent in both squares.

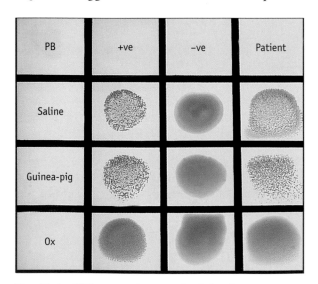

Fig. 22.1 Slide screening test for infectious mononucleosis. Upper: guinea-pig kidney. Lower: ox-cell suspension.

The reagents for the screening test are available commercially as diagnostic kits (e.g. *Monospot (Meridian Diagnostics)* and *IM Absorption kit (Microgen)*. Other commercially available kits are based on antigen-coated latex particles to which IM antibody binds, e.g. *Monolatex (Bio-Stat)* and *IM kit (Unipath)*, or agglutination of stabilized horse red cells, e.g. *Serascan; IM Quick test (Bio-stat)*. An extensive evaluation of 14 such slide tests has shown them to be sensitive and specific with an overall accuracy (positive and negative) in the order of 91.4 to 99.6%.[23] False-positive reactions occur in malaria,[24] toxoplasmosis and cytomegaloid virus infection, more commonly in patients with IgG antibodies to rheumatoid factor or other auto-immune diseases, and even occasionally without any apparent underlying disease.[25] False-negative reactions occur if the test is carried out before the level of heterophile antibody has risen or conversely when it has declined. False-negative reactions may also occur in the very young and the very old. Screening tests are also available based on enzyme-linked immunosorbent assay (ELISA) and immuno-chromatographic assay. These tests are more elaborate than the slide screening test described above, but they are less likely to give a false result.

The specific VCA-antibody reaction in EBV infection is to the nuclear antigen-1 (anti-EBNA-1).[26] Immunofluorescent antibody tests have been developed* which demonstrate the presence of these antibodies and are thus highly specific and sensitive they distinguish IgM antibody which occurs at high titre in the early phase of infection, diminishing during convalescence, from IgG antibody which persists at high titre for years after infection.[27,28]

QUANTITATIVE PAUL–BUNNELL TEST

When the screening test is positive or doubtful, a quantitative test with differential absorption should be carried out. The technique described below is based upon that of Barrett[29] and uses sheep red cells, but horse red cells, as recommended by Lee et al[30] can equally well be used.

---

*E.g. Gull Diagnostics/Launce Diagnostics Product 487003.

Reagents

Patient's serum and positive control serum. 1 ml, previously inactivated by heating at 56°C for 30 min.

Guinea-pig kidney emulsion. See page 535.

10% autoclaved ox red cell suspension. See page 535.

Sheep red cells. 0.4% suspension in 9 g/l NaCl (saline). The sheep blood should preferably be not more than 7 days old. If stored red cells are used instead, they should be washed three times in saline immediately before the test.

Absorption of serum

Deliver three 0.25 ml volumes of patient's inactivated serum into three small glass or plastic tubes, A, B and C. Add 1.0 ml of saline to Tube A, 0.75 ml of saline and 0.3 ml of guinea-pig kidney emulsion to Tube B, and 0.75 ml of saline and 0.25 ml of 10% ox-cell suspension to Tube C. Mix the contents of the three tubes and place them at 4°C for at least 2 h or overnight. Then centrifuge the tubes and retain the supernatants. 1 in 5 dilutions in saline of unabsorbed serum and of the serum absorbed with guinea-pig kidney and ox red cells, respectively, are thus obtained.

Method

Make serial dilutions of the sera from tubes A, B and C in saline; 0.15–0.2 ml volumes are suitable. Nine 75×8 mm tubes and a control tube to contain saline are usually sufficient. Add equal volumes of the 0.4% sheep (or horse) cell suspension to each tube, giving final serum dilutions of from 1 in 10 (tube 1) to 1 in 2560 (tube 9). After mixing their contents, incubate the tubes for 2 h at 37°C before reading the results. A standardized method of reading the end-point should be adopted. Macroscopic reading using a concave mirror is recommended (p. 447). A serum known to contain Paul–Bunnell antibody provides a control for the potency of the absorbents and the agglutinability of the red cells.

The Paul–Bunnell antibody of IM reacts well at 37°C; but agglutination is enhanced at lower temperatures and higher titres are obtained if the tests are carried out at 4°C. At this temperature, however, the test is less specific.

Interpretation

The following figures are given as examples of typical results with sheep cells:

1. Unabsorbed serum, end-point tube 7; titre 640. Guinea-pig kidney absorbed serum, end-point tube 7; titre 640.
   Ox-cell absorbed serum, end-point tube 4; titre 80.

   Such a result would be positive for IM, the antibody being not absorbed by guinea-pig kidney and significantly absorbed by ox cells. Naturally occurring antibody is absorbed by guinea-pig kidney, but not by ox cells, and that of serum sickness is absorbed by both reagents.

2. Uabsorbed serum, end-point tube 3; titre 40. Guinea-pig kidney absorbed serum, end-point tube 3, titre 40.
   Ox-cell absorbed serum, no agglutination in tube 1.

   In spite of the low titre in the unabsorbed serum, this result would also be positive for IM, the antibody being not absorbed by the guinea-pig kidney but absorbed by the ox cells.

3. Unabsorbed serum, end-point tube 3; titre 40. Guinea-pig kidney absorbed serum, no agglutination in tube 1.
   Ox-cell absorbed serum, end-point tube 3; titre 40.

   This is a normal result, and the screening test would have been negative. Caution is needed in interpreting the results when they are weakly positive or when there is only partial absorption by guinea-pig kidney.

   Lack of complete absorption with guinea-pig kidney is not in itself diagnostic of IM, as this may occasionally be observed with normal serum.[29] A positive test requires at least a two-tube difference in titre before and after absorption with ox cells.

   The antibodies normally present in human sera which agglutinate sheep red cells are of the Forssman type, i.e. they react against an antigen widely spread in animal tissues. Antibodies of this type are formed by rabbits injected with an emulsion of guinea-pig kidney. The antibodies react with dog, cat and mouse tissues as well as with sheep and horse red cells, but not with the tissues of man, ox or rat.[31] The antibody formed in IM is of a different nature and is not absorbed by red cells or tissues containing the Forssman antigen; hence the use, as absorbing agents, of guinea-pig kidney, rich in the antigen, and ox red cells, deficient in the antigen but capable of absorbing the Paul–Bunnell antibody.

The antibodies are lytic as well as agglutinating, and it is possible to read the results by recording lysis, if titrations are carried out in the presence of complement. Fresh ox red cells may be used instead of an autoclaved suspension, although less conveniently. The use of horse kidney instead of guinea-pig kidney as an absorbing agent has also been recommended because of the ease with which a large amount of a standard stable reagent can be prepared.[32]

Clinical value of the Paul–Bunnell test
Specific tests have been developed to demonstrate the IgG EBNA-1 (see above). However, tests for the heterophile antibody were developed before the EB virus was identified and they remain a useful aid to the diagnosis of the disease. The Paul–Bunnell test is not infallible. Most authors, have reported 80–90% of positive results in patients thought to be suffering from IM.[33,34] Antibodies are often present as early as the 4th to 6th day of the disease and are almost always found by the 21st day. They disappear as a rule within 4 to 5 months. There is no unanimity as to how frequently negative reactions are found in 'true' IM. Occasionally, the characteristic antibodies develop very late in the course of the disease, perhaps weeks or even months after the patient becomes ill, and it is also known that a positive reaction may be transient and that the antibodies may be present at such low titres that they may be missed or may produce anomalous agglutination reactions when associated with the naturally occurring antibody at similar titres. For all the above reasons, it is difficult to state categorically that any particular patient has not or will not produce antibodies. EBV-specific antibody has been demonstrated in the serum of 86% of patients with clinical and/or haematological features of IM.[35]

As far as false-positive reactions are concerned, there is no substantial evidence that sera containing agglutinins in high concentration giving the typical reactions of IM are ever found in other diseases uncomplicated by IM. In particular, the heterophile-antibody titres in the lymphomas are similar to those found in unselected patients not suffering from IM.[36] In virus hepatitis, although one-fifth of the patients in one series had antibody titres greater than normal, in only one patient did the result of absorption tests suggest the presence of the Paul–Bunnell antibody.[37]

Preparation of guinea-pig kidney suspension and heated or red cell suspension (after Barrett[29])
Guinea-pig kidney suspension
Strip the capsules and perirenal fat from at least two pairs of kidneys. Then wash them well in running water. Homogenize the tissue in 9 g/l NaCl (saline) in a blender for 2 min, sterilize it at 121°C (by autoclaving at 15 lb pressure for 20 min) and blend it again so as to obtain a fine suspension. Then centrifuge the suspension in saline and wash the deposit in two changes of saline. Finally, add to the deposit about four times its volume of 5 g/l phenol in saline. After resuspension, centrifuge the sample in a haematocrit tube in order to estimate its concentration. Then add sufficient phenol-saline to the remainder to produce a 1 in 6 suspension. Use it without further dilution. Its absorbing power must be tested with known positive and negative sera. The reagent will remain potent for at least 1 year if stored at 4°C.

Ox red cell suspension
Wash ox cells in several changes of 9 g/l NaCl (saline) and make a 30% suspension. Then sterilize it at 121°C (by autoclaving at 15 lb pressure for 20 min). When cool, adjust the PCV to 0.20 with saline and add an equal volume of 10 g/l phenol-saline to give a 10% suspension.

The ability of the suspension to absorb the IM antibody must be tested with known positive sera. It should remain potent for several years if stored at 4°C.

DEMONSTRATION OF ANTINUCLEAR FACTORS

Antinuclear antibodies, or antinuclear factors (ANF), occur in the serum in a wide range of auto-immune disorders, including systemic lupus erythematosus (SLE). The antibodies may be specific for DNA, soluble nucleoprotein or an extract of cell nuclei (Sm antigen). A characteristic of SLE is the presence of 7S IgG antibodies to double-stranded DNA (ds-DNA);[38] they can be detected and measured quantitatively by indirect immuno-fluorescence with fluorochrome-labelled anti-serum, ELISA and other immunological methods; these are sensitive and specific. There is also a rapid and simple qualitative screen test for detecting the presence of antinuclear antibodies; this is based on the ability of the serum to aggregate polystyrene latex particles coated with the appropriate nuclear components. Thus, the antinuclear antibody can be demonstrated fairly reliably and rapidly with a reagent comprising latex-bound deoxyribonucleo-protein. This is available as a kit from a number of suppliers.

LE-cell test

Antinuclear antibodies can also be detected by the LE-cell test. This is based on reaction between the patient's auto-antibodies and nuclear antigens, with subsequent phagocytosis by neutrophils. For many years, this was the standard criterion for diagnosing SLE, and the method of Zinkham & Conley[39] was described in previous editions of this book. It was considered to be a useful method as the facilities to carry it out are readily available in any haematology laboratory. However, it has been superseded by the immunological tests referred to above.

ERYTHROPOIETIN

Erythropoietin (Epo) regulates red cell production. It is a heat stable glycoprotein with a molecular weight of about 34 kDa. It is produced mainly in the kidney. Only a small quantity is demonstrable in normal plasma or urine.

The original method for measuring plasma Epo was an in-vivo biological assay, based on the uptake of ^{59}Fe by laboratory animals (usually rats) following the injection of test plasma or extract. A pure form of human erythropoietin from recombinant DNA (r-HuEpo) is now available; this has opened up a number of diagnostic and therapeutic uses and has led to more reliable and sensitive assay methods by ELISA, enzyme immuno-assay (EIA) and radio-immune assay (RIA). Commercial kits are available, but they are relatively expensive and there is inter-method variability.[40-42]

It is impractical to undertake the assay in laboratories where the test is required only occasionally; it is preferable to send the serum sample to a reference centre. In the UK, the test is carried out by a national erythropoietin assay service* where it is carried out by ELISA.

Results are expressed in international units by reference to an international (WHO) standard. This was originally a urinary extract, and a preparation is available with a potency of 10 iu per ampoule.[43] A standard has also been established for r-HuEpo with a potency of 86 iu per ampoule.[44]

Reference range

The normal reference range in plasma or serum has varied considerably according to the method of assay.[40] The original immuno-reactive method gave a normal range of 18–35 iu/l.[45] For the ELISA method used by the UK national erythropoietin service,* the normal range is 9.1–30.8 iu/l. With test kits, in the steady state without anaemia, it is usually given as 5–25 iu/l or slightly higher. In normal children, the levels are the same as in adults, except for infants under 2 months when the level is low.[46]

There is a diurnal variation, with the highest values at night.[47] In pregnancy, Epo concentration increases with gestation.[48]

Significance

Increased levels of Epo are found in the plasma in various anaemias[49] and there is normally an inverse relationship between haemoglobin and Epo.[50] In thalassaemia, it is lower than in iron deficiency with the same degree of anaemia, but there is a close inverse correlation with the red cell count.[51] In renal disease, there is a progressive decline in the Epo response to anaemia, and in end-stage renal failure, the concentration is normal or even lower than normal despite increasing anaemia. Some impairment of production of Epo may also occur in the anaemia of neoplastic and chronic inflammatory diseases.[50]

Raised concentrations of Epo occur in secondary polycythaemia owing to respiratory and cardiac disease, in the presence of abnormal haemoglobins with high oxygen affinity, in association with hypernephroma and Epo-secreting tumours such as hepatoma, uterine fibroma, ovarian carcinoma and some other rare tumours.[52]

In primary proliferative polycythaemia ('polycythaemia vera'), the plasma level is usually lower than normal even when the haemoglobin has been reduced by venesection.[53,54] In secondary polycythaemia, the level of Epo is never suppressed below normal. Assay is particularly useful in patients with erythrocytosis of undetermined cause. However, in such cases there may be an intermittent increase in Epo secretion. Thus, determining the Epo level in a single sample of plasma may be misleading.[45,53] Low levels have been found in some cases of primary (essential) thrombocythaemia.[54,55]

Autonomous in-vitro erythropoiesis

When bone marrow of mononuclear cells from blood are cultured, erythroid colonies (CFU-E) will normally develop only when Epo is present in the culture medium. However, growth will occur in erythropoietin-free medium in primary polycythaemia.[56] This provides a method for distinguishing primary from secondary polycythaemia.[57,58]

Mononuclear cells are collected from a blood sample by density separation, e.g. wtih Ficoll (p. 58) and added to an appropriate serum-free liquid culture medium which is then divided into two portions. To one portion is added 1 IU/ml of Epo. Both portions are plated and incubated for 7 days at 37°C. They are then stained with benzidene and examined directly under an inverted microscope or after spreading onto slides. The numbers of benzidene-positive cell clusters in the Epo-free and Epo-containing samples are counted and compared. A diagnosis of primary polycythaemia is indicated if there is an approximately equal growth in both samples. A method has been described in which flow cytometry with immunofluorescence is used to detect growth of the erythroid cells after only 2 to 5 days of culture.[59]

Thrombopoietin

Thrombopoietin regulates megakaryocyte development and platelet production. It is a protein produced by the liver and has been purified from serum.[60] It is considerably larger than erythropoietin with molecular weight of about 335 kDa. A recombinant human thrombopoietin (rhTPO) has been produced and used to prepare a monoclonal antibody and develop a sensitive and specific ELISA test. This has been used to measure TPO in normal serum and serum from patients with various blood disorders.[61] The normal range (mean and 2 SD) was 0.79±0.35 fmol/ml for men; 0.70 ± 0.26 fmol/ml for women. It was increased in thrombocytopenias, especially high at 18.5 ± 12.4 fmol/ml in aplastic anaemia with severe thrombocytopenia. In essential thrombocythaemia, it was in the range 1.01–4.82 fmol/ml.[61]

DIAGNOSIS OF MALARIA

In addition to examination of stained thick and thin blood films by conventional microscopy, as described in Chapter 4, there are a number of other methods for screening for the presence of malaria.[62,63]

Fluorescent microscopy

Red cells containing malaria parasites fluoresce when examined by fluorescent microscopy after staining with acridine orange. This has a sensitivity of about 90% in acute infections, but only 50% at lower levels of parasitaemia, and false-positive readings may occur with Howell–Jolly bodies and reticulocytes.[62] When positive, it is necessary to examine a conventionally stained blood film to identify the species.

Quantitative buffy coat method

The quantitative buffy coat (Becton Dickinson) is another method for detection of parasites by fluorescent microscopy. The blood is centrifuged in capillary tubes which are coated with acridine orange. It is fairly sensitive but requires expensive equipment and has the disadvantage of false-positive results in the presence of Howell–Jolly bodies and reticulocytes. When positive, identification of species will require examination of a stained blood film, but it is useful as an initial screening test.[62,64]

Antigen detection

Simple screening methods have been developed for *Plasmodium falciparum* which are based on binding of monoclonal antibody to histidine rich protein 2 (HRP-2) which occurs specifically in the red cells of *P. falciparum*.

ParaSight F (Becton Dickinson) is an ELISA-based dipstick method with a sensitivity of 95%, but less sensitive in low levels of parasitaemia.[62,65] It is negative when only gametocytes are present.[64] It is unhelpful in the immediate post-treatment follow-up as it remains positive for 1 to 2 weeks after clinical cure and disappearance of parasites from the blood.[62]

ICT Malaria Pf is a card test based on immunochromatographic demonstration of the HRP-2 which is reported to have a sensitivity of 100% and specificity of 96.2%.[66] A cheap version of the immunochromatographic method, *Falciparum Malaria IC Strip*, is manufactured by Program for Appropriate Technology for Health (PATH), especially as a diagnostic tool in malaria-endemic areas.[67] There are also kits which are capable of demonstrating *P. vivax* infection by combining the *P. falciparum* specific HRP-2 antibody with antibody against parasite lactic dehydrogenase which occurs in other types of malaria.[62,68]

With any of the screening tests, it must be borne in mind that it is always necessary to confirm a positive result by microscopy. Moreover, for clinical management of patients with *P. falciparum* infection, it is essential to examine a blood film to obtain an estimate of the percentage of red cells which are infected.

Polymerase chain reaction

This provides highly sensitive and specific results; it is especially useful for epidemiological studies, but it is impractical as a routine diagnostic tool when results are required rapidly.[69,70]

CYTOGENETIC ANALYSIS

Cytogenetic analysis is generally performed in specialist cytogenetics laboratories. Techniques employed are outside the scope of this book and the reader is referred to a specialized textbook.[71] It is, however, necessary for the haematologist to know the indications for such analysis and how to collect appropriate specimens, to understand the terminology and to be able to interpret the results. The term 'cytogenetic analysis' encompasses both classical cytogenetic analysis, in which stained chromosomes in metaphase preparations are examined, and fluorescent in situ hybridization (FISH), in which chromosomes, or parts of chromosomes, are labelled with fluorochrome-bound oligonucleotides that are complementary to specific sequences on a chromosome; examination is by fluorescence microscopy. FISH can be applied to both metaphase and interphase preparations. Cytogenetic analysis may be supplemented by molecular genetic analysis for (i) the investigation of specific oncogenes and cancer-suppressing genes and (ii) the demonstration of clonality by showing rearrangement of T-cell receptor or immunoglobulin genes (see Ch. 14 and 21).

Indications for cytogenetic analysis

Cytogenetic analysis may be carried out for the following reasons:

1. detection of an inherited or constitutional abnormality that may be responsible for a haematological disorder, e.g. the detection of trisomy 21 for the confirmation of Down's syndrome in patients with acute lymphocytic leukaemia (ALL), acute myeloid leukaemia (AML) or transient abnormal myelopoiesis in the neonatal period or diagnosis of Fanconi's anaemia by demonstration of increased breakage on exposure to a clastogenic agent;
2. confirmation that a condition is neoplastic when this is not otherwise certain, e.g. in some cases of myelodysplastic syndrome (MDS), natural killer (NK) cell leukaemia or eosinophilic leukaemia;

3. confirmation of a specific diagnosis, e.g. by the demonstration of t(9;22)(q34;q11) in chronic granulocytic leukaemia, t(14;18)(q32;q21) in follicular lymphoma, t(11;14)(q13;q32) in mantle cell lymphoma or inv(14)(q11q32) in T-lineage prolymphocytic leukaemia;

4. provision of prognostic information which is likely to influence choice of therapy, e.g. in ALL, AML and possibly MDS and multiple myeloma;

5. monitoring response to treatment, e.g. in chronic granulocytic leukaemia.

Cytogenetic analysis is important in the classification of haematological neoplasms such as AML, ALL, non-Hodgkin's lymphoma (NHL) and the chronic myeloid leukaemias. The proposed WHO classification incorporates some of the more common cytogenetic categories of AML as discrete entities and considers characteristic cytogenetic abnormalities in the classification of non-Hodgkin's lymphoma.[72] The necessity to incorporate the results of molecular genetic analysis, alongside the results of cytogenetic and other investigations (see Chs 13 and 14) has been recognized and a MIC-M (Morphological-Immunophenotypic-Cytogenetic-Molecular Genetic) classification of acute leukaemias has been proposed;[73–75] this approach means that some important entities that cannot be recognized by cytogenetic analysis, e.g. ALL associated with a cryptic t(12;21)(p12;q22), can be included in the classification. The MIC-M approach could be extended to the chronic myeloid leukaemias and myeloproliferative disorders where molecular mechanisms of neoplasia are increasingly being recognized.

Collection of specimens

Fibroblast cultures, phytohaemagglutinin (PHA)-stimulated lymphocytes or bone marrow cells can be used for the investigation of inherited and other constitutional abnormalities. Conventional cytogenetic analysis for the investigation of haematological neoplasms is usually best performed on bone marrow cells although peripheral blood cells can sometimes be used if there are large numbers of immature circulating cells. Cytogenetic samples should be anticoagulated with preservative-free heparin and transported rapidly to the cytogenetic laboratory. Refrigeration is not necessary. It is important that the cytogenetic laboratory knows the suspected diagnosis as optimal culture conditions differ for different conditions.

Terminology and interpretation of results[76]

Standard cytogenetic terminology and abbreviations are shown in Table 22.3. It should be noted that in describing a translocation, e.g. t(8;21)(q22;q22), the chromosomes involved in

Table 22.3 Abbreviations and terminology used in describing chromosomes and their abnormalities (reproduced with permission from Bain[76])

p	short arm of a chromosome
q	long arm of a chromosome
p+, q+	addition of chromosomal material to the short arm or long arm respectively
p−, q−	loss of chromosomal material from the short arm or long arm respectively
+	addition of a chromosome
−	loss of a chromosome
add	additional material of unknown origin
band	chromosomal region which, after staining, is distinguished from adjoining regions by appearing lighter or darker
c	constitutional anomaly
del	deletion
der	derivative chromosome, an abnormal chromosome derived from two or more chromosomes; it takes its number from the chromosome which contributes the centromere
dic	dicentric, a chromosome with two centromeres
dm	double minute (see minute)
dup	duplication, extra copy of the segment of a chromosome

Table 22.3 *(continued)*

hsr	homogeneously staining region, indicative of amplification (multiple copies) of a small segment of a chromosome
inv	inversion, i.e. a segment of a chromosome has been inverted or rotated through 180°
ins	insertion, movement of a segment of a chromosome to a new position on the same or another chromosome; may be direct (dir) or inverted (inv)
iso or i	isochromosome, a chromosome formed by duplication of the long arm or the short arm
mar	marker chromosome, an abnormal chromosome which cannot be characterized and is therefore of unknown origin
min	minute, an acentric fragment smaller than the width of a single chromatid; may be single or double
r	ring chromosome
t	translocation, movement of a segment of one chromosome to form part of another chromosome; a translocation is often reciprocal; a translocation may be described as balanced (no loss of chromosomal material) or unbalanced (a segment of chromosome has been lost)
aneuploid	cells having an abnormal number of chromosomes which is neither half nor a multiple of 46
centromere	the junction of the short arm (p) and the long arm (q)
diploid	cells having the normal complement of 46 chromosomes (23 pairs)
haploid	cells with 23 (unpaired) chromosomes; near haploid = 23–34 chromosomes
hypodiploid	cells having fewer than 46 chromosomes, usually 35–45
karyotype	written description of the chromosomal make-up of a cell and, by extension, of a clone of cells (or an individual)
karyogram	systematized array of the chromosomes of a cell and, by extension, of a clone of cells (or an individual); chromosomes are displayed in decreasing order of size which corresponds to increasing chromosome number; the sex chromosomes, X and Y, are displayed last
monosomy	loss of an entire chromosome so that there is only a single copy, indicated by '–' before the chromosome number, e.g. –7
paracentric inversion	inversion of a segment of a chromosome that is confined to one arm
pericentric inversion	inversion of a segment of a chromosome composed of part of both arms and the centromere
pseudodiploid	cells having 46 chromosomes but with structural abnormalities being present
tetraploid	cells having 92 chromosomes (four sets); near tetraploid = 81–103 chromosomes
triploid	cells having 69 chromosomes (three sets); near triploid = 58–80 chromosomes
trisomy	three copies of a chromosome, indicated by '+' before the chromosome number, e.g. +8

the translocation are listed in numerical order within one set of brackets, separated by a semicolon; the breakpoints involved in the translocation are listed, within a second set of brackets, in the same order and separated by a semicolon. In the case of an inversion, e.g. inv(16)(p13q22), the chromosome involved is designated within a first set of brackets and the breakpoints that define the inverted segment are listed within a second set of brackets without a semicolon. Conventionally a clone is considered to be present if two cells show the same structural abnormality or additional chromosome or if three cells show the same missing chromosome. However, it should be noted that loss of a Y chromosome from a significant proportion of cells is a normal, age-related phenomenon and –Y is therefore not usually an indication of a neoplastic clone. When following up a patient, e.g. a patient with chronic granulocytic leukaemia on interferon therapy, a single cell with the appropriate abnormality is indicative of persistence of the neoplastic clone.

REFERENCES

1 International Committee for Standardization in Haematology 1988 Guidelines on the selection of laboratory tests for monitoring the acute-phase response. Journal of Clinical Pathology 41:1203–1212.

2 Lowe GDO 1994 Annotation: Should plasma viscosity replace the ESR? British Journal of Haematology 86:6–11.

3 International Council for Standardization in Haematology 1993 ICSH recommendations for

measurement of erythrocyte sedimentation rate.
Journal of Clinical Pathology 46:198–203.

4 National Committee for Clinical Laboratory
Standards 1993 Methods for the erythrocyte
sedimentation rate (ESR) test (H2–A3). NCCLS,
Wayne, PA.

5 Westergren A 1921 Studies of the suspension
stability of the blood in pulmonary tuberculosis.
Acta Medica Scandinavica 54:247–282.

6 Stuart J, Lewis SM 1993 Recommendations for
standardization, safety and quality control of
erythrocyte sedimentation rate: Document
WHO/LBS/93.1. World Health Organization,
Geneva.

7 Kallner A, Engervall P, Björkholm M 1994 Kinetic
measurement of the erythrocyte sedimentation
rate. Upsala Journal of Medical Science
99:179–186.

8 Caswell M, Stuart J 1991 Assessment of Diesse
Ves-matic automated system for measuring
erythrocyte sedimentation rate. Journal of Clinical
Pathology 44:946–949.

9 Garvey BJ, Mahon A, Parker-Williams J, et al 1999
An evaluation of ESR-Chex control material for
erythrocyte sedimentation rate determination
(MDA 99/28). Medical Devices Agency,
Stationery Office, Norwich NR3 IPD.

10 Bull BS 1981 Clinical and laboratory implications
of present ESR methodology. Clinical and
Laboratory Haematology 3:283–298.

11 Froom P, Margaliot S, Caine Y, et al 1984
Significance of erythrocyte sedimentation rate in
young adults. American Journal of Clinical
Pathology 82:198–200.

12 Bain BJ 1983 Some influences on the ESR and the
fibrinogen level in healthy subjects. Clinical and
Laboratory Haematology 5:45–54.

13 Huisman A, Aarnoudse JG, Krans M, et al 1988
Red cell aggregation during normal pregnancy.
British Journal of Haematology 68:121–124.

14 Dintenfass L 1976 Rheology of blood in
diagnostic and preventive medicine. Butterworth,
London.

15 Harkness J 1971 The viscosity of human plasma;
its measurement in health and disease. Biorheology
8:171–193.

16 International Committee for Standardization in
Haematology 1984 Recommendation for selected
method for the measurement of plasma viscosity.
Journal of Clinical Pathology 37:1147–1152.

17 International Committee for Standardization in
Haematology 1986 Guidelines for measurement of
blood viscosity and erythrocyte deformability.
Clinical Hemorheology 6:439–453.

18 Paul JR, Bunnell WW 1932 The presence of
heterophile antibodies in infectious mononucleosis.
American Journal of Medical Science 183:90.

19 Huh J, Cho K, Heo DS, et al 1999 Detection of
Epstein–Barr virus in Korean peripheral T-cell
lymphoma. American Journal of Haematology
60:205–214.

20 Klein G 1994 Epstein–Barr virus strategy in normal
and neoplastic B cells. Cell 77:791–793.

21 Davidsohn I, Lee CL 1964 Serologic diagnosis of
infectious mononucleosis. A comparative study of
five tests. American Journal of Clinical Pathology
24:115–125.

22 Lee CL, Davidsohn I, Panczyszyn O 1968 Horse
agglutinins in infectious mononucleosis: II The
spot test. American Journal of Clinical Pathology
49:12–18.

23 Garvey BJ, Mahon A, Parker-Williams J, et al 1998
Evaluation report: fourteen commercial IM
screening kits (MDA 98/63). Medical Devices
Agency, Stationery Office, Norwich NR3 1PD.

24 Reed RE 1974 False-positive monospot tests in
malaria. American Journal of Clinical Pathology
61:173–174.

25 Horwitz CA, Henle W, Henle G, et al 1979
Persistent falsely positive rapid tests for infectious
mononucleosis. Report of five cases with four–six
year follow-up data. American Journal of Clinical
Pathology 72:807–811.

26 Strand BC, Schuster TC, Hopkins RF, et al 1981
Identification of an Epstein–Barr virus nuclear
antigen by fluoro-immuno-electrophoresis and
radioimmuno-electrophoresis. Journal of Virology
38:996–1004.

27 Edwards JMB, McSwiggen DA 1974 Studies on
the diagnostic value of an immunofluorescence test
for EB virus-specific IgM. Journal of Clinical
Pathology 27:647–651.

28 Henle W, Henle GE, Horwitz CA 1974
Epstein–Barr virus specific diagnostic tests in
infectious mononucleosis. Human Pathology
5:551–565.

29 Barrett AM 1941 The serological diagnosis of
glandular fever (infectious mononucleosis): a new
technique. Journal of Hygiene (Cambridge)
41:330–343.

30 Lee CL, Davidsohn I, Slaby R 1968 Horse
agglutinins in infectious mononucleosis. American
Journal of Clinical Pathology 49:3–11.

31 Mühlradt PF 1998 Forssman antigen. In: Delves
PJ, Roitt IM (eds) Encyclopedia of immunology,
2nd edn. Academic Press, London, p 953–955.

32 Davidsohn I, Goldin M 1955 The use of horse
kidney in the differential test of infectious

mononucleosis. Journal of Laboratory and Clinical Medicine 45:561–567.

33 Bernstein A 1940 Infectious mononucleosis. Medicine (Baltimore) 19:85–159.

34 Kaufman RE 1944 Heterophile antibody in infectious mononucleosis. Annals of Internal Medicine 21:230–251.

35 Evans AS, Niederman JC 1982 EBV-IgA and new heterophile antibody tests in diagnosis of infectious mononucleosis. American Journal of Clinical Pathology 77:555–560.

36 Goldman R, Fishkin BG, Peterson E 1950 The value of the heterophile antibody reaction in the lymphomatous diseases. Journal of Laboratory and Clinical Medicine 35:681–687.

37 Leibowitz S 1951 Heterophile antibody in normal adults and in patients with virus hepatitis. American Journal of Clinical Pathology 21:201–211.

38 Hughes GRV 1973 The diagnosis of systemic lupus erythematosus (Annotation). British Journal of Haematology 25:409–413.

39 Zinkham WH, Conley CL 1956 Some factors influencing the formation of L. E. cells. A method for enhancing L. E. cell production. Bulletin of the Johns Hopkins Hospital 98:102–119.

40 Marsden JT, Sherwood RA, Peters TJ 1995 Evaluation of six erythropoietin kits. (MDA 95/57) Medical Devices Agency, Stationery Office, Norwich NR3 1PD.

41 Cotes PM, Tam RC, Reed P, et al 1989 An immunological cross-reactant of erythropoietin in serum which may invalidate EPO radioimmunoassay. British Journal of Haematology 73:265–268.

42 Bechensteen AG, Lappin TRJ, Marsden J, et al 1993 Unreliability in immunoassays of erythropoietin: anomalous estimates with an assay kit. British Journal of Haematology 83:663–664.

43 Annable L, Cotes PM, Mussett MV 1972 The second international preparation of erythropoietin, human, urinary, for bioassay. Bulletin of the World Health Organization 47:99.

44 Storring PL, Gaines Das RE 1992 The international standard for recombinant DNA-derived erythropoietin: collaborative study of four recombinant DNA-derived erythropoietins and two highly purified human erythropoietins. Journal of Endocrinology 134:459–484.

45 Cotes PM, Doré CJ, Liu Yin JA, et al 1986 Determination of serum immunoreactive erythropoietin in the investigation of erythrocytosis. New England Journal of Medicine 315:283–287.

46 Hellebostad M, Haga P, Cotes MP 1988 Serum immunoreactive erythropoietin in healthy normal children. British Journal of Haematology 70:247–250.

47 Wide L, Bengtsson C, Birgegard G 1988 Circadian rhythm of erythropoietin in human serum. British Journal of Haematology 72:85–90.

48 Cotes PM, Canning CE, Lind T 1983 Changes in serum immunoreactive erythropoietin during the menstrual cycle and normal pregnancy. British Journal of Obstetrics and Gynaecology 90:304–311.

49 Winearls CG 1992 Erythropoietin. Proceedings of the Royal College of Physicians of Edinburgh 22:426–443.

50 Pippard MJ, Hughes HRT, Cotes PM 1992 Erythropoietin. In: Hoffbrand AV, Brenner MK (eds) Recent advances in haematology, No. 6. Churchill Livingstone, Edinburgh, p 1–18.

51 Tassiopoulos T, Konstantopoulos K, Tassiopoulos S, et al 1997 Erythropoietin levels and microcytosis in heterozygous beta-thalassaemia. Acta Haematologica 98:147–149.

52 Alexanian R 1977 Increased erythropoietin production in man. In: Fisher JW (ed) Kidney hormones, vol II: Erythropoietin. Academic Press, London, p 531.

53 Messinezy M, Westwood NB, Woodcock SP, et al 1995 Low serum erythropoietin – a strong diagnostic criterion of primary polycythaemia even at normal haemoglobin levels. Clinical and Laboratory Haematology 17:217–220.

54 Carneskog J, Kutti J, Wadenvik H, et al 1998 Plasma erythropoietin by high detectability immunoradiometric assay in untreated and treated patients with polycythaemia vera and essential thrombocythaemia. European Journal of Haematology 60:278–282.

55 Carneskog J, Safai-Kutti S, Wadenvik H, et al 1999 The red cell mass, plasma erythropoietin and spleen size in apparent polycythaemia. European Journal of Haematology 62:43–48.

56 Prchal JF, Axelred AA 1974 Bone marrow responses in polycythemia vera. New England Journal of Medicine 290:1382.

57 Lemoine F, Najman A, Baillou C, et al 1986 A prospective study of the value of bone marrow erythroid progenitor cultures in polycythemia. Blood 68:996–1002.

58 Beckman BS, Anderson WF, Beltran GS, et al 1983 Diagnostic use of CFU-E formation from peripheral blood in polycythemia vera. American Journal of Clinical Pathology 79:496–499.

59 Manor D, Rachmilewitz EA, Fibach E 1997 Improved method for diagnosis of polycythemia

vera based on flow cytometric analysis of autonomous growth of erythroid precursors in liquid culture. American Journal of Hematology 54:47–52.

60 Kaushansky K 1995 Thrombopoietin: the primary regulator of platelet production. Blood 86:419–431.

61 Tahara T, Usuki K, Sato H, et al 1996 A sensitive sandwich ELISA for measuring thrombopoietin in human serum: serum thrombopoietin levels in healthy volunteers and in patients with haemopoietic disorders. British Journal of Haematology 93:783–788.

62 Hänscheid T 1999 Diagnosis of malaria: a review of alternatives to conventional microscopy. Clinical and Laboratory Haematology 21:235–245.

63 British Committee for Standards in Haematology 1997 The laboratory diagnosis of malaria. Clinical and Laboratory Haematology 19:165–170.

64 Craig MH, Sharp BL 1997 Comparative evaluation of four techniques for the diagnosis of *Plasmodium falciparum* infections. Transactions of the Royal Society of Tropical Medicine and Hygiene 91:279–282.

65 Chiodini PL, Cooke AH, Moody AH, et al 1996 MDA evaluation of the Becton Dickinson ParaSight F test for the diagnosis of *Plasmodium falciparum*. (MDA 96/33). Medical Devices Agency, Stationery Office, Norwich NR3 1PD.

66 Garcia M, Kirimoama S, Marlborough D, et al 1996 Immunochromatographic test for malaria diagnosis. Lancet 347:1549.

67 Mills CD, Burgess DCH, Taylor HJ, et al 1999 Evaluation of a rapid and inexpensive dipstick assay for the diagnosis of *Plasmodium falciparum* malaria. Bulletin of the World Health Organization 77:553–558.

68 Durrheim DN, la Grange JJP, Govere J, et al 1998 Accuracy of a rapid immunochromatographic card test for *Plasmodium falciparum* in a malaria control programme in South Africa. Transactions of the Royal Society of Tropical Medicine and Hygiene 92:32–33.

69 Seesod N, Nopparat P, Hedrum A, et al 1997 An integrated system using immunomagnetic separation polymerase-chain-reaction and colorimetric detection for diagnosis of *Plasmodium falciparum*. American Journal of Tropical Medicine and Hygiene 56:322–328.

70 Hang VT, Be TV, Thanh CT, et al 1995 Screening donor blood for malaria by polymerase chain reaction. Transactions of the Royal Society of Tropical Medicine and Hygiene 89:44–47.

71 Rooney DE (ed) 2001 Human cytogenetics, vol 2, 2nd edn. Oxford University Press, Oxford.

72 Harris NL, Jaffe ES, Diebold J, et al 1999 World Health Organization Classification of Neoplastic Disease of the Hematopoietic and Lymphoid Tissues: Report of the Clinical Advisory Committee Meeting, November 1997. Journal of Clinical Oncology 17:3835–3839.

73 Bain BJ 1998 Classification of acute leukaemia. Journal of Clinical Pathology 51:420–423.

74 First MIC Cooperative Study Group 1986 Morphologic, immunologic and cytogenetic (MIC) working classification of the acute lymphoblastic leukaemias. Cancer Genetics and Cytogenetics 23:189–197.

75 Second MIC Cooperative Study Group 1988 Morphologic, immunologic and cytogenetic (MIC) working classification of the acute myeloid leukaemias. British Journal of Haematology 68:487–494.

76 Bain BJ 1999 Leukaemia diagnosis, 2nd edn. Blackwell Science, Oxford.

23

Laboratory organization and management

S. Mitchell Lewis

The essential function of a haematology laboratory is to obtain reliable and reproducible data and to make observations which will provide clinicians with timely, unambiguous and meaningful reports to assist in diagnosing disease and monitoring patient response to treatment. Advancing technology and increasing health-care legislation have both added to the complexity of modern laboratory practice. Laboratory organization and management are essential factors in good laboratory practice. The principles outlined in this chapter apply to small as well as to large departments despite the more complex management issues that arise in the latter.[1]

MANAGEMENT STRUCTURE AND FUNCTION

Management structure

The management structure of a haematology laboratory requires a clear line of accountability of each member of staff to the head of department. In turn, the head of department may be managerially accountable to a clinical director (of laboratories) and thence to a hospital or health authority executive. The head of department is responsible for departmental leadership, for ensuring that the laboratory has effective political representation within the hospital, and for ensuring that managerial and administrative tasks are performed efficiently. Management requires an integrated team effort with individual members of staff contributing managerial skills to specified aspects. All staff should receive some training in laboratory management. Where the head of department delegates managerial tasks to others, these responsibilities must be clearly defined and stated.

Management of a department requires an executive committee, and under this executive, answerable to the head of department, there should be a number of managerial appointments to implement the functioning of the department (Table 23.1). Clearly the activities of the various members of staff overlap, and there must be adequate effective communication between them. There should be regular briefing at meetings of technical heads with their section staff. All members of staff must be told of any plans which might have a bearing on their

Table 23.1 Suggested components of a management structure

Executive committee
Head of department
Business manager
Consultant haematologists
Principal Scientific Officer
Sectional technical heads
Cytometry
Blood film morphology
Immuno-haematology
Haemostasis
Blood transfusion
Special investigations, etc.
Safety officer
Quality control officer
Clerical supervisor
Computer and data processing supervisor

careers and their working practices. Unauthorized "leakage" of confidential information from policy-making committees must be avoided.

Because of the demands from regulatory agencies who inspect and accredit laboratories (see p. 559) and the plethora of guideline documents from standards-setting authorities, there may be a need for a special sub-committee of the executive whose duty is to keep abreast of these matters and interrelate with the different sections in the same way as the safety officer.

Staff appraisal

All members of staff should receive training to enhance their skills and to develop their careers. This requires setting of goals and regular appraisal of progress for both management and technical ability. The appraisal process should cascade down from the head of department, and appropriate training must be given at successive levels to each appraiser. It is useful for the appraiser, in advance, to provide a short list of proposed topics to the person to be interviewed, who should be encouraged to add to the list so that each understands the topics to be covered. An appraisal interview usually requires about 1 hour, and should be a constructive dialogue of the present state of development and the progress made to date. Ideally, the staff members

should leave the interviews with the knowledge that their personal development and future progress are of importance to the department, that priorities have been identified, that an action plan with milestones and a time-scale has been agreed, and that progress will be monitored. Formal appraisal interviews (annually for senior staff and more often for others) should be complemented by informal follow-up discussions to monitor progress. Documentation of formal interviews can be limited to a short list of agreed objectives.

Performance appraisal can have lasting value in the personal development of individuals,[2] but the process can easily be mishandled and it requires training to acquire the ability to hold appraisal interviews successfully.

Continuing professional development

Continuing professional development (CPD), linked with continuing medical education (CME), is a process of systematic learning which enables health workers to be constantly brought up to date on developments in their profession and thus ensure their competence to practise throughout their entire career. Policies and programmes have already been established in a number of countries, and in some participation may become a mandatory requirement for the right to practise.[3] It must not be confused with accreditation which concerns the performance (and licensing) of the laboratories themselves. CPD schemes are run by national professional bodies who are responsible for the practice standards of their members. In the UK, schemes relevant to haematology are the responsibility of the Royal College of Pathologists[4,5] for doctors, and Institute for Biomedical Science[6] for scientists/technologists. The process is based on obtaining 'credits' for various activities which qualify such as attendance at specified lectures, workshops and conferences, giving lectures and writing books or journal articles, using computer-based and journal-based programmes and taking part in peer review discussions. The credit points accumulate towards an annual required score.

STRATEGIC AND BUSINESS PLANNING

The head of department is responsible for determining the long-term (usually up to 5 years) strategic direction of the department. This requires awareness of any national and local legislation that may affect the laboratory and of changes in local clinical practice that may alter workload. It is conventional to perform an analysis of the internal *strengths* and *weaknesses* of the laboratory and its ability to respond to external *opportunities* and *threats* (SWOT analysis). Expansion of a major clinical service, such as organ transplantation, or the opportunity to compete for the laboratory service of other hospitals and clinics may pose both an external opportunity and threat to the laboratory depending on its ability to respond to the consequential increase in workload. Internal strengths may include technical or scientific expertise, whereas a heavy workload that precludes any additional developmental work would be a weakness.

A business plan is primarily concerned with determining short-term objectives that will allow the strategy to be implemented over the next financial year or so. It requires prediction of future work level and expansion. Planning of these objectives should involve all staff as this will heighten awareness of the issues and will develop 'ownership' of the strategy. In all but the smallest laboratory, a business manager is required to coordinate such planning and to liaise with the equivalent business managers in other clinical and laboratory areas. Business planning also requires a sophisticated laboratory accounting process with an up-to-date record of workload and costs so that the price of tests can be established.

Workload assessment and costing of tests

Health-care legislation determines the extent to which a laboratory needs to monitor workload and to cost its tests for clinical users. Even when this is not a legislative requirement, all laboratories should maintain accurate records of workload and costs in order to apportion resources to each section. Computerization of laboratories has greatly facilitated this process.

Methods for determining the workload of individual laboratory sections, adjusted for test complexity, include those of the College of American Pathologists,[7] the Canadian Workload Measurement System,[8] and the Welcan system as used in the UK.[9] In the Welcan system, one unit of workload corresponds to 1 minute of productive (excluding waiting) time of technical, clerical and aide staff. Examples are given in Table 23.2.

Table 23.2 Examples of Welcan units for haematological tests

Test	Unit value
Venepuncture	8
Automated blood count	3
Semi-automated blood count	9
Haemoglobin (manual method)	5
Packed cell volume by micro-haematocrit	3
Platelet count by microscopy	9
Reticulocyte count (automated)	3
Reticulocyte count (microscopic)	9
Prothrombin time (manual method)	5
Coagulation factor (one-stage, manual, clotting assay)	60
Blood film morphology	5
with differential white cell count	10
Bone marrow preparation and report	25
Vitamin B_{12} assay	10
Ferritin assay	8
Haemoglobin electrophoresis	25
ABO and Rh(D) blood group (manual method)	5
Blood volume	180
Red cell survival	180

Welcan units encompass the total time taken from receipt of a specimen to issue of the report and are based on timing studies from a range of laboratories, but continuous refinement of the method for assessing workload is necessary with changing technical procedures, particularly for tests that are performed in high volume with automated methods.

Financial control

Efficient budgeting requires regular monitoring, at least monthly. Computer spreadsheets are a useful means to obtain an easily comprehended view of the financial state and the likely outcome. Full costing of tests includes all overheads (Table 23.3), but the apportionment of such indirect costs remains highly variable. Using Welcan units has limitations,[10] as they exclude training time and the

Table 23.3 Factors contributing to cost of laboratory tests

Direct costs
Staff salaries
Laboratory equipment purchases
Reagents and other consumables
Equipment maintenance
Indirect costs
Depreciation of capital assets
Building repairs and routine maintenance
Lighting, heating and waste disposal
Personnel services
Cleaning services
Transport and portering
Laundry services
Telephone and fax
Postage

absence of staff for annual leave or sickness and when different departments are compared, there is no standardized method of determining and apportioning overhead costs. The approach can, however, facilitate comparison of the relative labour costs between different sections of a department which share common overhead costs. When preparing a budget, the following formula provides a reasonably reliable estimate of the total annual costs:

$$[L \times T] + [C \times T] + E + M + O + A;$$

where
L = labour costs for each test from estimate of time taken and the salary rate of the staff member(s) performing the tests
C = cost of consumables per test (including controls)
T = number of tests in the year
E = annual equipment cost* based on initial cost divided by expected life of the item
M = annual maintenance and servicing of equipment
O = laboratory overheads (see Table 23.3)
A = laboratory administration, including salaries of clerical and other non-technical staff.

If savings become necessary, they can be achieved in a variety of ways, but large savings usually necessitate a reduction in staff as employment costs can account for 70–80% of total expenditure. Possible initiatives include:

---

*Either a proportion of the original cost or the annual cost of leasing, as discussed below.

- rationalization of service with other local hospitals to eliminate duplication
- restructuring within a hospital laboratory for cross-discipline working, e.g. between haematology and clinical chemistry
- sub-contracting of labour-intensive tests to a specialist laboratory
- employment of part-time contract staff, e.g. for overnight and week-end emergency service or for the phlebotomy service
- sharing common emergency service between local hospitals; turnaround time, safety of blood transfusion practice, and other quality measures of the emergency service must be maintained.

Increasing use of automated systems will also allow staff reduction,[11] although an estimate of savings must take account of capital and running costs of the equipment and whether it can be used to high capacity and ideally throughout a 24-h service.

Purchasing expensive equipment outright adds to the capital assets of the laboratory, with the consequential cost of depreciation (usually 8–10% per annum). Leasing equipment may be a better alternative and, in some countries, most equipment is obtained in this way. Careful calculation of the lease cost is required, as this can be up to 20% higher than outright purchase. Advantages of leasing include flexibility to upgrade equipment should workload increase or technology change. Inclusion of consumables and maintenance costs in the lease agreement allows total cost to be known for the duration of the lease.[1]

When automation is coupled with centralization of the service to another site, care must be taken to maintain service quality. Failure to do so will encourage clinicians to establish independent satellite laboratories. Loss of contact between clinical users and laboratory staff may compromise the pre-analytical phase of the test process and may lead to inappropriate requests, excessive requests, and test samples that are of inadequate volume or are poorly identified. When services are centralized, attention must be paid to all phases (pre-analytical, analytical and post-analytical) of the test process, including the need for packaging the specimens and the cost of their transport to the laboratory.

TEST SELECTION

Methods are selected for their reliability in terms of accuracy and precision (see p. 550). On the other hand, the selection of tests will be guided by their clinical utility, i.e. by their impact on diagnostic reasoning, their influence on treatment of patients, their reliability for screening asymptomatic individuals to detect occult disease and their usefulness for surveillance studies for disease prevalence. Economic aspects also need to be considered, with the least costly option for the same outcome being identified.

To evaluate the diagnostic utility and predictive value of an individual laboratory test, it is necessary to calculate test sensitivity and specificity.[12] Sensitivity is the percentage of true positive results when a test is applied to patients known to have the relevant disease or when results have been obtained by a reference method. Specificity is the percentage of true negative results when the test is applied to normals.

Diagnostic sensitivity $= \dfrac{TP}{(TP + FN)} \times 100\%$

Diagnostic specificity $= \dfrac{TN}{(TN + FP)} \times 100\%$

Positive predictive value $= \dfrac{TP}{(TP + FP)} \times 100\%$

Negative predictive value $= \dfrac{TN}{(TN + FN)} \times 100\%$

where TP = true positive; TN = true negative; FP = false positive; FN = false negative.

Sensitivity and specificity should be near 100% if the test is used to make a specific diagnosis. It is not usually possible to have both 100% sensitivity and 100% specificity as they tend to counter each other but a lower level of sensitivity or specificity may still be acceptable if the results are interpreted in conjunction with other tests as part of an overall pattern with sensitivity and specificity expressed as fractions.

Likelihood ratio

The ratio of positive results in disease to the frequency of false-positive results in normals gives a statistical measure of the discrimination by the test between disease and normality. It can be calculated in two different ways:

1. $\dfrac{\text{Sensitivity}}{1-\text{Specificity}}$.[13] The higher the ratio, the greater is the probability of disease, whilst a ratio <1 makes the possibility of the disease much less likely.

2. Sensitivity + Specificity – 1.[14] Values range between –1 and +1. There is an increasing probability of the disease with a positive ratio rising towards +1 and decreasing likelihood when the ratio falls from 0 to –1.

INSTRUMENTATION

Equipment evaluation

Evaluation of equipment to match the nature and volume of laboratory workload is a very important exercise. Protocols for evaluating blood cell counters and other haematology instruments have been published by the International Committee (now Council) for Standardization in Haematology.[15-17] The following are usually included in such evaluations:

1. Verification of instrument requirements for space and services.
2. Extent of technical training required to operate the instrument.
3. Clarity and usefulness of instruction manual.

4. Assessment of safety (mechanical, electrical, microbiological and chemical).
5. Determination of:
    a. linearity
    b. precision and imprecision*
    c. carry-over
    d. extent of inaccuracy by comparison with measurement by definitive or reference methods
    e. comparability with an established method used in the laboratory

---

*Precision refers to agreement between replicate measurements. It has no numerical values as it is recognized only in terms of imprecision which is the standard deviation/coefficient of variation of a set of replicate measurements.

f. sensitivity (i.e. determination of the smallest change in analyte concentration which gives a measured result)

g. specificity (i.e. extent of errors caused by interfering substances).

6. Throughput time and number of specimens that can be processed within a normal working day

7. Cost per test.

8. Reliability of the instrument when in routine use and adequacy of service and maintenance provided.

9. Staff acceptability, impact on laboratory organization and level of technical expertise required to operate the instrument.

As a rule, this type of evaluation is carried out by a reference laboratory on behalf of a national consumer organization or government health agency such as the Medical Devices Agency of the United Kingdom Department of Health, who list a large number of such reports in their catalogue.* After an instrument has been purchased and installed, however, a less extensive check of performance with regard to precision, linearity, carry-over and comparability is often useful and details are given below.

Precision

Carry out appropriate measurements 10 times consecutively on three or more specimens selected in the pathological range so as to include a low, a high and a normal concentration of the analyte. Calculate the replicate standard deviation (SD) and coefficient of variation (CV) as derived on page 613. The degree of precision which is acceptable depends on the purpose of the test (Table 23.4). To check between-batch precision, measure three samples in several successive batches of routine tests; calculate the SD and CV in the same way.

Linearity

This demonstrates the effects of dilution. Prepare a specimen with a high concentration of the analyte to be tested and, as accurately as possible, make a series of dilutions in plasma so as to obtain 10 samples with evenly spaced concentration levels between 10% and 100%. Measure each sample three times and calculate the means. Plot results on arithmetic graph paper. Ideally, all points

Table 23.4 Test precision for different purposes

Purpose of test	Expected CV% (automated counters)		
	Hb	RBC	WBC
Scientific standard State of art	<1	1	1–2
best performance	1.5	2	3
routine laboratories	2–3	3	5–6
Clinical needs	5–10	5	10–15

Hb, haemoglobin concentration; RBC, red cell count; WBC, white cell count.

should fall on a straight line which should pass through the zero of the horizontal and vertical axes. In practice, the results should lie within 2SD limits of the mean calculated from the CVs which have been obtained from analysis of precision (see above). Inspection of the graph will show whether there is linearity throughout the range or whether it is limited to part of the range.

Carry-over

This indicates the extent to which measurement of an analyte in a specimen is likely to be affected by the preceding specimen. Measure a specimen with a high concentration in triplicate, immediately followed by a specimen with a low concentration of the analyte, also in triplicate.

$$\text{Carry-over (\%)} = \frac{l_1 - l_3}{h_3 - l_3} \times 100$$

where l_1 and l_3 are the results of the first and third measurements of the samples with a low concentration and h_3 is the third measurement of the sample with a high concentration.

Accuracy and comparability

These test whether the new instrument (or method) gives results which agree satisfactorily with those obtained with an established procedure and with a reference method. Test specimens should be measured alternately, or in batches, by the two procedures. If results by the two methods are analysed by correlation coefficient (r), a high correlation does not mean that the two methods agree. Correlation coefficient is a measure of relation and not agreement. It is better to use the limits of agreement method.[18]

For this, plot the differences between paired results on the vertical axis of linear graph paper

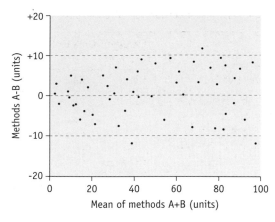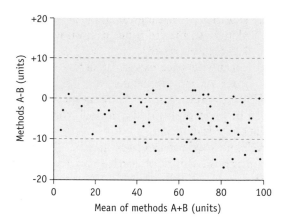

Fig. 23.1 Limits of agreement method. Shows mean values for paired results by two methods A plus B (horizontal axis) plotted against the differences (A minus B) between the paired results (vertical axis). Horizontal lines represent equality with range of ±10 units (mean ±SD). Left figure shows no bias between methods A and B, whereas right figure shows false high results (negative values) for method B or false low results for method A.

against the means of the pairs on the horizontal axis (Fig. 23.1); differences between the methods are then readily apparent over the range from low to high values. If the scatter of differences increases at high values, logarithmic transformed data should be plotted.

It is also useful to check for bias by including the instrument or method under test in the laboratory's participation in an external quality assessment scheme (p. 574). Bias is expressed by:

$$\frac{R - M}{M} \times 100\%$$

where R = measurement by the device/method being tested and M = target EQAS result.

Maintenance logs

All laboratory equipment should be inspected regularly and specific maintenance procedures carried out. Each item of laboratory equipment should have a maintenance log to document what maintenance is required, the desired frequency and when it was last carried out. The log includes servising and repairs by the manufacturer. Equipment used to test biological specimens must be cleaned thoroughly before a maintenance procedure is carried out to reduce the biohazard. The procedure for such cleaning must be documented (as a standard operating procedure) together with the name of the responsible worker and the date.

DATA PROCESSING

It is essential that accurate records of laboratory results are kept for whatever period is stipulated by national legislation. Computer-assisted data handling is essential for all but the smallest laboratory. For long-term storage of data, possibilities include a printed (hard) copy, a floppy disk, and the newer compact disc read-only memory (CD-ROM) or write once, read-many (WORM) systems that are read using a modified personal computer.

Laboratory results are usually issued as numerical data with abnormal results highlighted for the clinician. Report forms should be reader friendly. Serial data are particularly useful to illustrate any trend with time and may be in

the form of a cumulative numerical display or a graph. The latter is widely used to facilitate adjustment of dosage of drugs that affect haemopoiesis. An arithmetical scale should be used to display haemoglobin, red cell count and reticulocyte count, while platelet and leucocyte counts are best displayed on a logarithmic scale (Fig. 23.2).

LABORATORY COMPUTERS

Developments in computer technology have made available powerful microcomputers and sophisticated computer software at moderate

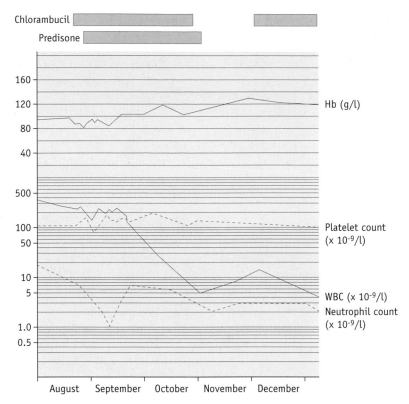

Fig. 23.2   Haematological chart for plotting blood count data on a time-related graph. This illustrates the course in a patient with chronic lymphocytic leukaemia. Haemoglobin is recorded arithmetically, the other parameters on a logarithmic scale. If reticulocytes are included, they should be recorded arithmetically.

prices. Such computers may be an integral part of an analytical instrument or interfaced to it by cable. A modem is required to link the computer to the telephone network for access to the internet and electronic mail. Stand-alone personal computers have wide application in haematology laboratories (Table 23.5).

When purchasing a personal computer for use in the laboratory, it should have adequate memory and speed, with room for expansion to run sophisticated programs. There is considerable attraction in interconnecting computers within a local area network to allow flexibility and data inter-change, and to enable multiple workers to use a common database. Larger computer systems catering for all the pathology disciplines require a larger RAM (e.g. 30–60 megabytes) and the purchase or lease of such systems requires considerable planning as to the necessary specification. Much time and effort are involved in the procurement process and expert advice is needed.

Table 23.5   Some uses of laboratory personal computers

Statistics

Graphics

Word processing

Creating lecture slides

Desktop publishing

Database files

Spreadsheets

Workload recording

Test costing and invoicing

Managing budgets

Stock control

Quality control procedures

Audit systems

Internet information

Electronic mail

Teaching/training materials, including morphology

Expert systems – clinical decision support

Helpful advice on the use of personal computers is provided in *ABC of Medical Computing* by Lee Millman[19] and there are also monographs specifically dealing with applications of the internet for health professionals.[20]

The internet provides access to a vast amount of information. Medline and other libraries provide citations and abstracts of articles from almost every medical journal in the world; many journals now provide full articles which can be read directly on the computer or printed out. The major publishers allow free or low cost access to these in developing countries. Many experts have their own web-sites for commentaries on their specialities, whilst manufacturers provide up-to-date information on their products.

It is impractical to provide a comprehensive index of the ever expanding list of relevant web-sites; Table 23.6 indicates some which are of particular interest to laboratory haematology.

Table 23.6 Some web-sites of haematological interest

National Library of Medicine for Medline database
www.ncbi.nlm.nih.gov/PubMed

Medline from British Medical Association (for registered members)
www.medline@bma.org.uk

British Medical Journal – electronic version of the weekly publication
www.bmj.com

The Lancet – electronic version of the weekly publication
www.thelancet.com

British Journal of Haematology
www.blacksci.co.uk/products/journals/toc/bjh.htm

Health information on the Internet with details of various sources
www.wellcome.ac.uk/healthinfo

World Health Organization (WHO) general information and library resources
www.who.ch or *www.who.int*

WHO Blood safety, clinical and laboratory technology; also includes links to ISH, ICSH, ISBT
www.who.int/bct/main areas of work

International Society of Haematology
www. *ish-ead.org*

International Council for Standardization in Haematology
www. *icshaem.org*

International Society on Thrombosis and Hemostasis
www.med.unc.edu/isth/welcome.htm

Royal College of Pathologists
www.rcpath.org

Institute of Biomedical Science
www.ibms.org

British Society for Haematology
www.blacksci.co.uk/uk/society/bsh/default.htm

Malaria diagnosis training programme
www.rph.wa.gov.au

J.O. Westgard's 'Lesson of the month' and other tutorials on quality assurance
www.westgard.com

The Hammersmith web journal of laboratory haematology
www.haem.net

PRE-ANALYTICAL AND POST-ANALYTICAL STAGES OF TESTING

The haematology laboratory should be concerned with the pre-analytical stage (test requesting, blood sample collection and transport to the laboratory) as well as the post-analytical stage (return of results to the clinician).

Test requesting

There is considerable variation between clinicians in their test-ordering patterns and the laboratory has historically exerted little influence on test-request pattern; sustained educational programmes have sometimes achieved more selective testing.[21] Unnecessary requests are often due to inappropriate request forms, such as where clinicians are able to tick from a list instead of requesting specific tests. Innovations in modifying requesting patterns have included use of problem-orientated request forms[22,23] and computer-assisted ordering of tests according to protocols written by specialist clinical teams.[24]

Sample collection and delivery

Blood sample collection by phlebotomists and manual delivery of specimen tubes to the laboratory by porters are traditionally performed by different work teams whose activities are not coordinated. Blood samples may therefore remain in clinical areas awaiting collection by porters who then follow a fixed circuit of other hospital areas before eventually reaching the laboratory. Once responsibility for blood collection and transport is held by the laboratory, however, these separate activities can be coordinated. Alternative and faster means of specimen delivery to laboratories include rail track or pneumatic tube conveyor systems.[25]

Return of results

Computer-assisted reporting of results to linked printers located in clinical areas is an ideal, but most hospitals rely on manual transport of result sheets and this can significantly prolong request completion times. Pneumatic tube and rail track conveyor systems used for the pre-analytical stage can also be used for rapid return of results to wards and clinics. Return of results is, of course, no guarantee that ward or clinic staff will react in a timely way to change a patient's treatment or even file report forms in the patient's medical record. Audit trials of selected test results are helpful in determining whether the sequence from requesting a test to taking clinical action has been completed.

Test turnaround time

Test turnaround time is most easily measured as the time lapse between arrival of a blood specimen in the laboratory and issue of the validated result. It is possible, but tedious, to use a date/time stamp to record manually the arrival and issue times for each request/report form. In a computerized laboratory, it is relatively easy to record these times and then to analyse the data to calculate the median time and the 95th percentile for completing each test; the percentage of tests completed within a pre-selected time is also of value.[26,27] Computer-assisted graphical presentation of the frequency distribution of completed tests is a useful way of displaying turnaround times for individual tests (Fig. 23.3).

Test turnaround time, as defined above, refers to the analytical stage of testing and excludes the time delay of the pre-analytical and post-analytical stages of testing. When the laboratory has responsibility for all three stages, it becomes possible to extend the measurement of analytical turnaround time to the more meaningful parameter of request completion time (total time from initiation of the request to delivery of the result to a clinician). This is becoming an increasingly important criterion of laboratory quality.[28,29] The speed with which modern systems perform reduces the need for interrupting the routine specimens for urgent ('stat') tests, but they still require an effective way to convey the urgent results to the clinician.[30]

POINT-OF-CARE TESTING

Point-of-care testing (POCT), also known as near-patient testing (NPT), functions at two levels, i.e. either as an adjunct to the laboratory within a hospital, or for primary health care outside the hospital.

Specialist clinical areas within hospitals have an increasing need for a customized laboratory service to meet their particular requirements. When rapid results are especially important, laboratory testing within the clinical area may be the

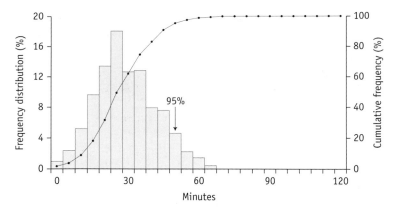

Fig. 23.3   Frequency histogram, cumulative percentage (■ – ■ – ■), and 95th percentile (arrow) showing analytical completion time for non-urgent prothrombin times.

best arrangement. Intensive care units have a long established need for near-patient monitoring of blood gases, but other clinicians use laboratory tests for monitoring ill patients and for making rapid decisions on treatment, e.g. in oncology out-patient clinics, and this has increased demand for a rapid results service. Instrument manufacturers are now developing haematology analysers for this market so that demand for haematology testing nearer the patient will increase.

Diagnostic laboratories are often located in areas of the hospital that are remote from critical care and out-patient areas. Rapid transit systems, including pneumatic tubes (see above), may be the preferred alternative to multiple satellite testing areas, particularly when the main laboratory already offers a 24-h rapid results service. Knowledge of test turnaround time (see Fig. 23.3) is required to make an informed decision on the need for NPT in satellite areas. When POCT is the preferred option, the running of the satellite laboratory and maintenance of its equipment must be the responsibility of the appropriate pathology discipline. This is essential for quality control, safety and accreditation whether the satellite is staffed by laboratory staff, as a full-time job in a busy location, or used by medical staff or nurses as a marginal activity. A designated member of laboratory staff should supervise this service, visiting each test location daily and ensuring that all results and quality control data are integrated into the main laboratory computer system. Some instruments designed for POCT will store quality control data on a computer floppy disk which can be removed

and taken to the main laboratory. Essential criteria for satisfactory near-patient working are described by Marks[31] and guidelines have been published by the *British Committee for Standards in Haematology*[32] and by the *Joint Working Group on Quality Assurance.*[33]

Laboratory services for general practitioners

The customers of a haematology laboratory include primary health care general practitioners/family doctors who have different priorities from hospital practitioners. Close attention to the general practitioner's needs is an important demonstration of the quality of the laboratory and this will encourage continued referral of patients after the initial use of the laboratory services. The customized service should include the following.

Quality assurance

General practitioners are not specialists in laboratory medicine and require evidence that a haematology laboratory provides a service of high quality. This may be based on accreditation of the laboratory, its participation in external quality control schemes, a good local reputation amongst other laboratory users, and a willingness to collaborate with general practitioners in a mutually beneficial audit programme.

Pre-analytical service

Education of the general practitioner is important. This may include a users' handbook or wallchart (to show the correct specimen container and volume of blood required), reference ranges, requirements for patient preparation (e.g. fasting), the timing of any medication that may affect the test result, and the turnaround time for each test. The latter is important so that patients can be given a follow-up appointment to be told the result. Handbooks should be of loose-leaf format to facilitate updating. An occasional laboratory news-sheet may also be of value, particularly when a new test or service is introduced. Education should also cover safety aspects, such as how to deal with blood spillage or a needlestick injury.

Efficient specimen collection and transport are also of high priority. A general practitioner may require health centre staff to be trained and accredited for collecting blood samples. A specimen transport system at an agreed time of day is particularly important so that patients can be given a suitable appointment for blood collection. Request forms should, as far as possible, be standardized, with one request form for all pathology requests.

Post-analytical service

The general practitioner needs a fast report service for abnormal test results to a direct telephone number or, preferably to the telefax at the health centre. To facilitate contact with the laboratory, there should be a direct dial help-line to the haematologist of the day. With transmission of results by telefax, there is a problem with confidentiality unless a computer-assisted call-back system is used to identify the correct recipient number before the data are transmitted. Direct transfer of encoded data by electronic mail from the laboratory computer to that of the practice may be justified for major users.

Point-of-care testing

This is increasingly popular in some countries, and it is particularly useful when patients live a distance away from a hospital laboratory. Instrument manufacturers are becoming aware of this market; they are now producing table-top or hand-held analysers which are simple to use, auto-calibrated and require minimum maintenance. The haematology tests which are commonly undertaken include haemoglobin, blood cell counting by simple analysers, erythrocyte sedimentation rate and prothrombin time for oral anticoagulation control.[34–37] In the UK, guidelines have been issued by the *Joint Working Group on Quality*

Assurance to assist health service managers and staff on the use of devices suitable for POCT.[33] But POCT may be applied more widely; as an example, studies on the management of anticoagulation control have shown that with appropriate training and cooperation from the laboratory, pharmacists are able to provide as reliable a service as the hospital-based one, and with more convenience for the patient.[38]

The laboratory should encourage the doctors and clinics to seek advice and help with the selection of appropriate instruments, their calibration and quality control, including a link into the external quality assessment scheme in which the laboratory participates. Harmonization of reports with laboratory records is helpful when a patient is referred to the hospital. A major source of error in POCT outside the hospital is faulty specimen collection; clinic staff who undertake this procedure should be given supervised training (see Ch. 1).

Patient self-testing

There is an increasing trend towards self-testing by patients, and glucose checks for self-management of diabetes mellitus are now routine practice. Simple portable precalibrated coagulometers which use capillary blood to measure prothrombin time and international normalized ratio are now available.[35] It has been shown that patients are able to use their instruments correctly and once their treatment has been established, the individual patients can be relied on to maintain their anticoagulation within the therapeutic range.[39] There are European standards to ensure that such instruments are reliable and that the instructions for their use are clear, unambiguous and written for the layperson.*

HEALTH AND SAFETY

Safety practice is essential in all aspects of the laboratory's work, including satellite near-patient test areas and satellite storage refrigerators for blood and blood products. Each haematology laboratory should designate a safety officer of sufficient seniority, and with authority to implement departmental safety policy in all sections of the labor-

---

*Instructions for use of in-vitro diagnostic instruments for self-testing (EN592); Information supplied by the manufacturer with in vitro diagnostic reagents for self-testing (EN376); General requirements for in vitro diagnostic medical devices for self-testing.

atory. The safety officer should be responsible for day-to-day management of safety issues and should be directly accountable to the head of department. Departmental safety policy should be documented as a booklet which is readily accessible in each section of the laboratory. A loose-leaf format facilitates updating. It must provide a comprehensive account of departmental safety policy and draw attention to known and potential hazards in relation to infection, fire, radiation and mechanical injury. Where a hazard cannot be eliminated, the risk should be reduced so far as is reasonably practicable, e.g. by reducing the frequency and period of exposure. The safety booklet should refer to relevant local, national and international safety legislation. In the UK, the Health Services Advisory Committee has set out rules for prevention of infections in clinical laboratories;[40] WHO has published comprehensive manuals on safety in health-care laboratories[41,56] and an international standard on safety management for medical laboratories is in preparation (ISO 15190). Aspects of safety policy relevant to a haematology laboratory are listed in Table 23.7.

There must be an established protocol for handling needlestick injury to a member of staff, with immediate referral to the appropriate hospital department of occupational health which should provide a 24-h advisory service.

The safety officer must have the training and time to do the job well and provide training for other staff who must not be allowed to handle potentially hazardous materials until they have completed training in accordance with the safety requirements. The safety officer should represent the laboratory on relevant safety committees and work closely with hospital occupational health, control of infection, and radiation protection officers. Within the department, a statutory safety committee should be established as a useful forum for safety audit.

HANDLING BIOHAZARDOUS SPECIMENS

All material of human origin should be regarded as capable of transmitting infection and handled accordingly in the laboratory. However, particular care is needed with material from patients suffering from hepatitis or human immunodeficiency virus (HIV) infection or patients from a high-risk group, e.g. haemophilia unit, liver unit, or from

Table 23.7 Some aspects of laboratory safety policy

Blood collection from high-risk patients

Labelling, transport and reception of specimens

Handling and containment of high-risk specimens

Location of protective equipment

Needlestick injury

Sharps disposal

Blood spillage

Hazard risk assessment for all substances in the laboratory

Near-patient testing

Protective clothing

Health records of staff, including immunization

Equipment maintenance and log books

Visitors to the department

Waste disposal including access to an autoclave

Electrical equipment testing

Recording of accidents

Safety cabinet monitoring

Laboratory cleaning policies

Laboratory security, including out-of-hours working

Policy for postal specimens

Radiation protection

Fire precautions

Training in safety

Safety inspections

Advisory service to general practitioners

countries with a high prevalence of infection. The laboratory safety policy must define the special precautions required when blood is collected from such patients and when specimens are handled in the laboratory.

Universal precautions for good safety practice include:

1. Personal hygiene precautions to be adopted in areas where specimens are handled and analytic work is carried out:
   — eating, drinking and applications of cosmetics absolutely forbidden

— staff should not wear jewellery, and ideally watches and rings should be removed
— gloves should be worn during sample handling and analytic work
— personal clothing should not be allowed to protrude beyond the sleeves of the protective clothing
— any exposed cuts or abrasions must be kept covered with waterproof dressings
— hands must be washed when leaving analytic areas.

2. Venepuncture to be performed wearing disposable thin plastic or rubber gloves. Care must be taken to prevent injuries when handling syringes and disposing of the needles. Do not recap used needles by hand; do not detach the needle from the syringe or break, bend, or otherwise manipulate used needles by hand. Used disposable syringes and needles, lancets and other sharp items such as glass slides, must be placed in a puncture-resistant plastic 'sharps' container for disposal. Care must be taken to avoid blood contamination of tourniquets as a potential cause of cross-infection.

3. As far as possible only disposable syringes, needles and lancets to be used. Disposable syringes and lancets must never be re-used on a different person.

4. Centrifugation to be performed in sealed centrifuge buckets.

5. Blood and bone marrow slides to be handled in the same way as blood samples until they are fixed in methanol, stained and covered with a cover glass.

6. Used material must be placed in designated biohazard plastic bags awaiting disposal (see below).

Additional precautions with high-risk material include:

1. Only experienced staff to perform procedures.
2. Specimens to be handled in a microbiological safety cabinet (if the procedure involves generation of an aerosol) or in a clearly segregated and designated area of the laboratory.
3. Specimens to be handled using protective clothing (close-fitting disposable plastic or thin rubber gloves, disposable plastic apron, glasses or goggles, face mask).

4. Disposable plastic to be used instead of glass-ware, and sharp-pointed instruments (e.g. scissors) should not be used.

5. On completion of the work, the laboratory bench must be disinfected immediately using freshly prepared 1% w/v sodium hypochlorite solution (10 000 p.p.m. available chlorine). Disposable pipettes should be used but, if re-usable pipettes are essential, they must be soaked in this solution for 30 min or longer. A 10% solution must be used for cleaning up spilled material. The diluted sodium hypochloride solution should be freshly made each day. It is helpful to add detergent to the solution as disinfectants are most active on clean surfaces.

6. Some automated equipment can be disinfected by flushing several times with 10% w/v sodium hypochlorite, or with 2% w/v glutaraldehyde, followed by several flushes with water. Only glutaraldehyde should be used in instruments with a metal surface as hypochlorite causes corrosion. Other instruments have special requirements for decontamination; always refer to the manufacturer's instructions.

Laboratory centrifuges require particular attention. Any spillage of blood should be dealt with immediately and the bowl, head and buckets (including rubber pads) should be disinfected regularly with 2% w/v glutaraldehyde solution. Centrifuges should never be cleaned using hypochlorite solution or other metal corrosives. Special care is required when a glass or plastic tube breaks in a centrifuge (Table 23.8).

Waste disposal

Blood and other potentially infected body fluids can safely be poured down a drain provided that the drain is connected to a sanitary sewer. Laboratory waste, such as specimen containers, used syringes, swabs and tissues, should be collected in special colour-coded bags for subsequent incineration or autoclaving before being disposed of in a rubbish dump. 'Sharps' containers should be incinerated without opening.

Soiled laundry must be placed in leak-proof labelled bags for transport to the laundry where the items should be washed in hot water (>70°C) with detergent for 25–30 min before being rinsed,

Table 23.8 Recommended procedure for decontaminating a centrifuge after breakage of a tube

1. Switch off centrifuge motor and do not open lid for 30 min. Inform the safety officer.
2. When breakage involves a known high-risk specimen in a sealed bucket, gloves, goggles and a protective apron must be worn and the bucket opened in a safety cabinet.
3. Strong gloves must be worn and forceps used when removing solid debris. All broken tubes, fragments of glass or plastic, buckets, trunnions and rotor should be placed in 2% w/v glutaraldehyde solution for 24 h.
4. The centrifuge bowl should be washed with 2% w/v glutaraldehyde solution, left to dry, and washed again.
5. All contaminated disposable material must be placed in appropriate bags for autoclaving.

or alternatively soaked in disinfectant (see above) before being washed by hand.

Toxic or carcinogenic reagents

Manufacturers' product safety data sheets must be checked for advice on safe handling of any potentially hazardous substances. Such reagents must be stored in a secure place with restricted access; they should be handled only by experienced staff wearing protective clothing, and weighing should be carried out in a fume cupboard whose air flow is regularly monitored (face velocity of around 0.8 m/s).

Specimen transport

There are strict national and international regulations about packaging and shipment of patients' specimens and other biological material.[42-44]

STANDARD OPERATING PROCEDURES

Standard operating procedures (SOPs) are written instructions which are intended to maintain optimal consistent quality of performance in the laboratory. They should cover all aspects of work, some relating to test procedures, others to specimen collection, laboratory safety, handling urgent requests, data storage, telephone reporting policy, etc. They may be based on standard textbook descriptions or an instrument manufacturer's instruction manual, but they should reflect daily practice and each laboratory must prepare its own individual set of SOPs. They should be reviewed once a year and any revisions must be highlighted with the date. A suggested format for an SOP is given in Table 23.9.

LABORATORY AUDIT AND ACCREDITATION

Audit

Laboratory audit is the systematic and critical analysis of the quality of the laboratory service. The essence of audit is that it should be continuous and designed to achieve incremental improvement in quality of the day-to-day service. It should encompass the pre-analytical, analytical, and post-analytical stages of laboratory practice; some examples are given in Table 23.10.

The first stage of audit is to define the standard to be achieved and this may be in the form of a SOP for an analytical procedure, a protocol for test ordering, pre-surgery blood transfusion order schedule, or a target turnaround time. These standards will have been agreed within the laboratory in conjunction with relevant users of the laboratory. Clinical input is invaluable in discussing the clinical significance of analyser-generated results,

effectiveness of laboratory reports, advantages and disadvantages of POCTs.[45,46] To monitor performance against the agreed standards, each laboratory section should form its own audit group or, if there is an audit group for the whole department, it should be open to all grades of staff to allow peer review and to take advantage of the educational value of audit. Laboratory staff should lead the audit process rather than having it imposed upon them. It is good practice to make a short report of each audit meeting, recording attendance, the items identified for improvement, and an action list.

The audit process improves quality simply by examining and questioning established standards and guidelines. The ever increasing need for cost effectiveness is likely to forge closer working relationships between the different pathology

Table 23.9 Format for a standard operating procedure (SOP)

Cover page
Title, reference number, date of preparation; name of composer

Scope
Purpose of the SOP; principles of procedure or test; grade(s) of staff permitted to undertake the task(s)

Specimen requirements
Type and amount; delivery arrangements; storage conditions and any time or temperature restrictions

Specimen reception
Registration and check of request form; criteria for rejecting a specimen

Safety precautions
Obligatory protection requirements
Handling 'high-risk' samples

Equipment and reagents
Lists of equipment, apparatus, reagents, controls, calibrators, forms and other stationery

Test procedure
Step-by-step details of method; calculation of results; quality control checks

Reporting
Procedure for reporting results for routine and urgent requests

Clinical significance
An understanding of the clinical reason for the test and significance of abnormal results;
Reference range for healthy subjects

Test limitations
How to recognize errors and steps to avoid or correct them

Maintenance of equipment
List of schedule for routine in-house maintenance (daily, weekly), and servicing

Specimen storage post-test
Period of retention and conditions for storage; instructions for disposal of specimens and diluted sub-samples

List of relevant literature

disciplines, as well as between laboratories within the same discipline. This changing laboratory environment highlights the need for continuous training of haematology staff in good laboratory management and the importance of audit.

Accreditation

The purpose of laboratory accreditation schemes is to allow external audit of a laboratory's organization, management, quality assurance programme, and level of user satisfaction. The advantage to the accredited laboratory is that this indicates to clinical users that it has a defined standard of practice which has been independently confirmed by external peer review. Such review should include assessment of basic functional structure (laboratory facilities such as staff and equipment), processes (test analyses), outcome (quality of test results including timeliness and interpretation), interaction with clinical users and optimal use of resources. The International Standards Organization (ISO) has established guidelines for quality management and quality standards (ISO 9000 series, ISO 17025 and ISO/IEC Guide 25). In some countries, certification of conformity to these requirements is undertaken by government-authorized bodies such as the UK Accreditation Service (UKAS) and the European Accreditation of Laboratories (EAL), while in the USA there is legislation known as the Clinical Laboratories Improvement Act (CLIA 1988). In the UK, the majority of clinical laboratories are accredited by a professional authority, Clinical

Table 23.10 Examples of laboratory audit

Education of laboratory users

Appropriateness of test requests

Test menu in response to clinical needs

Appropriateness of blood samples (e.g. adequate volume)

Interpretation of abnormal results

Timeliness of reports

Internal quality control results

External quality assessment scheme performance

Cost effectiveness of specialist tests

Reporting of abnormal results

Compliance with safety policies

Use of blood and blood products

Frequency and cause of transfusion reactions

Turnaround time for emergency requests

Satisfaction of out-patients undergoing venepuncture

Satisfaction of laboratory users

Pathology Accreditation (CPA Ltd), which undertakes a similar activity but with less checking on test performance provided that the laboratories participate in an approved external quality assessment scheme.[47-50] Descriptions of the requirements for national accreditation programmes are available for the USA,[49-52] Australia,[53] and the UK.[47] Overviews of how various laboratory accreditation schemes function have been published.[48,54,55] An important component of all accreditation programmes is participation in proficiency testing/external quality assessment schemes. These schemes are required to conform to standards which are specified in ISO/IEC Guide 43 and by the International Laboratory Accreditation Co-operative in the ILAC Guidance document G13/2000 (*Requirements for the competence of providers of proficiency testing schemes*).

REFERENCES

1 Stuart J, Bull BS 1995 Laboratory organization management and economics. In: Lewis SM, Koepke JA (eds) Haematology laboratory management and practice. Butterworth Heinemann, Oxford, ch 7.

2 Stuart J, Hicks JM 1991 Good laboratory management: an Anglo-American perspective. Journal of Clinical Pathology 44:793–797.

3 Peck C, McCall M, McLaren B, et al 2000 Continuing medical education and continuing professional development: international comparisons. British Medical Journal 320:432–435.

4 Royal College of Pathologists 1999 Continuing professional development. Royal College of Pathologists, London.

5 Du Boulay C 1999 Continuing professional development: some new perspectives. Journal of Clinical Pathology 52:162–164.

6 Institute of Biomedical Science 2000 Continuing professional development for biomedical scientists. IBMS, London.

7 College of American Pathologists Workload and Personnel Management Committee 1992 Workload recording method and personnel management manual. College of American Pathologists, Northfield, Ill.

8 Statistics Canada 1998 Canadian workload measurement system. A schedule of unit values for clinical laboratory procedures. Canadian Government Publishing Centre, Ottawa.

9 Bennett CHN 1991 Welcan UK: its development and future. Journal of Clinical Pathology 44:617–620.

10 Tarbit IF 1990 Laboratory costing system based on number and type of test: its association with the Welcan measurement system. Journal of Clinical Pathology 43:92–97.

11 Macdonald AJ, Bradshaw AE, Holmes WA, et al 1996 The impact of an integrated haematology screening system on laboratory practice. Clinical and Laboratory Haematology 18:271–276.

12 Galen RS, Gambino S 1975 Beyond normality: the predictive value and efficiency of medical diagnoses. Wiley, New York.

13 Griner PF, Nayawski RJ, Mushlin AI, et al 1981 Selection and interpretation of diagnostic tests and procedures: principles and applications. Annals of Internal Medicine 94:553–563.

14 Youden WJ 1950 Index for rating diagnostic tests. Cancer 3:32–35.

15 International Committee for Standardization in Haematology 1978 Protocol for type testing equipment and apparatus used for haematological analysis. Journal of Clinical Pathology 31:275–279.

16 International Council for Standardization in Haematology 1994 Guidelines for the evaluation of blood cell analysers including those used for differential leucocyte and reticulocyte counting and

cell marker applications. Clinical and Laboratory Haematology 16:157–174.

17 International Council for Standardization in Haematology 1993 ICSH recommendations for measurement of erythrocyte sedimentation rate. Journal of Clinical Pathology 46:198–203.

18 Bland JM, Altman DG 1986 Statistical methods for assessing agreement between two methods of clinical measurement. Lancet i:307–310.

19 Lee N, Millman A 1996 ABC of medical computing. BMA Publishing, London.

20 Kiley R 1996 Medical information on the internet: a guide for health professionals. Churchill Livingstone, Edinburgh.

21 Bareford D, Hayling A 1990 Inappropriate use of laboratory services: long term combined approach to modify request patterns. British Medical Journal 301:1305–1307.

22 Fraser CG, Woodford FP 1987 Strategies to modify the test-requesting patterns of clinicians. Annals of Clinical Biochemistry 24:223–231.

23 Wong ET, Lincoln TL 1983 Ready! Fire! ... Aim! An inquiry into laboratory test ordering. Journal of the American Medical Association 250:2510–2513.

24 Mutimer D, McCauley B, Nightingale P, et al 1992 Computerised protocols for laboratory investigation and their effect on use of medical time and resources. Journal of Clinical Pathology 45:572–574.

25 Keshgegian AA, Bull GE 1992 Evaluation of a soft-handling computerized pneumatic tube specimen delivery system. Effects on analytical results and turnaround time. American Journal of Clinical Pathology 97:535–540.

26 Westgard JO, Burnett RW, Bowers GN 1990 Quality management science in clinical chemistry: a dynamic framework for continuous improvement of quality. Clinical Chemistry 36:1712–1716.

27 Valenstein PN 1996 Laboratory turnabout time. American Journal of Clinical Pathology 105:676–688.

28 Hilbourne LH, Oye RK, McArdle JE, et al 1989 Use of specimen turnaround time as a component of clinician expectations with laboratory performance. American Journal of Clinical Pathology 92:613–618.

29 Winkelman JW, Tansijevic MJ, Wynbenga DR, et al 1997 How fast is fast enough for clinical laboratory turnabout time: measurement of the interval between result entry and inquiries for reports. American Journal of Clinical Pathology 108:400–405.

30 Hillbourne L, Lee H, Cathcart P 1996 STAT testing? A guideline for meeting clinical turnaround time requirements. American Journal of Clinical Pathology 105:671–675.

31 Marks V 1988 Essential considerations in the provision of near-patient testing facilities. Annals of Clinical Biochemistry 25:220–225.

32 England JM, Hyde K, Lewis SM, et al 1995 Guide-lines for near patient testing: haematology. Clinical and Laboratory Haematology 17:301–310.

33 Joint Working Group on Quality Assurance 1999 Guidelines: Near to patient or point of care testing. Clinical and Laboratory Haematology 21 (Supplement – Advancing Laboratory Haematology):31–34.

34 Baer DM, Belsey RE 1995 Physician's office testing. In: Lewis SM, Koepke JA (eds) Haematology laboratory management and practice. Butterworth Heinemann, Oxford, ch 5.

35 Machin SJ, Mackie IJ, Chitolie A, et al 1996 Near patient testing (NPT) in haemostasis – a synoptic review. Clinical and Laboratory Haematology 18:69–74.

36 Cachia PG, McGregor E, Adlakha S, et al 1998 Accuracy and precision of the TAS analyzer for near-patient INR testing by non-pathology staff in the community. Journal of Clinical Pathology 51:68–72.

37 Rose PE, Fitzmaurice D 1998 New approaches to the delivery of anticoagulant services. Blood Reviews 12:84–90.

38 Radley AS, Hall J, Farrow M, et al 1995 Evaluation of anticoagulant control in a pharmacist operated anticoagulant clinic. Journal of Clinical Pathology 48:545–547.

39 Ansell JE, Patel N, Ostrovsky D, et al 1995 Long term patient self-management of oral anticoagulation. Archives of Internal Medicine 155:2185–2189.

40 United Kingdom Health and Safety Executive 1991 Safe working and the prevention of infections in clinical laboratories. Stationery Office, Norwich NR3 1GN.

41 World Health Organization 1997 Safety in health-care laboratories – Document LAB/97.1. WHO (Blood Safety and Clinical Technology), Geneva.

42 National Committee for Clinical Laboratory Standards 1994 Procedures for handling and transport of diagnostic specimens and etiological agents H5-A3. NCCLS, Wayne, PA.

43 United Nations 1993 Recommendations on the transport of dangerous goods, 8th edn. United Nations, New York.

44 European Committee for Standardization 1996 Transport packages for medical and biological specimens – requirements, tests EN 829. CEN, Brussels.

45 Gray TA, Freedman DB, Burnett D, et al 1996 Evidence based practice: clinicians use and attitudes to near patient testing. Journal of Clinical Pathology 49:903–908.

46 Klee GG, Spackman KA, Habermann TM 1995 Targeting the usage and reporting of haematological laboratory tests to help streamline patient care. In: Lewis SM, Koepke JA (eds) Haematology laboratory management and practice. Butterworth Heinemann, Oxford, ch 17.

47 Advisory task force on standards to the audit steering committee of the Royal College of Pathologists 1991 Pathology department accreditation in the United Kingdom: a synopsis. Journal of Clinical Pathology 44:798–802.

48 Bachner P, Hamlin WB 1995 Regulatory and professional standards affecting clinical laboratories. In: Lewis SM, Koepke JA (eds) Haematology laboratory management and practice. Butterworth Heinemann, Oxford, ch 20.

49 Batjer JD 1990 The College of American Pathologists laboratory accreditation programme. Clinical and Laboratory Haematology 2 (Suppl. 1):135–138.

50 College of American Pathologists 1998 Standards for laboratory accreditation. College of American Pathologists, Northfield, Ill.

51 National Committee for Clinical Laboratory Standards 1996 Clinical laboratory technical procedures manual – third edition; approved guideline GP2-A3. NCCLS, Wayne, PA.

52 National Committee for Clinical Laboratory Standards 1995 Training verification for laboratory personnel; approved guideline GP21-A. NCCLS, Wayne, PA.

53 Hynes AF, Lea AR, Hailey DM 1989 Pathology laboratory accreditation in Australia. Australian Journal of Medical Laboratory Science 10:12–16.

54 Burnett D 1993 Laboratory accreditation – an overview. Journal of the International Federation of Clinical Chemistry 5:146–151.

55 Phillips PK, Voak D, Smith K, et al. 1994 The illusion of quality in quality management systems: meaningful accreditation. Transfusion Medicine 4:179–183.

56 World Health Organization 1993 Laboratory Biosafety Manual 2nd edn. WHO, Geneva.

Quality assurance

S. Mitchell Lewis

Quality assurance in the haematology laboratory is intended to ensure the reliability of the laboratory tests. The objective is to achieve reliable test results by precision and accuracy. *Accuracy* refers to the closeness of the estimated value to that considered to be true. *Precision* refers to the reproducibility of a result, but a test can be precise without being accurate. Inaccuracy and/or imprecision occur as a result of using unreliable standards or reagents, incorrect instrument calibration, or poor technique, e.g. consistently faulty dilution or the use of a method that gives a reaction that is incomplete or not specific for the test.

Precision can be controlled by replicate tests and by repeated tests on previously measured specimens. Accuracy can, as a rule, be checked only by the use of reference materials which have been assayed by reference methods

A quality assurance programme includes internal quality control, external quality assessment and standardization. It must also ensure adequate control of the pre- and post-analytic stages from specimen collection (see Ch. 1) to the timely despatch of an informative report (see p. 554).

Internal quality control is based on monitoring the haematology test procedures that are performed in the laboratory. It includes measurements on specially prepared materials, and repeated measurements on routine specimens, as well as statistical analysis, day by day, of data obtained from the tests which have been routinely carried out. There is thus continual evaluation of the reliability of the work of the laboratory with validation of tests before reports are released.

External quality assessment (EQA) is evaluation by an outside agency of the performance by a number of laboratories on specially supplied samples. Analysis of performance is retrospective. The objective is to achieve between-laboratory and between-method comparability, but this does not necessarily guarantee accuracy unless the specimens have been assayed by a reference laboratory alongside a reference preparation of known value. Schemes are usually organized on a national or regional basis. National schemes are usually known by the acronym NEQAS. Proficiency testing is the term used mainly in the USA to describe the procedures by which EQAS functions.

Standardization refers to both materials and methods. A *material standard* or *reference preparation* is used to calibrate analytic instruments and to assign a quantitative value to calibrators. Where possible it must be traceable to a defined physical or chemical measurement based on the metrological units of length (metre), mass (kilogram), amount of substance (mole) and time (seconds). A *reference method* is an exactly defined technique which provides sufficiently accurate and precise data for it to be used to assess the validity of other methods. The main international authority concerned with material standards (reference preparations) in haematology is the World Health Organization (WHO).[1,2] In the European Union, the Institute for Reference Materials and Measurements has produced a number of standards of '*certified reference materials*' for haematology and clinical chemistry (see p. 607). *International standards* are not freely available and are not intended for routine use but serve as standards for assigning values to commercial (or laboratory produced) '*secondary standards*' or *calibrators. Controls* are preparations which are used for either internal quality control or external quality

assessment. Some control preparations have assigned values (see below) but they must not be used as standards as the assigned values are usually only approximations.

Standardization of methods and devices are the concern of the *International Council for Standardization in Haematology* (ICSH)[3] whose recommendations are published in haematological journals. Increasingly, the *International Organization of Standardization* (ISO) and the *Comité Européen de Normalisation* (CEN) are also establishing standards for medical laboratory practice.[4] In the UK, the *British Committee for Standards in Haematology* (BCSH)* publishes guidelines in journals and as monographs;[5] in the USA, a wide range of practice guidelines have been published by the *National Committee for Clinical Laboratory Standards* (NCCLS).**

In this chapter, principles of quality assurance are described and the blood count is used as an illustrative model. Method and/or material standards which are available for various tests are referred to in the sections of this book where these tests are described.

REFERENCE PREPARATIONS

HAEMOGLOBIN AND BLOOD COUNT STANDARDS

The availability of an international reference preparation (see p. 607)[6] has contributed to improved accuracy of Hb measurement. In several countries, working standards are prepared which conform to the international standard and the appropriate national authority certifies that this is so. A limited quantity of the international standard can be obtained from WHO† and a comparable certified reference material is available in Europe.†† A method for preparing a lysate is described on page 568.

As whole blood can be kept only for a short time, it cannot be used as an alternative to a

haemiglobincyanide (HiCN) standard for calibration purposes except by an indirect procedure (p. 23). However, both whole blood and lysates are of use in quality assurance as differences in results obtained with these preparations help to distinguish errors owing to incorrect dilution from those owing to inadequate mixing or failure of a reagent to bring about complete lysis. Whole blood reference samples should be introduced into a batch of blood samples and all the samples assayed together. This is applicable to both automated and manual methods.

---

† WHO International Laboratory for Biological Standards, see p. 609.

†† EC Institute for Reference Materials and Measurements, see p. 609.

*A list of the publications is available from the British Society of Haematology, 2 Carlton House Terrace, London SW1 5AF; Fax: +44 20 7770 0933 or from www.blacksci.co.uk/society/bsh.

**Catalogue from NCCLS, 940 West Valley Road, Wayne PA 19087–1898, USA; Fax: +1-610 688 0700; www.nccls.org.

Blood cells

Standard preparations are essential for the calibration of electronic particle counters, especially automated systems which can be adjusted arbitrarily. This means that to obtain a true result the machine has to be calibrated using a reference preparation with assigned values of known accuracy.

Natural blood, collected into EDTA, is of no value as a reference preparation because of its short life in the laboratory. Various methods to preserve blood without affecting the blood count parameters have been tried,[7–9] and commercial products using preserved blood are now available. Blood will keep for a few weeks at 4°C if acid-citrate-dextrose (ACD) or citrate-phosphate-dextrose (CPD) has been added to it. Even so, the mean cell volume (MCV) slowly increases and some of the red cells lyse, with the result that the blood cannot be regarded as a reference material, although it can be used as a control preparation to check the precision and reliable functioning of a cell counting system over relatively short periods of time.[7,8]

Attempts have been made to provide suitably sized particles in stable suspension as substitutes for normal blood cells. These include fixed red cells and spherical latex particles.[3,10] The cells can be permanently stabilized by fixation, especially in glutaraldehyde solution. The glutaraldehyde causes red cells to shrink in size immediately, and the shrinking process continues for 3 to 4 days. Thereafter, the cells remain constant in size and shape, and the results of cell counts and cell size distribution remain the same for months or even years. The drawback in their use as a reference standard is that fixed red cells are inflexible biconcave discs with flow properties which differ from that of fresh blood in analytic systems, so that they cannot be used to calibrate an instrument for subsequent measurement of natural blood.[11,12] Latex spheres are available in defined sizes and may be used as primary reference materials for sizing platelets and red cells provided that a reliable 'shape factor' can be established for the latter.[10]

For total leucocyte counts, two types of material have been used successfully as standard reference materials, at least with simple analysers, but these fixed preparations may not be suitable for use with modern systems.

1. Leucocytes concentrated from human blood and fixed in the following solution:[13]

glacial acetic acid 42 mg; sodium sulphate 7 g; sodium chloride 7 g; water to 1 litre.

2. Glutaraldehyde-fixed erythrocytes suspended in leucocyte-free mammalian whole blood.[14] Turkey or chicken blood is suitable for the total leucocyte count. Different animal species can provide cells of sizes comparable to those of the differential leucocytes count; however, other physical properties of the different types of leucocyte are not paralleled in the reference materials, so that such preparations are unsuitable as direct standards for automated differential counts based on identifying cells by their various physical properties.

Assigning values

Methods used for assigning values to reference materials must be as accurate and precise as is practical. Standardized reference methods have been described for haemoglobin,[6] RBC and WBC[15] and packed cell volume (PCV).[16]

QUALITY CONTROL MATERIALS

There are problems in preparation of control material for any tests. Stored plasma for chemical or serological analysis may, for example, be affected by unstable enzymes in plasma, interference in immunological reactions by added preservatives, and effects of plasma turbidity. With the blood count, there are especially difficult problems because of the need to ensure homogeneity in aliquot samples and the instability of blood cells, whilst procedures that enhance the stability of blood samples distort the behaviour of the cells, so that control material is not strictly analogous to fresh blood. Nonetheless, provided attention is paid to these difficulties, preserved or stabilized blood provides suitable material for internal quality control procedures for haemoglobin, red cell counts and leucocyte counts. Blood collected into ACD or CPD (see p. 603) and passed through a blood-infusion set to remove any clots is suitable. For lysates, blood in EDTA or heparin is also suitable. Care should be taken at all stages to avoid contamination. Where possible, sterile glassware and reagents should be used and aseptic handling procedures adopted. To help maintain sterility, broad-spectrum antibiotics should be added to the product, e.g. 1 mg of penicillin together with 5 mg of gentamycin per 100 ml.

When human blood is used, it should be handled in the same way as a patient's sample (see p. 557), and where possible, it should first be checked to ensure that it is negative for hepatitis B and C and HIV.

Preparation of preserved blood[14,17]

1. Collect blood into a sterile container (e.g. a blood transfusion donor bag) with ACD or CPD anticoagulant (p. 603). Leave for 2 to 3 days at 4°C.
2. Centrifuge the blood for 20 min at c 2000 g. Separate (and keep) the supernatant plasma but discard the buffy coat. Transfer the red cell concentrate into 500 ml bottles.
3. Mix 3 volumes of the red cells with 1.5 volumes of 9 g/l NaCl, centrifuge for 20 min at c 2000 g and remove the supernatant and upper layer of the red cells by suction.
4. Repeat step 3.
5. Dilute 5 volumes of the plasma with 2 volumes of 9 g/l NaCl and add antibiotic.
6. Add the diluted plasma from step 5 to the red cell concentrate at an appropriate ratio to obtain a preparation suitable for use as a red cell count control.
7. Mix well and, with continuous mixing, dispense in aliquot volumes into clean sterile vials, and cap tightly. Store at 4°C.

Assign values for Hb, red cell count and PCV by at least 5 replicate measurements, using the counter on which the subsequent tests will be performed. Before analysis, mix the sample on a roller mixer or continuously by hand for 5 min before opening. The between-test coefficient of variation (CV) should not exceed 2%. Check between-sample homogeneity of dispensing by repeated counts on five randomly selected vials. Unopened vials of human blood should keep in good condition for about 3 weeks at 4°C, equine blood for up to 2 months.[17] Equine blood has an added advantage that it can be used to simulate microcytic human blood as horse red cells have an MCV of c 50 fl.[7]

Preparation of lysate

1. Collect blood as described above, e.g. into a blood transfusion donor bag. Out-of-date donor blood can be used provided that it is not lysed. Centrifuge at c 2000 g for 20 min and discard the plasma and buffy coat.
2. Add an equal volume of 9 g/l NaCl, mix well, transfer to a sterile centrifuge bottle and re-centrifuge; discard the supernatant. Repeat the saline wash three times to ensure complete removal of the plasma, leucocytes and platelets.
3. To each 10 ml volumes of the washed cells, add 6 volumes of water and 4 volumes of toluene, cap and shake vigorously on a mechanical shaker or vibrator for 1 h. Then keep overnight at 4°C to allow the lipid/cell debris to form a semi-solid surface between the toluene and lysate.
4. On the following day, centrifuge at c 2000 g for 20 min, remove the lysate layers and pool them in a clean bottle.
5. Using gentle vacuum suction, e.g. by water-pump, filter the lysate through coarse filter paper (e.g. Whatman No. 1) in a Buchner funnel. Repeat filtration using 0.22 μm micropore or fine filter paper (e.g. Whatman No. 42), changing the paper whenever the filtration slows down. It is important not to overload the funnel with lysate.
6. To each 70 ml of lysate, add 30 ml of glycerol and broad-spectrum antibiotic (see above). If a lower Hb is required, add 30% glycerol in saline. Mix well, dispense into sterile containers and cap tightly.
7. Assign a value for Hb concentration by the spectrophotometric method (p. 23); carry out 10 replicate tests, taking samples at random from several vials of the batch. The CV should be less than 2%. Stored at 4°C, the product should retain its assigned value for at least several months, or for 1 to 2 years if kept at −20°C.

PREPARATION OF STABILIZED WHOLE BLOOD CONTROL[18]

Reagent

Formaldehyde 37–40%   6.75 ml
Glutaraldehyde 50%   0.75 ml

Trisodium citrate	26 g
Water to	100 ml.

Method

1. Obtain whole blood in CPD or ACD. This should be as fresh as possible and never more than 48 h old. Filter through a 40 µm blood filter into a series of plastic bottles.
2. If an increased red cell count is required, centrifuge one (or more) of the samples and remove part of the plasma; if a lower red cell count is required, add to another sample the plasma which was removed. If paired bottles are gently centrifuged (c 1500 g) for 15 min to produce buffy coats, these can then be manipulated in a similar way to provide different levels of leucocyte and platelet counts. Add broad-spectrum antibiotic (see above) to each sample.
3. Mix well and add 1 volume of reagent to 50 volumes of the cell suspension. Mix on a mechanical mixer for 1 h at room temperature and leave for 24 h at 4°C.
4. With continuous mixing, dispense into sterile containers; cap tightly and seal with plastic tape. Refrigerate at 4°C until needed. Unopened vials should keep in good condition for several months at 4°C.

For analysis, samples should be gently mixed on a roller mixer or by hand before opening. Assign values for Hb and cell counts by at least five replicate tests and check between-sample homogeneity by repeated counts on five randomly selected vials. CV should not exceed 2%. Note, however, that the PCV by centrifugation will be c 10% lower than the haematocrit obtained by automated counters.

Simple method for blood count quality control preparations

The method described below provides a suitable preparation for control of total red cell, leucocyte and platelet counting by some semi-automated blood cell counters, but it is not suitable for some automated systems. It should be stable for c 3 weeks if kept at 4°C.

Method

Collect a unit of human blood into CPD anticoagulant (p. 603). Carry out the subsequent procedure no later than 1 day after collection.

Filter the blood through a blood transfusion recipient set into a 500 ml glass bottle.

Add 1 ml of fresh 40% formaldehyde. Mix well by inverting and then leave on a roller mixer for 1 h.

Leave at 4°C for 7 days, mixing by inverting a few times each day. At the end of this period of storage, mix well on a roller mixer for 20 min and then, with constant mixing by hand, dispense in 2 ml volumes into sterile containers.

PREPARATION OF SURROGATE LEUCOCYTES[15]

Chicken and turkey red blood cells are nucleated, and when fixed their size is within the human leucocyte range as recognized on electronic cell counters. They are thus suitable to serve as surrogate leucocytes. However, such material may not be suitable for the newer counting systems which are based on technologies other than impedance cell sizing.

For use as a white blood cell control, 25 ml of blood collected into any anticoagulant will suffice; after processing, an appropriate amount is added to preserved whole blood. Sterility must be maintained throughout the procedure.

Method

1. Centrifuge blood at c 2000 g for 20 min and remove the plasma aseptically.
2. Add an equal volume of 0.15 mol/l phosphate buffer, pH 7.4 (p. 605); mix and transfer to a sterile centrifuge bottle; recentrifuge and discard the supernatant and buffy coat.
3. Repeat the wash and centrifugation twice. To the washed cells, add 10 times their volume of glutaraldehyde fixative (0.25% in 0.15 mol/l phosphate buffer, pH 7.4). Leave overnight at 4°C.
4. On the next day, shake vigorously to ensure complete resuspension. Mix on a mechanical mixer for 1 h. To check that fixation has been complete, centrifuge 2–3 ml of the suspension, discard the supernatant and add water to the deposit. If lysis occurs, the stock glutaraldehyde requires replacement.
5. When fixation is complete (i.e. after 18 h exposure), centrifuge the suspension at c 2000 g for 10 min and discard the supernatant. Add an equal volume of water to the fixed cell deposit, resuspend and mix by stirring and shaking;

recentrifuge at c 2000 g for 10 min and discard the supernatant; repeat twice.

6. Resuspend the fixed cells to c 30% concentration in 9 g/l NaCl. Mix well with vigorous shaking. Add antibiotic (see p. 568), cap tightly, seal with a plastic seal and store at 4°C.

Before use, stand at room temperature for 10–20 min; then resuspend by vigorous shaking by hand or on a vortex mixer until no clumps remain at the base of the container, and then mix on a rotary mixer for at least 20 min before opening the vial.

For use as a WBC surrogate, after resuspension as described above, transfer an appropriate amount to a volume of preserved blood from which the leucocytes have been depleted by passing through a leucocyte filter. Establish the count by 5 to 10 replicate measurements on three vials and check intersample homogeneity by counts on three random vials from the batch. The CV should be not more than 5%.

An occasional batch may be found to be unsatisfactory and should be discarded.

QUALITY CONTROL PREPARATION FOR PLATELET COUNTS[14]

Reagents

Alsever's solution. (A) Trisodium citrate, 16 g; NaCl, 8.2 g to 1 litre with water; (B) Dextrose, 41 g to 1 litre with water.

Store at 4°C. Immediately before use, mix equal volumes of A and B; filter through 0.2 μm micropore filter.

EDTA solution. 100 g/l of K_2 EDTA in the Alsever's solution; stable for 6 months at 4°C.

Method

1. Collect a unit of blood into ACD or CPD anticoagulant. Centrifuge for 10 min at 200 g and collect the platelet suspension into a plastic container.
2. Add 1 ml of EDTA solution. Mix well and leave at 37°C for 2 h to allow the platelets to disaggregate.
3. Add 200 ml of glutaraldehyde fixative (0.25% in 0.15 mol/l phosphate buffer, pH 7.4). Shake vigorously by hand to ensure complete platelet distribution and leave for 48 h at room temperature with occasional shaking.
4. Centrifuge for 30 min at 3500 g. Wash the deposit twice in Alsever's solution and finally resuspend in 15–20 ml of Alsever's solution.
5. Carry out a rough platelet count to determine the approximate concentration and add an appropriate amount of the suspension to preserved blood (p. 568). Mix well for 20 min and, with continuous mixing, dispense into sterile containers. Cap and seal. At 4°C, the preparation should have a shelf life of 3 to 4 months. Before use, resuspend by thorough hand shaking followed by mechanical mixing for c 15 min.

A simpler method for preserving platelets by adding prostaglandin E_1 to blood in ACD provides a control preparation with stability of about 14 days.[19]

ANALYSIS OF DATA

STANDARD DEVIATION OF CONTROLS

Control material may be prepared by the individual laboratory as described above or obtained from commercial sources. To ensure homogeneity, the stock should be dispensed into vials with continuous mixing; this is conveniently undertaken by means of a rotating flask. A mixing unit which is suitable has been designed specifically for this.[20] Inter-tube homogeneity should then be checked by measuring the relevant analytes in at least three (preferably 10) vials taken at random from the batch. Their results should be within

2SD of 5 to 10 replicate measurements on one sample from the batch. The SD is calculated as shown on page 613. Calculating the CV provides an alternative way of expressing the dispersion of results. The advantage of CV is that it describes the significance of SD irrespective of the measured value.

CONTROL CHARTS

The use of control charts, originally described for industry by Shewhart,[21] was first applied in clinical

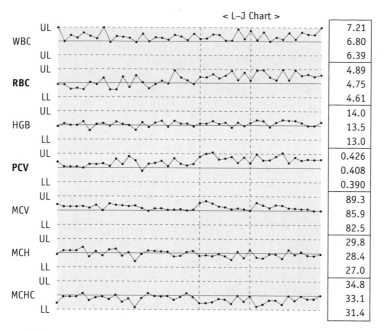

WBC	UL	7.21
		6.80
	UL	6.39
RBC	UL	4.89
		4.75
	LL	4.61
HGB	UL	14.0
		13.5
	LL	13.0
PCV	UL	0.426
		0.408
	LL	0.390
MCV	UL	89.3
		85.9
	LL	82.5
MCH	UL	29.8
		28.4
	LL	27.0
MCHC	UL	34.8
		33.1
	LL	31.4

< L–J Chart >

Fig. 24.1 Control chart (Levey–Jennings chart) with automated blood count analyser. The mean value for each component of the blood count is shown on the right together with the upper and lower limits for satisfactory performance which have been set at +2SD and –2SD, respectively.

chemistry by Levey & Jennings.[22] They are now widely used in haematology for both automated and manual procedures.

Samples of the control specimen are included in every batch of patients' specimens and the results checked on a control chart. To check precision, it is not necessary to know the exact value of the control specimen. If, however, its value has been determined reliably by a reference method, the same material can also be used to check accuracy or to calibrate an instrument. If possible, controls with high, low and normal values should be used. It is advisable to use at least one control sample per batch even if the batch is very small. As the controls are intended to simulate random sampling, they must be treated exactly like the patients' specimens. The results obtained with the control samples can be plotted on a chart as described below.

The mean value and SD of the control specimen should first be established, as described above, in the laboratory where the tests on specimens are performed. Using arithmetical graph paper, a horizontal line is drawn to represent the mean (as a base) and on an appropriate scale of quantity and unit, lines representing +2SD and –2SD are drawn

above and below the mean. The results of successive control sample measurements are plotted. If the test is satisfactory, sequential results will oscillate about the mean value and less than 5% of the results will fall outside 2SD. Figure 24.1 illustrates a control chart from an automated system; a similar principle can be used for simple methods (Fig. 24.2).

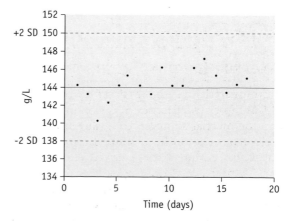

Fig. 24.2 Control chart for haemoglobinometry by manual method. The limits for satisfactory performance have been set at ±2SD

The following indicate a fault in technique or in the instrument or reagent used:

One widely deviant result outside 3SD = a gross error or 'blunder'

Two or more results on or outside the +2SD or −2SD limits = random error

Several consecutive values on one side of the mean = calibration fault

Consecutive values constantly rising (or falling) = continuing bias error.

The fault may be in the reagents or the laboratory ware, or caused by incorrect adjustment/calibration of the instrument, technical error or even to clerical error in transcribing the results. Before an intensive investigation, the test should be repeated with another sample, and the possibility must also be considered that the inconsistency may be due to deterioration or infection of the batch of material.

CUMULATIVE SUM METHOD (CUSUM)[23]

The CUSUM is an alternative way of expressing the results on control numerically. It is the cumulative sum obtained by adding together differences between the present measurement and the original value in consecutive tests, taking the positive and negative signs into account. When this sum reaches a pre-determined value, the test is out of control. The main advantage of CUSUM is that it is sensitive to slight progressive drift away from the original mean; also, it is readily computerized in a busy laboratory with successive batches of tests requiring several control checks during the day.

DUPLICATE TESTS ON PATIENTS' SPECIMENS

This provides another way of checking the precision of routine work.[24] Test 10 consecutive specimens in duplicate under careful conditions. Calculate the differences between the pairs of results and derive the SD (p. 613). Subsequent duplicate tests should not differ from each other by more than 2SD. This method will detect random errors but it is not sensitive to gradual drift nor will it detect incorrect calibration. If the test is always badly done or has an inherent fault, the SD will be wide. This procedure is suitable for both manual and automated methods; it is,

however, impractical for routine blood counts in a busy laboratory. In this case, a few consecutive specimens in a batch should be tested in duplicate from time to time as a rough check.

Another method is to repeat measurement on a few specimens which have been measured originally in an earlier batch. The two tests should agree with each other within 2SD in the majority of cases.[25] This procedure will detect any deterioration of apparatus and reagents which may have developed between tests, if it is certain that the earlier specimen has not altered on standing.

USE OF NORMAL HAEMATOLOGICAL DATA FOR QUALITY CONTROL

In healthy individuals, the blood count remains virtually constant day by day, subject only to the physiological changes already discussed (p. 13). It is possible to use observations on healthy individuals for quality control in routine laboratory work by analyzing the results of blood counts from five or more selected healthy subjects at intervals and calculating means and SD for MCV, MCH and MCHC (p. 613). On each occasion, the mean should not vary by more than 2SD, and the SDs themselves should remain constant. A significant difference in mean indicates a constant error, e.g. incorrect calibration; random errors will result in an increase in SD although the mean may be unaffected. This method is more appropriate for a small laboratory using manual or semi-automated methods rather than for a large laboratory with a fully automated system.

USE OF PATIENT DATA FOR QUALITY CONTROL

In hospitals with at least 100 patients investigated each day, there should be no significant day-to-day variability in the means of their red cell indices obtained by an automated blood counter provided that the population of patients remains stable and that samples from a particular clinical source are not processed all in the same set, thus disproportionately influencing the mean. Assuming that the sample population is stable, any significant change in the means of the red cell indices will indicate a change in instrument calibration or a drift owing to a fault in its function.

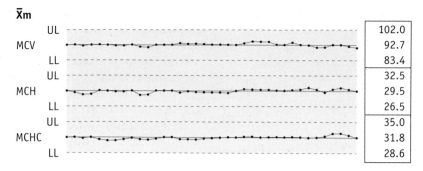

Fig. 24.3 Quality control based on patients' data. Control of automated blood counts by mean results for red cell indices (MCV, MCH, MCHC). The predetermined means are shown together with the upper limits (UL) and lower limits (LL) for satisfactory control.

A robust application of this principle was developed by Bull[26–28] who developed a computer program to estimate the daily patient means of absolute values (MCV, MCH and MCHC). To start this program, it is first necessary to assay samples from at least 300 to 500 patients in an automated blood counter and to establish the means of MCV, MCH and MCHC. Then, using the algorithm proposed by Bull, it is possible to analyse the results in successive batches of 20 specimens. By plotting these results (X_B) on a graph, any drift from the three indices can be readily recognized and used to identify instrument faults. To ensure that each batch is representative, the samples must be randomized before analysis and within any batch of 20, no more than seven should come from one clinical source or have the same clinical condition.

The method is now incorporated in some automated blood counters (Fig. 24.3). In laboratories using manual methods, a simple adaptation of the same principle can be applied, confined to MCHC and excluding results from any special clinic that are likely to be specifically biased. From the daily means for all measurements on 10 consecutive working days, an overall daily mean and SD are established. The mean MCHC is then calculated at the end of each day If the test does not vary by more than 2SD, it is considered to be satisfactory, but may be misleading if there is an error in the same direction simultaneous in both Hb and PCV. The results may be displayed graphically as illustrated in Figure 24.4. It is useful in validating successive batches of calibrators.

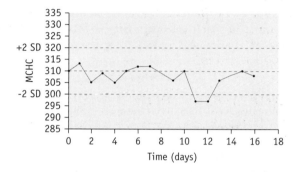

Fig. 24.4 Quality control based on patients' data. Control of manual blood counts using MCHC as indicator.

Correlation check

This implies that any unexpected result of a test must be checked to see whether it can be explained on clinical grounds or whether it correlates with other tests. Thus, for example, an unexpectedly higher or lower haemoglobin might be explained by a blood transfusion or a haemorrhage, respectively. A low MCHC should be confirmed by demonstrating hypochromic red cells on a Romanowsky-stained blood film; a high MCV must correlate with macrocytosis; similarly the blood films should be examined to confirm leucocytosis or leucopenia, thrombocytosis or thrombocytopenia, or to distinguish between platelets and red cell fragments – but be careful as the blood film itself may be misleading if not correctly made and stained.

Recording blood count data on cumulative report forms is good clinical practice as well as providing an inbuilt quality control system by making it easy to detect an aberrant result when compared with a previously determined baseline. This is especially useful in detecting the occasional wild errors caused by incorrect labelling, inadequate mixing, partial clotting of a blood sample or deterioration on storage.

A formal way of testing for aberrant results is known as the 'delta check'. The blood count parameters should not differ from recent tests in the previous 2–3 weeks by more than a certain amount which takes into account both test CV and physiological variation. With automated counters, the differences should generally be not more than 10% for Hb and RBC, 20–25% for WBC and 50% for the platelet count, assuming that the patient's clinical condition has not altered significantly.

EXTERNAL QUALITY ASSESSMENT[17,29–31]

External quality assessment (EQA) is an important complement to internal control. Even when all precautions are taken to achieve accuracy and precision in the laboratory, errors arise which are only detectable by objective external assessment. The principle is that the same material is sent from a national or regional centre to a large number of laboratories. It is important that surveys should be performed at regular intervals, although their frequency may vary, depending on the diagnostic importance of the particular test, how frequently they are requested and their technical reliability. Thus, for example, in the UK NEQAS for haematology, specimens are distributed at 4-weekly intervals for blood counts and every 3 months for most other tests. Results are analysed at the NEQAS centre and interpreted by one of several procedures.

Deviation index

From the results returned by the participants the median or mean and SD are calculated. An individual laboratory can then compare its performance in the survey with that of other laboratories and with its own previous performance from the *deviation index (DI)* (or *z-score* as it is sometimes called). This is calculated as the difference between the individual laboratory's result and the median or mean relative to the SD. Thus,

$$DI = \frac{[\text{Actual results for test} - \text{Adjusted mean or median}]}{\text{Trimmed SD}}$$

Note.

a. The mean is adjusted after excluding results which are outside ±3SD in a preliminary calculation.

b. When distribution of results is non-Gaussian, median should be used rather than mean, and in this case outliers are not excluded; SD is then calculated as: Central 50% spread ÷ 1.349. This applies, especially, to the blood count.

c. There are several ways of trimming the SD:
   — use SD of best performance, i.e. by reference laboratories
   — calculate SD of results from a selected group of the participants, e.g. first 30 results to be returned
   — calculate from a predetermined constant CV which takes account of technical variance of the method, clinical utility of the test and the critical range of measurement for diagnostic discrimination.

In this method, a DI (score) of less than 0.5 denotes excellent performance; a score between 0.5 and 1.0 is satisfactory, and a score between 1.0 and 2.0 is still acceptable. A score above 2.0 suggests that the analyser calibration should be checked, whilst DI >3.0 indicates a serious defect requiring attention.

Persistent unsatisfactory performance

It is essential to monitor EQA results in consecutive surveys, noting any fluctuations in the DI. A convenient way for quantifying this is to add together six recent DI scores, e.g. from the two samples in the last three surveys; any values >3.5 are rounded down to 3.5 to avoid an isolated very high value having an excessive effect on the calculation. The total is then multiplied by 6. A score of 100 or more indicates persistent unsatisfactory performance.

It is, however, to be hoped that participants will have corrected any problems before this stage is reached.

Target values and bias

The true value for a test may usually be assumed to be the result obtained by best performance of selected participants in the survey or by experts using reference methods. This is the target value (TV) to be aimed for by all the participants. The percent bias by an individual participant's result (R) can then be calculated as:

$$[R-TV] \div TV \times 100$$

The pattern of bias in successive surveys will indicate whether there is a constant calibration error or a progressive fault, or whether the original defect has been corrected.

Youden (xy) plot

This is a useful method for relating measurements on two samples in a survey to provide a graphic display and, when a participant's results are unsatisfactory, for distinguishing between a consistent bias and random error. Results for the two samples are plotted on the horizontal (x) and the vertical (y) axis, respectively, and the standard deviations (2SD or 3SD) for the two sets are drawn, as shown in outline in Figure 24.5.

Results which fall in the central block are satisfactory; those in blocks B indicate a consistent bias which may be positive (to right) or negative (to left), while results in other areas indicate random errors (inconsistency) in the two samples.

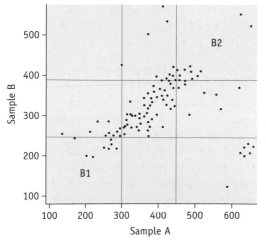

Fig. 24.5 Youden (xy) graph. The SDs of the results with the two samples are drawn on the x and y axis, respectively, and individual paired results are plotted. Results in the central square are satisfactory; those in B demonstrate a consistent bias with measurements that are too low (B1) or too high (B2), while results in other areas indicate random errors.

Technique check

It is sometimes useful to check separate components of a method. Thus, appropriate samples can be used to check adequacy of mixing to ensure sample homogeneity, the reliability of dilution and the use of an instrument. As an example, a survey might include a pair of identical whole blood samples and lysates from the same specimen for measuring haemoglobin, together with a diluted haemiglobincyanide solution to be measured on the spectrometer at A^{540} and A^{504}.

Clinical significance

In assessing performance, using limits based on the SD will, in some cases, be too rigid, and, in others, be too lenient. To ensure that results are clinically reliable, they should be within a certain percentage of the assigned value. This must take account of unavoidable imprecision of the method as well as normal diurnal variations. The following limits are adequate to meet these requirements in practice:

Hb and RBC (by counter)	3–4%
PCV, MCV, MCH, MCHC	4–5%
Leucocyte count	8–10%
Platelet count	10–15%
Vitamin B_{12}, folate, iron, ferritin	20%
HbA_2 and HbF quantitation	5–10%

In addition to providing guidance on the laboratory's general level of performance, an important function of EQA is to achieve harmonization or concordance between laboratories. However, some blood cell counters handle preserved blood differently from routine specimens and, even if correctly calibrated, different types of counter may differ in their responses to EQA samples.[32–33] It may thus be necessary to analyse results separately for different groups of instruments. When there are unexplained differences in counts on EQA samples with different instruments in a laboratory, counts should be made on fresh EDTA blood samples with the different instruments in order to check their comparability.

In assessing qualitative or interpretative tests (e.g. blood film morphology), results are compared with the consensus obtained from a panel of referees or by concordance of 75% or more of the participants. Performance can be based on either a *penalty* system for incorrectly reported features (false-positive) and missed features (false-negative) or an *award* system for correctly observed abnor-malities. The features are graded for scoring according to their diagnostic significance.

ROUTINE QUALITY ASSURANCE PROTOCOL[34-35]

The procedures which should be included in a quality assurance programme will vary with the tests undertaken, the instruments used and (especially if these include a fully automatic counting system) the size of the laboratory and the numbers of specimens handled, the computer facilities available and the amount of time which can be devoted to the programme. At least some form of internal quality control must be undertaken and also participation in an external quality assessment scheme where one is available. Some control procedures should be performed daily, and other performance checks at appropriate intervals. The latter is particularly important when there is a change in staff and after a maintenance service or repair has been carried out on equipment. The comprehensive protocol is summarized in Table 24.1.

All laboratory staff require training in these various aspects of quality assurance. A useful training manual from WHO describes the principles and methods together with practical exercises to illustrate these.[14]* Another good teaching source is J.O. Westgard's internet web-site (*www.westgard.com*); this includes a *Lesson of the month*, and other current topics which are regularly updated.

*Available on request to Diagnostic Imaging and Laboratory Technology Unit (DIL), WHO, 1211 Geneva 27, Switzerland.

Table 24.1 Quality assurance procedures

Calibration with **reference standards**
Instruments: At 6-month intervals; also if control chart or EQA indicates bias or fluctuation in results, and after any repair/service
Diluting systems: Initially and at 1 to 2-week intervals
Control chart with **control material**
Daily or with each batch of specimens
Delta check on **patients' samples**: daily
Duplicate measurements on **patients' samples** (2–3): if control chart or delta check shows discrepancies
Analysis of **patients' results**
Constancy of mean MCV, MCH, MCHC: daily
Correlation assessment of **test reports**
Cumulative results: following previous tests
Blood film: if unusual test results and/or counter flags appear
Clinical state
EQAS

REFERENCES

1 World Health Organization 1991 Biological substances: international standards reference preparations and reference reagents. WHO, Geneva.

2 World Health Organization 1998 Expert committee on biological standardization 47th report. WHO Technical Report 878. WHO, Geneva.

3 International Council for Standardization in Haematology 1995 Standards, reference materials and reference methods. In: Lewis SM, Koepke JA (eds) Haematology laboratory management and practice. Butterworth Heinemann, Oxford, ch 13.

4 Shinton NK 1999 Standardization of quality management in the medical laboratory. Accreditation and Quality Assurance 4:442–445.

5 British Committee for Standards in Haematology 2000 Standard haematology practice, vol 3. Blackwell Science, Oxford. [Also vol 1:1991; vol 2:1996].

6 International Council for Standardization in Haematology 1996 Recommendations for reference methods of haemoglobinometry in human blood (ICSH Standard 1995) and specifications for international haemiglobincyanide standard, 4th edn. Journal of Clinical Pathology 49:271–274.

7 Lewis SM 1975 Standards and reference preparations. In: Lewis SM, Coster JF (eds) Quality control in haematology. Academic Press, London, ch 6.

8 International Council for Standardization in Haematology 1988 The assignment of values to fresh blood used for calibrating automated blood cell counters. Clinical and Laboratory Haematology 10:203–212.

9 Springer W, Prohaska W, Neukammer J, et al 1999 Evaluation of a new reagent for preserving fresh blood samples and its potential usefulness for internal quality controls of multichannel haematology analyzers. American Journal of Clinical Pathology 111:387–396.

10 Lewis SM, England JM, Rowan RM 1991 Current concerns in haematology 3: blood count calibration. Journal of Clinical Pathology 44:881–884.

11 Richardson Jones A 1982 Counting and sizing of blood cells using aperture-impedance systems. In: van Assendelft OW, England JM (eds) Advances in hematological methods: the blood count. CRC Press, Boca Raton, Fl, ch 5.

12 Thom R 1972 Hemocytometry: method and results by improved electronic blood-cell sizing. In: Izak G, Lewis SM (eds) Modern concepts in hematology. Academic Press, New York, p 191–200.

13 Torlontano G, Tata A 1972 Stable standard suspension of white blood cells suitable for calibration and control of electronic counters. In: Izak G, Lewis SM (eds) Modern Concepts in hematology. Academic Press, New York, p 230–234.

14 Lewis SM 1998 Quality assurance in haematology: document LAB/98.4. World Health Organization, Geneva.

15 International Council for Standardization in Haematology 1994 Reference method for the enumeration of erythrocytes and leucocytes. Clinical and Laboratory Haematology 16:131–138.

16 International Council for Standardization in Haematology 2000 Recommended method for the determination of packed cell volume by centrifugation: document LAB/00. World Health Organization, Geneva.

17 Deom A, El Aouad R, Heuck CC, et al 2000 Requirements and guidance for external quality assurance programmes for health laboratories: document LAB/2000. World Health Organization, Geneva.

18 Reardon DM, Mack D, Warner B, et al 1991 A whole blood control for blood count analysers, and source material for an external quality assessment scheme. Medical Laboratory Sciences 48:19–26.

19 Zhang Z, Tatsumi N, Tsuda I, et al 1999 Long-term preservation of platelet count in blood for external quality control surveillance using prostaglandin E_1. Clinical and Laboratory Haematology 21:71.

20 Ward PG, Chappel DA, Fox JGC, et al 1975 Mixing and bottling unit for preparing biological fluids used in quality control. Laboratory Practice 24:577–583.

21 Shewhart WA 1931 Economic control of quality of manufactured products. Van Nostrand, New York.

22 Levey S, Jennings ER 1950 The use of control charts in the clinical laboratory. American Journal of Clinical Pathology 20:1059–1066.

23 Cavill I 1990 Intralaboratory quality confirmation using control samples. Methods in Haematology 22:154–171.

24 Carstairs KC, Peters E, Kuzin EJ 1977 Development and description of the 'random duplicates' method of quality control for a hematology laboratory. American Journal of Clinical Pathology 67:379–385.

25 Cembrowski GS, Lunetsky ES, Patrick CC, et al 1988 An optimized quality control procedure for hematology analyzers with the use of retained patient specimens. American Journal of Clinical Pathology 89:203–210.

26 Korpman RA, Bull BS 1976 The implementation of a robust estimator of the mean for quality control on a programmable calculator or a laboratory computer. American Journal of Clinical Pathology 65:252–253.

27 Bull BS, Hay KL 1990 Interlaboratory quality control using patients' data. Methods in Haematology 22:172–192.

28 Smith FA, Kroft SH 1996 Exponentially adjusted moving mean procedure for quality control: an optimized patient sample control procedure. American Journal of Clinical Pathology 105:44–51.

29 Lewis SM 1995 External quality assessment. In: Lewis SM, Koepke JA (eds) Haematology laboratory management and practice. Butterworth Heinemann, Oxford, ch 19.

30 International Council for Standardization in Haematology 1998 Guidelines for organization and management of external quality assessment using proficiency testing. International Journal of Haematology 68:45–52.

31 International Organization for Standardization 1997 Guide 43–1 Proficiency testing by interlaboratory comparisons Part I: Development and operation of proficiency testing schemes. ISO, Geneva.

32 Wardle J, Ward PG, Lewis SM 1985 Response of various blood counting systems to CPD-A1 preserved whole blood. Clinical and Laboratory Haematology 7:245–250.

33 Leyssen MHJ, DeBruyere MJG, van Druppen VJM, et al 1985 Problems related to CPD preserved blood used for NEQAS trials in haematology. Clinical and Laboratory Haematology 7:239–243.

34 International Organization for Standardization 1990 ISO/IEC Guide 25 General requirements for the technical competence of testing laboratories. ISO, Geneva.

35 International Organization for Standardization 1999 ISO/DIS 15189 Quality management in the medical laboratory. ISO, Geneva.

25

Approach to the diagnosis of blood diseases

Imelda Bates

COMMON PRESENTATIONS OF HAEMATOLOGICAL DISEASES

An abnormal blood count or blood cell morphology do not necessarily indicate a primary haematology problem, as they may reflect an underlying non-haematological condition or may be the result of therapeutic interventions. Anaemia is common in many conditions but a primary blood disease should be considered when a patient has splenomegaly, lymphadenopathy, a bleeding tendency, thrombosis and/or non-specific symptoms of malaise, sweats or weight loss.

As with any clinical problem, the first steps in determining the diagnosis include a careful clinical and drug history, and thorough physical examination. The result of these, in combination with the patient's age, sex, ethnic origin, social and family history and a knowledge of the locally prevalent diseases, will determine subsequent laboratory investigations.

INITIAL SCREENING TESTS

Although the range of haematological tests available to support clinical and public health services is broad, it is often the simplest investigations which are most useful in indicating the diagnosis. Even poorly resourced laboratories are usually able to provide an initial panel of tests such as haemoglobin, white cell and platelet counts (Chapter 3), and examination of a peripheral blood smear for differential white cell count and cellular morphology (Chapter 5). These screening tests will often enable the underlying pathological processes to be suspected promptly and point to a few key diagnostic tests. The investigation of specific haematological problems is covered in detail in Chapters 7 (iron-deficiency anaemia), 8 (megaloblastic anaemia), 9, 10 and 11 (haemolytic anaemias), 12 (haemoglobinopathies) and 16 and 17 (coagulation disorders).

Interpretation of screening tests

Results of laboratory screening tests should always be interpreted with an understanding of the limitations of the tests and the physiological variations in reference ranges that occur with sex, age and conditions such as pregnancy and exercise. Physiological variations in cell counts are detailed in Chapter 2 (p. 13). Abnormalities of red cells, white cells or platelets may be quantitative (increased or reduced numbers) or qualitative (abnormal appearance and/or function).

QUANTITATIVE ABNORMALITIES OF BLOOD CELLS

INCREASED NUMBERS OF CELLS

1. Increases affecting more than one cell line

A simultaneous increase in the cells of more than one cell line suggests that the overproduction of cells originates in an early precursor cell. This occurs in myeloproliferative disorders in which one cell type may predominate, e.g. platelets in essential thrombocythaemia and red cells in polycythaemia vera (primary proliferative polycythaemia) but there are often increases in other cell lines. The diagnosis will depend on which cell line expansion is dominant.

2. Erythrocytosis

Increases in red cells may be:

- 'primary' (polycythaemia vera) as part of the spectrum of myeloproliferative disorders (see above)
- 'relative' (pseudopolycythaemia) owing to reduced plasma volume
- 'secondary' to chronic hypoxia (e.g. chronic lung disease, congenital heart disease, high affinity haemoglobins) and aberrant erythropoietin production.

Secondary polycythaemia can generally be excluded by the clinical history and examination, assessment of erythropoietin secretion, arterial oxygen saturation, haemoglobin electrophoresis and abdominal ultrasound. The presence of splenomegaly is suggestive of polycythaemia vera and this can be confirmed by demonstrating an absolute increase in total red cell volume and excluding other causes of erythrocytosis.

3. Leucocytosis

Neutrophilia. Neutrophils are commonly increased in acute infections, inflammation, intoxication, corticosteroid therapy and acute blood loss or destruction. Increased neutrophils with heavy cytoplasmic granulation ('toxic' granulation) are a common finding in severe bacterial infections. In the absence of any underlying cause, a high neutrophil count with immature myeloid cells suggests chronic granulocytic leukaemia: cytogenetic and molecular studies to look for chromosomal translocations and the *BCR–ABL* fusion gene may be helpful.

Lymphocytosis. Lymphocytosis is a feature of infection, particularly in children. It may be especially marked in pertussis, infectious mononucleosis, cytomegalovirus infection, infectious hepatitis, tuberculosis and brucellosis. In the elderly, lymphoproliferative disorders, including chronic lymphocytic leukaemia and lymphomas, often present with lymphadenopathy and a lymphocytosis. Morphology and immunophenotyping of the cells combined with histological examination of bone marrow trephine biopsies are used to classify these disorders and to give an indication of management and prognosis. It is occasionally difficult to differentiate between a reactive and a neoplastic lymphocytosis. In this situation, immunophenotyping, evidence of light chain restriction and polymerase chain reaction for immunoglobulin or T-cell receptor gene rearrangements may point towards the presence of a monoclonal population of lymphocytes, thereby supporting a diagnosis of neoplastic, rather than reactive, lymphoproliferation. If lymph nodes are enlarged, a fine needle aspirate or node biopsy for immunophenotyping and histology may be helpful in diagnosis.

Monocytosis. A slight to moderate monocytosis may be associated with some protozoal, rickettsial and bacterial infections including malaria, typhus and tuberculosis. High levels of monocytes ($>1 \times 10^9/l$) in an elderly patient suggest chronic myelomonocytic leukaemia. As this is in the myeloproliferative and myelodysplastic spectrum of disorders, the diagnosis would be supported by finding splenomegaly, quantitative and qualitative abnormalities in other cell lines and cytogenetic derangements.

Eosinophilia. Eosinophilia is typically associated with allergic disorders including drug sensitivity, skin diseases and parasitic infections. In most cases, the cause is ascertainable from the clinical history, which should include details of all medications and foreign travel, and by examination of the stool and urine for parasites and ova. Idiopathic hypereosinophilic syndrome is an unusual cause of eosinophilia in which release of the contents of eosinophil granules results in damage to the heart, lungs and other tissues.

Basophilia. Basophilia as an isolated finding is unusual. However, it is a common feature of myeloproliferative disorders and basophils may be particularly prominent in chronic granulocytic leukaemia. In this condition, an increasing basophil count may be the first indication of transformation to a more malignant course.

4. Thrombocytosis

Thrombocytosis is often associated with infectious and inflammatory conditions such as osteomyelitis and rheumatoid arthritis. Haematological causes of thrombocytosis include chronic blood loss, red cell destruction, splenectomy and rebound following recovery from marrow suppression. Under these circumstances, a moderately raised platelet count (e.g. $400–800 \times 10^9/l$) does not usually have any pathological consequences. Primary (essential) thrombocythaemia belongs to the spectrum of myeloproliferative diseases and is characterized by a persistently high platelet count (often defined as greater than $600 \times 10^9/l$), and thrombotic or haemorrhagic complications. Further investigations to confirm primary thrombocythaemia include bone marrow examination for increased and abnormal megakaryocytes, and cytogenetic analysis.

REDUCED NUMBERS OF CELLS
Reductions in more than one cell line

A reduction in cell numbers occurs because of increased destruction or reduced production. A common cause of a global reduction in circulating cells is pooling of the cells in a grossly enlarged spleen (hypersplenism) which may be secondary to conditions such as myelofibrosis and portal hypertension. Reduced production of cells may be due to aplastic anaemia, a lack of haematinics such as folate

or vitamin B_{12}, or interference with normal haemopoiesis by infiltration (e.g. leukaemia, lymphoma, multiple myeloma, secondary or 'idiopathic' myelofibrosis), infection (e.g. HIV infection, tuberculosis, leishmaniasis), or exposure to toxins (e.g. alcohol) or myelosuppressive drugs (e.g. hydroxyurea, busulphan). Examination of a bone marrow aspirate and trephine biopsy specimen is therefore helpful in determining the cause of bi- or pancytopenias for which no obvious cause can be found.

Anaemia

There are many causes of anaemia and the choice of further investigations must be guided by the mean cell volume (MCV) and red cell morphology. Despite a degree of overlap, anaemia can be broadly divided into three categories:

microcytic (low MCV)
macrocytic (high MCV)
normocytic (normal MCV).

Figures 25.1–25.3 are flow charts which provide an orderly sequence of investigations for the different types of anaemia on the basis of these indices. Examination of a blood film will usually suggest the quickest route to the diagnosis; confirmation may require the more specific tests which are given in the text.

Microcytic anaemia (Fig. 25.1)

The commonest cause of anaemia worldwide is iron deficiency. It can be suspected from a low MCV and the presence of hypochromic, microcytic red cells. Laboratory confirmation of iron deficiency may include measurements of serum iron, total iron-binding capacity, serum ferritin, transferrin assay, red cell protoporphyrin and staining of bone marrow aspirates for iron (see Ch. 7). A search for the cause of iron deficiency should include specific questions relating to blood loss and dietary insufficiency, and may require stool examination for parasites and occult blood, and endoscopic examination of the gastrointestinal tract to exclude occult malignancy. The thalassaemias may produce similar morphological changes to iron deficiency but the clinical setting and further investigations, such as haemoglobin electrophoresis, measurement of Hb A_2 and Hb F, 'H' body preparation and globin chain and DNA studies, may help to confirm the diagnosis. α-thalassaemia trait may be particularly

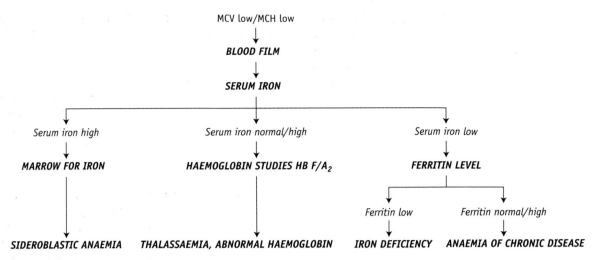

Fig. 25.1 Investigation of a microcytic hypochromic anaemia. Tests are shown in bold capitals, results in italics and the diagnosis in capitals.

difficult to diagnose and referral to a specialist centre may be necessary.

Macrocytic anaemia (Fig. 25.2)

A high MCV with oval macrocytes and hypersegmented neutrophils suggests folate or vitamin B_{12} deficiency; subsequent investigations could include malabsorption studies and a Schilling test to detect pernicious anaemia (p. 139) and small bowel disease. A high MCV may also be associated with alcohol excess and liver disease, or drugs such as hydroxyurea. Immature red cells appear slightly larger and more purple than normal red cells on a Romanowsky-stained peripheral blood film (poly-

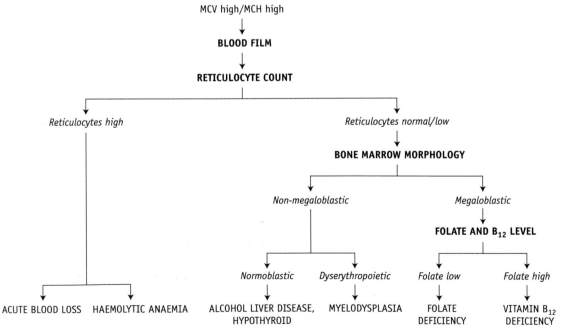

Fig. 25.2 Investigation of a macrocytic anaemia. Tests are shown in bold capitals, results in italics and the diagnosis in capitals.

chromasia p. 86). Supravital stains (p. 27) can be used to confirm that these cells are reticulocytes. Anaemia associated with polychromasia is likely to indicate blood loss or haemolysis. The combination of red cell fragments, thrombocytopenia and polychromasia indicates microangiopathic haemolytic anaemia and should trigger further tests such as coagulation studies, assessment of renal function and a search for infection or neoplastic disease.

Normocytic anaemia (Fig. 25.3)

Normochromic, normocytic anaemia is frequently due to an underlying chronic, non-haematological disease. Investigations should include screening for renal disease, subclinical infections, auto-immune diseases and neoplasia. In the presence of anaemia, a lack of polychromasia, confirmed by reticulocytopenia, points towards a primary failure of erythropoiesis, or blood loss or haemolysis without compensatory red cell production. Examination of the bone marrow may be helpful in demonstrating haematological causes for the normochromic, normocytic anaemia such as aplastic anaemia or early myelodysplastic syndrome. Staining for iron may

also show that there is a block in iron metabolism suggestive of anaemia associated with chronic disorders.

Leucopenia

Neutropenia. Once physiological variation, ethnicity and familial or cyclical neutropenia have been excluded, the non-haematological causes of isolated neutropenia include overwhelming infection, auto-immune disorders such as systemic lupus erythematosus, irradiation and drugs, particularly anti-cancer agents. Bone marrow examination may assist in determining whether the problem is due to peripheral destruction (increased marrow myeloid precursors) or stem-cell failure (lack of narrow myeloid precursors). Typical marrow appearances occur in drug-induced neutropenia in which there is a relative paucity of mature neutrophils and in Kostmann's syndrome (infant genetic agranulocytosis) where there is maturation arrest at the promyelocytic stage.

Reduced lymphocytes, monocytes, eosinophils and basophils. Lymphocytes, eosinophils and basophils may all be reduced by stress such as

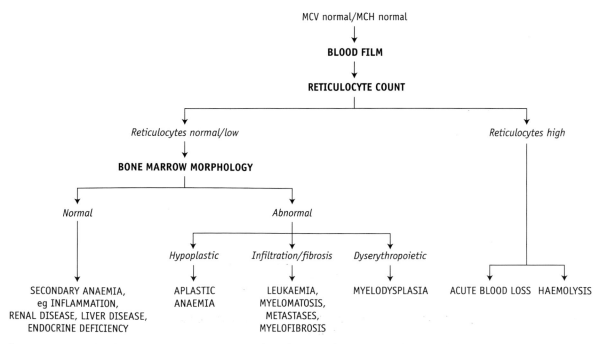

Fig. 25.3 Investigation of a normocytic, normochromic anaemia. Tests are shown in bold capitals, results in italics and the diagnosis in capitals.

surgery, trauma and infection. Lymphopenia especially affecting the CD4 cells, may occur in HIV infection and renal failure. Monocytopenia ($<0.2 \times 10^9/l$) is typically found in hairy cell leukaemia which is also associated with pancytopenia, typical bone marrow histology and lymphocytes with a characteristic cytology and immunophenotype.

Thrombocytopenia

Thrombocytopenia is a common isolated finding and it is important to ensure that the laboratory result reflects a true reduction in platelet count before embarking on further diagnostic tests. Frequent causes of spurious thrombocytopenia include blood clots in the sample, platelet agglutination and platelet satellitism. Platelet aggregation, which can be seen on the blood film, may occur in vitro as the result of a temperature or anti-coagulant-dependent auto-antibody. Small platelet aggregates are also seen in slides which have been made directly from a finger prick sample. True thrombocytopenia is most frequently due to auto-antibodies ('idiopathic' auto-immune thrombocytopenic purpura), drugs (such as thiazide diuretics) and, in the elderly, myelodysplastic syndromes. The clinical circumstances and platelet antibody studies, combined with a bone marrow examination, enable these conditions to be differentiated. Thrombocytopenia associated with other complications, such as thromboses, disturbed renal or hepatic function and haemolytic anaemia, should prompt investigations for other diseases such as thrombotic thrombocytopenic purpura, haemolytic uraemic syndrome or the HELLP (Haemolysis + Elevated Liver enzymes + Low Platelet count) syndrome. A bone marrow examination is often carried out early in the investigation of thrombocytopenia as it is helpful in excluding conditions such as acute leukaemia, which may present with isolated thrombocytopenia.

QUALITATIVE ABNORMALITIES OF BLOOD CELLS

In health, only the most mature forms of cells appear in the peripheral blood. Early, immature cells, such as polychromatic red cells or myelocytes and metamyelocytes, may be released from the bone marrow in conditions where the bone marrow is overactive, such as acute haemolytic states or recovery after suppression, or functionally abnormal. Their presence in the peripheral blood indicates that active haemopoiesis is taking place.

Abnormalities of all cell lines

The combination of anisopoikilocytosis, mild macrocytosis, hypogranular neutrophils with abnormal nuclear morphology and platelet anisocytosis, often with quantitative abnormalities, is virtually pathognomonic of a myelodysplastic syndrome. These features are reflected in the bone marrow with disturbance of the normal developmental pathway and nuclear:cytoplasmic asynchrony. Cytogenetic studies are not a prerequisite but can confirm the diagnosis and assist in determining the prognosis.

Abnormalities of individual cell lines
Red cells
Congenital abnormalities of the red cell affecting the structure (e.g. spherocytosis, elliptocytosis) and content (e.g. haemoglobinopathies, enzymopathies) produce typical morphological changes (see Chapter 5). These will guide further investigations towards analysis of structural proteins, haemoglobin electrophoresis and enzyme assays. Acquired red cell abnormalities may also help to indicate underlying pathology. For example, target cells may prompt investigation of liver function whereas rouleaux may indicate the need for investigations for multiple myeloma or inflammatory conditions such as rheumatoid arthritis.

White cells
Congenital abnormalities of neutrophils are unusual but similar morphological abnormalities (e.g. Pelger–Huët cells) may be seen in acquired conditions such as myelodysplastic syndrome. Reactive changes in mononuclear cells, including basophilic, faceted cytoplasm, are typically seen in infectious mononucleosis, which can be diagnosed using the Paul–Bunnell or equivalent test (p. 532). These cells may sometimes be difficult to differentiate from circulating lymphoma cells (p. 95). Bone marrow histology, combined with immunophenotyping studies and determination of lymphocyte clonality by gene rearrangement molecular studies, may be needed to reach a firm conclusion.

Platelets

Platelets that function poorly may not necessarily appear morphologically abnormal. Disorders of platelet function are characterized by a normal platelet count with a prolonged bleeding time. Hereditary disorders of platelet function are uncommon and usually present as a bleeding diathesis. They can broadly be divided into two categories: abnormalities of the platelet membrane (e.g. Bernard–Soulier syndrome, Glanzmann's thrombasthenia) and of platelet secretory function (e.g. α- and δ-storage pool diseases). In comparison, acquired disorders of platelet function are common. Haematological conditions associated with platelet dysfunction include myeloproliferative and myelodysplastic disorders and dysproteinaemias. Many widely prescribed drugs can interfere with platelet function, including aspirin and non-steroidal anti-inflammatory agents, whilst systemic conditions, particularly chronic renal failure and cardiopulmonary bypass, are associated with a bleeding tendency as a result of qualitative platelet defects.

SPECIFIC TESTS FOR COMMON HAEMATOLOGICAL DISORDERS

Common haematological disorders are outlined below with suggestions for investigations which may be helpful in confirming the diagnosis. The investigations discussed are those which are likely to be available within a general haematology department; the lists are not intended to be exhaustive as the range of tests provided locally will depend on the availability of expertise and technology.

RED CELL DISORDERS

Microcytic hypochromic anaemias (see Chs 7 and 12)

- Measurement of serum ferritin or iron, total iron-binding capacity, transferrin assay, red cell protoporphyrin
- Bone marrow aspirate with staining for iron
- Stool examination for occult blood; blood loss studies with ^{51}Cr-labelled red cells
- Tests for malabsorption
- Endoscopic examination with biopsy.

If thalassaemia is suspected:

- Haemoglobin electrophoresis plus Hb A_2 and Hb F measurements
- Haemoglobin 'H' body preparation
- Family studies
- Tests for unstable haemoglobin
- DNA analysis
- Globin chain synthesis.

Macrocytic anaemias (see Ch. 8)

Where macrocytic, megaloblastic erythroid maturation is demonstrated, further investigations should be undertaken as described in Chapter 8. Macrocytosis may also be secondary to common conditions such as alcohol excess, liver disease, myelodysplastic syndrome and hypothyroidism. Reticulocytosis from any cause can also increase the MCV.

Aplastic anaemia

- Bone marrow aspirate and trephine biopsy
- Acidified serum (Ham's) test for PNH (urine examination for haemosiderin and neutrophil alkaline phosphatase if Ham's test is positive)
- Vitamin B_{12} and folate assays
- Viral studies, particularly Epstein–Barr and hepatitis viruses.

If Fanconi's anaemia is suspected:

- Studies of sensitivity of chromosomes to breakage by DNA cross-linking agent
- Radiology of hands and forearms.

Haemolytic anaemias (see Chs 9, 10 and 11)

A haemolytic process may be suspected by the presence of a falling haemoglobin, a reticulocytosis and jaundice with an increase in unconjugated bilirubin level.

WHITE CELL DISORDERS

The blood may appear entirely normal in some patients with white cell disorders (e.g. lymphoma, myelomatosis, immune deficiency, neutrophil dysfunction). Changes in white cell numbers or morphology may occur rapidly in response to local or systemic disorders. The investigation of white cell disorders is more likely than investigation of red cell disorders to require marrow examination, especially when a primary marrow disorder is suspected. In chronic leukaemias, bone marrow examination may add little to the diagnosis but the pattern of infiltration may have prognostic significance as in chronic lymphocytic leukaemia. The distribution of white cells is better appreciated in trephine biopsies, which are particularly important in lymphomas.

Acute leukaemia

- Bone marrow aspirate
- Cytochemical stains
- Blood and marrow immunophenotyping
- Cytogenetic analysis
- Molecular studies for rearrangements of specific oncogenes and for oncogene products.

Neutropenia

- Bone marrow aspirate and trephine biopsy
- Serial neutrophil counts for cyclic neutropenia
- Tests for anti-neutrophil antibodies
- Auto-antibody screen and investigations for systemic lupus erythematosus
- Vitamin B_{12} and folate assays
- Acidified serum (Ham's) test.

Chronic granulocytic leukaemia

- Bone marrow aspirate
- Neutrophil alkaline phosphatase
- Cytogenetic analysis
- Molecular studies for *BCR–ABL* rearrangement.

Chronic lymphoproliferative disorders/ lymphadenopathy

- Bone marrow aspirate and trephine biopsy (for lymphocyte distribution)
- Immunophenotyping
- Serum protein electrophoresis and immunoglobulin concentrations
- Lymph node biopsy (fine needle or surgical)
- Serum urate, calcium and lactate dehydrogenase (LDH)
- Radiological studies (X-ray, ultrasonography, CT scan, MRI)
- Serological screening for infectious mononucleosis, cytomegalovirus and toxoplasmosis (if infectious cause suspected).

Myelomatosis

- Bone marrow aspirate
- Serum protein electrophoresis and immunoglobulin concentrations
- Serum albumin and calcium measurements
- B_2-microglobulin
- Urine (random and 24 h) for Bence–Jones protein detection and quantitation
- Tests of renal function
- Radiological skeletal survey.

OTHER DISORDERS

Myeloproliferative disorders

- Blood volume measurement and red cell mass (for polycythaemia)
- Bone marrow aspirate and trephine biopsy
- Arterial oxygen saturation and carboxyhaemoglobin level
- Abdominal ultrasound
- Neutrophil alkaline phosphatase
- Vitamin B_{12} (or B_{12}-binding capacity)
- Serum urate.

Myelodysplasia

- Bone marrow aspirate and trephine biopsy
- Cytogenetic analysis.

'Idiopathic' myelofibrosis

- Bone marrow trephine biopsy
- Red cell folate assay
- Urate.

   If splenectomy is contemplated:

- Ferrokinetic and red cell survival studies
- Spleen scan and red cell pool measurement.

Pancytopenia with splenomegaly

- Bone marrow aspirate and trephine biopsy
- Bacterial culture of marrow for tuberculosis
- Marrow examination for amastigotes of *Leishmania donovani*
- Biopsy of palpable lymph nodes (aspiration or surgical)
- Vitamin B_{12} and folate assays
- Liver biopsy

- Splenic aspirate
- Acidified serum (Ham's) test
- Serum rheumatoid factor and auto-antibody screen
- Laparotomy and splenectomy.

The rationale behind these tests, and details of more specialized investigations outside general haematology practice, can be found in current, comprehensive haematology textbooks or from electronic databases and websites.

26

Haematology in under-resourced laboratories

Imelda Bates

TYPES OF LABORATORY FACILITIES

In most countries, there are likely to be some laboratories with limited resources. In low-income countries, there are few laboratories with sophisticated equipment and highly trained technologists and it is not unusual for laboratory tests to be carried out by nurses and orderlies in outpatient consulting rooms and corridors, and in rural health centres. Understaffing, poor morale, inadequate equipment and erratic supplies of reagents are chronic problems in laboratories in poorer countries and these factors have a huge impact on the range and quality of services that can be offered. Many smaller laboratories are multifunctional, performing haematology, parasitology, clinical chemistry and microbiology tests. A blood transfusion service is usually available at the larger institutions and, unless there is a national blood service, laboratory staff will be involved in both donor selection and venesection, and issuing of blood. In low-income countries, there may be no institutionalized system of public health laboratories, so routine laboratories are required to provide high-quality health surveillance data for epidemiological and public health monitoring.

The purpose of this chapter is to point towards an effective haematology service which can be provided despite serious limitations. In planning such a service, it is necessary to identify what facilities are needed and to plan a network for referral when a clinical problem requires investigations beyond the facilities and expertise that are available locally.

In this context, clinical laboratory facilities in poorer countries can conveniently be divided into three levels (Fig. 26.1) according to their size, staff complement and the services they provide:

A. sub-district facilities including health centres
B. district hospitals
C. central, regional and teaching hospitals.

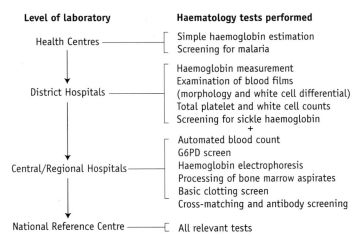

Fig. 26.1 Network of laboratories.

STAFFING AND EQUIPMENT AT EACH LEVEL

Level A. Sub-district facilities including health centres

The level A 'laboratory' generally acts as a resource for helping to determine whether a patient should be referred to the local hospital. The laboratory facilities may comprise a side room or simply be an 'on-the-spot' haemoglobin estimation during the clinical consultation. Laboratory tests are often carried out by nurses, assistants or orderlies with no technical qualifications. The haematology equipment available may include a simple method for measuring haemoglobin, and a microscope for examination of slides for tuberculosis or malaria. However, maintenance of microscopes in the rural areas is often poor and this can significantly compromise the quality of results.

Level B. District hospitals

District hospital laboratories are usually multipurpose and carry out microbiological and biochemical investigations in addition to haematological tests. Laboratory staff consist of one or two qualified technicians supported by assistants who often have minimal or no training. The minimum equipment available at level B is a microscope and centrifuge, and possibly a simple colorimeter for haemoglobin estimation.

Level C. Central and teaching hospitals

Although laboratory staff receive multidisciplinary training, each laboratory at this level generally has a specialist technical head and many of the more senior staff will have received postgraduate training in their chosen discipline. Even in low-income countries, automated haematology analysers may be found in such laboratories. In many cases, these have been supplied by donor agencies. Long-term funding to support maintenance and training for these systems is often lacking and consequently they may function poorly, if at all, owing to a shortage of reagents and inadequate maintenance and staff training. Additional equipment generally found at this level includes centrifuges, colorimeters, microscopes, haemoglobin electrophoresis equipment and possibly blood bank centrifuges for the separation of blood components.

AVAILABILITY OF HAEMATOLOGY TESTS AT EACH LEVEL

The haematology tests which are available at different levels of health-care facility in resource-poor countries are very variable and depend on the clinical need, the equipment available and the number and skills of laboratory staff. The following is a general description of the tests which are likely to be required, but may not necessarily be available at each level in a malaria-endemic area.

Level A

- Haemoglobin estimation by simple method (p. 593)
- Malaria screen on peripheral blood thick films (p. 55)

Level B

- Haemoglobin measurement (p. 20)
- Peripheral blood morphology, especially to identify the cause of anaemia (Chapter 5)*
- Platelet and total white cell counts (p. 595)
- Differential white cell count (p. 25)
- Malaria screening thick and thin peripheral blood smears (p. 58) or rapid immunological test for *Plasmodium falciparum* and possibly other species (p. 537)
- Screening test for sickle haemoglobin in areas where this is relevant (p. 255).

Level C

In addition to tests carried out at level B, the haematology services offered by level C might include:

- Automated Hb, MCV, MCH, MCHC, platelet and white cell counts and white cell differential (p. 30)
- Haemoglobin electrophoresis (p. 241)
- Haemoglobin A$_2$ and F measurements (pp. 256 and 261)
- Glucose-6-phosphate dehydrogenase screen (by fluorescent spot or methaemoglobin reduction method) (p. 179)
- Staining of bone marrow smears for morphological assessment (p. 105) and estimation of iron status (p. 270)
- Blood grouping (p. 472)
- Identification of blood group antibodies (p. 478)
- Basic clotting screen (prothrombin time, thrombin time and activated partial thromboplastin time) (p. 353)
- Oral anticoagulant control (p. 416)
- Separation of whole blood into packed cells, plasma and, occasionally, platelets (p. 24).

DETERMINING 'ESSENTIAL' HAEMATOLOGY TESTS[2]

Despite the relatively high cost of running a laboratory service and the low per capita health-care budget in poorer countries, there is very little data available on which to base rational decisions about 'essential' laboratory tests. The need for such information has become urgent in many countries as a result of the overwhelming burden placed on the health service by the HIV/AIDS epidemic.

In determining which tests are 'essential,' it is important to have reliable information concerning the clinical and public health needs of the local community, and to collaborate with health planners in projecting the medium- and long-term trends. It is therefore not possible to draw up a list of 'essential' tests which will be applicable to all countries or even to different regions within a country. However, the process by which essential tests are defined can be generally applied and will be outlined in this section.

THE PROCESS FOR DETERMINING ESSENTIAL TESTS

The final determinant of whether a test can be introduced or not will be its cost-effectiveness.

The major factors that influence cost-effectiveness are:

- cost/test
- quality and predictive values of test
- clinicians' use of test.

Cost/test

Often the cost of a test is calculated from the price of reagents divided by the number of tests performed. However, this oversimplifies the situation and is not accurate enough to form the basis for national policy decisions and budget allocation. In laboratories with computerized data collection systems, complex analyses of factors which influence the cost of tests can be performed and used to develop rational internal policies for the laboratory (see p. 547). Details of some of the factors which need to be taken into account when calculating the total annual costs for a laboratory, including a formula for the calculation, are given on page 592.

Quality and predictive values of test

The quality of all tests carried out by a laboratory should be regularly monitored and systems for doing this are well established (see Ch. 24). It is also important to know the sensitivity and specificity of the test and its predictive value. Details of

---

*A Bench-aid on morphology is available from WHO.[1]

how to perform these calculations are given in Chapter 23 (p. 549). However, in many poorer countries, it is difficult to obtain these figures because the 'gold standard' diagnostic services needed to determine 'true positive' and 'true negative' results are lacking.

Clinicians' use of test

Data on the clinicians' use of a test are difficult to obtain as they are highly subjective and vary with the level of clinical training and supervision. Any test, however inexpensive and well performed, will be ineffective if it is not used appropriately to guide patient management or for public health surveillance.

CALCULATING COST-EFFECTIVENESS OF LABORATORY TESTS IN LOW-INCOME COUNTRIES

In many poorer countries, decisions for the laboratories are made at central level by health-care planners whose interests are wider that those of the laboratory manager. The planners need to take into account, not only the cost of tests, and their quality, but also whether the tests appropriately support public health needs, whether laboratory results are utilized effectively by clinicians, and whether the tests serve any purpose if resources for treatment are not available.

For laboratories without access to computerized data systems and for whom the formulae in Chapter 23 are impractical, the true cost-effectiveness of tests can be assessed from the following formula which takes account of their contribution to patient management:[3]

$$\frac{A \times 100}{C} \times \frac{100}{B}$$

where A = cost/test; B = quality of test; C = clinical usefulness of test.

A. Cost/test

The cost for a test is not simply reagent cost, but should include:

— staff salaries for the hours of staff time required based on workload units for each test which have been documented[4]

— equipment, with an annual amount for annual depreciation
— supplies and reagents, including quality control materials
— supervision
— transport and communications
— overheads, general maintenance and building costs.

As an example of the effect of these factors on costs, in a typical district hospital laboratory in Africa, malaria and tuberculosis microscopy may each comprise 20% of the total number of tests performed, but when the various factors outlined above are taken into account, tuberculosis smears actually account for 43% and malaria microscopy for 9% of the basic test cost.

B. Quality of test

The quality of the test will influence its utility. For example, if the result of a test in routine practice is only correct 80% of the time, then 1 in 5 tests will be wasted, reducing the effectiveness of the test by 20%. Furthermore, the inaccurate test may result in a patient receiving inappropriate treatment.

C. Clinical usefulness

An assessment of the clinical usefulness of a test should be carried out by an independent clinician who is familiar with local diseases and the diagnostic support services which are available. This assessor needs to compare actual clinical practice with locally agreed 'best practice' or, if available, local guidelines. From observation of a range of clinical interactions, the percentage of times that ideal practice is followed can be calculated. For example, transfusion guidelines may recommend that transfusions are given routinely to children with Hb less than 5 g/dl. The assessor can record how many children with Hb below this level failed to receive a transfusion, and how many transfusions were given without waiting for the Hb result, or at an inappropriate Hb. For each test, the assessor needs to judge whether appropriately requested and are used to influence patient management or public health decisions. The percentage of tests which are not used to guide clinical decisions will provide a figure for 'clinical wastage' of the test and this can be entered into the formula.

MAINTAINING THE QUALITY OF TESTS

Paradoxically, it is in under-resourced laboratories, where equipment and supplies are limited, and training and supervision may be minimal, that the level of skills and motivation required to maintain quality of service need to be highest. Even the most basic of laboratories should ensure that procedures are in place to monitor quality (see Ch. 24). In addition to monitoring the technical quality of each test, the quality of the whole service must be assured both within the laboratory (internal) and between laboratories (external). Standard operating procedures should be drafted for every method. In addition to providing standardized techniques, these are excellent teaching resources and adherence to these procedures will minimize errors. They need to be regularly reviewed and updated to keep pace with technical developments and changes in local circumstances (e.g. non-availability of reagents, technical limitations).

Quality control of individual test methods (technical quality)

Each test should include an internal quality control. For example, each batch of sickle screening tests should include known positive and negative samples; for monitoring haemoglobin estimations, the same high and low value samples can be re-measured several times during the day. Methods for internal quality control for each haematology test are described in Chapter 24 but these may need to be adapted to suit local circumstances in resource-poor countries.

Internal quality assurance

This is system within an individual laboratory for ensuring that the whole test process, rather than just one technical element, is of acceptable quality. Measures such as the introduction of standard operating procedures, in-service training and equipment maintenance schedules are designed to improve, and prevent problems with, quality assurance. Monitoring of quality by the use of controls which are put through the whole process will highlight problems with the system. For example, an inaccurate white cell differential count may point towards problems with sample collection and handling, slide preparation, fixing and staining, morphological interpretation and microscope quality as well as inadequate microscopy technique.

External quality assurance

Poor communications and transport facilities make this the most difficult type of quality monitoring for underresourced laboratories to establish. While linkage to an international or even, national, external quality assurance system may be beyond the capabilities of a small rural laboratory, it should be possible for them to link with neighbouring facilities. Rural laboratories can take advantage of programmes with established communications between the districts, to exchange materials and results between different laboratories. Such programmes might include district medical officer supervisory visits, or national vertical programmes such as tuberculosis monitoring or health education visits. A rural laboratory, which detects a problem with its results, needs to have a clearly defined reporting system to a higher level facility which is in turn, responsible for addressing the problem. Accreditation schemes (p. 559), either national or local, can be set up to formally recognize laboratories which are performing well and to assist those which are not.

BASIC HAEMATOLOGY TESTS

MEASUREMENT OF HAEMOGLOBIN CONCENTRATION

Various methods for the measurement of haemoglobin concentration are given in Chapter 3. The most accurate method which may be available in under-resourced laboratories is the haemiglobincyanide (cyanmethaemoglobin) method. However, this requires a power source and considerable technical expertise in order to carry out accurate dilutions and to prepare the standard curve.

Methods for measuring the haemoglobin concentration that are robust, accurate and can be used by unskilled health workers include the HemoCue Blood Hemoglobin system, the DHT haemoglobin meter and the haemoglobin colour scale.

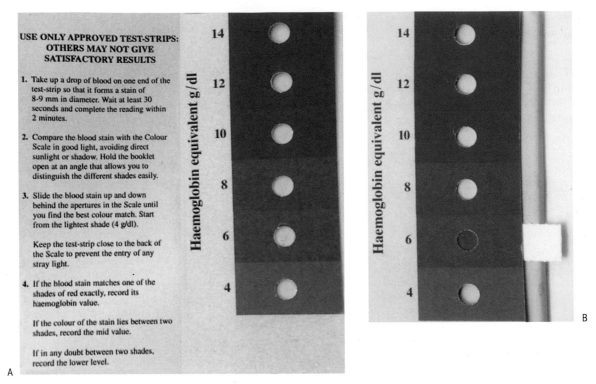

Fig. 26.2 Haemoglobin colour scale. The stained test-strip being read on the right (B) indicates a severe anaemia with haemoglobin value of about 6 g/dl.

HemoCue Blood Hemoglobin system (see p. 23)*

This is a battery or mains operated portable, direct read-out machine that uses disposable dry-chemistry cuvettes. It is precise and accurate and unlike most other systems, does not require pre-dilution of the sample. Although the use of disposable cuvettes makes this method relatively expensive, it is very simple to use so that the cost may be offset by savings on training and supervision.

DHT Haemoglobinmeter**

This is a portable, battery/mains operated, tropicalised, direct read-out machine. It has been specifically designed for use in poorer tropical countries. It uses a stable, inexpensive diluting fluid and has low power consumption. It is simple to use as the diluted sample is placed in a cuvette that is inserted into the

machine. This automatically initiates the reading and display of the haemoglobin value

Haemoglobin colour scale

Many colour comparison methods have been developed in the past but these have become obsolete because they were not sufficiently accurate or the colours were not durable. A new low-cost haemoglobin colour scale has been developed for diagnosing anaemia which is reliable to within 10 g/l (1 g/dl).[5] It consists of a set of printed colour shades representing haemoglobin levels between 4 and 14 g/dl. The colour of a drop of blood collected onto a specific type of absorbent paper is compared to that on the chart (Fig. 26.2). Evaluation studies have shown 96% sensitivity and 86% specificity for classifying haemoglobin levels as normal when Hb is $\geq$ 12 g/dl (i.e. 120 g/l), and anaemia as mild, moderate, marked and severe.[6] The utility of the scale in clinical practice has been demonstrated by field trials in rural antenatal clinics and peripheral health centres.[7,8] However, care must be taken to follow the instructions exactly as poor lighting, allowing the blood spot to dry out

*available from HemoCue AB, Box 1204, SE-262 23, Angelholm, Sweden. Tel: +46 431 45 82 00.

**available from Developing Health Technology, Bridge House, Worlington Road, Barton Mills, IP28 7DX, U.K. Tel: +44 (0) 1603 416058.

and using the incorrect type of absorbent paper can have detrimental effects on the results.**

MANUAL CELL COUNTS USING COUNTING CHAMBERS

Visual counting of blood cells is an acceptable alternative to electronic counting for white cell and platelet counts. It is not recommended for routine red cell counts because the number of cells which can be counted within a reasonable time in the routine laboratory (e.g. about 400) will be too few to ensure a precise result (see below).

Microscopes

The microscope is the most important piece of equipment in laboratories in under-resourced countries. It is essential for the diagnosis of anaemia, tuberculosis, malaria and other blood parasites, and for performing absolute and differential cell counts. Reliable assessment of these morphological features requires that the microscope is clean and set up to ensure clear images at high magnification. Failure to maintain the quality of microscopes to a high standard by routine maintenance and regular professional servicing can lead to inaccurate diagnoses and inefficient use of technician time.[9,10] Routine maintenance of the microscope is described on page 619.

Counting chambers

The visibility of the rulings in the counting chamber is as important as the accuracy of calibration, so that chambers with a 'metallized' surface and Neubauer or Improved Neubauer ruling are recommended. These have nine 1 mm × 1 mm ruled areas which, when covered correctly with the special thick cover-glass, each contain a volume of 0.1 µl of diluted blood (Figs 26.3 and 26.4). Cover slips designed for mounting of microscopy preparations are not suitable for use with counting chambers. The sample is introduced between the chamber and the cover-glass using a pipette or capillary, and the preparation is viewed using a ×40 objective and ×6 eyepieces. With Neubauer and Improved Neubauer

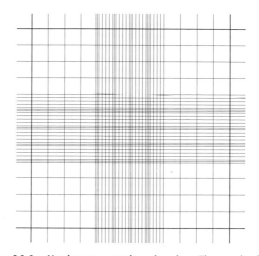

Fig. 26.3 Neubauer counting chamber. The total ruled area is 3 mm × 3 mm; the central ruled area is 1 mm × 1 mm. In the central area, 16 groups of 16 small squares are separated by triple rulings.

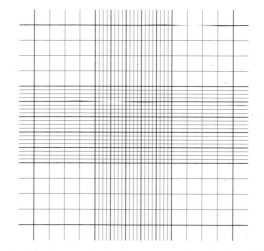

Fig. 26.4 Improved Neubauer counting chamber. The central area consists of 25 groups of 16 small squares separated by closely ruled triple lines (which appear as thick black lines in the photograph).

chambers, count the cells in 4 or 8 horizontal rectangles of 1 mm × 0.05 mm (80 or 160 small squares) or in 5 or 10 groups of 16 small squares, including the cells which touch the bottom and left-hand margins of the small squares.

Total white blood cell count

To make the counting of white cells easier, diluted whole blood is mixed with a fluid to lyse the red cells and stain the white cell nuclei deep violet-black.

**Information on availability of the Hb Colour Scale can be obtained from: Division of Blood Safety and Clinical Technology, WHO, 1211 Geneva 27; *Fax*: +41 22 791 4836.

Method

Make a 1 in 20 dilution of blood by adding 0.1 ml of well-mixed blood (lack of adequate mixing is a major source of error) to 1.9 ml of lysing fluid* (2% (20 ml/l) acetic acid coloured pale violet with gentian violet) in a 75×10 mm glass or plastic tube. After sealing the tube with a lid or tightly fitting bung, mix the diluted blood in a mechanical mixer or by hand for at least 2 min by tilting the tube through an angle of about $120°$ combined with rotation, thus allowing the air bubble to mix the suspension. Fill a clean dry counting chamber, with its cover-glass already in position, without delay. This is simply accomplished with the aid of a Pasteur pipette or a length of stout capillary glass tubing which has been allowed to take up the suspension by capillarity. Care should be taken that the counting chamber is filled in one action and that no fluid flows into the surrounding moat.

Leave the chamber undisturbed on a bench for at least 2 min for the cells to settle, but not much longer, for drying at the edges of the preparation initiates currents which cause movement of the cells after they have settled. The bench must be free of vibrations and the chamber not exposed to draughts or to direct sunlight or other sources of heat. It is important that the cover-glass should be of a special thick glass and perfectly flat, so that when laid on the counting chamber, diffraction rings are seen. The cover-glass should be of such a size that when placed correctly on the counting chamber the central ruled areas lie in the centre of the rectangle to be filled with the cell suspension.

If any of the following filling defects occur, the preparation must be discarded and the filling procedure repeated using another clean dry chamber:

● overflow into moat
● chamber area incompletely filled
● air bubbles anywhere in chamber area
● any debris in chamber area.

To obtain a coefficient of variation of 5%, it is necessary to count about 400 cells; in practice, it is reasonable to count 100 white cells. To minimize distribution errors, count the cells in the entire ruled area (i.e. 9×0.1 μl areas in an Improved Neubauer counting chamber).

---

* or a proportionately, smaller volume: 20 μl of blood in 0.38 ml of lysing fluid.

Calculation

White blood cell count per litre (WBC/l) =
$$\frac{\text{No. of cells counted}}{\text{Volume counted (μl)}} \times \text{Dilution} \times 10^6$$

Thus, if N cells are counted in 0.1 μl, then the WBC/l is:
$$\frac{N}{0.1} \times 20 \times 10^6 = N \times 200 \times 10^6$$

e.g. if 115 cells are counted, the WBC is $115 \times 200 \times 10^6/l = 23 \times 10^9/l$

Range of WBC in health
See pages 12 and 13.

Platelet count

Manual counts are used routinely in under-resourced laboratories and they are still needed even in well-equipped laboratories for blood samples with a significant proportion of giant platelets. However, for all other samples, automated full blood counters produce platelet counts with a precision which is much superior to that of manual platelet counts.

Platelet counts are best performed on EDTA-anticoagulated blood which has been obtained by clean venepuncture. They can also be carried out on blood obtained by skin prick but the results are less satisfactory than those on venous blood. Skin-prick platelet counts are significantly lower than counts on venous blood and less constant;[11] a variable number of platelets are probably lost at the site of the skin puncture. Manual platelet counts are performed by visual examination of diluted, lysed whole blood using a Neubauer or Improved Neubauer counting chamber as for total white cell counts.[12,13]

Method

The diluent consists of 1% aqueous ammonium oxalate in which the red cells are lysed. This method is recommended in preference to that using formal-citrate as diluent, which leaves the red cells intact and is more likely to give incorrect results, when the platelet count is low.

Before diluting the blood sample, examine it carefully for the presence of blood clots. If these are present, a fresh specimen should be requested as clots will cause the platelet count to be artificially low. Make a 1 in 20 dilution of well-mixed blood in the diluent by adding 0.1 μl of blood to 1.9 ml of ammonium oxalate diluent (10 g/l).

Not more than 500 ml of diluent should be made at a time, using scrupulously clean glassware and fresh glass-distilled or deionized water. If possible, the solution should be filtered through a micropore filter (0.22 μm) and kept at 4°C. For use, a small part of the stock is refiltered and dispensed in 1.9 ml volumes in 75 × 12 mm tubes.

Mix the suspension on a mechanical mixer for 10–15 min. Fill a Neubauer counting chamber with the suspension, using a stout glass capillary or Pasteur pipette. Place the counting chamber in a moist Petri dish and leave untouched for at least 20 min to give time for the platelets to settle.

Examine the preparation with the ×40 objective and ×6 or ×10 eyepieces. The platelets appear under ordinary illumination as small (but not minute) highly refractile particles, if viewed with the condenser racked down; they are usually well separated and clumps are rare if the blood sample has been skilfully collected. To avoid introducing dirt particles into the chamber which might be mistaken for platelets, all equipment must be scrupulously clean. Platelets are more easily seen with the phase-contrast microscope. A special thin-bottomed (1 μm) counting chamber is best for optimal phase-contrast effect. The number of platelets in one or more areas of 1 mm² should be counted. The total number of platelets counted should always exceed 200 in order to ensure a coefficient of variation of 8–10%.

Calculation

Platelet count per litre =

$$\frac{\text{No. of cells counted}}{\text{Volume counted (μl)}} \times \text{Dilution} \times 10^6$$

Thus, if N is the number of platelets counted in an area of 1 mm² (0.1 μl in volume), the number of platelets per litre of blood is:

$$N \times 10 \times 20 \text{ (dilution)} \times 10^6 = N \times 200 \times 10^6$$

Range of platelet counts in health
See pages 12 and 13.

Errors in manual cell counts

The errors associated with manual cell counts are *technical* and *inherent*.

Technical errors can be minimized by avoiding the following:

- poor technique in obtaining the blood specimen
- insufficient mixing of the blood specimen
- inaccurate pipetting and the use of badly calibrated pipettes or counting chambers
- inadequate mixing of the cell suspension
- faulty filling of the counting chamber
- careless counting of cells within the chamber.

Standardized counting chambers. To reduce errors, it is important to have a good quality counting chamber. The exact chamber depth depends also on the cover-glass, which should be free from bowing and sufficiently thick so as not to bend when pressed on the chamber. It must be free from scratches, and even the smallest particle of dust may cause unevenness in its lie on the chamber. The *British Standard for Haemocytometer and Particle Counting Chambers (BS 748: 1982)* has specified a tolerance of dimensions for counting chambers which provides reasonable accuracy.

Accurate dilutions. Bulb-diluting pipettes are not recommended; they are difficult to calibrate and easily broken. The volumes of blood used are unnecessarily small and it is difficult to fill the counting chamber so that the exact amount of fluid is delivered. 0.1 ml and 20 μl pipettes are relatively inexpensive and easy to calibrate. With a 2 ml volume in a glass or plastic tube provided with a tightly fitting rubber or plastic bung, a suspension easy to label and handle is obtained, and, with a little practice, a perfect filling of the counting chamber can regularly be accomplished with the aid of a fine plastic Pasteur pipette or stout glass capillary.

Automatic diluter units are useful. These consist of a dual metering system which enables a volume of diluent and the appropriate volume of blood to be dispensed consecutively into a tube (see p. 617). A variety of automatic diluting systems are now available which have good accuracy and precision. Hand-held semi-automatic microsamplers with a detachable tip are designed to operate as 'to deliver' pipettes but a regular supply of the disposable tips may be too expensive and difficult to maintain for poorer laboratories.

Pipetting errors apply to all tests which involve dilution of the blood sample and they also occur with autodiluters which are liable to error with viscid fluids and when the delivery volume of the unit is not correctly adjusted.

Microscopy artefacts. Dirt or clumped red cell debris may be mistaken for white cells or particularly for platelets. Clumping of white cells occurs particularly in heparinized blood, especially when the concentration of heparin exceeds 25 iu per ml of blood. The clumps are most frequently seen in blood which has been allowed to stand for several hours before undertaking the count.

Inherent errors are due to uneven distribution of cells in the counting chamber, and no amount of mixing will minimize this inherent variation in numbers between areas. Inherent error can only be reduced by counting more cells in a preparation. In theory, the count varies in proportion to the square root of the number of cells counted, i.e. if four times the number of cells are counted, the variation is halved. For example, when performing a manual white cell count, 95% of observed counts on a sample of true value 5.0×10^9 cells per litre would lie within the range 4.0–6.0. In practice, the difference between 5.0 and 6.0×10^9 cells per litre is of little clinical significance.

It is also important for the observer not to bias the count by foreknowledge of what result might be expected, or by selecting certain areas in the chamber for counting.[14]

LABORATORY-ASSOCIATED TRAINING

In poorer countries, there is often no system for regular supervision of an individual's performance in the laboratory, and many staff never receive any regular, broad-based education between graduation and retirement. Professional education and monitoring of standards should continue for the whole professional life of laboratory staff in order to ensure high quality results. For under-resourced countries, training is often delivered in association with vertical health programmes such as HIV or TB control. The need for training in basic haematological techniques is often overlooked because tests such as haemoglobin estimation and white cell counts are usually not linked to specific diseases and are therefore not amenable to incorporation in a vertical programme. However, the importance of accurate haemoglobin measurements cannot be overemphasized. Anaemia is the most prevalent disorder worldwide and is often the first sign of underlying disease. Continuing education should consequently be based on the whole range of tests offered by the laboratory rather than concentrating on those that are used to support the diagnosis of specific diseases.

Laboratory staff
Individuals need to keep their own training record, perhaps in the form of a log book, and to have their training achievements and plans regularly reviewed by their line managers. Central records of all training should also be maintained for monitoring purposes and to ensure equitable and appropriate distribution of training between different cadres of staff. Regular monitoring of the quality of results from individual laboratories will enable specific problems to be identified and issues such as equipment failures, discontinuity of supplies and communication breakdowns brought to the attention of regional management teams. In addition, this quality monitoring will allow discrete training needs to be identified, enabling limited teaching resources to be specifically targeted.

Laboratory users
Appropriate clinical use of the laboratory has a direct impact on the cost-effectiveness of the service (p. 592). Laboratory tests may be initiated by nurses, health field workers and public health institutions as well as doctors. Many of these cadres have had little or no training in how to request appropriate tests, provide timely and suitable samples and how to use the results for maximal benefit. Training for laboratory users needs to be incorporated into laboratory training programmes and closely monitored. In poorer countries, there is often a dearth of clinicians with both clinical and laboratory experience who are qualified to provide such training. Under these circumstances, the relationship between the laboratory and clinical staff can be enhanced, and use of the laboratory optimized, by using a clinician/ technologist team to provide training across both disciplines.

Health management teams
Local health management teams are often responsible for ensuring that their laboratories are provided with the necessary tools to deliver a high quality service. As a rule, these teams do not

include members of the laboratory profession who instead are represented by other allied professions such as pharmacists. Staff in under-resourced laboratories are therefore not always responsible for purchasing supplies and equipment for the laboratory and this results in wastage through the purchase of inappropriate or poor quality equipment and reagents. In addition to encouraging adequate representation of laboratory professionals at management level, it is important to ensure that non-laboratory personnel responsible for making decisions about under-resourced laboratories, are educated about the needs of their laboratory service.

HEALTH AND SAFETY ISSUES

Details of these issues are described in Chapter 23 (p. 556). Awareness of safety issues should be constantly promoted within all laboratories and the working environment needs to be made as safe as possible. A *Code of Safe Laboratory Practice* should be prepared which is affordable and relevant to the local circumstances. It should include:

- identification of the potential workplace hazards and the risk they pose to individuals working or visiting the laboratory (i.e. risk assessment)
- education about safe working practices
- monitoring of adherence to health and safety regulations
- prompt reporting and investigation of laboratory accidents.

BLOOD COLLECTION

Disposable syringes are available for single-use only. They cannot withstand sterilization and should never be re-used.

Needles are generally intended for single use. Similarly, disposable lancets for skin puncture must never be re-used. The practice of using a single lancet on several patients consecutively, and cleaning it with alcohol between use, is totally unacceptable.

REFERENCES

1 Lewis SM, Bain BJ, Swirsky DM 2001 Bench-aid for the morphological diagnosis of anaemia. WHO, Geneva.

2 World Health Organization 1998 Laboratory services for primary heath care: requirements for essential clinical laboratory tests. Document: LAB/98.1. WHO, Geneva.

3 Floyd K, Gilks C, Kadewele G, et al 1997 A baseline assessment of laboratory services in Ntcheu District. The Essential Medical Laboratory Services Project (EMLS) – Phase 1. Available from: HIV Work Programme, Liverpool School of Tropical Medicine, Pembroke Place, Liverpool L3 5QA, UK.

4 Welcan UK 1990 Workload measurement system for pathology, manual with schedule of units, 1990 edition. ISBN 0750400722.

5 Stott GJ, Lewis SM 1995 A simple and reliable method for estimating haemoglobin. Bulletin of the World Health Organization 73:369–373.

6 Ingram CF, Lewis SM 2000 Clinical use of WHO haemoglobin colour scale: validation and critique. Journal of Clinical Pathology 53:933–937.

7 Van den Broek NR, Ntonya C, Mhanga E, et al 1999 Diagnosing anaemia in pregnancy in rural clinics: assessing the potential of the haemoglobin colour scale. Bulletin of the World Health Organization 77:15–21.

8 Montressor A, Albonico M, Khalfan N, et al 2000 Field trial of a haemoglobin colour scale: an effective tool to detect anaemia in pre-school children. Tropical Medicine and International Health 5:129–133.

9 Mundy C, Ngwira M, Kadawele G, et al 2000 Transactions of the Royal Society of Medicine and Hygiene 94:583–584.

10 Opoku-Okrah C, Rumble R, Bedu-Addo G, et al 2000 Transactions of the Royal Society of Medicine and Hygiene 94:582.

11 Brecher G, Schneiderman M, Cronkite EP 1953 The reproducibility and constancy of the platelet count. American Journal of Clinical Pathology 23:15.

12 Brecher G, Cronkite EP 1950 Morphology and enumeration of human blood platelets. Journal of Applied Physiology 3:365.

13 Lewis SM, Wardle J, Cousins S, et al 1979 Platelet counting – development of a reference method and a reference preparation. Clinical and Laboratory Haematology 1:227.

14 Sanders C, Skerry DW 1961 The distribution of blood cells on haemocytometer counting chambers with special reference to the amended British Standards Specification 748 (1958). Journal of Clinical Pathology 48:298.

USEFUL PUBLICATIONS NOT SPECIFICALLY REFERRED TO IN THE TEXT
Laboratory organization and management
World Health Organization 1990 Primary health care – towards the year 2000. WHO/SHS/901. WHO, Geneva.

Houng L, El-Nageh MM 1993 Principles of management of health laboratories. WHO Regional Publications, Eastern Mediterranean Series No. 3.

World Health Organization 1993 Laboratory equipment preventative maintenance programme. In: Principles of management of health laboratories. WHO Regional Publications, Eastern Mediterranean Series No 3.

World Health Organization 1994 Health laboratory facilities in emergency and disaster situations. WHO Regional Publications, Eastern Mediterranean Series No. 6.

World Health Organization 1999 Health laboratory services in support of primary health care in South East Asia. WHO South East Asia Regional Office (SEARO), Publication No. 24 (2nd edn).

Health and safety
World Health Organization 1993 Laboratory biosafety manual, 2nd edn. WHO Distribution and Sales, Geneva.

Centers for Disease Control and National Institutes for Health 1993 US Department of Health and Human Services: Biosafety in microbiological and biomedical laboratories, 3rd edn. Government Printing Office, Washington DC.

World Health Organization 1997 Safety in health care laboratories. WHO/LAB/97.1. WHO, Geneva.

Practical methods
World Health Organization 1986 Methods recommended for essential clinical chemical and haematological tests for intermediate hospital laboratories. WHO/LAB/86.3. WHO, Geneva.

Carter JY, Lema OE 1994 Practical laboratory manual for health centres in Eastern Africa. African Medical and Research Foundation, PO Box 31025, Nairobi, Kenya.

World Health Organization 1995 Production of basic diagnostic laboratory reagents. WHO Regional Publications, Eastern Mediterranean Series No. 2.

World Health Organization 2000 Manual of basic techniques (revised 2nd edn). WHO Distribution and Sales, Geneva.

Quality assurance
World Health Organization 1992 Basics of quality assurance for intermediate and peripheral laboratories. WHO Regional Publications, Eastern Mediterranean Series No. 2.

World Health Organization 1993 Quality assurance related to health laboratory technology. WHO, Geneva.

World Health Organization 1995 Quality systems for medical laboratories: Guidelines for implementation and monitoring. WHO Regional Publications, Eastern Mediterranean Series No. 14.

Lewis SM 1998 Quality Assurance in Haematology WHO Document: LAB/98.4. WHO, Geveva.

Preventive maintenance of equipment
World Health Organization 1992 Calibration and maintenance of semi-automated haematology equipment: Document: LBS/92.8. WHO, Geneva.

World Health Organization 1994 Maintenance and repair of laboratory, diagnostic imaging, and hospital equipment. WHO Distribution and Sales, Geneva.

Training for laboratories
Abbott FR 1992 Teaching for better learning: a guide for teachers of primary health care staff. WHO, Geneva.

World Health Organization 1992 Technical training requirements: Report of meeting on development of appropriate technology to support primary health care. WHO, Geneva.

WHO addresses
The WHO documents on this list are generally available, without charge, from Blood Safety and Clinical Technology Division, WHO, 1211 Geneva 27 (Fax: +41 22 791 4836) or from the appropriate Regional Office:
- Eastern Mediterranean: PO Box 1517, Alexandria 21511, Egypt.
- South-east Asia: World Health House, Indraprastha Estate, New Delhi, 110002, India.

Material from WHO Distribution and Sales is available at reduced prices in developing countries.

Sources of teaching material and equipment for underresourced laboratories
ECHO JOINT MISSION HOSPITAL EQUIPMENT BOARD
Ullswater Crescent, Coulsdon, Surrey, CR3 2HR, UK
Telephone: +44 (0) 208 660 2220;
Fax: +44 (0) 208 668 0751;
e-mail; cs@echohealth.org.uk

DEVELOPING HEALTH TECHNOLOGY
Bridge House, Worlington Road, Barton Mills, IP28 7DX, UK

TROPICAL HEALTH TECHNOLOGY
14 Bevill's Close, Doddington, March, Cambridgeshire
PE15 0TT, UK
Telephone: +44 (0) 1354 740825;
Fax: +44 (0) 1354 740013
e-mail: thtbooks@tht.ndirect.co.uk

TEACHING AIDS AT LOW COST (TALC)
P.O Box 49, St Albans, Herts. AL1 5TX, UK

Telephone: +44 (0) 727 853869;
Fax: +44 (0) 727 846852
e-mail: talcuk@btinternet.com
web page: www.talcuk.org

TALC Library/Resource Centre:
Institute of Child Health
30 Guilford Street, London, WC1N 1EH, UK
Telephone: +44 (0) 207 242 9789, ext. 2424

Appendices

S. Mitchell Lewis

1. PREPARATION OF COMMONLY USED REAGENTS, ANTICOAGULANTS AND PRESERVATIVE SOLUTIONS

Water

For most purposes, still-prepared distilled water or deionized water is equally suitable. Throughout this text, this is implied when 'water' is referred to. When doubly-distilled or glass-distilled water is required this has been specially indicated, and when tap-water is satisfactory or indicated, this, too, has been stated.

Acid–citrate–dextrose (ACD) solution – NIH-A

Trisodium citrate, dihydrate (75 mmol/l)	22 g
Citric acid, monohydrate (42 mmol/l)	8 g
Dextrose (139 mmol/l)	25 g
Water	to 1 litre

Sterilize the solution by autoclaving at 121°C for 15 min. Its pH is 5.4. For use, add 10 volumes of blood to 1.5 volumes of solution. For use in red cell survival studies, see page 328.

Acid–citrate–dextrose (Alsever's) solution

Dextrose (114 mmol/l)	20.5 g
Trisodium citrate, dihydrate (27 mmol/l)	8.0 g
Sodium chloride (72 mmol/l)	4.2 g
Water	to 1 litre

Adjust the pH to 6.1 with citric acid (c 0.5 g) and then sterilize the solution by micropore filtration (0.22 μm) or by autoclaving at 121°C for 15 min. For use, add 4 volumes of blood to 1 volume of solution.

Citrate–phosphate–dextrose (CPD) solution, pH 6.9

Trisodium citrate, dihydrate (102 mmol/l)	30 g
Sodium dihydrogen phosphate, monohydrate (1.08 mmol/l)	0.15 g
Dextrose (11 mmol/l)	2 g
Water	to 1 litre

Sterilize the solution by autoclaving at 121°C for 15 min. After cooling to c 20°C, it should have a brown tinge and its pH should be 6.9.

Citrate–phosphate–dextrose (CPD) solution, pH 5.6–5.8

Trisodium citrate, dihydrate (89 mmol/l)	26.30 g
Citric acid, monohydrate (17 mmol/l)	3.27 g

Sodium dihydrogen phosphate
monohydrate (16 mmol/l)   2.22 g
Dextrose (142 mmol/l)   25.50 g
Water   to 1 litre

Sterilize the solution by autoclaving at 121°C for
15 min. For use as an anticoagulant-preservative,
add 7 volumes of blood to 1 volume of solution.

Citrate–phosphate–dextrose–adenine (CPD-A) solution, pH 5.6–5.8

Trisodium citrate, dihydrate
(89 mmol/l)   26.30 g
Citric acid, monohydrate (17 mmol/l)   3.27 g
Sodium dihydrogen phosphate,
monohydrate (16 mmol/l)   2.22 g
Dextrose (177 mmol/l)   31.8 g
Adenine (2.04 mmol/l)   0.275 g
Water   to 1 litre

Sterilize the solution by autoclaving at 121°C for
15 min. For use as an anticoagulant-preservative,
add 7 volumes of blood to 1 volume of solution.

Low ionic strength solution[1]

Sodium chloride (NaCl) (30.8 mmol/l)   1.8 g
Disodium hydrogen phosphate
(Na_2HPO_4) (1.5 mmol/l)   0.21 g
Sodium dihydrogen phosphate
(NaH_2PO_4) (1.5 mmol/l)   0.18 g
Glycine (NH_2CH_2COOH)
(240 mmol/l)   18.0 g
Water   to 1 litre

Dissolve the sodium chloride and the two phosphate salts in c 400 ml of water; dissolve the glycine separately in c 400 ml of water; adjust the pH of each solution to 6.7 with 1 mol/l NaOH. Add the two solutions together and make up to 1 litre. Sterilize by Seitz filtration or autoclaving. The pH should be within the range of 6.65–6.85, the osmolality 270–285 mmol, and conductivity 3.5–3.8 mS/cm at 23°C.

EDTA

Ethylenediamine tetra-acetic acid,
dipotassium salt   100 g
Water   to 1 litre

Allow appropriate volumes to dry in bottles at c 20°C so as to give a concentration of 1.5 ± 0.25 mg/ml of blood.

Neutral EDTA, pH 7.0, 110 mmol/l

Ethylenediamine tetra-acetic acid,
dipotassium salt   44.5 g
or disodium salt   41.0 g
1 mmol/l NaOH   75 ml
Water   to 1 litre

Neutral buffered EDTA, pH 7.0

Ethylenediamine tetra-acetic acid,
disodium salt (9 mmol/l)   3.35 g
Disodium hydrogen phosphate
(Na_2HPO_4) 26.4 mmol/l   3.75 g
Sodium chloride (NaCl) (140 mmol/l)   8.18 g
Water   to 1 litre

Saline

Sodium chloride (NaCl)
(154 mmol/l)   9.0 g
Water   to 1 litre

Trisodium citrate ($Na_3C_6H_5O_7.2H_2O$), 109 mmol/l

Dissolve 32 g* in 1 litre of water. Distribute convenient volumes (e.g. 10 ml) into small bottles and sterilize by autoclaving at 121°C for 15 min.

Heparin

Powdered heparin (lithium salt) is available with an activity of c 160 iu/mg. Dissolve it in water at a concentration of 4 mg/ml. Sodium heparin is available in 5 ml ampoules with an activity of 1000 iu/ml. Add appropriate volumes of either solution to a series of containers and allow to dry at c 20°C so as to give a concentration not exceeding 15–20 iu/ml of blood.

---

* or 38 g of $2Na_3C_6H_5O_7.11H_2O$.

2. BUFFERS

Barbitone buffer, pH 7.4

Sodium diethyl barbiturate ($C_8H_{11}O_3N_2Na$) (57 mmol/l)	11.74 g
Hydrochloric acid (HCl) (100 mmol/l)	430 ml

Barbitone buffered saline, pH 7.4

NaCl	5.67 g
Barbitone buffer, pH 7.4	1 litre

Before use, dilute with an equal volume of 9 g/l NaCl.

Barbitone buffered saline, pH 9.5

Sodium diethyl barbiturate ($C_8H_{11}O_3N_2Na$) (98 mmol/l)	20.2 g
Hydrochloric acid (HCl) (100 mmol/l)	20 ml
NaCl	5.67 g

Before use, dilute the buffer with an equal volume of 9 g/l NaCl.

Barbitone–bovine serum albumin (BSA) buffer, pH 9.8

Sodium diethyl barbiturate ($C_8H_{11}O_3N_2Na$) (54 mmol/l)	10.3 g
NaCl (102 mmol/l)	6.0 g
Sodium azide (31 mmol/l)	2.0 g
Bovine serum albumin	5.0 g
Water	to 1 litre

Dissolve the reagents in c 900 ml of water. Adjust the pH to 9.8 with 5 mol/l HCl. Make up the volume to 1 litre with water. Store at 4°C.

Citrate-saline buffer

Trisodium-citrate ($Na_3C_6HO_7.2H_2O$) (5 mmol/l)	1.5 g
NaCl (96 mmol/l)	5.6 g
Barbitone buffer, pH 7.4	200 ml
Water	800 ml

Glycine buffer, pH 3.0

Glycine (NH_2CH_2COOH) (82 mmol/l)	6.15 g
NaCl (82 mmol/l)	4.80 g
Water	820 ml
0.1 mol/l HCl	180 ml

HEPES buffer, pH 6.6

4-(2-Hydroxyethyl)-1-piperazine-ethane sulphonic acid (100 mmol/l)	23.83 g

Dissolve in c 100 ml of water. Add a sufficient volume of 1 mol/l NaOH (c 1 ml) to adjust the pH to 6.6. If the buffer is intended for use with Romanowsky staining (p. 53), then add 25 ml of dimethyl sulphoxide (DMSO). Make up the volume to 1 litre with water.

HEPES–saline buffer, pH 7.6

HEPES (4-(2-Hydroxyethyl)-1-peperazine-ethane sulphonic acid (20 mmol/l)	4.76 g
NaCl	8.0

Dissolve in c 100 ml of water. Add a sufficient volume of 1 mol/l NaOH to adjust the pH to 7.6. Make up volume to 1 litre with water.

Imidazole buffered saline, pH 7.4

Imidazole (50 mmol/l)	3.4 g
NaCl (100 mmol/l)	5.85 g

Dissolve in c 500 ml of water. Add 18.6 ml of 1 mol/l HCl and make up the volume to 1 litre with water. Store at room temperature (18–25°C).

Phosphate buffer, iso-osmotic

(A) $NaH_2PO_4.2H_2O$ (150 mmol/l)	23.4 g/l
(B) Na_2HPO_4 (150 mmol/l)	21.3 g/l

pH	Solution A	Solution B
5.8	87 ml	13 ml
6.0	83 ml	17 ml
6.2	75 ml	25 ml
6.4	66 ml	34 ml
6.6	56 ml	44 ml
6.8	46 ml	54 ml
7.0	32 ml	68 ml
7.2	24 ml	76 ml
7.4	18 ml	82 ml
7.6	13 ml	87 ml
7.7	9.5 ml	90.5 ml

Normal human serum has an osmolality of 289 ± 4 mmol. Hendry[2] recommended slightly different concentrations of the stock solution, namely, 25.05 g/l $NaH_2PO_4.2H_2O$ and 17.92 g/l Na_2HPO_4 for an iso-osmotic buffer.

Phosphate buffered saline

Equal volumes of iso-osmotic phosphate buffer and 9 g/l NaCl.

Phosphate buffer, Sörensen's

Stock solutions:

	66 mmol/l	100 mmol/l	150 mml/l
(A) KH_2PO_4	9.1 g/l	13.8 g/l	20.7 g/l
(B) Na_2HPO_4	9.5 g/l	14.4 g/l	21.6 g/l
or $Na_2HPO_4.2H_2O$	11.9 g/l	18.0 g/l	27.1 g/l

To obtain a solution of the required pH, add A and B in the indicated proportions:

pH	A	B
5.4	97.0	3.0
5.6	95.0	5.0
5.8	92.2	7.8
6.0	88.0	12.0
6.2	81.0	19.0
6.4	73.0	27.0
6.6	63.0	37.0
6.8	50.8	49.2
7.0	38.9	61.1
7.2	28.0	72.0
7.4	19.2	80.8
7.6	13.0	87.0
7.8	8.5	91.5
8.0	5.5	94.5

This buffer is not iso-osmotic with normal plasma (see above).

Tris–HCl buffer (200 mmol/l)

Tris (Hydroxymethyl)aminomethane (24.23 g/l)	250 ml

To obtain a solution of the required pH, add the appropriate volume of 1 mol/l HCl and then make up the volume to 1 litre with water.

pH	Volume
7.2	44.5 ml
7.4	42.0 ml
7.6	39.0 ml
7.8	33.5 ml
8.0	28.0 ml
8.2	23.0 ml
8.4	17.5 ml
8.6	13.0 ml
8.8	9.0 ml
9.0	5.0 ml

100 mmol/l, 150 mmol/l, 300 mmol/l and 750 mmol/l stock solutions may be similarly prepared with an appropriate weight of Tris and volume of acid.

Tris–HCl bovine serum albumin (BSA) buffer, pH 7.6, 20 mmol/l

Tris (hydroxymethyl) aminomethane (20 mmol/l)	2.42 g
EDTA, disodium salt (10 mmol/l)	3.72 g
NaCl (100 mmol/l)	5.85 g
Sodium azide (3 mmol/l)	0.2 g

Dissolve the reagents in c 800 ml of water. Adjust the pH to 7.6 with 10 mol/l HCl. Add 10 g of bovine serum albumin and make up to 1 litre with water.

Buffered formal acetone

Dissolve 20 mg Na_2HPO_2 and 100 mg KH_2PO_4 in 30 ml distilled water. Add 45 ml acetone and 25 ml 40% formalin. Mix well and store at 4°C. Use cold. Make up new fixative every 4 weeks.

3. COAGULATION REAGENTS

Rabbit brain thromboplastin

Freeze-dried rabbit brain thromboplastins are now widely available commercially with a shelf-life of at least 2 to 5 years. Usually, they are calibrated against the WHO International Reference Preparation of thromboplastin and are supplied with an International Sensitivity Index (ISI) and a table converting prothrombin times to International Normalized Ratios (INR).

If a commercial preparation is not available, it is possible to prepare a home-made substitute using rabbit brain which does not require freeze drying and which is relatively stable.

Acetone-dried brain powder

Strip the membrane off freshly collected rabbit brain, wash free from blood and place in about 3 times its volume of cold acetone. Macerate for 2–3 min and then filter through absorbent lint (BP or USP grade) on a Büchner funnel. Repeat the extraction 7 times; after two extractions increase the time of exposure to acetone to *c* 20 min for each subsequent extraction. The material should become 'gritty' by the fourth or fifth extraction. After the last extraction, spread the acetone-dried brain on a piece of paper and allow to dry in air for 30 min. Rub through a 1-mm mesh nylon sieve to produce a coarse powder. Dispense into a batch of screw-capped bottles and dry over phosphorus pentoxide in a vacuum dessicator. After drying, screw down the caps tightly and store at 4°C or –20°C. At –20°C, the material should be stable for at least 5 years. 100 g of whole brain yield *c* 15 g of dried powder.

Preparation of liquid suspension

Dissolve 0.9 g of NaCl and 0.9 g of phenol in 100 ml of water. Suspend 3.6 g of the acetone-dried brain in 100 ml of this phenol–saline solution at 15–20°C and allow to stand at this temperature for 4–5 h, mixing at 30-min intervals. Transfer to a 4°C refrigerator for 24 h with occasional mixing. Thereafter, leave undisturbed at 4°C for 3 h and then decant the supernatant carefully through fine muslin or similar material. The ISI should be not more than 1.4 (see p. 416) and the mean normal prothrombin time 12–13 s. Store the suspension at 4°C. At this temperature, it will be stable for at least 6 months, and for at least 7 days at room temperature. It must not be allowed to freeze as freezing results in flocculation of the smooth suspension with deterioration of thromboplastic activity.

APTT phospholipid reagent

Acetone-dried rabbit brain is suitable for preparing a APTT reagent. Bovine brain may also be used.

Prepare acetone-dried brain powder as described above. Suspend 5 g of the powder in 20 ml of chloroform (analytic grade) in a covered beaker for 1–2 h. Filter through filter paper to obtain a clear filtrate. Wash the brain deposit on the filter paper with 20 ml of chloroform and pool the clear filtrate with the previous filtrate. Evaporate the filtrate to dryness in a beaker of known weight in a water-bath at 60–70°C and weigh the residual deposit: 5 g of dried brain should yield *c* 1.5 g of phospholipid deposit. Emulsify in saline to give a 5% emulsion; 1.5 g of deposit should provide 30 ml of emulsion. Distribute the emulsion in small volumes in stoppered tubes. At –20°C it should be stable for at least 1 year.

For use, dilute 1 in 100 in saline and mix with an equal volume of 2.5 mg/ml kaolin suspension in imidazole buffer.

4. REFERENCE STANDARDS AND REAGENTS

A wide range of international reference materials has been established by the World Health Organization and these are held at designated institutions. The majority of the materials of haematological interest which are listed below are held at the National Institute for Biological Standards and Control (NIBSC). Those indicated by an asterisk are held at the WHO International Laboratory for Biological Standards, Central Laboratory of the Netherlands Red Cross Blood Transfusion Service (CLB). A comprehensive catalogue is available[3] and details can also be found on the WHO* and NIBSC** websites.

General haematology

Erythropoietin, human, urinary
Erythropoietin, rDNA-derived
Ferritin, human, recombinant
Haemiglobincyanide
Hb A_2
Hb F
Vitamin B_{12} in human serum

Folate, whole blood
C-reactive protein (CRP)
Human serum protein for immuno-assay: includes transferrin*

Immunohaematology
Anti-A blood-typing serum*
Anti-B blood-typing serum*
Anti-D (anti-Rh_0) incomplete blood-typing serum*
Anti-D (anti-Rh_0) complete blood-typing serum*
Anti-E complete blood-typing serum*

Immunology
Human serum immunoglobulins IgG, IgA and IgM
Human serum immunoglobulin IgE
Antinuclear factor, homogeneous*
Horseradish peroxidase-conjugated sheep anti-human IgG*
Human serum complement components C1q, C4, C5, factor B and functional CH_{50}*

Coagulation
Ancrod
Anti-thrombin, plasma
Anti-thrombin concentrate
Factors II, VII, IX, X, plasma
Factors II and X concentrate
Factor VIII and von Willebrand factor, plasma
Factor VII concentrate
Factor VIII concentrate
Factor IX concentrate
Factor IXa concentrate
Heparin, low molecular weight
Plasma fibrinogen
Plasmin
Plasminogen activator inhibitor
Tissue plasminogen activator, recombinant
Streptokinase
α-Thrombin
β-Thromboglobulin
Anti-human platelet antigen-1a

Platelet factor 4
Protein S, plasma
Protein C, plasma
Protamine
Urokinase, high molecular weight
Thromboplastin, bovine, combined*
Thromboplastin, human, recombinant*
Thromboplastin, rabbit, plain*

The following Certified Reference Materials have been established by the European Union (BCR).

Haemiglobincyanide
Monosized latex particles:
CRM165: 2.2 μm (5.7 fl); CRM166: 4.8 μm (60.0 fl); CRM167: 9.5 μm diameter
Thromboplastin, bovine (CRM148)
Thromboplastin, rabbit, plain (CRM149)
Human serum proteins (CRM470), including haptoglobin

Contact addressess

National Institute for Biological Standards and Control (NIBSC):
Blanche Lane, South Mimms, Herts EN6 3QH, England
Tel: 44 1707 646399
Fax: 44 1707 646977
Email: standards@nibsc.ac.uk

Central Laboratory of Netherlands Red Cross Blood Transfusion Service (CLB):
125 Plesmanlaan, 1066 AD Amsterdam Netherlands
Tel: 31 20 512 9222
Fax: 31 20 512 3252

European Union (BCR)
Institute for Reference Materials and Measurements (IRMM)
Retieseweg B2440, Geel, Belgium
Fax: 32 14 590 406
Email: bcr.sales@irmm.jrc.be

5. PREPARATION OF GLASSWARE

Flask for defibrination of blood
Provide a 100 ml conical flask with a central glass rod to the bottom end of which are fused pieces of glass capillary (Fig. 1.2, p. 4). The rod is kept in position with a cotton-wool plug. Deliver 10–50 ml of blood into the flask and, after reinserting the central rod, hold the flask by the neck and rotate it by hand. The blood is usually successfully defibrinated within 5 min, the fibrin forming on the glass

rod, usually in one piece. Little or no lysis is caused, and the blood is as a rule completely free from small clots.

Siliconized glassware

Use c 2% solution of silicone (dimethyldichlorosilane) in solvent. Immerse the clean glassware or syringes to be coated in the fluid and allow to drain dry. (Rubber gloves should be worn and the procedure should be performed in a fume cupboard provided with an exhaust fan.) Then rinse the coated glassware thoroughly in water, and allow to dry in an oven at 100°C for 10 min or overnight in an incubator.

6. METHODS OF CLEANING SLIDES AND APPARATUS

New slides

Boxes of clean, grease-free slides are available commercially. If these are not available, the following procedure should be carried out. Leave the slides overnight in a detergent solution. Then wash well in running tap-water, rinse in distilled or deionized water and store in 95% ethanol or methanol until used. Dry with a clean linen cloth and carefully wipe free from dust before they are used.

Dirty slides

When discarded, place in a detergent solution, heat at 60°C for 20 min and then wash in hot, running tap-water. Finally, rinse in water before being dried with a clean linen cloth.

Chemical apparatus and glassware

Wash in running tap-water and then boil in a detergent solution, rinse in acid and wash in hot, running tap-water, as described above. Alternatively, the apparatus can be soaked in 3 mol/l HCl.

For the removal of deposits of protein and other organic matter, 'biodegradable' detergents are recommended. Decon 90 (Decon Laboratories Ltd, Hove BN3 3LY, UK) is suitable but a number of similar preparations are also available.

Iron-free glassware

Wash in a detergent solution, then soak in 3 mol/l HCl for 24 h and finally rinse in deionized, double-distilled water.

7. SIZES OF TUBES

The sizes of tubes recommended in the text have been chosen as being appropriate for the tests described. The dimensions given are the length and external diameter (in mm). The equivalent in inches, as given in some catalogues, and certain corresponding internal diameters, are as follows:

75 × 10 mm
(internal diameter 8 mm) $= 3 \times \frac{3}{8}''$

75 × 12 mm
(internal diameter 10 mm) $= 3 \times \frac{1}{2}''$
65 × 10 mm $= 2\frac{1}{2} \times \frac{3}{8}''$
38 × 6.4 mm $= 1\frac{1}{2} \times \frac{1}{4}''$ ('precipitin tubes')
100 × 12 mm $= 4 \times \frac{1}{2}''$
150 × 16 mm $= 6 \times \frac{5}{8}''$
150 × 19 mm $= 6 \times \frac{3}{4}''$

8. SPEED OF CENTRIFUGING

Throughout the book, the unit given is the relative centrifugal force (g). Conversion of this figure to rpm (rev/min) depends upon the radius of the centrifuge; it can be calculated by reference to the nomogram illustrated in Figure 27.1, or from the formula for relative centrifugal force:

$$RCF = 118 \times 10^{-7} \times r \times N^{-2}$$

where r = radius (cm) and N = speed of rotation (rpm).

The following centrifugal forces are recommended:

'Low-spun' platelet-
rich plasma   150–200 g (for 10–15 min).
'High-spun' plasma   1200–1500 g (for 15 min).
Packing of red cells 2000–2300 g (for 30 min).

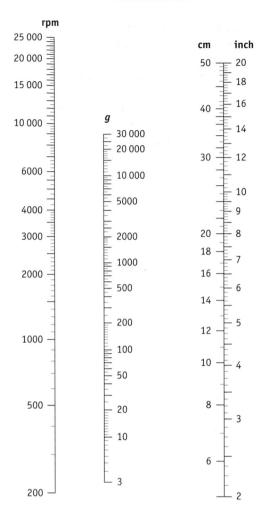

Fig. 27.1 Nomogram for computing relative centrifugal forces.

9. UNITS OF WEIGHT AND MEASUREMENT IN COMMON USE IN HAEMATOLOGY

Throughout the book, measurements have been expressed in SI units, in accordance with international recommendations.[4] These units are derived from the metric system. The base units are shown below and the abbreviated forms are indicated alongside.

Weight – unit: gram (g)
$\times 10^3$ = kilogram (kg)
$\times 10^{-3}$ = milligram (mg)
$\times 10^{-6}$ = microgram (μg)
$\times 10^{-9}$ = nanogram (ng)
$\times 10^{-12}$ = picogram (pg)

Length – unit: metre (m)
$\times 10^{-1}$ = decimetre (dm)

$\times 10^{-2}$ = centimetre (cm)
$\times 10^{-3}$ = millimetre (mm)
$\times 10^{-6}$ = micrometre (μm)
$\times 10^{-9}$ = nanometre (nm)

Volume – unit: litre (l or L) = dm^3
$\times 10^{-1}$ = decilitre (dl) (fomerly 100 ml)
$\times 10^{-3}$ = millilitre (ml) = cm^3 (formerly cc)
$\times 10^{-6}$ microlitre (μl) = mm^3
$\times 10^{-9}$ = nanolitre (nl)
$\times 10^{-12}$ = picolitre (pl)
$\times 10^{-15}$ femtolitre (fl)

Amount of substance – unit: mole (mol)
$\times 10^{-3}$ = millimole (mmol)
$\times 10^{-6}$ = micromole (μmol)

Substance concentration – unit: moles per litre (mol/l) (formerly M)

$\times 10^{-3}$ = millimole per litre (mmol/l)
$\times 10^{-6}$ = micromole per litre (μmol/l)

Mass concentration – unit: gram per litre (g/l)

$\times 10^{-3}$ = milligram per litre (mg/l)
$\times 10^{-6}$ = microgram per litre (μg/l)

When preparing a small amount of a reagent, it is more appropriate to express its concentration per ml or dl.

To convert a measurement from mass concentration to molar concentration, divide by the molecular mass. Thus, for example, the molecular mass of human Hb (as 4Fe tetramer) is 64 458 (see p. 21) or 16 114 as the Fe monomer. Then, when Hb is 160 g/l this is equivalent to 160 ÷ 16 114 mol/l, i .e. 9.9 mmol/l.

10. ATOMIC WEIGHTS AND MOLECULAR CONCENTRATIONS

The concentration of a substance in solution can be expressed either in g/l or in mol/l. The latter is also indicated by M; thus, e.g. 0.1M HCl = 0.1 mol/l. A mole (mol) is the molecular weight or relative molecular mass (RMM) of the substance (including water of crystallization if present). Thus, e.g.

RMM of NaCl $= 58.5$
$\therefore$ 1 mol/l $\quad = 58.5$ g/l
$\quad$ 9 g/l $\quad\quad = 9 \div 58.5 = 0.154$ mol/l
$\quad\quad\quad\quad\quad = 154$ mmol/l

The atomic weights of some chemicals which are commonly used in preparation of reagents are as follows:

Calcium	40
Carbon	12
Chlorine	35
Chromium	52
Hydrogen	1
Iron	56
Magnesium	24
Nitrogen	14
Oxygen	16
Phosphorus	31
Potassium	39
Sodium	23
Sulphur	32

11. RADIATION DOSES

When using radionuclides, account must be taken of their potential risk for the recipient and for the laboratory workers. The extent of radiation hazard in relation to the small amount of radionuclide employed in diagnostic work depends on a number of factors, namely, the energy and range of the radiations; whether the radionuclide is widely distributed in the body or becomes localized in specific organs; the physical half-life of the radionuclide and its biological half-time in the body.

Formerly, radioactivity was expressed in curies (Ci); 10^{-3} Ci = 1 mCi and 10^{-6} = 1 μCi. The preferred SI unit of radioactivity is the Bequerel (Bq). 1 Bq corresponds to one disintegration per second, so that 1 Ci = 3.7×10^{10} Bq, 1 millicurie (mCi) = 3.7×10^{7} Bq or 37 megabequerels (MBq), and 1 microcurie (μCi) = 3.7×10^{4} Bq or 0.037 MBq; 10^{3} MBq = 1 gigabequerel (GBq).

The effect of radiation on the body depends, essentially, on the amount of energy deposited. This is expressed in grays (Gy). 1 Gy is the dose of radiation which deposits 1 joule of energy per kg of tissue. In the past, this has been expressed in rads (1 Gy = 100 rad). The reaction of the body to the radiation is also affected by the type of the particular ionizing ray. The biological effect of the radiation is calculated from the amount of Gy (or rad) multiplied by an ionization quality factor; this factor varies with the type of ray and it is 20 times more for α-rays than for β- and γ-rays. The unit for describing biological effect of radiation, i.e. the unit of 'effective dose', is the Sievert (Sv). The annual dose limit for the whole body for somebody working with radionuclides is 50 mSv, with a larger amount for individual organs. Lower dose limits, of 5 mSv, apply to members of the public.

12. CHEMICAL DISINFECTANTS[5]

Sodium hypochlorite (chlorine)

This is the most commonly used disinfectant in the laboratory as it is very active against all microorganisms, although less active against fungi than other compounds described below. Its disadvantage is that it is corrosive to metal. As hypochlorite solutions gradually lose their strength, fresh dilutions must be made daily. For general use a concentration of 1 g/l (1000 ppm) as available chlorine is required; a stronger solution containing 5 g/l (5000 ppm) is necessary for dealing with blood spillage.

Household bleaches usually contain 50 g/l as available chlorine, and should thus be diluted 1:50 for general use and 1:10 for blood contamination. Other chlorine-containing compounds can be prepared as follows:

Calcium hypochlorite (70% available chlorine) 1.4 g/l; 7 g/l for blood contamination.
Sodium dichloroisocyanurate (NaDCC) (60% available chlorine) 1.7 g/l; 20 g/l for blood contamination.
Chloramine (25% available chlorine) 20 g/l in all conditions.

Formaldehyde

Formaldehyde is active against all organisms, but is less effective at temperatures below 20 °C. A solution of 5% formalin in water is recommended for use against hepatitis B virus and also Ebola virus.

Gluteraldehyde

Active against all microorganisms at a concentration of 20 g/l (2%). It is especially useful for decontaminating equipment with metal components. Before use, the solution must be activated by addition of bicarbonate to make it alkaline, and it must be used within 2 weeks. It must be handled with caution, avoiding contact with skin, eyes and respiratory tract.

Phenolic compounds

Several common disinfectants are based on phenolic compounds. They are active against fungi and all vegetative bacteria but not against spores, and they vary in their activity against viruses.

Alcohols

Ethanol and isopropyl alcohol have similar disinfectant properties at a concentration of 70% in water; higher or lower concentrations reduce their germicidal effectiveness. They are active against vegetative bacteria, and lipid viruses but not against spores or fungi. Their effect on nonlipid viruses is variable. Alcohol is especially effective when mixed with other agents, e.g. 70% alcohol with 100 g/l of formaldehyde or with 2 g/l (2000 ppm) available chlorine.

13. STATISTICAL PROCEDURES

Mean ($\bar{x}$) is the sum of all the measurements (Σ) divided by the number of measurements (n).

Median (m) is the point on the scale that has an equal number of observations above and below.

Mode is the most frequently occurring result.

Gaussian distribution describes events or data which occur symetrically about the mean (see Fig. 2.1, p. 10); with this type of distribution, mean, median and mode will be approximately equal. The extent of spread of measurements about the mean is expressed as the standard deviation (SD). Its calculation is described below. 68% of all the measurements will be within the ±1 SD range, 95% within ±2 SD and 99% within ±3 SD.

Log normal distribution describes events which are asymetrical (skewed) with a larger number of observations towards one end. The mean will thus be nearer that end; the mean, median and mode may differ from each other. To calculate geometric mean and SD, the data are first converted to their logarithms and after calculating the mean and SD of the logarithms, the results are reconverted to the antilog.

Poisson distribution describes events which are random in their occurrence. This will be the case, for example, when blood cells are counted in a diluted suspension. The number of cells which are counted in a given volume will vary on each occasion; this count variation (σ) is $0.92 \sqrt{\lambda}$, where λ = the total number of cells counted (see p. 598). It is an estimate of the standard deviation of the entire population whereas SD denotes the standard deviation of the items that were actually measured.

Coefficient of variation (CV) is another way of indicating standard deviation, related to the actual measurement so that variation at different levels can be compared. It is expressed as a percentage.

Standard error of mean (SEM) is a measure of dispersion of the mean of a set of measurements. It is used to compare means of two sets of data.

CALCULATIONS

Variance $(s^2) = \dfrac{\sum (x - \bar{x})^2}{n - 1}$

Standard deviation (SD) $= \sqrt{s^2}$

Coefficient of variation (CV) $= \dfrac{SD}{\bar{x}} \times 100\%$

Standard error of mean (SEM) $= \dfrac{SD}{\sqrt{n}}$

Standard deviation of paired (duplicate) results =

$$\sqrt{\frac{\sum d^2}{2n}}$$

Where   d = difference between duplicates,

n = number of duplicate measurements.

Standard deviation of median =

$$\frac{\text{Central } 50\% \text{ of results*}}{1.35}$$

(*i.e. between 25% and 75%)

ANALYSIS OF DIFFERENCES BY T-TEST

This is a method for comparing two sets of data, e.g. to assess the accuracy of a new method against a reference method.

Calculation

(1) Variance $(s^2) = \dfrac{\sum (d - \bar{d})^2}{n - 1}$

where   d = differences between paired measurements

$\bar{d}$ = mean of the differences

n = number of paired measurements

(2) $t = \bar{d} \div \sqrt{\dfrac{s^2}{n}}$

From the t-test chart (Table 27.1) read the value of t for the appropriate degree of freedom (i.e. $n - 1$). Express results as the level of probability (p) that there is *no* significant difference between the sets of data that are being compared.

ANALYSIS OF VARIANCE BY F-RATIO

This is a method to assess the relative precision of two sets of measurements.

Calculation

Variance $(s^2) = \dfrac{\sum (x - \bar{x})^2}{n - 1}$

for set A and for set B, respectively:

$F\text{-ratio} = \dfrac{s^2 \text{ of set A}}{s^2 \text{ of set B}}$

As the ratio must not be less than 1, use the higher variance as the numerator. Then, from the chart (Table 27.2), read the value at either 95% or 99% probability (i.e. $p = 0.05$ or $p = 0.01$) for the appropriate degrees of freedom (i.e. $n - 1$) for the two sets of data.

Interpretation

There is a significant difference in variance between the two sets when the calculated ratio is greater than the value read from the chart.

14. AUTOMATED (MECHANICAL) PIPETTES

Accurate pipetting is an essential requirement for all quantitative tests. A variety of automated hand-held pipettes are available, many of which incorporate a disposable tip with an ejector mechanism which allows the user to remove it without hand contact. Some pipettes have a fixed capacity, in others a range of volumes can be obtained by means of an adjusting screw and

Table 27.1 Critical values of t-test

df	% Probability level						
	50 (0.5)	40 (0.4)	30 (0.3)	20 (0.2)	10 (0.1)	5 (0.05)	1 (0.01)
1	1.000	1.376	1.963	3.078	6.314	12.706	63.657
2	0.816	1.061	1.386	1.886	2.920	4.303	9.925
3	0.765	0.978	1.250	1.638	2.353	3.182	5.841
4	0.741	0.941	1.190	1.533	2.132	2.776	4.604
5	0.727	0.920	1.156	1.476	2.015	2.571	4.032
6	0.718	0.906	1.134	1.440	1.943	2.447	3.707
7	0.711	0.896	1.119	1.415	1.895	2.365	3.499
8	0.706	0.889	1.108	1.397	1.860	2.306	3.355
9	0.703	0.883	1.100	1.383	1.833	2.262	3.250
10	0.700	0.879	1.093	1.372	1.812	2.228	3.169
11	0.697	0.876	1.088	1.363	1.796	2.201	3.106
12	0.695	0.873	1.083	1.356	1.782	2.179	3.055
13	0.694	0.870	1.079	1.350	1.771	2.160	3.012
14	0.692	0.868	1.076	1.345	1.761	2.145	2.977
15	0.691	0.866	1.074	1.341	1.753	2.131	2.947
16	0.690	0.865	1.071	1.337	1.746	2.120	2.921
17	0.689	0.863	1.069	1.333	1.740	2.110	2.989
18	0.688	0.862	1.067	1.330	1.734	2.101	2.878
19	0.688	0.861	1.066	1.328	1.729	2.093	2.861
20	0.687	0.860	1.064	1.325	1.725	2.086	2.845
21	0.686	0.859	1.063	1.323	1.721	2.080	2.831
22	0.686	0.858	1.061	1.321	1.717	2.074	2.819
23	0.685	0.858	1.061	1.321	1.717	2.074	2.819
24	0.685	0.857	1.059	1.318	1.711	2.064	2.797
25	0.684	0.856	1.058	1.316	1.708	2.060	2.787
26	0.684	0.856	1.058	1.315	1.706	2.056	2.779
27	0.684	0.855	1.057	1.314	1.703	2.052	2.771
28	0.683	0.855	1.056	1.313	1.701	2.048	2.763
29	0.683	0.854	1.055	1.311	1.699	2.045	2.756
30	0.683	0.854	1.055	1.310	1.697	2.042	2.750
40	0.681	0.851	1.050	1.303	1.684	2.021	2.704
50	0.680	0.849	1.048	1.299	1.676	2.008	2.678
60	0.679	0.848	1.046	1.296	1.671	2.000	2.660
120	0.677	0.845	1.041	1.289	1.658	1.980	2.617
∞	0.674	0.842	1.036	1.282	1.645	1.960	2.576

the delivery volume is displayed on a digital readout.

As the designs are varied, the specific manufacturer's instructions must be carefully adhered to. The following important points are common to all:

1. Always use the specified tip.
2. Never wash and re-use tips.
3. Ensure that the tip is fitted firmly to the pipette.
4. Keep the pipette clean of dirt and grease.
5. Always pipette in a vertical position.
6. Never leave the pipette on its side with liquid in the tip.
7. Return the pipette to its stand after use.
8. Operate by a slow, smooth consistent procedure, avoiding bubbles or foaming.
9. Use 'reverse pipetting' for plasma, high viscosity fluids and/or very small volumes. With the plunger pressed all the way down (2nd

Table 27.2 F Distribution tables
(a) 99% Probability (p = 0.01)

df Numerator

df Numerator	1	2	3	4	5	6	7	8	9	10	12	15	20	24	30	40	60	120	∞
1	4052	4999.5	5403	5625	5764	5859	5928	5981	6022	6056	6106	6157	6209	6235	6261	6287	6313	6339	6366
2	98.50	99.00	99.17	99.25	99.30	99.33	99.36	99.37	99.39	99.40	99.42	99.43	99.45	99.46	99.47	99.47	99.48	99.49	99.50
3	34.12	30.82	29.46	28.71	28.24	27.91	27.67	27.49	27.35	27.23	27.05	26.87	26.69	26.60	26.50	26.41	26.32	26.22	26.13
4	21.20	18.00	16.69	15.98	15.52	15.21	14.98	14.80	14.66	14.55	14.37	14.20	14.02	13.93	13.84	13.75	13.65	13.56	13.46
5	16.26	13.27	12.06	11.39	10.97	10.67	10.46	10.29	10.16	10.05	9.89	9.72	9.55	9.47	9.38	9.29	9.20	9.11	9.02
6	13.75	10.92	9.78	9.15	8.75	8.47	8.26	8.10	7.98	7.87	7.72	7.56	7.40	7.31	7.23	7.14	7.06	6.97	6.88
7	12.25	9.55	8.45	7.85	7.46	7.19	6.99	6.84	6.72	6.62	6.47	6.31	6.16	6.07	5.99	5.91	5.82	5.74	5.65
8	11.26	8.65	7.59	7.01	6.63	6.37	6.18	6.03	5.91	5.81	5.67	5.52	5.36	5.28	5.20	5.12	5.03	4.95	4.86
9	10.56	8.02	6.99	6.42	6.06	5.80	5.61	5.47	5.35	5.26	5.11	4.96	4.81	4.73	4.65	4.57	4.48	4.40	4.31
10	10.04	7.56	6.55	5.99	5.64	5.39	5.20	5.06	4.94	4.85	4.71	4.56	4.41	4.33	4.25	4.17	4.08	4.00	3.91
11	9.65	7.21	6.22	5.67	5.32	5.07	4.89	4.74	4.63	4.54	4.40	4.25	4.10	4.02	3.94	3.86	3.78	3.69	3.60
12	9.33	6.93	5.95	5.41	5.06	4.82	4.64	4.50	4.39	4.30	4.16	4.01	3.86	3.78	3.70	3.62	3.54	3.45	3.36
13	9.07	6.70	5.74	5.21	4.86	4.62	4.44	4.30	4.19	4.10	3.96	3.82	3.66	3.59	3.51	3.43	3.34	3.25	3.17
14	8.86	6.51	5.56	5.04	4.69	4.46	4.28	4.14	4.03	3.94	3.80	3.66	3.51	3.43	3.35	3.27	3.18	3.09	3.00
15	8.68	6.36	5.42	4.89	4.56	4.32	4.14	4.00	3.89	3.80	3.67	3.52	3.37	3.29	3.21	3.13	3.05	2.96	2.87
16	8.53	6.23	5.29	4.77	4.44	4.20	4.03	3.89	3.78	3.69	3.55	3.41	3.26	3.18	3.10	3.02	2.93	2.84	2.75
17	8.40	6.11	5.18	4.67	4.34	4.10	3.93	3.79	3.68	3.59	3.46	3.31	3.16	3.08	3.00	2.92	2.83	2.75	2.65
18	8.29	6.01	5.09	4.58	4.25	4.01	3.84	3.71	3.60	3.51	3.37	3.23	3.08	3.00	2.92	2.84	2.75	2.66	2.57
19	8.18	5.93	5.01	4.50	4.17	3.94	3.77	3.63	3.52	3.43	3.30	3.15	3.00	2.92	2.84	2.76	2.67	2.58	2.49
20	8.10	5.85	4.94	4.43	4.10	3.87	3.70	3.56	3.46	3.37	3.23	3.09	2.94	2.86	2.78	2.69	2.61	2.52	2.42
21	8.02	5.78	4.87	4.37	4.04	3.81	3.64	3.51	3.40	3.31	3.17	3.03	2.88	2.80	2.72	2.64	2.55	2.46	2.36
22	7.95	5.72	4.82	4.31	3.99	3.76	3.59	3.45	3.35	3.26	3.12	2.98	2.83	2.75	2.67	2.58	2.50	2.40	2.31
23	7.88	5.66	4.76	4.26	3.94	3.71	3.54	3.41	3.30	3.21	3.07	2.93	2.78	2.70	2.62	2.54	2.45	2.35	2.26
24	7.82	5.61	4.72	4.22	3.90	3.67	3.50	3.36	3.26	3.17	3.03	2.89	2.74	2.66	2.58	2.49	2.40	2.31	2.21
25	7.77	5.57	4.68	4.18	3.85	3.63	3.46	3.32	3.22	3.13	2.99	2.85	2.70	2.62	2.54	2.45	2.36	2.27	2.17
26	7.72	5.53	4.64	4.14	3.82	3.59	3.42	3.29	3.18	3.09	2.96	2.81	2.66	2.58	2.50	2.42	2.33	2.23	2.13
27	7.68	5.49	4.60	4.11	3.78	3.56	3.39	3.26	3.15	3.06	2.93	2.78	2.63	2.55	2.47	2.38	2.29	2.20	2.10
28	7.64	5.45	4.57	4.07	3.75	3.53	3.36	3.23	3.12	3.03	2.90	2.75	2.60	2.52	2.44	2.35	2.26	2.17	2.06
29	7.60	5.42	4.54	4.04	3.73	3.50	3.33	3.20	3.09	3.00	2.87	2.73	2.57	2.49	2.41	2.33	2.23	2.14	2.03
30	7.56	5.39	4.51	4.02	3.70	3.47	3.30	3.17	3.07	2.98	2.84	2.70	2.55	2.47	2.39	2.30	2.21	2.11	2.01
40	7.31	5.18	4.31	3.83	3.51	3.29	3.12	2.99	2.89	2.80	2.66	2.52	2.37	2.29	2.20	2.11	2.02	1.92	1.80
60	7.08	4.98	4.13	3.65	3.34	3.12	2.95	2.82	2.72	2.63	2.50	2.35	2.20	2.12	2.03	1.94	1.84	1.73	1.60
120	6.85	4.79	3.95	3.48	3.17	2.96	2.79	2.66	2.56	2.47	2.34	2.19	2.03	1.95	1.86	1.76	1.66	1.53	1.38
∞	6.63	4.61	3.78	3.32	3.02	2.80	2.64	2.51	2.41	2.32	2.18	2.04	1.88	1.79	1.70	1.59	1.47	1.32	1.00

Table 27.2 F Distribution tables (contd.)
(b) 95% Probability (p = 0.05)

df Numerator / df Numerator	1	2	3	4	5	6	7	8	9	10	12	15	20	24	30	40	60	120	∞
1	161.4	199.5	215.7	224.6	230.2	234.0	236.8	238.9	240.5	241.9	243.9	245.9	248.0	249.1	250.1	251.1	252.2	253.3	254.3
2	18.51	19.00	19.16	19.25	19.30	19.33	19.35	19.37	19.38	19.40	19.41	19.43	19.45	19.45	19.46	19.47	19.48	19.49	19.50
3	10.13	9.55	9.28	9.12	9.01	8.94	8.89	8.85	8.81	8.79	8.74	8.70	8.66	8.64	8.62	8.59	8.57	8.55	8.53
4	7.71	6.94	6.59	6.39	6.26	6.16	6.09	6.04	6.00	5.96	5.91	5.86	5.80	5.77	5.75	5.72	5.69	5.66	5.63
5	6.61	5.79	5.41	5.19	5.05	4.95	4.88	4.82	4.77	4.74	4.68	4.62	4.56	4.53	4.50	4.46	4.43	4.40	4.36
6	5.99	5.14	4.76	4.53	4.39	4.28	4.21	4.15	4.10	4.06	4.00	3.94	3.87	3.84	3.81	3.77	3.74	3.70	3.67
7	5.59	4.74	4.35	4.12	3.97	3.87	3.79	3.73	3.68	3.64	3.57	3.51	3.44	3.41	3.38	3.34	3.30	3.27	3.23
8	5.32	4.46	4.07	3.84	3.69	3.58	3.50	3.44	3.39	3.35	3.28	3.22	3.15	3.12	3.08	3.04	3.01	2.97	2.93
9	5.12	4.26	3.86	3.63	3.48	3.37	3.29	3.23	3.18	3.14	3.07	3.01	2.94	2.90	2.86	2.83	2.79	2.75	2.71
10	4.96	4.10	3.71	3.48	3.33	3.22	3.14	3.07	3.02	2.98	2.91	2.85	2.77	2.74	2.70	2.66	2.62	2.58	2.54
11	4.84	3.98	3.59	3.36	3.20	3.09	3.01	2.95	2.90	2.85	2.79	2.72	2.65	2.61	2.57	2.53	2.49	2.45	2.40
12	4.75	3.89	3.49	3.26	3.11	3.00	2.91	2.85	2.80	2.75	2.69	2.62	2.54	2.51	2.47	2.43	2.38	2.34	2.30
13	4.67	3.81	3.41	3.18	3.03	2.92	2.83	2.77	2.71	2.67	2.60	2.53	2.46	2.42	2.38	2.34	2.30	2.25	2.21
14	4.60	3.74	3.34	3.11	2.96	2.85	2.76	2.70	2.65	2.60	2.53	2.46	2.39	2.35	2.31	2.27	2.22	2.18	2.13
15	4.54	3.68	3.29	3.06	2.90	2.79	2.71	2.64	2.59	2.54	2.48	2.40	2.33	2.29	2.25	2.20	2.16	2.11	2.07
16	4.49	3.63	3.24	3.01	2.85	2.74	2.66	2.59	2.54	2.49	2.42	2.35	2.28	2.24	2.19	2.15	2.11	2.06	2.01
17	4.45	3.59	3.20	2.96	2.81	2.70	2.61	2.55	2.49	2.45	2.38	2.31	2.23	2.19	2.15	2.10	2.06	2.01	1.96
18	4.41	3.55	3.16	2.93	2.77	2.66	2.58	2.51	2.46	2.41	2.34	2.27	2.19	2.15	2.11	2.06	2.02	1.97	1.92
19	4.38	3.52	3.13	2.90	2.74	2.63	2.54	2.48	2.42	2.38	2.31	2.23	2.16	2.11	2.07	2.03	1.98	1.93	1.88
20	4.35	3.49	3.10	2.87	2.71	2.60	2.51	2.45	2.39	2.35	2.28	2.20	2.12	2.08	2.04	1.99	1.95	1.90	1.84
21	4.32	3.47	3.07	2.84	2.68	2.57	2.49	2.42	2.37	2.32	2.25	2.18	2.10	2.05	2.01	1.96	1.92	1.87	1.81
22	4.30	3.44	3.05	2.82	2.66	2.55	2.46	2.40	2.34	2.30	2.23	2.15	2.07	2.03	1.98	1.94	1.89	1.84	1.78
23	4.28	3.42	3.03	2.80	2.64	2.53	2.44	2.37	2.32	2.27	2.20	2.13	2.05	2.01	1.96	1.91	1.86	1.81	1.76
24	4.26	3.40	3.01	2.78	2.62	2.51	2.42	2.36	2.30	2.25	2.18	2.11	2.03	1.98	1.94	1.89	1.84	1.79	1.73
25	4.24	3.39	2.99	2.76	2.60	2.49	2.40	2.34	2.28	2.24	2.16	2.09	2.01	1.96	1.92	1.87	1.82	1.77	1.71
26	4.23	3.37	2.98	2.74	2.59	2.47	2.39	2.32	2.27	2.22	2.15	2.07	1.99	1.95	1.90	1.85	1.80	1.75	1.69
27	4.21	3.35	2.96	2.73	2.57	2.46	2.37	2.31	2.25	2.20	2.13	2.06	1.97	1.93	1.88	1.84	1.79	1.73	1.67
28	4.20	3.34	2.95	2.71	2.56	2.45	2.36	2.29	2.24	2.19	2.12	2.04	1.96	1.91	1.87	1.82	1.77	1.71	1.65
29	4.18	3.33	2.93	2.70	2.55	2.43	2.35	2.28	2.22	2.18	2.10	2.03	1.94	1.90	1.85	1.81	1.75	1.70	1.64
30	4.17	3.32	2.92	2.69	2.53	2.42	2.33	2.27	2.21	2.16	2.09	2.01	1.93	1.89	1.84	1.79	1.74	1.68	1.62
40	4.08	3.23	2.84	2.61	2.45	2.34	2.25	2.18	2.12	2.08	2.00	1.92	1.84	1.79	1.74	1.69	1.64	1.58	1.51
60	4.00	3.15	2.76	2.53	2.37	2.25	2.17	2.10	2.04	1.99	1.92	1.84	1.75	1.70	1.65	1.59	1.53	1.47	1.39
120	3.92	3.07	2.68	2.45	2.29	2.17	2.09	2.02	1.96	1.91	1.83	1.75	1.66	1.61	1.55	1.50	1.43	1.35	1.25
∞	3.84	3.00	2.60	2.37	2.21	2.10	2.01	1.94	1.88	1.83	1.75	1.67	1.57	1.52	1.45	1.39	1.32	1.22	1.00

stop), dip the tip well below the surface of the fluid and release the plunger knob slowly. Remove the pipette, wipe the outside of the tip carefully with a tissue and then, with the tip against the inside wall of the receiving container, deliver its contents by depressing the plunger knob to the 1st stop. Then discard the tip with its residual contents.

10. For blood dilution, fill and empty the tip with the blood 2–3 times, then depress the plunger to the 1st stop and with the tip well below the surface of the specimen, release the plunger to fill the tip with blood. Withdraw the pipette from the specimen, wipe the outside of the tip carefully with a tissue, dip the tip into the diluent well below the surface, and press the plunger knob repeatedly to fill and empty the tip until the interior wall is clear. Then depress the plunger to the 2nd stop to empty the tip completely.

11. At intervals, monitor the reliability of the pipette by checking its accuracy and precision.

Quality control of pipette reliability

1. Ensure that all the items to be used are at ambient room temperature.
2. Record the weight of a weighing beaker using a precision balance sensitive to 0.1 mg.
3. Record the temperature of a tube of distilled water, fill the pipette with the water, wipe the outside of the tip and dispense the water into the weighing beaker with the tip touching the side of the beaker.

Table 27.3 Ambient temperature factor for correction of weight:volume ratio

Temp °C	Volume factor
18	0.9986
19	0.9984
20	0.9982
21	0.9980
22	0.9978
23	0.9976
24	0.9973
25	0.9971
26	0.9968
27	0.9965
28	0.9963
29	0.9960
30	0.9957

4. Record the weight of the beaker plus water and calculate the weight of the water.
5. Calculate the volume (in μl) from the weight (in mg) ÷ the ambient temperature factor (Table 27.3).
6. Repeat the procedure ten times, changing the tip each time.
7. Calculate the mean, SD and CV of the dispensed volume (see p. 613). From the mean, calculate the percentage deviation from the expected volume by the formula:

$$\frac{\text{Expected volume} - \text{Delivered volume}}{\text{Expected volume}} \times 100.$$

For routine purposes, this should not differ by more than 1.5%. The CV should be <1%.

15. AUTODILUTERS

Autodiluter systems provide a constant dilution of blood in reagent by a single process. To check their accuracy, a calibrated 0.2-ml pipette and 50-ml volumetric flask are required. Equipment which is certified as conforming to these measurements in accordance with national standards is available commercially, or their accuracy can be checked by the procedure described above.

Mix well a 2–3 ml specimen of fresh whole blood and lyse (see p. 240). Then dilute manually 1/251 in haemiglobincyanide reagent (see p. 20) using the calibrated pipette and volumetric flask. At the same time, dilute a sample of the blood in haemiglobin-cyanide solution, in duplicate, by means of the autodiluter. Read the absorbance of each solution at 540 nm in a spectrophotometer. The dilution by the autodiluter is obtained from the formula:

$$A_1 \times \frac{\text{dilution (i.e. 1:251)}}{A_2}$$

where A_1 = absorbance at 540 nm of manual dilution and A_2 = absorbance at 540 nm of autodiluted sample.

If indicated, an appropriate adjustment should be made to the autodiluter in accordance with the manufacturer's instructions or a correction factor should be applied whenever the autodiluter is used.

16. MICROSCOPY

Microscope components

The main components of most routine microscopes are illustrated in Figure 27.2. The objectives are usually marked with their magnifying power, but older lenses may be marked by their focal length instead. The approximate equivalents are as follows:

Focal length (mm)	Magnification
2	× 100
4	× 40
16	× 10
40	× 4

The working distance of the objective is the distance between the objective and the object to be visualized. The greater the magnifying power of the objective, the smaller the working distance:

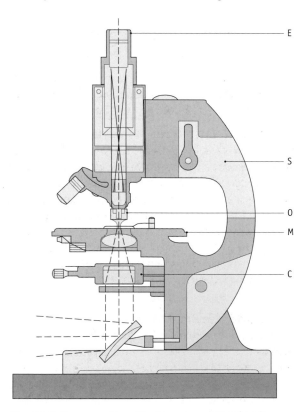

Fig. 27.2 Cross-section of microscope, showing its components. E, eyepiece; S, stand; O, objective; M, mechanical stage; C, condenser. The broken lines indicate the light path. Note that this shows an external light source being directed into the microscope. In most modern microscopes there is an inbuilt lamp in the base.

Objective	Working distance
× 10	5–6 mm
× 40	0.5–1.5 mm
× 100	0.15–0.20 mm

These specifications mean that when a cover-glass is used, if it is too thick it will not be possible to focus at high magnification. Thus, the cover-glass should be no more than 0.15 mm thick for examination of covered preparations by the ×100 oil-immersion. Furthermore, if the glass slide is too thick, this may prevent correct focus of the light path through the condenser to the object, as described below.

Setting up the microscope illumination

1. If the microscope requires an external light source, using the mirror at the base direct the light into the condenser. If the illumunation is built in make sure that the lamp voltage is turned down before switching on the microscope; then turn up the lamp until it is c 70% of maximum power.
2. Place a slide of a blood film with a cover-glass on the stage.
3. Lower the condenser, open the iris diaphragm fully and bring the preparation on the slide into focus with the ×10 objective.
4. Check that the eyepieces are adjusted to the operator's inter-pupillary width and that the specimen is in focus for each eye by rotating the focusing mechanism on the adjustable eyepiece.
5. Close the diaphragm and raise the condenser slowly until the edge of the circle of light comes into sharp focus.
6. Using the condenser centering screws, adjust its position so that the circle of light is in the centre of the field.
7. Open the diaphragm completely so that light fills the whole field of view.
8. Remove the eyepieces, so that the upper lens of the objective is seen to be filled with a circle of light. Close the diaphragm slowly until the circle of light occupies about two-thirds of the surface.

9. Replace the eyepieces, refocus the specimen and if necessary re-adjust the condenser aperture and lamp brightness to obtain the sharpest possible image.

Examination of slides

Low power (×10). Start with the objective just above the slide preparation. Then raise the objective with the coarse adjustment screw until a clear image is seen in the eyepiece. If there is insufficient illumination, rack up the condenser slightly.

High power (×40). Rack the condenser halfway down; lower the objective until it is just above the slide preparation. Use the coarse adjustment to raise the objective very slowly until a blurred image appears. Then bring into focus using the fine adjustment. If necessary, raise the condenser to obtain sufficient illumination.

Oil immersion (×100). Place a small drop of immersion oil on the part to be examined. Rack up the condenser as far as it will go. Lower the objective until it is in contact with the oil. Bring it as close as possible to the slide, but avoid pressing on the preparation. Look through the eyepiece and turn the fine adjustment very slowly until the image is in focus.

After using the oil-immersion objective, to avoid scratching the lens or coating the ×40 lens with oil, first swing the ×10 objective (or an empty lens space on the nosepiece) into place before removing the slide. As far as possible, use oil only when essential, e.g. for determining malaria species, and examine blood films for morphology or differential leucocyte count with the ×40 lens without oil.

17. ROUTINE MAINTENANCE OF MICROSCOPE

The microscope is a delicate instrument which must be handled gently. It must be installed in a clean environment away from chemicals, direct sunlight, heating source or moisture. If the stage is contaminated with saline, it must be cleaned immediately to avoid corrosion. Even in a temperate climate humidity and high temperatures cause growth of fungus which can damage optical surfaces. As storage in a closed compartment encourages fungal growth, do not store it in its wooden box, but keep it standing on the bench protected by a light plastic cover.

Optics. After use, wipe the immersion objective with lens tissue, absorbent paper, soft cloth or medical cotton wool. If other lenses are smeared with oil, wipe them with a little toluene or a solution of 40% petroleum ether, 40% ethanol and 20% ether.

Lenses must never be soaked in alcohol as this may dissolve the cement.

Clean non-optical parts with mild detergent and remove grease or oil with petroleum ether, followed by 45% ethanol in water. Remove dust from the inside and outside of the eyepieces with a blower or soft camel-hair brush.

Condenser and iris. Clean the condenser in the same way as the lenses with a soft cloth or tissue moistened with toluene, and the mirror (if present) with a soft cloth moistened with 5% alcohol. The iris diaphragm is very delicate and if damaged or badly corroded it is usually beyond repair.

Mechanical parts. Never force the controls. If movement of the focusing screws or mechanical stage becomes difficult, lubricate them with a small drop of machine oil. All accessible moving parts should be cleaned occasionally and given a touch of oil to protect against corrosion. Do not use vegetable oils as they become dry and hard. Always keep the surface of the fixed stage dry as moving wet slides requires increased force which may damage the mechanical stage.

Hot humid climates

In hot humid climates, if no precautions are taken, fungus may develop on the microscope, particularly on the surface of the lenses, in the grooves of the screws and under the paint, and the instrument will soon be useless. This can be prevented as follows.

Every evening fit the microscope into an airtight dust cover together with silica gel. When necessary, the silica is dried out and re-used. An alternative method is to place the microscope in a warm cupboard. This is a cupboard with a tight-fitting door, heated by a 40-watt light bulb.

Check that the temperature inside the cupboard is at least 5°C warmer than that of the laboratory but take care that it does not overheat.

Hot dry climates

In hot dry climates, the main problem is dust. Fine particles work their way into the threads of the screws and under the lenses. This can be avoided as follows:

1. Always keep the microscope under a dust proof plastic cover when not in use.
2. At the end of the day's work, clean the microscope thoroughly by blowing air on it from a rubber bulb.
3. Finish cleaning the lenses with a lens brush or fine paintbrush. If dust particles remain on the surface of the objectives, remove with clean paper.

18. BLOOD SAMPLES FOR COAGULATION TESTS

For coagulation tests, as a rule 9 volumes of blood are added to 1 volume of trisodium citrate. When the haematocrit is abnormal with either polycythaemia or severe anaemia it is necessary to adjust the blood:citrate ratio as shown in Table 27.4.

Table 27.4 Amount of citrate required with 5 ml blood samples

Haematocrit	Citrate (ml)
0.2	0.70
0.25	0.65
0.30	0.61
	0.55
0.55	0.39
0.60	0.36
0.65	0.31
0.70	0.27

REFERENCES

1 Moore HC, Mollison PL 1976 Use of a low-ionic-strength medium in manual tests for antibody detection. Transfusion 16:291.
2 Hendry EB 1961 Osmolarity of human serum and of chemical solutions of biological importance. Clinical Chemistry 7:156.
3 World Health Organization Expert committee on Biological Standardization 2000 International biological reference preparations. Technical Report Series No. 897 p. 75–100.. WHO, Geneva.
4 World Health Organization 1977 The SI for the health professions. WHO, Geneva.
5 World Health Organization 1993 Laboratory biosafety manual, 2nd edn. WHO, Geneva.

Index